Profound Deafness and Speech Communication

Edited by
Geoff Plant and Karl-Erik Spens

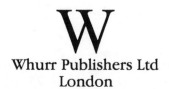

Whurr Publishers Ltd
London

© 1995 Whurr Publishers Ltd
Whurr Publishers Ltd
19b Compton Terrace, London N1 2UN, England

British Library Cataloguing in Publication Data
A catalogue record for this book is available from the British Library.

ISBN 1-897635-45-1

Photoset by Stephen Cary
Printed and bound in the UK by Athenaeum Press Ltd, Gateshead, Tyne & Wear

Contents

Contributors

Evelyn Abberton
Department of Phonetics and Linguistics, University College London, Gower Street, London WC1, UK

Lynne E. Bernstein
Center for Auditory and Speech Sciences, Gallaudet University, 800 Florida Avenue, NE, Washington, DC 20002, USA

Peter J. Blamey
The Bionic Ear and Hearing Institute, The University of Melbourne, 384–388 Albert Street, East Melbourne, Victoria 3002, Australia

Arthur Boothroyd
City University of New York, 33 West 42nd Street, New York, NY 10036, USA

Teresa Ching
National Acoustic Laboratories, 126 Greville St., Chatswood, NSW 2067, Australia

Graeme M. Clark
Department of Otolaryngology, The University of Melbourne, 384–388 Albert Street, East Melbourne, Victoria 3002, Australia

Birgit Cook
Department of Speech Communication and Music Acoustics, Hearing Technology Group, Royal Institute of Technology, Box 70014, S-100 44, Stockholm, Sweden

Robert S.C. Cowan
The Bionic Ear and Hearing Institute, The University of Melbourne, 384–388 Albert Street, East Melbourne, Victoria 3002, Australia

Roddy Cowie
School of Psychology, Queen's University, Belfast BT7 1NN, Northern
Ireland, UK

Harvey Dillon
National Acoustic Laboratories, 126 Greville St., Chatswood, NSW 2067,
Australia

Ellen Douglas-Cowie
School of English, Queen's University, Belfast BT7 1NN, Northern
Ireland, UK

Richard C. Dowell
Department of Otolaryngology, The Royal Victoria Eye and Ear
Hospital, 32 Gisborne Street, East Melbourne, Victoria 3002, Australia

Rebecca E. Eilers
Mailman Center for Child Development, University of Miami, PO Box
016820, Miami, FL 33101, USA

Gunnar Fant
Department of Speech Communication and Music Acoustics, Royal
Institute of Technology, Box 70014, S-100 44, Stockholm, Sweden

Adrian Fourcin
Department of Phonetics and Linguistics, University College London,
Gower Street, London WC1, UK

Karyn L. Galvin
The Bionic Ear and Hearing Institute, The University of Melbourne,
384–388 Albert Street, East Melbourne, Victoria 3002, Australia

Linda Gottermeier
National Technical Institute for the Deaf, Rochester Institute of
Technology, 1 Lombe Memorial Drive, Rochester, NY 14623, USA

David House
Department of Linguistics and Phonetics, Lund University,
Helgonabacken 12, S-223 62 Lund, Sweden

Harry Levitt
Graduate School and University Center, City University of New York, 33
West 42nd Street, New York, NY 10036, USA

James Mahshie
Centre for Auditory and Speech Sciences, Gallaudet University, 800
Florida Avenue, NE, Washington DC 20002, USA

D. Kimbrough Oller
Mailman Center for Child Development, University of Miami, PO Box
016820, Miami, FL 33101, USA

Mary Joe Osberger
Advanced Bionics, 45 Normandy Village Apt 26, Nanuet, NY 10954, USA

Anne-Marie Öster
Department of Speech Communication and Music Acoustics, The
Hearing Technology Group, Royal Institute of Technology, Box 700 14,
S-100 44, Stockholm, Sweden

James M. Pickett
Professor Emeritus (Gallaudet University), Windy Hill Lab, Morgan Bay
Road, PO Box 198, Surry, ME 04684, USA

Geoff Plant
46 Chandler Street, Arlington, MA 02174, USA

Adele Proctor
Department of Speech and Hearing Science, University of Illinois at
Urbana, Champaign, IL 61820-6206, USA

Charlotte M. Reed
Research Laboratory of Electronics, Massachusetts Institute of
Technology, 77 Massachusetts Avenue, Cambridge MA 02139, USA

Jerker Rönnberg
Department of Education and Psychology, Linköping University, S-581
83, Linköping, Sweden

Donald G. Sims
National Technical Institute for the Deaf, Rochester Institute of
Technology, 1 Lombe Memorial Drive, Rochester, NY 14623, USA

Gustaf Söderlund
Audiological Department, Academic Hospital, University of Uppsala,
S-751 85 Uppsala, Sweden

Karl-Erik Spens
Department of Speech Communication and Music Acoustics, The
Hearing Technology Group, Royal Institute of Technology, Box 700 14,
S-100 44, Stockholm, Sweden

Kathleen Vergara
Mailman Center for Child Development, University of Miami, PO Box 016820, Miami, FL 33101, USA

Anita Wallin
Eriksbergsvägen 32, S-751 85, Uppsala, Sweden

Akira Watanabe
Department of Electrical Engineering and Computer Science, 39-1, Kurokamicho 2-chome, Kumamoto-shi, Kumamoto 860, Japan

Foreword

This volume is dedicated to Arne Risberg to honour him on the occasion of his retirement. It is, therefore, fitting to recall some of the highlights of his academic career.

Arne graduated from the school of Electrical Engineering at the Royal Institute of Technology (KTH) in Stockholm in 1957. For the previous two years he had been working part-time at KTH's Speech Transmission Laboratory, which had been established in 1951, and later became the Department of Speech Communication and Music Acoustics. Arne has spent almost all of his working life working with us at KTH. In 1957–1958 he had a temporary position at the Research Institute of the National Defense followed by a year as a teacher at a Folk High School. In 1969–1972 Arne again left us to take up a position at the Swedish Handicap Institute were he was in charge of planning and coordination of research and technical development for the hearing impaired.

When Arne joined us we already had a background in auditory research. At that time our laboratory was a part of the Department of Telegraphy and Telephony. Another member of the Department, Bertil Johansson, had already started his surveys of transposer techniques and hearing aids which expanded later into more general auditory research. Bertil's group, funded by Karolinska Institutet (Stockholm's medical university), became the Unit of Technical Audiology but remained close to our quarters at KTH. Professor Georg von Békésy, the famous auditory physiologist, had also worked with us in 1945–1947. Some of my own early work was oriented towards speech perception, language statistics and audiometry. Our contacts with the Manilla school for the Deaf in Stockholm were well established and we had started work on visual and tactile aids for the deaf when Mac Pickett joined us in 1962. This period is described in more detail in his contribution to this volume.

The contribution of Arne and the research group he established to audiology and auditory rehabilitation in Sweden was recognized in 1986 when the Swedish government appointed him Professor in Hearing Technology. This is a regular chair which will be retained after Arne's retirement.

Arne is an ideal promoter of interdisciplinary work. He has a solid base of knowledge in communication theory and engineering, audiology and speech sciences. In the early part of his career he made important contributions to voice fundamental tracking techniques and to speech processing for synthesis.

Arne has always insisted on searching for integrated holistic views of auditory disability and of the function of communication aids. He has thus performed multiparameter analysis of auditory and cognitive processes which he relates to basic information bearing structures in speech. Examples of this approach include measures of periodic/non-periodic discrimination, stop gap detection and noise interference tests supplementing frequency discrimination tests and pure tone and speech audiometry.

Arne has also worked extensively on the practical applications of his findings. He has pursued and stimulated development of aids for severely and profoundly hearing-impaired people. In his work he has favoured a multisensory approach supplementing lipreading with technically enhanced residual hearing, visual and tactile aids or cochlear implants. He has also been involved in investigations of speech development by severely and profoundly hearing-impaired children. This work has implications for all involved in the education of deaf children and is an important contribution to the ongoing discussion concerning the use of speech and/or sign language with deaf children. A minor study in this domain that Arne and I have pursued is the possible use of a phonetically based Cued Speech system.

This volume reflects the widespread international recognition of Arne's work and his ability to stimulate new ideas and new developments within the field. Arne is a true internationalist and much of his time is devoted to coordinating international projects. A recent example of his commitment in this area has been the strong support he has given to the establishment of an auditory rehabilitation centre in Leningrad run by Ludmilla Chistovich and her daughter Elena.

Arne has a warm, strong personality that engages and stimulates friends and colleagues. He is an idealist in his goals and he combines scientific curiosity with a critical mind. Beside his specific scientific and technical achievements he has effectively contributed to closer ties between research oriented specialists in various disciplines and professionals in several applied fields. This is technology for the benefit of humanity – an example of bringing together what C.P. Snow coined the Two Cultures. He is indeed cultivating a wide and expanding growth in his scientific garden. We wish him all success in a continued role as a gardener, not only at home but also in contact with us all.

Gunnar Fant

Preface

This book is to mark the retirement of Arne Risberg from his position as Professor of Hearing Technology at Stockholm's Royal Institute of Technology. We decided to celebrate Arne's many achievements and contributions to our field by putting together a book on the 'state of the art' in his areas of research interest. Once that decision was made, we realized that this would cover all areas of research concerning speech perception and production by profoundly deaf children and adults. We wrote to a large number of researchers asking them to contribute to this book and were overwhelmed by their positive responses. Almost all of those asked agreed to contribute because they saw Arne as one of the preeminent researchers in their specific area of expertise. Coupled with this recognition of Arne's many scientific achievements, was the great personal regard in which he is held internationally. Arne has been one of the world's leading researchers in the field of profound deafness for over thirty years, but he has always willingly shared his ideas and provided advice to a new generation of researchers.

We both feel very privileged to have known and worked closely with Arne over many years. He has been a great influence on our work through his ideas, encouragement, and his probing and insightful questioning. Presented with an idea he will carefully consider it and then quietly offer suggestions *re* further areas of investigation or alternative analyses. This is the persona which so many researchers throughout the world respect and value, but there is another side to Arne Risberg. Outside his work Arne is a very private man with a great love of family and the simple pleasures of life. Arne spent his early childhood living in a forest to the north of Stockholm, and he has retained his love of the outdoors throughout his life. He is never happier than when he is walking in the forest searching for mushrooms or wild strawberries with his beloved wife Svjetlana. We are lucky enough to have shared some of these times with him. Arne is a great researcher but even more importantly, he is a great friend.

Arne is also a humanitarian, with a strong sense of social justice. His willingness to provide advice and assistance to programs in the developing world is one manifestation of his humanity. His generous personal support of the early childhood intervention center in St. Petersburg is another. Arne is deeply committed to helping establish better programs for deaf people in all countries, and we are sure that his work in this area will continue despite his retirement.

Arne, this book reflects the high regard in which you are held throughout the world. You have earned our great respect through your research, and our deep personal affection through your friendship. Enjoy your retirement doing all of the things that you love. We know that this includes your work, so we are confident that your contributions will continue for many years to come.

Geoff and Karl-Erik

1

Sensory Aids for Deaf People: Past, Present and Future

HARRY LEVITT

Introduction

Arne Risberg, in his long and distinguished career, was deeply involved in many facets of sensory aids research and, in so doing, helped push the field forward on a broad front. His early work on visual aids for speech training soon evolved into pioneering studies on optimal supplements for speechreading as well as basic studies of tactile aids for both speech reception and speech production. This work was followed by an interest in cochlear implants and underlying theories as to why these devices worked so well for some, but not all, implantees. The pattern of these evolving interests is not surprising. He instinctively focused on the most promising approach which, as shown by his publications, laid the groundwork for the successful development of several practical sensory aids.

The path followed by Arne Risberg in his research is also not surprising from another perspective. There are subtle, yet substantial barriers to the successful development of sensory aids for hearing impairment. These include limitations of human cognition, learning and adaptation, as well as limitations of a technological nature. These limitations impose conflicting constraints on the development of effective sensory aids. Arne was quick to recognize the nature of the limitations governing the development of practical sensory aids and, with considerable insight, he chose a path of investigation that provided a practical compromise between conflicting constraints, almost invariably leading to positive results.

It is the purpose of this chapter to identify these basic constraints and the potential for practical solutions. Many of the ideas developed in the discussion that follows are based on findings obtained by Arne

1

and his research team over the years and it is with a debt of gratitude that this chapter has been written.

Classifying Sensory Aids

An obvious way of classifying sensory aids (for hearing impairment) is by their mode of stimulation. The four basic modes of stimulation are auditory, visual, tactile and direct electrical stimulation of the auditory system. It is possible to subdivide these modes of stimulation further; for example, tactile stimulation may be subdivided into stimulation by mechanical means or by electro-tactile means. For the purpose of this discussion the four basic modes of stimulation noted above are sufficient.

A more subtle classification is according to the degree of speech processing. The importance of this classification is evident from the history of sensory aids research. Early attempts at developing sensory aids focused initially on making acoustic signals perceptible; i.e. audible, visible or feelable, depending on the mode of stimulation. It was soon realized, however, that perceptibility was a necessary but insufficient requirement for a sensory aid. Improved signal processing was soon introduced in which perceptually important characteristics of the speech signal, such as the frequency spectrum, were taken into account. Further refinements in signal processing followed, leading to a large number of different speech analysing aids.

Signal processing techniques used with modern sensory aids can be subdivided into four broad categories: (1) non-speech specific, (2) spectrum based, (3) speech feature extraction, and (4) automatic speech recognition. Further subdivision of these categories is, of course, possible. The category of speech feature extraction, for example, can be subdivided into phonetic feature extraction and articulatory feature extraction. Similarly, processing for automatic speech recognition can be further subdivided into discrete word recognition, sentence recognition and automatic recognition of conversational speech. For the purposes of this discussion, four broad categories of classification are sufficient.

Table 1 provides a breakdown of the many different types of sensory aid that have been developed or experimented with in terms of these two dimensions. Note that the two dimensions are independent of each other and that, as a consequence, the cells in the matrix identify non-overlapping sets of sensory aids. It is also interesting to note that, with one exception, there is an entry for every cell in the matrix. The one exception is the use of automatic speech recognition with cochlear implants. There is also reason to believe that this cell will not remain unfilled for much longer, at least in terms of experimental devices of this type.

Table 1. Categories of sensory aids

Type of processing	Modality			
	Auditory	Visual	Tactile	Direct electrical
Non-speech specific	Early hearing aids	Oscilloscope envelope displays	Single-channel vibrator	Single-channel stimulation
Spectrum analysis	Modern hearing aids	Spectrographic displays	Tactile vocoder	Multichannel stimulation
Feature extraction	Speech-feature translation	Feature displays	Feature displays	Feature extraction prior to stimulation
Speech recognition	Speech recoding	Captioning, TTY	Speech to Braille	–

Other possible dimensions of classification are: (1) cognitive complexity of the display, (2) whether the sensory aid is intended to supplement or bypass the impaired auditory system, (3) whether the device functions as an aid to speech reception or speech production (e.g., as a speech training aid), or incorporates both functions, (4) earliest age at which the sensory aid can be used, (5) amount of learning required in order to use the aid effectively, (6) accessibility of the sensory aid, e.g., at all times, as in a personal hearing aid, or for only limited periods of time, as in a classroom-based speechtraining aid, (7) accuracy and reliability of the displays, (8) convenience of use, and (9) cost. A multi-dimensional matrix could be constructed incorporating all of the above factors, but the result would be both unduly complex and not very helpful since the factors are not independent of each other. The two-way classification shown in Table 1 is both concise and simple to comprehend, but it is important not to lose sight of the many other factors affecting the form and function of sensory aids.

Identification of Trends

The first row of Table 1 identifies the earliest sensory aids that were developed for each modality. Also covered in this row are several simple, but very useful non-speech-specific sensory aids, such as alerting devices (e.g. visual or tactile displays signalling the ringing of a doorbell or telephone, and important warning signals such as a fire alarm). Simple visual or tactile displays of sound intensity have also been found to be useful in speech training and as a supplement to lipreading. Perhaps the most advanced non-speech-specific displays are single-channel cochlear implants. Although early cochlear implants of this type did not include speech-specific preprocessing of the signal, remarkable improvements in face-to-face communication were obtained with several patients using these single-channel implants. Modern single-channel cochlear implants now include some form of preprocessing that takes into account the average temporal and spectral characteristics of speech.

The second row of Table 1 identifies sensory aids in which the average characteristics of the speech signal, such as the power-frequency spectrum, are taken into account. Most of the sensory aids currently in use today involve signal processing of this type. Modern hearing aids, for example, take into account the shape of the speech spectrum. In addition, hearing aids with amplitude compression also take into account the intensity-temporal characteristics of speech. Another highly successful spectrum-based sensory aid is the multichannel cochlear implant in which signals representing different portions of the speech spectrum are delivered to corresponding regions of the cochlea. A recent variation of this approach is to limit the information transmitted to only the peaks of the short-term speech spectrum. Some success has also been obtained with wearable tactile vocoders. Visual spectrum displays have not been as successful. The Visible Speech Translator, for example, was found to be of limited value as an aid to speech reception, although a modified version of the device was found to be useful as a speech training aid. Modern spectrum-based visual displays have yielded similar results and practical implementations of these displays can be found primarily in computer-based speech training aids.

The third row of Table 1 covers speech analysing aids in which important phonetic and/or articulatory features are displayed. Some of these devices have found practical application although most are still at the experimental stage of development. It has been shown experimentally (due in large measure to Arne's pioneering research) that the addition of the voice fundamental frequency (F0), auditorially, produces a significant improvement in speechreading ability. An experimental hearing aid that extracts F0 from the acoustic speech signal and delivers it to the user so as to best match his/her residual hearing characteristics has been developed and is currently being evaluated.

Another type of speech-feature hearing aid is that in which the high frequency components of voiceless fricatives are transposed to a lower frequency region where there is a greater amount of residual hearing. It is also possible to provide an additional, small improvement in intelligibility by a moderate amount of frequency lowering for voiced sounds. A behind-the-ear hearing aid incorporating both of these methods of signal processing has recently been introduced and is currently being used clinically.

Visual aids displaying one or more speech features have been employed successfully as speech training aids. Computer-based speech-feature displays are now widely used for this purpose. Visual speech-feature displays for speech reception have been less successful. Whereas displays for speech training can focus on one feature at a time, speech reception displays are more complex in that several features may need to be displayed simultaneously and in synchrony with a rapidly varying speech signal. On the other hand, many hearing-impaired individuals do remarkably well with speechreading although the visual cues in speechreading are complex and vary rapidly in time.

In principle, it should be possible to develop a simple visual supplement that will help disambiguate many of the complex cues available in speechreading. Experimental speechreading eyeglasses have been developed in which supplementary speech cues are superimposed (by optical means) on the listener's view of the speaker's face. Although the concept is promising, laboratory evaluations of experimental sensory aids of this type have not been entirely positive, possibly because of the complexity of the rapidly changing visual display and errors in extracting and displaying the designated speech features.

Wearable tactile aids are more convenient to use than wearable visual aids and some success has been achieved with aids of this type. Wearable spectrum-based tactile aids have proven to be quite practical and experimental speech-feature displays, such as a wearable F0 display, have already been developed with promising results. It remains to be seen whether sensory aids of this type will be commercially viable.

One of the most successful speech-feature sensory aids is the Nucleus-22 cochlear implant in which F0, the first two formants and the voiced/voiceless distinction in continuants are encoded and delivered to the impaired cochlea. Although good results were obtained with this cochlear implant system, the method of signal processing has been replaced by one in which the peaks of the short-term speech spectrum are identified and delivered to the cochlea. This type of processing bears some similarity to formant extraction in that the major spectrum peaks are similar to formant frequencies.

Improved performance has been claimed for the spectrum peak-picking strategy as opposed to the older formant-extraction technique. This observation highlights a particularly important issue. Increasing the speech processing capabilities of a sensory aid offers greater potential for improving the effectiveness of the device, but in order to achieve this goal the method of signal processing must be both accurate and reliable. An inherent problem with all speech-feature sensory aids is that the algorithms used to extract speech features are not always accurate, particularly in a noisy or reverberant acoustic environment. In sensory aids of this type, misleading cues are more damaging to intelligibility than missing cues, i.e. cues that are lost as a result of the hearing impairment.

The last row of Table 1 involves devices at the cutting edge of technology. Recent advances in the field of automatic speech recognition (ASR) have been substantial and ASR devices for discrete word recognition are now available which allow for reasonably accurate recognition of speech (greater than 95% correct word recognition) for vocabularies of relatively large size (over 20 000 words). Significant advances in continuous speech recognition are also being made, although for much smaller vocabularies.

The great potential of ASR technology in developing communication aids for deaf people is evident from the great success of semi-automatic speech transcription systems. In systems of this type, the spoken word is converted to symbols by a stenographer using a shorthand typewriter. The keystrokes of the typewriter are transmitted electronically to a computer which converts the shorthand symbols to text which is then displayed on a screen. A large screen is typically used for meetings in auditoria whereas smaller computer screens, as in a laptop computer, are convenient for individual use. Semi-automatic speech transcription is now widely used for lectures and professional meetings involving a deaf audience. Telephone relay services and television captioning have similarly met with a high degree of success.

A major problem with television captioning, telephone relay services and semi-automatic transcription is the relatively high cost of providing these services because of the intensive use of skilled personnel. An ASR system that operates reliably on continuous speech offers a possible solution but, at present, the state of the art has not yet reached a satisfactory level of performance for this application.

The most obvious application of ASR technology for sensory aids is that of visual displays in which the spoken word is displayed as text. There are, however, other applications that are being experimented with. These include a tactile Braille output for deaf–blind individuals as well as a speech–recognition hearing aid in which the speech is first recognized and then regenerated so as to render the speech more intelligible to a person with a severe hearing impairment. The application of ASR technology in cochlear implant systems has yet to be investigated.

Conclusions

The preceding discussion has identified several significant trends. Whereas the earliest sensory aids did not employ speech-specific processing, the vast majority of sensory aids currently in use incorporate some degree of speech processing. Whereas most of these sensory aids use relatively simple spectrum-based speech processing, a number of practical speech-feature sensory aids have been developed. Speech-to-text displays have also met with considerable success (television captioning, telephone relay services and real-time transcription) although, at present, the speech–recognition process is not automated and provision of these services is expensive.

In short, the underlying trend is towards increased levels of speech processing in modern sensory aids for hearing impairment. Further, sensory aids with more advanced signal processing appear to be more effective, provided the resulting displays are both simple and reliable. In particular, speech-feature and speech-recognition sensory aids appear particularly promising, but a major limitation to their practical implementation is their lack of accuracy under everyday conditions of use, e.g. with background noise and reverberation.

A characteristic of almost every successful sensory aid is that of ease of use. Accessibility and long-term use are also important characteristics of these aids. The most widely used sensory aid of all, the hearing aid, is relatively easy to use. It is also wearable, readily accessed at any time and is typically used over long periods of time. The cochlear implant and wearable tactile displays have similar characteristics and have proven to be relatively successful.

Another significant trend is that speech analysing aids which utilize an auditory input of some kind (when possible) have proven to be more effective than sensory aids that are entirely non-auditory. The use of F0 as a supplement to speechreading, for example, is far more effective when presented auditorially than when presented by tactile or visual means. There is a close, symbiotic relationship between speech and hearing and there are advantages to utilizing the auditory system as far as possible in the development of sensory aids for speech communication.

An important issue closely related to the above is that many deaf children have great difficulty learning to read. As a consequence, there are substantial numbers of deaf adults whose reading skills are relatively poor and who are unable to make effective use of television captioning or other real-time text displays. These individuals rely primarily on the use of signing in order to communicate. Recent advances in video technology, particularly computer-interactive video displays of high resolution, have provided a new impetus to the development of communication aids in which information is conveyed by means of signs or pictures. Research on these techniques is likely to expand rapidly as the marriage between video and computer technology provides greater and more convenient access to visual means of communication, whether by sign language, speechreading, or pictorial representations of language. Hopefully, the lessons learned and insights gained in the development of sensory aids for speech communication will be of value in the development of effective visual aids for language communication. Arne's approach to the problem of finding practical solutions within the conflicting constraints imposed by both human and technological limitations should serve as a model for this new area of research.

Part 1
Tactile Aids

2
Tactile Aids: A Personal Perspective

JAMES M. PICKETT

Introduction

I am sincerely honoured to contribute to this celebration of our colleague, Arne Risberg. Obviously, since I have been retired for more than a criterion-length time (> 5 years), I am well-qualified to write on this occasion. Our Editors qualify me as the 'pioneer American', a sort of catalyst to latent Swedish projects to aid the hearing-impaired that began around 1947. Arne's career, with his many contributions to theory and practice in aids for the hearing-impaired, and his guidance at the Swedish Handicap Institute, represents the attainment of some of those early goals. Gunnar Fant, in his Foreword, might have noted that he was either the father or uncle of the KTH programme on aids for the deaf, into which I more or less inserted myself, as a SpeechCom cousin from the optimistic post-WWII scene in US technology. We, together with the Swedes, could design electronics to solve any problem in speech communication.

How it will all come out, I do not know, of course, so here I will simply tell the informal story of how, with the help of Gunnar and Arne, our field of speech technology for the hearing-impaired started to expand. I cannot cover any details but I will describe some general strategies that we followed and include some notes about the zeitgeist, our colleagues, and various influences on us.

Background

Here is how I came to be part of that renaissance of research for sensory aids in Stockholm near the turn of the 1960s. I had been working in post-war research on speech communication problems for the US Air Force and Navy and, although I learned quite a bit of acoustics, it was

11

not very basic speech acoustics. I really wanted to be an acoustic pho-
netician. At the 1959 International Congress on Acoustics in Stuttgart I
heard Bertil Johansson's (1961) paper on his transposer hearing aid. I
also met Gunnar and János Mártony (Note 1). Fortunately this led me
toward my phonetics goal: I could use my early student interest in phonetics for the deaf, sparked by the pioneer of motor phonetics, R.H.
Stetson, to work at KTH. Gunnar's Speech Transmission Laboratory
(STL) was one of the three most sophisticated in the world; the other
two were at Bell Labs and MIT, but they had no on-going projects on
aids for the deaf. STL had built and tested a 10-channel speech-spec-
trum display, Lucia (Note 2), that included a tactile output to the fingertips on an array of vibrators. Furthermore, the Technical Audiology
Laboratory directed by Bertil Johansson and adjacent to STL offices,
had built and field-tested an ear-level frequency-transposing hearing
aid. I applied to Gunnar and our National Institutes of Health, for a fellowship to work primarily on extended testing of the tactile display.
The NIH Special Fellow award for 1961 put me directly into the
advanced speech research atmosphere that Gunnar had fostered.

The Swedish Experience

Arriving in Stockholm, and checking into the laboratory, you seem to
be entering the most serious, studious, competent place in the world
for communication research. Indeed it was. Every Saturday morning
was spent in reading and discussing an unknown spectrogram. This
was one way for me to learn basic speech acoustics. Another way was
to join others who knew little, e.g. linguists, in tutorials, generously
offered to us by János Mártony, on the application of Laplace transforms to spectrum analysis. Everything was done to help you understand speech analysis and perception problems, including Swedes
always switching into English discussion whenever I entered the room.

I was really excited to be able to feel speech for my first time, on the
vibrator array of Lucia. I spoke some test syllables into the system. My
hopes were quickly dashed by the very diffuse impressions I felt. The
sensations seemed to provide mainly amplitude envelope cues and
some movement of a very diffuse spectral centre. Instead of distinct formant locations, I felt mainly a single area of vibration that changed
position as the mean between the formants moved in frequency. I was
so certain the skin could do better that I suspected there was something wrong with the spectrum analyser.

The first thing Arne did for me was to have the system and filter
responses checked, because Lucia had originally been built as a 1955
student project (Lövgren and Nykvist, 1959) and might need to be
improved. Everything checked out OK. Furthermore, tactile threshold

checks to a frequency sweep, one finger at a time, confirmed the correct band limits to which each vibrator was actually responding.

The problem obviously was the cross-spread of sensation and masking between fingers and even between hands. I still did not like to believe that. It happened that there was a psychophysicist, Günter Rösler, who had worked with Békésy in our same lab area, across our hallway from the venerable first Békésy audiometer. Günter assured me that tactile spread and masking was substantial and gave me a reprint to prove it (Rösler, 1957).

I was very depressed, but Arne consoled me with the suggestion that at least we probably had a better representation of amplitude envelope at our fingertips than what was available in the ear canal, via the vibration of a high-powered hearing aid. And in addition we had a chance of using the speech information available in motions of vibrations across our array.

Arne was quite busy as the Assistant Director of STL, which was rapidly building up its basic speech research capabilities. Sometimes I needed to interrupt him for help and advice. These were usually occasions for some deep thinking together about why and how speech aids for the deaf would or should work. This basic theoretical approach has always been one of Arne's most important qualities. For myself at that time, I liked to think that I was non-theoretical and need not be seriously concerned about speech perception theory or communication theory in general; my attitude toward speech perception theories was that they were too crude and based on too little data for such highly complex phenomena, to be of much value. However, Arne pointed out that most of our communication research designs were actually structured according to a communication model although usually the model was not explicitly acknowledged. Arne always insisted on thinking as deeply as possible on initial assumptions and what might be going on in experiments: not simply grinding out the results. Some early examples of this theoretical bent appear in his paper for our 1967 Conference at Gallaudet (Risberg, 1968): fully 20% of that text is devoted to a review of the latest theories in psychology of sensory learning; all that theory came before his presentation of seven visual speech training devices, each in terms of its intended function according to the theoretical concepts developed. For an engineer, Arne is one of the most thorough psychologists I have encountered.

For transmission tests of the vibrators, it seemed to us that we shouldn't worry about attainable word-scores, or anything that easy to assess or explain to clinicians or teachers. Rather we decided it would be more useful to run tests that would be 'diagnostic' of what types of speech information could be transmitted with such a system. Without such basic information it would be difficult to know how to change the system for better performance. It would also help in knowing how to use the system. The strategy was to first use the simplest speech stimuli that would shed some light on the spectral resolution of the analyser/skin system. Thus the stimuli for the first tests were chosen to be single nonsense syllables with well-known acoustic vowel differences and gross changes in spectrum between consonants . Vowel stimulus-pair discrimination was first tested and then identification within two six-vowel sets, one chosen to be easy to identify (long, well-discriminated vowels with large formant differences) and a second, more-difficult set (short, with small formant differences). The results would not tell us what percentage of words could be transmitted, but we might be able to find out something about the capacities of the acoustic-to-tactile transform.

I attribute this strategy to a corollary of what I am going to call Stetson's Dictum, which he usually pronounced about speech training for deaf speakers, as follows: To teach speech you need to know exactly how it works. In other words you need a correct motor model of speaking (Note 3). A corollary by implication is: If your treatment of a communication deficiency does not work do not suspect your procedure; recheck your underlying theory for hidden assumptions. If your study is correctly designed to check assumptions, their validity will be apparent in the results. A benefit of this approach, for you grant writers, is that you can satisfy basic-science reviewers if you construct your treatment experiments as tests of a basic theoretical model. Thus, if you design your experiment on a good model, the results are a test of the model as well as a test of the device operation or training methods. Furthermore the results stand a good chance of being diagnostic of how the system works or doesn't work, telling what functions in the perception or learning model are supported and to what degree.

The results of the testing of the six-vowel sets indicated that the set of long acoustically distinct vowels were identified tactually with only fair accuracy (60% correct) and the short acoustically more compact set of vowels rather poorly (42%) (Pickett and Pickett, 1963).

My next question was how we might get some performance data that would be of practical use. The original study by Lövgren and Nykvist used deaf children as subjects and was based on the assumption that the tactile vocoder would be valuable primarily as an aid to lipreading. So my next study was designed to expand on this theme. Gunnar had established a connection with the State School for the Deaf (called 'Manilla' because the building was formerly the Philippines Embassy). The supervising teacher, Rut Madebrink, and her colleague, Göte Hanson, both had an intense interest in applications of speech science, so they arranged for me to use a room dedicated to the study, and assigned two young teachers to serve as assistants and Swedish translators to work with the children. Since all children had a daily communication training session of speaking and lipreading, assigned outside of the classroom, it was no disruption for some of these appointments to be scheduled by Rut to do their lipreading as a subject in our study. I was also allowed to lunch at the staff buffet.

I don't suppose any foreign researcher had ever been so generously and neatly supported in a school. Midway in the work, however, the School Director suddenly felt my arrangements were too costly in space and people. Appeals by Rut and Göte were of no avail. Gunnar had to intercede to keep me going.

The study tested some types of vowel and consonant discrimination and identification, with children lipreading vs tactile reception, vs combined (Pickett, 1963). Now we were getting a little closer to practice. There was even the possibility that the Director would look in to check our operation. Still the study design dealt with speech-sound categories and a prosodic variable of number of syllables in the test word. Results were reasonably encouraging but from both studies I came away with the opinion that the skin sense was probably never going to afford easy speech perception (Pickett and Pickett, 1963); still our results suggested many interesting questions about informationally redundant sensory sources on speech and how to combine them.

Surprisingly, one somewhat discouraging experience was a talk with Georg von Békésy. He won a Nobel Prize during our year. Gunnar got tickets for us and we rented full evening dress to see the King honour our shy, modest von Békésy; I had met him earlier in his lab at Harvard when I was a student on a visit to C.V. Hudgins (Note 4); he seemed very nice but rather abstracted and simply pointed to his tactile cochlea model on a huge work table that virtually filled the centre of the small lab room. Just after the Award ceremony Bertil Johansson reintroduced me. I told Békésy all about our tactile speech study and asked what he thought, because at that time he probably knew more than anyone about complex tactile perception. In effect he said, somewhat bluntly, 'It won't work.' Well, his tactile experiments showed how a cyclic wave of skin pressure, spread along the surface, actually felt like a single locus of stimulation while we were trying to do the opposite. Of course, now we know the tactile vocoder can work, with a tremendous amount of practice (Brooks and Frost, 1983; Frost et al., 1983). Still, most people who knew Békésy say he was full of insightful remarks, if you know how to bring them out. That night I didn't know how.

The insights came in Békésy's Nobel Lecture the next day, 'Concerning the pleasures of observing and the mechanics of the middle ear' (Békésy, 1961). The theme of the Lecture he presented was that truly incisive scientific inquiry seeks to discover natural commonalities, much as does fine art. He began with slides of his own objects of ancient art and described their simple unity and the organic aspects of their beauty. He then talked about some of his experimental approaches which had always been strikingly direct and simple in concept. Good experiments, like good art objects, developed concepts that were organic wholes, with inescapable, neat conclusions: no loose ends. Can we apply this art to research on aids for the hearing-impaired? When I do so it seems that some of our approaches may be too unnatural ever to result in organically pleasing functions. But it would be very satisfying to discover some new commonalities between auditory and tactile perception.

There are some loose ends in audiovisual speech phenomena which suggest that research on lipreading and tactile speech might contribute to models of speech perception (Summerfield, 1991). Good lipreaders tend to have very fast evoked cortical responses to light; on the other hand, the viewer of a talker tolerates very large temporal leads or lags between visual and auditory tracks. Experiments with rhythmic pacing precursors (Kidd, 1989), together with staggered audio vs visual vs tactile tracks, might shed some light that would organize these discrepancies into a meaningful model and at the same time help us design better lipreading aids (Summerfield, 1992).

Subsequent Tactile Research

Because of my Manilla School experience and all I had learned about speech acoustics at STL I felt I was highly qualified to set up a research group in the area of technology for the deaf. I wrote to the Director of the Hearing and Speech programme at Gallaudet, D. Robert Frisina, and proposed myself. He politely turned me down. So when I returned to the US after my fellowship year I did a year of basic speech research in Weiant Wathen-Dunn's Speech Research Branch of the Air Force Cambridge Research Laboratories at Bedford, MA (Note 5). Then I needed to return to Washington, where I found a position in vocoder research at Melpar, Inc. I could then visit D. Robert Frisina in person and soon was able to get a research professorship there in 1964. Support by Gallaudet and via NIH grants was superb for nearly twenty years. That research group, the Center for Auditory and Speech Science, now has a staff of 15 people. Gunnar and Arne's support of my Swedish experience can now be seen as a direct cause of the beginning of our Gallaudet development.

At about the same time, 1964, Gunnar decided to set up a research group on 'Medical and Pedagogical Speech Research', with Arne as Director and János Mártony as his Assistant. First they focused on small speech-teaching visual aids that used simple electronics and simple criterion indicators, with adjustable thresholds. This type of design, according to the KISS principle ('keep it simple, stupid'), was followed up in later tactile research by others. Visual devices were described in considerable number in 1967 at our first international Conference on Speech-Analyzing Aids for the Deaf (Conference, 1968). There was only one paper on a tactile device (Kringlebotn, 1968).

Research on tactile aids languished for a few years. Arne and János concerned themselves with classroom training devices to find out what problems would arise there. The tactile vocoder was impractical to submit as a device for extensive field testing as compared with the simple speech trainers. A one-hand, electronically simple, array of vibrators, however, was spawned from Arne's group, designed and tested by a Norwegian visiting research engineer (Kringlebotn, 1968). Arne also conceived a tactile 'speech wand' that would be gripped in the hand with a thumb vibrator as a rhythm or voice pitch indicator and four finger vibrators for the spectrum. I don't believe this was actually built. Wearability of aids for field tests was needed and tactile stimulators were too power-hungry, needed too much alimentation, to be easily wearable and remain sufficiently nourished all day. Then Arne was called away to work on the research and development plans at the new Handikappinstitutet. Alas, when funding of future developments is being planned, current research must be held in abeyance for many discussions and much writing.

After the 1967 Conference at Gallaudet, János remained with us to work on describing the residual hearing of moderate-to-severely deaf listeners for low-frequency speech formants (Pickett and Mártony, 1970). At present, residual hearing for speech cues and the enhancement of these cues remains the primary emphasis of our Center at Gallaudet, under the direction of Sally Revoile.

In the interim, Kirman (1974) had published a thorough review of tactile speech communication which was much more optimistic than our 1963 papers; he pointed out a number of promising ideas for tactile speech. Orrin Cornett, our Gallaudet Vice President, developed the Cued Speech System and was making some reception tests with an electrotactile array of stimulators coded in Cued Speech categories to present stimulus patterns intended to disambiguate lipreading (Conference, 1977).

About 1975, Arne and János came back to Gallaudet to help us plan a further conference on speech-aids technology developments and needs, the 1977 Research Conference on Speech-Processing Aids for the Deaf. Although we were not able to produce a conference publication that could be distributed widely, selected papers were eventually bound and distributed to all participants (Conference, 1977). Now with hindsight I think the most notable paper was the description and results with the Discourse Tracking Procedure by De Filippo and Scott (1978), from the Central Institute for the Deaf. This method, the first to conveniently measure lipreading in meaningful communication, is still being refined and used, as we see in the paper below by Spens and Gnosspelius. Many of the researchers reporting at the 1977 Conference were from institutions for the deaf. Several of the engineer participants, besides those from Sweden, were US. research engineers, including groups on tactile aid research at Johns Hopkins and MIT, respectively under Moise Goldstein and Nathaniel Durlach. We also received the unique contributions of three scientists with personal experience of communication handicap: James Linvill who developed the Optacon tactile print-scanner for his blind daughter, Frank Saunders' electrotactile vocoder for his deaf daughter, and Hubert Upton who built an eyeglass speech display for himself. A tactile review monograph by the MIT group appeared as Reed, Durlach, and Braida (1982).

Other groups or individuals who entered tactile speech research during the 1970s were Arthur Boothroyd and Nancy McGarr at CUNY and Lexington School, Rebecca Eilers and Kim Oller at the Mailman Center, Frank Saunders at the Smith-Kettlewell Institute, David Sparks at the University of Washington, Brian Scott and Carol De Filippo at the Central Institute for the Deaf, T.R. Willemain at Northeastern University, and Engelmann and Rosov at the Oregon Research Institute. References and discussions on some of these authors' reports will be found in our implant-tactile review paper (Pickett and McFarland,1985).

For our part at Gallaudet, a programme was designed in 1980 to take advantage of new developing technology via our Rehabilitation Engineering Center (REC) grant from our government's Institute for Handicapped Research. Three of our Center projects were on tactile aid research, one on cochlear implants plus tactile aid, one on visual indicators of speech activity for deaf speech trainees, and one on residual hearing cues for speech perception. The tactile research was carried out at CUNY/Lexington, MIT, and Johns Hopkins. Our REC lasted only as long as the initial 3-year grant, 1981–1983, but the work of these three tactile research groups is still progressing.

Advent of the Cochlear Implant

Although some well-controlled experimental implant work was reported as early as 1966 together with an excellent history of earlier attempts (Simmons, 1966), there seems to have been little effect on speech-aids research until the late 1970s when W.F. House (1976) began implanting a substantial number of adult deaf patients with a single electrode using a very simple surgical approach. For example, I do not recall any extensive discussion of implants during the 1977 Conference, although Robert Bilger presented a summary of his performance measures on the first House implantees; the measured benefits were minimal, although implantees were often enthusiastic about hearing at least some type of sound.

When the implant clinical trials were starting, about 1980, I was very negative because I felt the nature and cochlear distribution of stimulation was not well-controlled, certainly not well enough to tell even approximately, how implants might work. Following the corollary: if you didn't know how and why they achieved minimal speech transmission, how could you prescribe and adjust them? Some of my colleagues in the Gallaudet Audiology Department were not too happy with my attitude; we applied for a grant but did not get it, possibly because I was not very enthusiastic. It seemed to me that the more-simple implants were not based on principles of acoustic analysis via cochlear function and no scientific conclusions could be drawn from a simple 'how much benefit' study. Positive results could easily be due merely to the well-known enthusiasm and new hope that accompany an advanced concept.

Simmons' (1966) procedures were eventually developed into a well-designed, theoretically motivated, single-electrode implant that was manufactured for a clinical trials programme. Bill McFarland, our new Audiology Department Head, had some first-hand experience in Simmons' projects. We then decided we could respond to the pressure for implants of Gallaudet late-deafened adults with some tests of this implant together with a wearable tactile aid from Audiological Engineering that had automatic compression and background control. Two patients were implanted. They appeared to enjoy their new 'hearing' and said they felt more in touch (!). They also responded positively to the tactile aid. The satisfaction these persons experienced in hearing was undeniable, but unfortunately this research could not be continued. Gallaudet's main contribution to current implant research is in the early research training of M.J. Osberger (see Chapter 11) who studied speech-cue hearing with E. Danaher and me before she went on to CUNY and Lexington School. In addition to our 1985 paper comparing implant and tactile results (Pickett and McFarland, 1985) we published a discussion of communication testing methods for implants and tactile aids (Pickett, 1983).

I still feel that auditory and speech scientists should carefully weigh the potential efficacy of their contributions to implant research compared to what they may accomplish in hearing-aid and tactile-aid research. One factor in favour of implants, in my opinion, is the probable existence of a natural alerting function of hearing. In addition, electronic hearing might offer more usable directional environmental impressions. One wonders whether these non-speech functions in daily life can be as well-served via touch or vision. To me this question is very interesting biologically, and perhaps equal in importance to speech communication functions.

The first published paper comparing implant vs hearing-aid use by the deaf is Owens and Telleen (1981). For our tactile vs implant review paper, through 1984, there were no published reports of tactile vs implant performance in the same subjects at the same time. The papers below on cochlear implants will present some new comparative studies that would help to quantify the trade-offs of inexpensive tactile aids with expensive implants. Have we reached the stage where predictions of best treatment methods and outcomes are meaningful? Perhaps it is far too early for this, as remarkable improvements are still taking place in technology and training methods (for example, see Fryauf-Bertschy, Kirk and Weiss, 1993).

Current tactile aids employ more efficient stimulators and may eventually be competitive in wearability with hearing aids and cochlear implant stimulators. However, I have often questioned whether vibratory tactile aids can ever compete with the more-natural avenue of hearing for speech transmission. In a 1978 workshop on prosthetic devices at the National Technical Institute for the Deaf, I presented some arguments for exploring tactile/kinaesthetic parameters that might be more natural than sensations of vibration (Pickett, 1978). The three following chapters in this book describe some 'natural' tactile research. Lynne Bernstein, from the Hopkins groups and now at Gallaudet, has developed new quantitative methods for measuring lipreading of meaningful communications. Chapter 8 describes new theoretical possibilities for 'haptic' communication.

Parting Thoughts

My final visit to KTH was in 1985 when Karl-Erik Spens had to defend his doctoral dissertation against my attacks as his opponent from the outside. This was a great honor for me, presumably bestowed by Arne, with Gunnar's blessing. Thankfully the tradition of full dress for these grillings had been dropped some time ago. Americans try to be very informal about these things, so I was not at all a formidable opponent, I think; for such an admirable, well-reasoned series of tactile studies, on such an eminently wearable device as the Optacon, how can one hope to obstruct progress? At the end of my summary of his defence I thought I was already conferring the doctorate on Karl-Erik when I shook his hand (as instructed), publicly offering my congratulations to 'Dr Spens'. Gunnar quietly informed me the Committee still had to judge the defense and decide.

When it became fairly clear by 1980 that most of the aids for the deaf were going to find their major use as lipreading aids, Arne decided lipreading was overdue for some serious analytic attention. In my final year at Gallaudet, 1986, he came to visit, and we had our usual deep thinking session about lipreading, a skill that I had given only occasional attention since my experiments at Manilla School. Arne came up with the theory that there might be two types of adult-deafened speech perceivers, prosodics-dependent and segmentals-dependent, during their normal-hearing lives, possibly due to different roles in life. Then when hearing-impairment develops, with decreases in auditory resolution in the middle and high frequencies, the prosodic person is not so

greatly affected but the segmental person is in more trouble, even
with amplification. If this were true it meant that provision of the segmental acoustic cues over the entire spectrum would be of limited
value to the prosodics-dependent and, if they cannot hear any usable
prosodic cues, they could be provided with prosodic cues by a very
simple implant. For the segmentals-dependent, lipreading would be of
more value and the aid should focus on cueing the invisible segmentals. I don't know if this has been followed up but it might be a further
set of productive Risbergian assumptions for an important series of
studies.

Acknowledgements

The research and experience described in this chapter were sponsored by the US
Air Force Cambridge Research Laboratories, the US Public Health Service (National
Institutes of Health), the US Office of Education (Institute of Handicapped
Research), Gallaudet University and my wife/collaborator Dr Betty Pickett.

Notes

Note 1. I heard about Gunnar via basic speech acoustic papers presented at
    Acoustical Society of America meetings, by MIT researchers, Kenneth Stevens,
    Arthur House, and John Heinz. I believe they first met, approximately at the
    turn of the 1950s, when Gunnar studied transmission line theory at MIT and all
    came together at Harvard with Morris Halle and Roman Jakobson in the semi-
    nars held by Jakobson's 'Russian' project. This project was a highly seminal
    meeting ground; in our field it resulted in the distinctive features theory under
    which many of us work or criticize (Jakobson, Fant and Halle, 1952).
Note 2. The Lucia display for speech training consisted of ten vertical glow-tubes of
    the type that was normally used as a signal amplitude indicator. Lucia was
    named after the secular Swedish winter celebration of Santa Lucia in which one
    tradition was for a pretty girl of the household, office, school, or laboratory to
    serve warm drinks wearing a crown of lighted candles.
Note 3. One of Stetson's proofs was the failure of the so-called 'elements' method
    of teaching speech to the deaf. This procedure was based on a simplistic ver-
    sion of linguistic theory that speech is merely a series of canonic sounds, the
    phonemes. Thus the elements method sought first to teach correct production
    of these elementary sounds and then teach how to string them to form words.
    Usually these elements were taught as isolated pronunciations. Thus the first
    word-attempts, and sometimes the final general result for the rest of the deaf
    pupil's life, were strings of vowels separated by syllabic consonants instead of
    words of syllable-coarticulated consonants and vowels. Such a result would be
    unthinkable under today's methods which train from the beginning with whole
    syllables and words and phrases.
        For those readers interested in Stetson's role in phonological theory and
    syllable theory, see Stetson (1945, 1951). His interests in phonetically-based
    speech-training aids for the deaf are typified by the papers of his student, C.V.
    Hudgins (Hudgins, 1935).
Note 4. Clarence V. Hudgins was a psychology student at Oberlin College where

Stetson was Head of the Department (1909–1939). Hudgins spoke with a slight stammer that had been corrected in lessons by Stetson, and thus came to work with Stetson on experimental phonetics problems while studying for his Master's Degree. After obtaining his PhD at Clark University (Worcester, MA), Hudgins became the first full-time scientist to head a research group in a US institution for the deaf, at Clarke School for the Deaf in Northampton, MA, in 1937. In 1947–1951, while I was at Brown University working on my Doctorate in brain function in sensory learning, I visited Hudgins' lab and home several times; he offered me a position but at that time I was convinced I could make greater contributions by working in neurobehaviour.

Note 5. As a member of Weiant's crew at the Speech Research Branch in 1962 I was exposed to two major influences on how to attack speech perception problems of the hearing-impaired. One was to anticipate automatic speech-processing hearing aids and the other was to use digital computers interactively to study the importance of various speech cues to hearing.

How to study the cues of real speech would be attacked by hands-on manipulation and alteration of speech wave segments using a digital computer. Far across our parking lot was MIT's Lincoln Laboratory which had built one of the first interactive computers, one of the 'TX' models, the immediate ancestor of Digital's PDP Series. Irv Pollack and I (Pollack and Pickett, 1964) were just beginning our experiments on the intelligibility of excerpts from fluent speech, so we arranged with Bernard (Ben) Gold, Lincoln Labs researcher on speech processing, to try out the TX as a digital processor for displaying the speech wave, marking it, listening, and making the excerpts. It worked beautifully, even at midnight when Ben had project-free access to the machine, and if we were awake enough to follow the power-up procedure and thus avoid tripping the alarm horn. But speech-excerpting was too low a task for such a high-powered experimental computer and our former Air Force boss in Washington, the late Fred Frick, who had become Director of Lincoln, could not see his way to 'allowing my million-dollar computer to be used as a tape-splicer'. Irv and I walked back across the parking lot and used a Kay spectrograph loop and electronic timing switches instead (designed and set up for us by Philip Lieberman doing his military service as a research engineer). Still, in my mind, the computer technique had been proven for our use, when 30 years later we had $1000 computers on our desks that were at least a million times better than the early interactive computers.

The possibility of automatic adjustment of speech spectra for hearing aids was suggested by the Air Force work on spectral processing to remove redundancies before vocoding for transmission. A large processing system had been developed at the Branch, by Caldwell P. Smith; it filled a small building with rack upon rack of processing. After visiting this building and hearing the remarkable quality of a very narrow-band system that worked with a statistical approach to spectral pattern-matching, it became apparent to me and Irv Pollack as we walked back across the parking lot, that this type of processing could conceivably be used to enhance speech signals for the hearing-impaired. We could certainly depend on the processing schemes to be designed and miniaturized, as we knew that powerful military and economic interests (Bell Labs) were behind these developments. The problem would be that so little was known about abnormal distortions of speech that we wouldn't know how to set the parameters of the processors. I decided that perceptual distortions of speech due to hearing impairments would be a very interesting and useful field for future research.

In addition to recent technical contributions resulting from military and economic interests it might be noted that Gunnar Fant's early research in modelling speech was based on his work on telephone transmission line theory under Professor Laurent of KTH. There has always been a strong beneficial interplay between the telephone industry and hearing problems, as exemplified in the careers of Harvey Fletcher and von Békésy, but I know of no formal history of this subject.

References

Békésy, G. von (1961) Concerning the pleasures of observing, and the mechanics of the inner ear. Nobel Prize Lectures, 1961-1962, Nobelstiftelsen, Stockholm.

Brooks, P.L. and Frost, B.J. (1983) Evaluation of a tactile vocoder for word recognition. Journal of the Acoustical Society of America 74: 34–9.

Conference (1968) Proceedings of the Conference on Speech-Analyzing Aids for the Deaf (1967). American Annals of the Deaf 113: 116–330.

Conference (1977) Papers from the Research Conference on Speech-Processing Aids for the Deaf, Center for Auditory and Speech Sciences, MTB, Gallaudet University, 800 Florida Ave. N.E., Washington, DC.

De Filippo, C. and Scott, B. (1978) A method for training and evaluating the reception of ongoing speech. Journal of the Acoustical Society of America 63: 1186–92.

Frost, B.J., Brooks, P.L., Gibson, D.M. and Mason, J.L. (1983) Identification of novel words and sentences using a tactile vocoder (abstract). Journal of the Acoustical Society of America, Suppl. 1, 74: S104–5.

Fryauf-Bertschy, H., Kirk, K.I. and Weiss, A.L. (1993) Cochlear implant use by a child who is deaf and blind: A case study. American Journal of Audiology 2: March, 38-47.

House, W.F (1976) Cochlear implants. Annals of Otology, Rhinology and Laryngology. 85 (Supplement 27), 93 pp.

Hudgins, C.V. (1935) Visual aids in the correction of speech. Volta Bureau, Washington, DC.

Jakobson, R., Fant, G. and Halle, M. (1952) Preliminaries to Speech Analysis: The Distinctive Features and Their Correlates. Cambridge MA: MIT Press.

Johansson, B. (1961) A new coding amplifier system for the severely hard of hearing. Proc. Third International Congress on Acoustics. Amsterdam: Elsevier.

Kidd, G.R. (1989) Articulatory-rate context effects in phoneme identification. Journal of Experimental Psychology: Human Perception and Performance 15: 736–48.

Kirman, J.H. (1974) Tactile communication of speech: A review and analysis. Psychological Bulletin, 80, 54–74.

Kringlebotn, M. (1968) Experiments with some visual and vibrotactile aids for the deaf. In Proceedings of the Conference on Speech-Analyzing Aids for the Deaf, American Annals of the Deaf 113: 311–17.

Lövgren, A. and Nykvist, O. (1959) Talöverforing och talträning med döva barn på visuell och taktil väg under utnyttjande av speciell apparatur (Speech transmission and speech training for the deaf child by visual and tactile means using special devices). Nordiska Tidskrift Dövundervisning 1959, 122–43.

Owens, E. and Telleen, C. (1981) Speech perception with hearing aids and cochlear implants. Archives of Otolaryngology 107: 160–3.

Pickett, J.M. (1963) Tactual communication of speech sounds to the deaf: Comparison with lipreading. Journal of Speech and Hearing Disorders 28: 315–30.

Pickett, J.M., and Pickett, B.H. (1963) Communication of speech sounds by a tactual vocoder. Journal of Speech and Hearing Research 6: 207–22.

Pickett, J. M. and Mártony, J. (1970) Low-Frequency vowel formant discrimination in deaf listeners. Journal of Speech and Hearing Research 13: 347-59.

Pickett, J.M. (1978) On somesthetic transforms of speech for deaf persons. In McPherson D and Davis M (Eds) Advances in Prosthetic Devices for the Deaf: A Technical Workshop. Rochester, NY: National Technical Institute for the Deaf, Rochester Institute of Technology. pp 184–8.

Pickett, J.M. (1983) Theoretical considerations in testing speech perception through electroauditory stimulation. Annals of the New York Academy of Sciences (proceedings of a conference on implants for hearing) 424–34.

Pollack, I. and Pickett, J.M. (1964) Intelligibility of excerpts from fluent speech: auditory vs structural context. Journal of Verbal Learning and Verbal Behavior 3: 79–84.

Pickett, J.M. and McFarland, W. (1985) Auditory implants and tactile aids for the profoundly deaf. Journal of Speech and Hearing Research 28: 134–50.

Reed, C.M., Durlach, N.I. and Braida, L.D. (1982) Research on Tactile Communication of Speech: A Review. ASHA Monographs, No. 20, American Speech-Language-Hearing Association, 10801 Rockville Pike, Rockville, MD.

Risberg, A. (1968) Visual aids for speech correction. American Annals of the Deaf 113: 178–94.

Rösler, G. (1957) Über die Vibrationsempfindung. Literaturdurchsicht und Untersuchungen im Tonfrequenzbereich. Zeitschrift für angewandte Psychologic. 4: 549–602.

Simmons, F.B. (1966) Electrical stimulation of the auditory nerve in man. Archives of Otolaryngology, 84, 2–54.

Stetson, R.H. (1951) Motor Phonetics: A Study of Speech Movements in Action, North-Holland, Amsterdam; reprinted with commentary as Motor Phonetics: A Retrospective Edition, J.A.S. Kelso and K.G. Munhall (Eds), Boston, MA: College-Hill Press, 1988.

Stetson, R.H. (1945) Bases of Phonology, Oberlin College, corrected edition 1954, Oberlin, OH.

Summerfield, Q. (1991) Visual perception of phonetic gestures. in Mattingly I and Studdert-Kennedy M. Modularity and the Motor Theory of Speech Perception. Hillsdale NJ: Erlbaum. pp 117–43

Summerfield, Q. (1992) Lipreading and audio-visual speech perception. Philosophical Transactions of the Royal Society of London, B 335: 71–8.

3
Tactiling and Tactile Aids: A User's Viewpoint

GUSTAF SÖDERLUND

What is Tactiling?

'Tactiling' is the name I have given to the method of tactile-visual speech communication that I have used for over 40 years. In tactiling, a deaf person places her/his hand on the speaker's throat or neck and uses the vibratory information as a supplement to lipreading. Although this is a very simple method of tactile supplementation, it is very successful. Testing has shown that my ability to understand speech improves by around 50% when I supplement lipreading with vibrator information from the speaker's neck. In real-life situations tactiling is probably even more effective. I find that tactiling contributes to much more relaxed communication. Tactiling also provides me with information about my own speech, allowing me to monitor my voice level so that I speak at an appropriate loudness level.

Despite these advantages, very few deaf people use this method. In this article I will consider some of the reasons for this situation. I will give some background about my development and use of the method, and tell of my almost fruitless search to find other 'tactilers'. I will also discuss current developments in tactile aid research and my own experiences in this area.

This chapter draws extensively from a number of sources. These include papers presented at the International Conferences on Tactile Aids and Cochlear Implants, the first held in Sydney (1990) and the second in Stockholm (1992) (Risberg et al., 1992). I have also used much information from Gunilla Öhngren's (1992) thesis 'Touching Voices'.

The Development of Tactiling

In mid-1945 I was 8 years old and attending a school in one of the outer suburbs of Stockholm. I had just completed my second year of schooling and was an average student. I could read and write at about the same level as the other children. I'm deliberately pointing this out because there seems to be a widespread belief that tactiling requires special gifts – that only a small number of specially talented children could benefit from the method. I still have my school reports from that time. If you saw these reports you would see that I was not really all that bright!

In June 1945 I contracted meningitis whilst on a visit to Copenhagen. I spent several weeks in hospital, and during that time it became apparent that I had lost my hearing. I slowly recovered over the summer, struggling with, and fairly quickly overcoming, some balance problems. That August I was taken to a Swedish clinic for observation and hearing testing. Unfortunately, they found there was nothing to test – I was totally deaf. My parents, as you would expect, were very anxious for me, but I really didn't understand the consequences of my hearing loss. I had tinnitus at this time and this concerned me a lot, but we all thought that maybe this was a sign that my hearing was recovering in some way. My parents were told that I would probably have to attend a special school for deaf children where I would be able to learn to sign. It was felt that this would be a better placement for me than my old school.

But then my parents met Erik Wedenberg who was developing a new form of oral training for deaf children. Wedenberg, who later became a Professor of Audiology, encouraged my parents to speak loudly and clearly in my ears to stimulate whatever residual hearing I had. Other cues were also available from this method – I could feel the breath stream and, on occasions, I could use lipreading information. Although my parents did not follow Erik Wedenberg's method fully he became a valued friend and adviser to us. To me the most important thing that Erik Wedenberg did was to encourage my parents to become directly involved in my rehabilitation.

My parents started daily training sessions with me. My father spent hours reading aloud to me from books. But I didn't perform as they had been led to expect. I couldn't hear anything, but I was irritated by the physical impact of my parents' voices. I wanted to maintain some distance between their lips and my ear, and I did this by putting my hand rather firmly on their necks. My parents also allowed me to watch their lips while they were reading. Sometimes I followed the written patterns, whilst at other times I watched my parents' lips. I think that this enabled me to make an immediate connection between lipreading and the tactual patterns I picked up from their necks. Using this method we made rapid progress. I experimented with different hand positions, and eventually found the one which seemed to be the best. At first I placed my hand directly on the throat, but soon found that it was much more comfortable if I put my hand on either the neck or shoulder.

The training period only lasted about a month, and after that I always placed my hand on the neck of a speaker. I performed so well using this method that when the summer vacation ended I was allowed to return to my old school. From that time on I lived as if I was hard-of-hearing rather than deaf. I learned to speak foreign languages without any great trouble, although I have never actually *heard* them being spoken. My tactual sense took over many of the functions that audition provides for normally-hearing people. I received almost no other rehabilitative training after that initial period. I was able to complete secondary schooling, and later attended university to study life science, eventually receiving a *filosifie licentiat*. At that time – the 1960s – there were no interpreting services available for deaf university students. But I was able to get by with assistance from my fellow students, my curiosity, and by reading.

I do not want to give the impression that my life has been without problems. There have been some, of course, but anyone who experiences a challenge has to overcome problems. But I can't recall ever experiencing any social problems. My method of communication has always been accepted. I have had a rather normal family life and have been employed in the same molecular biology research group for the last 30 years.

Lipreading and 'Inner Speech Memory'

What are the characteristics of a good lipreader? This is a topic which seems to be the subject of endless discussions. A few years ago it was examined in a discussion letter distributed among deaf adults in Sweden. Most of us were sure of one thing – drills and exercises will not make a good lipreader. This is something that you develop yourself, and will master as a consequence of your general communication ability. It does not seem to be related to other intellectual abilities nor to level of education. A number of respondents also expressed the opinion that when lipreading works well you can *hear* the words being pronounced inside your head. It would seem to me that all humans who have developed speech whilst they had normal hearing must have memories of the sounds of speech and the flow of connected discourse.

Professionals working in this area have made similar observations. Gunilla Öhngren (1992) gives several examples of this phenomenon in her thesis. Jerker Rönnberg, a Swedish psychologist with a special interest in lipreading, has tested some excellent lipreaders and he points out some characteristics of these persons. He believes that a very well developed 'working memory' must be present, and that there must be 'inner speech' mediated by a phonological coding system. He concludes that any technical aid developed for deafened adults must be compatible with this phonological coding. If this demand is not met then the capacity of the working memory will not be used effectively.

This aided phonological coding is, in my opinion, the ability to perceive and combine tactual and visual information to shape 'inner speech'. And now to what I believe is a very important point – I don't think that the brain can perform simultaneous decoding and recoding of more than a few different and unrelated sensory inputs. If you first have to register a coded signal on the skin – say Braille, morse code, or even special signals for different consonants – then you have a script related form which has to be recoded before it can be used to support lipreading. We see this when we watch small children learning how to read. They say each word aloud as they read them – they are recoding the written information!

It could be argued that the vibrations of speech also need to be recoded. I think, however, that this sensory input is very close to what we are used to receiving via our hearing. It is related to the basic verbal images that we have developed in learning speech by hearing.

When I am lipreading without any support from tactiling, I assume I find it more difficult to construct inner speech patterns. When I have the visual and the tactual information at the same time, however, I find the task much easier. I find that I depend less on guessing and that overall communication proceeds more comfortably. I am more relaxed, and this in turn makes communication so much easier. On the other hand when I am lipreading only, I have to rely on a lot more guessing and I start to feel tense and I am prone to frustration.

Some Special Attributes of Tactiling

I want to consider a number of factors which I hope will help parents who are faced with the same situation that confronted my parents in 1945. This information should also be useful to professionals giving advice to the parents of newly deafened children.

Tactiling is a method that places no special demands on the speaker

A number of systems, for example Cued Speech or Signing, have been developed or have evolved for use with deaf children and adults. Unfortunately, such systems require a trained user, and this limits the number of people with whom the deaf person can communicate. Some technical aids require the speaker to wear a microphone, and this can be annoying for some people. Trailing cords, switches, and fussy electronics may be unacceptable to some speakers no matter how well intentioned. Tactiling places no special demands on the speaker at all. Of course, the person who is used to talking to deaf people may be easier to understand, but this is not of great importance. I have found that most people speak a little slower and more clearly when they are talking to a deaf person. When I first meet someone I explain that I am deaf and tell them why I place my hand on the speaker's neck. This seems to put them at their ease and normal communication can then proceed.

Training should start very soon after the onset of deafness

There are reports from neurobiologists that indicate that the primate brain is flexible for some time after an accident. A study of apes (Fox, 1984) which had had one finger surgically removed found a reorientation of the corresponding area in the somatosensory cortex over time. This reorientation occurred 3 to 6 months after the ape had lost the finger, and restored the brain's 'tactual map' which had been showing a 'blank' area. The authors commented that this effect was not restricted to young individuals. Reorientation also occurred with older apes. I first read this paper about ten years ago, and I was excited by its findings. Maybe I learned tactiling so easily because my sensory system was predisposed to such learning soon after the onset of deafness.

Training should involve the simultaneous use of lipreading and tactiling

Some of my adult deaf friends have experimented with tactiling. They usually tell me that it is possible that they do receive a little more, but they find it hard to concentrate on combining lipreading and the tactile signal. Additionally, they dislike having to put their hands on unfamiliar people. These factors make them unwilling to use tactiling in their everyday lives. Interestingly, there also seems to be a negative effect if the performer is already a good lipreader. The short-term benefits of tactiling for such people is very small, and they may be unwilling to persevere with the system long enough to benefit from higher order cues.

When I tell people about tactiling they always want to try it for themselves. So what do they do? They put their hand on the speaker's neck and either close their eyes or look away. They don't look at the face of the speaker, yet lipreading is crucial to the success of tactiling.

There are many complex skills that we perform every day that require the simultaneous use of several senses. Riding a bike and swimming are just two examples of activities which require multi-sensory integration. When people have some residual hearing they use it to supplement lipreading. No one turns off their hearing aids when they are lipreading! In the same way no one should 'turn off' their visual input (lipreading) when they are tactiling.

Tactiling helps speech production as well as speech understanding

When I meet people for the first time they often comment on the naturalness of my speech. It seems that my voice quality is quite normal and when I speak foreign languages I sound the same as normal hearing Swedes. Having a normal sounding voice is a great help in social interactions – if you are afraid of making mistakes, being misunderstood, or sounding 'strange' you will become shy and insecure.

One of the most valuable attributes of tactiling for me is the feedback it provides of my own voice. I can feel my own voice and compare it to that of other speakers. I don't mean that I put my hand on my neck to feel my voice. I feel it through tactile receptors in my throat and neck. If you cannot hear there would seem to be no other way of maintaining good speech quality. You can, of course, have people listen to your speech and provide feedback, but this is not really feasible for day-to-day speech control and maintenance.

I find that tactiling helps me to speak at appropriate loudness levels. I feel the level that a speaker is using and try to copy it. In this way I can raise my voice in the presence of background noise, and lower it when everything, and everyone, around me is quiet. It is also a good idea to have someone willing to alert you if the situation suddenly changes. For example, if there is a sudden decrease in background noise when music stops, or someone rises to present an after dinner speech.

Tactile Tactics

The method described in this chapter is quite unknown to the general public. Accordingly, there are times when I need to explain why and what I am doing. This can be quite time consuming, and it helps to know a variety of strategies to use at different times.

My first rule is that in simple communicative situations I do nothing at all! If I am out buying the daily paper or a loaf of bread I can get by with just lipreading. If there are problems or misunderstandings my simplest solution is to tell the person that I am deaf and ask them to speak more slowly.

Sometimes a stranger stops me to ask for directions, and we become involved in a conversation. On these occasions I often use my 'pickpocket's' tactic. I will gently touch the person's shoulder whilst I am explaining something or asking them to 'Please repeat what you said because I don't hear very well'. If the discussion turns out to be more complex, however, I explain that my lipreading is greatly helped if I can pick up the vibrations of a speaker's voice. Then, I can ask if it is all right for me to put my hand on her/his shoulder so that I can receive the vibrations. It's at this point that I can put my hand more firmly on the speaker's shoulder and closer to her/his neck. I don't need to touch the throat as I can get strong enough cues from the bones of the shoulder. The best position that I've found is to rest my hand on the speaker's shoulder and lightly place my thumb on the side of the neck just under the jaw. The shoulder provides me with a firm platform, and the thumb is just in contact with the skin.

Clothes seldom interfere with my ability to pick up vibrations. Thick overcoats can be a problem but it's not really all that serious. One thing which some people find unusual is that I have very rarely received any negative responses to my use of tactiling. The opposite is usually the case, in fact. People are usually very interested, and will say things like – 'It's so interesting and practical. Do other deaf people use the same method as you?' The key seems to be that the stranger should first experience the difficult situation of communicating with a deaf person, and then be offered a way of making it so much easier.

When I am in an unfamiliar group of people, or in an unfamiliar situation, I always let people know that I'm deaf from the very beginning. I also try to find the person who knows about the group, the topic or even the milieu in which we are operating. I hope to find at least one person who can act as an 'interlocutor' for me. Part of being a successful deaf person seems to me to involve the ability to pick the right 'interlocutor' for a specific situation. Tactiling can also help bring people closer to you in unfamiliar surroundings. 'He's a nice guy. He really feels what you say!' This affective aspect is an important part of the success of tactiling. Finally, tactiling is a very positive reminder to people in the group that you are deaf.

Tactile Aids

About twelve years ago I had the opportunity to try out some newly developed tactile aids. I was very excited by this prospect. I had often thought about combining my practical experience as a deaf person with my knowledge of electronics and physics to build a tactile aid for myself.

The tactile devices I saw represented a number of different approaches. One of them was Hartmut Traunmüller's (1980) 'Sentiphone' which gave a strong signal via a cylindrical vibrator held in the hand. I liked this approach and found that it was similar in many ways to what I received from tactiling, although I thought that the 'Sentiphone's' signal was coarser. Its main drawback was in its resolution of the signals. The vibrator was not damped and, as a result, a strong, low frequency sound (a vowel, for example) effectively masked any higher frequency sounds with lower intensities. Further, the device was rather bulky and required a number of batteries. I found that I could perform better with natural tactiling, but wrote a report suggesting the need for a better vibrator. I am sorry to say that nothing came of it.

Not long after this I saw a much neater device which was also developed in the Department of Speech Communication and Music Acoustics at the Royal Institute of Technology in Stockholm. This was Karl-Erik Spens' 'Minivib' (Spens and Plant, 1983). I thought that the 'Minivib' had a good output but I had two basic objections to it. Firstly, the signal was a fixed frequency resulting in a buzzing sensation of varying intensities. I felt that it gave me less information than tactiling, an opinion confirmed in later testing (Plant and Spens, 1986; Öhngren, 1992). Secondly, in a noisy environment the output from the 'Minivib' was confusing. It has a built-in noise suppression circuit to depress continuous sounds, but this circuit interacted negatively with aspects of the speech signal that I wanted to interpret.

Despite these problems I found the 'Minivib' to be useful on some occasions. I was also encouraged by the fact that the Stockholm group was engaged in scientific research into the use of tactile aids. Since that time, I have had many valuable contacts with Arne Risberg and Karl-Erik Spens, and this has encouraged me to continue my own work with tactile aids.

It was not long after these first meetings that I asked about the development of a simple, straightforward tactile aid. I had in mind a relatively simple device that would pick up vibrations from the neck, amplify them, and present them through a hand-held vibrator. In this way I hoped that I would be able to receive a stronger signal than I received from tactiling. I mentioned the possibility of using a laryngeal microphone such as the ones that are used by pilots. If this wasn't feasible I thought that perhaps a directional microphone would provide me with the required signal. Unfortunately, it was a lot easier to have these ideas than to get the support necessary to realize them! I came into contact with a number of engineers and technicians who worked with hearing aids and they showed interest in the idea, but nothing came of this interest.

Until 1984 I had almost no contact with other hearing-impaired people. I was not totally aware that a hearing loss could be very disabling for many people. I thought that if you had established language skills it was not really much of a problem. I was only vaguely aware that tactiling was unknown to the vast majority of hearing-impaired people. I was far more involved with the trivial everyday problems that concern us all, regardless of whether or not we have a hearing loss – my family, my career, and my social life. At about that time a campaign was started in Sweden to identify the adult deaf 'community'. I was interested in this, and became somewhat involved. From this time on I became far more interested in finding out more about a suitable tactile aid. I was convinced that a good tactile aid would be very useful to very many deaf people, not just myself.

I attended a meeting of the International Federation of the Hard of

Hearing in Stockholm that year, and presented a paper about my thoughts on tactiling and tactile aids. I was hoping that through this meeting I would meet other tactilers, because I knew just how successful the approach had been for me. I was also hoping that maybe parents of deafened children would be interested in trying tactiling with their children. Unfortunately, this was all in vain. There are very few other deaf people who use tactiling in their daily lives. Gunnilla Öhngren (1992) mentions a few in her thesis, and I have met one other person who uses tactiling. This was a farmer's wife in Australia and she said that the only person she used it with was her husband. She was a good lipreader, and we were able to understand each other, but she refused to show me how good she was at tactiling. Maybe she was unaware that tactiling could enhance her communication abilities in general, rather than just the quality of her marriage!

Slowly, however, my efforts began to yield some results. I wasn't interested in doing any research work myself. I felt that I didn't have the right background for such an undertaking. I have my training in molecular biology and I am interested in a number of other areas of scientific research. My biggest problem that I could see, however, was that I was too intimately concerned with the subject. I wondered if I could be truly objective in any examination of tactiling. My aim was to find someone who was interested in the subject, preferably someone from the field of hearing research, and encourage them to initiate a study of tactiling. A breakthrough came in 1985 when Geoff Plant and Karl-Erik Spens invited me to take part in a study comparing two tactile aids and tactiling (Plant and Spens, 1986). After that study a number of other people from the field of cognitive psychology became interested in the subject. Gunilla Öhngren, who lives in my home town of Uppsala, started her thesis work to find out if the lipreading skills of other deafened adults would benefit from tactiling. She did some very fine work, and found a small but consistent improvement in performance for all of the subjects in her study.

Gunilla and I also considered how to develop a tactile aid which would provide the same information as tactiling. I had found that there was a small piezo-electric sensor used to pick up the nasal vibrations in the speech of deaf children. I asked Gunilla's colleagues in Stockholm whether they would be interested in building a device using a contact microphone of this type. They had previous experience with just this type of application, and in 1989 an experimental aid was built. Later I got some help from Jan Nordstrand, an audiological engineer in Uppsala. Jan and I received some grants to support this work and we worked on the development of an aid for everyday use. The aid proved to be very useful to me, and Gunilla also used it in some of her studies of deafened adults. She named it the 'Tactilator' and looked at its use as an aid to lipreading with 16 deafened subjects. Using De Filippo and

Scott's (1978) speech tracking procedure, Gunilla found that her subjects all improved when the 'Tactilator' supported lipreading. The degree of improvement varied from subject to subject with a range of 10–50% better tracking rates when lipreading was supplemented by the 'Tactiliator'. This was a very exciting finding, and it should be pointed out that these subjects had received no training in the use of the 'Tactilator'. Some people think that performance will not improve with long-term training. I believe, however, that long-term experience with tactiling and the use of strategies developed over time will lead to enhanced performance and a better quality of life.

I have already mentioned the recent study of Jerker Rönnberg which shows that there are special abilities a person must possess if she or he is to be an effective tactiler: For example, an effective working memory, and a large lexical 'library'. I do not want to argue about Jerker's findings concerning the wiring of my own neurons. He finds them extraordinary but I think they are, at least partially, the result of forty years experience with tactiling. There is also a considerable body of research on the use of Tadoma by deaf–blind people (see Charlotte Reed, Chapter 4). Tadoma is very similar in many ways to tactiling. When Tadoma users place their hands on a speaker's face they feel laryngeal vibrations as well as lip movements, jaw movement, and the breath stream. They understand speech astonishingly well with this method, and their speech production skills are also very well developed. I haven't seen any comments related to the need for Tadoma users to be highly intelligent. Perhaps one develops these intellectual capacities along the way. There is another way in which Tadoma and tactiling are very similar – there are very few users of either method. Current estimates put the number of Tadoma users in the United States at around ten people (Lorraine Delhorne, personal communication).

I have also tested some other tactile aids over the past ten or so years. Most of them use coding schemes that prevent me from using the skills I have developed from tactiling. Electrotactile aids I find interesting at an intellectual level, but I feel that their disadvantages are too great. They are simply not comfortable to use when you compare them with the alternatives.

Tactile Aids Versus Cochlear Implants

One of my best friends in the adult deaf community is Anita Wallin. She also lives in Uppsala and is an eminent researcher in a field related to my own in molecular and cell biology. Our families often get together, and we share many interests. Anita became deaf only a few years ago, and received her implant in 1990. Interestingly enough, she was amongst the first to receive training in the use of the 'Tactilator'. She performed very well with it, immediately scoring 40% better than her lipreading alone score when the Tactilator supplemented lipreading.

I have no doubt that Anita would have become a tactiler if she had not received her implant quite soon after she had first worked with the 'Tactilator'. What I find very interesting is that she seemed, unlike most cochlear implantees, to immediately derive benefit from her implant. At first her aided performance was just a little better than that which she had obtained with the 'Tactilator'. Over one year, however, her performance improved until her face-to-face tracking rates are close to those of a normal hearing person (Öhngren, 1990, personal communication). From this finding I conclude, albeit tentatively, that tactiling provides much the same speech information as the cochlear implant. The nerves involved in the output from the implant array are the same as those used for normal hearing, and the brain probably uses the sensations in a more effective way. Furthermore, the cochlear implant uses much more complex speech processing strategies, and with their widespread use and existing research resources, cochlear implants may seem to be a more promising area of development than tactile aids. But tactile aids are considerably more economical, and could be used as training devices before a cochlear implant is fitted. There are also a number of deaf people who, for a variety of reasons, cannot benefit from cochlear implantation. Elderly people make up the largest group of hearing-impaired people and many of them may not be suitable candidates for implantation. Tactile aids may represent an effective solution to the communication problems of many elderly people.

In following Anita's progress over time I have gained a number of insights into those things which are really important to those of us who are deafened. No one is better able to express these insights than Anita herself, and she has done so in this book (see Chapter 10). I warmly recommend her chapter to all readers. I especially agree that being unable to pick up environmental sounds has a great influence on deafened people. I often think that environmental sounds provide us with many different sensations. Consider this recent example from my own experience. Recently I used my portable 'Tactilator' at a musical stage show. I alternated between picking up the signal from a loop system and using the aid's directional microphone. I could get a lot of the music and singing, and was able to experience the emotions of what was a partly sad story. I couldn't pick up the words but that wasn't very important, as I had been told the story in advance. I think that this is a most important finding. It is simply not possible to understand every single word that is spoken. What is really important is to feel that you, the spectator, are a part of the performance. You are not a person sitting by yourself, heavily occupied with taking in the words that are spoken. Rather, you are surrounded by the sounds and the performance.

Towards the Ideal Tactile Aid

Recently I spent a week in Boston with Geoff Plant and David Franklin. We spent a lot of that time talking about tactile aids. It seems there are ways to process the information in speech that would make them very suitable for presentation to the skin. Over the week I tested a number of different approaches and found that I didn't receive the benefits from frequency cues that I expected. The frequency discrimination ability of the skin is relatively limited, and this is especially true for short signals, such as the time taken to produce a consonant (Geoff Plant, personal communication). I have always argued against processing speech vibrations as I am most familiar with the signal that I pick up from direct contact tactiling. In fact, we found that some processing, reducing voice pitch to a constant frequency for example, had no effect on my overall performance. The only difference that I could notice is that I had to concentrate a little harder to yield the same result.

A very interesting outcome of the visit was that I became aware of the Chorus – a multi-task aid developed by David Franklin. Originally designed for the hard-of-hearing, the Chorus has many of the features that deaf people also require. The Chorus can be adapted to receive signals from infra-red and FM transmitters, the output of an induction loop, and also has its own highly directional built-in microphone. David was able to adapt the Chorus as a tactile aid, and I now use it in conjunction with the 'Tactilator' microphone we developed in Uppsala. I think that it is a very effective aid, and we probably have a very good system to present voice vibrations. Further work does need to be done, however, before we have a truly practical aid.

I have already mentioned the importance of environmental sounds to those of us who are deafened. One woman I know in Uppsala has struggled with a progressive loss for many years and is now totally deaf. She is a rather poor lipreader and has little confidence in the ability of aids to improve her communication skills. Her text telephone and writing serve as her main sources of communication input. What she wants is an aid that will give her access to environmental sounds such as footsteps, passing cars and music. When cochlear implants were first introduced I heard people saying much the same thing. They wanted the implant to give them a more 'natural' picture of their environment. What sounds natural to one implantee, however, may sound quite unnatural to another. As a result, there is a need for flexibility in programming the implant. The APL system is a Canadian programming tool used with some cochlear implants which does allow such flexibility (Deslauriers, 1993). I think that we need such a system for tactile aids. Then it would be possible to adjust all available parameters freely for optimal performance and to meet the preferences of individual users. It might also be possible to take the output from the speech processor of a cochlear implant and present it to the skin.

As far as picking up the sounds of speech, I strongly recommend the use of contact microphones that only pick up the sounds of the speaker(s) you wish. If the use of contact microphones is not possible in a certain situation a conventional microphone, preferably one that is directional, could be used.

To me, the problem with tactile communication is not so much one of finding a suitable aid. Rather it seems to be a pedagogical problem. How do you best learn to use tactiling – direct contact or via an aid? This question is one which needs to be considered in any research into the area.

Who Are We Aiming At?

Who should have a tactile aid? In Sweden and many other countries there is a common belief that all deaf and deafened children should learn the sign language of their deaf community as their first language. The parents of hard-of-hearing children can choose between oral methods and signing, but the children also learn sign as their second language. Cochlear implants are not officially recommended for children in Sweden, but some individual parents have demanded them, and a few children are now implanted. All of these children and their parents appear to be quite satisfied with the outcome. Unfortunately, those parents whose children have had cochlear implants have severe problems in being accepted by the parents' organizations in Sweden.

I think that the parents' organizations would have a lot less trouble accepting a suitable tactile aid such as the 'Tactilator'. There are strong arguments in favour of the cochlear implant, but the 'Tactilator' should be comparatively cheap and should provide assistance in speech training and in lipreading. There is nothing about the 'Tactilator' which precludes its use whilst signing.

A report given at a meeting on paediatric audiology in June 1993 (Nordisk Barnaudiologisk Kongress, 1993) concluded that the typical deaf child is most happy when she or he is able to use a variety of communication methods. Children who derive no benefit from conventional hearing aids should be provided with a 'Tactilator' or some other tactile aid. The tactile aid may provide small children with an awareness of their parents' voices, and the knowledge that lip movements are accompanied by sound. This should also encourage the development of babbling patterns. The 'Tactilator' would also expose deaf children to environmental sounds such as dogs barking, door bells, etc. The tactile sense is extremely important to our exploration of the world. If we were deprived of it as a newborn infant we would grow up severely impaired, both behaviourally and emotionally. 'Touch is the core of sentience, the foundation for communication with the world around us.' (Sachs, 1988).

In considering the needs of deaf and deafened children I again come to the argument as to whether a tactile aid should, at least initially, present vibrator patterns in an unprocessed way. In this way the patterns will be compatible with the sound memories of the deafened user. Alternatively, Chomsky (1957) argues that our brains have pre-designed patterns for sound recognition. If this is so, we should present an unprocessed signal so as to best fit these patterns. If it can later be shown that processing does lead to improved speech recognition performance, these changes can be accommodated in the tactile aid's design.

With deafened adults it is more difficult to give an answer. Almost all of them have established communication skills, and will not readily accept a method which takes many years training before it is mastered. This group is quite heterogeneous, but those who are most active in the community are practising or developing signing in their own way. In Sweden we use a variant of the Deaf community's signing as an adjunct to lipreading. There are some who see signing as the way to go, the Golden Brick Road to success, but most of us, as deafened adults, believe that spoken language is our first language. We want to go on communicating orally as much as possible. Signing in this way is a complement to oral communication, not a separate language. The mastery of signing that members of the Deaf community attain is beyond most of us who are deafened.

Deafened people do have access to interpreters in Sweden, but we want other assistance as well. If we are attending a lecture we also want a written translation – in real time if it is possible! The same appears to be the case in the United States according to the Association of Late Deafened Adults (ALDA). With the 'Tactilator' it is possible to use an oral interpreter. The great advantage of oral interpreters is that only one interpreter is needed. The interpretation is much faster, easier, and less tiring, and no special equipment is needed. If the speaker at a meeting is 'readable' I will give her/him the microphone to use, but if there are questions or discussion I need an interpreter to help me keep up with what is being discussed around me. I would like to see a system developed for such situations which would simultaneously meet the needs of tactile aid users, hearing aid users, and cochlear implantees. We all have the same underlying needs, and the development of a universal tool would be of great assistance.

Many deafened adults get cochlear implants but, as Anita Wallin says, you're still a deafened adult. Not totally deaf but rather hard-of-hearing! The same will surely be true for well-trained users of tactile aids in the future. The aids will give better access to interpreting and communication, better speech, and an awareness of environmental sounds and, I hope, music.

Acknowledgements

This project, concerning the development of a wireless 'Tactilator', has been supported by grants from the Swedish National Board for Technical Development and from Tysta Skolans Stiftelse, Stockholm, Sweden.

References

Chomsky, N. (1957) Syntactic Structures. The Hague: Mouton.

DeFilippo and Scott (1975) A method for training and evaluating the reception of ongoing speech. Acoustic Society of America 63: 1186–92.

Deslauriers, V. (1993) APL helps the deaf to hear again. APL Quote Quad, APL93, pp 63–8.

Fox, J.L. (1984) The brain's dynamic way of keeping in touch. Science 225: 820–1.

Nordisk Barnaudiologisk Kongress (1993) Örebro, Sweden, 13–16 June.

Öhngren, G. (1992) Touching voices: Components of direct tactually supported speech reading. Acta Univ. Ups. Compr. Summ. of Uppsala Diss. from the Faculty of Social Sciences 32. Uppsala. 44 pp.

Öhngren, G. (1992) Tracking tests. In Proceedings from the 2nd International Conference on Tactile Aids, Hearing Aids and Cochlear Implants in Stockholm, June 9-11, 1992, Eds. A. Risberg, S. Felicetti, G. Plant and K.-E. Spens.

Plant, G. and Spens, K-E. (1986) An experienced user of tactile information as a supplement to lipreading. An evaluation study. STL-QPSR 1: 87–110.

Rönnberg, J. (1993) Cognitive characteristics of skilled tactiling. European Journal of Cognitive Psychology 5, 1: 19–33.

Sachs, V. (1988) The intimate sense; understanding the mechanics of touch. The Sciences January/February, pp 28–34.

Spens, K-E. and Plant, G. (1983) A tactual hearing aid for the deaf. STL-QPSR 1: 52–6.

Traunmueller, H. (1980) The Sentiphone, a tactual speech communication aid. Journal of Comm. Dis. 13: 183–93.

4

Tadoma: An Overview of Research

CHARLOTTE M. REED

History and Current Use of Tadoma

The earliest use of a natural approach to the tactual reception of speech is attributed to a Norwegian teacher by the name of Hofgaard in the last decade of the 19th century (Hansen, 1930). In working with a deaf–blind adolescent, Hofgaard placed the student's hand on his face to enable her to feel the various articulatory actions that occur while speech is being produced. Apparently this child was successful in learning both to speak and to understand speech. An American teacher of the deaf, named Sophia Alcorn, became aware of Hofgaard's method in the 1920s and adapted and refined the technique in the teaching of two young deaf–blind children (Alcorn, 1932). The name by which this method is now commonly referred (Tadoma) is derived from the names of Alcorn's first two students. Through Alcorn's influence, the use of the Tadoma method spread to schools for the deaf and deaf–blind throughout the United States in the 1920s and 1930s. For several decades (up until the 1960s) the method was used both in the education of the deaf (for speech production) and the deaf–blind (for both speech production and speech reception).

Guidelines were developed for the teaching of speech reception and speech production using the Tadoma method (e.g., see Vivian, 1966; Stenquist, 1974). Training began with a series of tasks designed to develop the child's ability to control gross and fine motor movements, to imitate movements, and to attend to tactual stimulation. Speechreading was introduced by placing the child's hand on the teacher's face while she was talking. The child thus became aware of the general movements and actions taking place on the face as the teacher spoke. By presenting simple commands or the names of concrete objects, the teacher attempted to help the child develop an association between the actions being felt on the face and the movement or object in the environment that it represented. This method was used to develop the child's vocabulary while at the same time the teachers talked to the children 'at every opportunity, using natural language' (Stenquist, 1974: 29). Training on speech production was generally delayed for 6 months after initiation of speech-reception work and was based on an imitation procedure. The student first attended to the teacher's model production of a given utterance by placing a hand on the teacher's face. Then, the student's hand was transferred to his or her own face while he or she attempted to reproduce the actions felt on the teacher's face. The speech training began with isolated speech elements (beginning with the vowels /u/ and /ɑ/ and the consonants /hw/, /p/, /f/, and /t/) which were then used to form words. As the training progressed, the full set of isolated speech sounds was eventually introduced and the length of speech utterances increased from single words to phrases to sentences to nursery rhymes and stories. Speech-production training was closely related to the ongoing work on speech reception. One of the primary educational goals was to 'bring the child in contact with the outside world by giving him speech as a means of self-expression' (Inis B. Hall as quoted in Stenquist: 25). The child's education was conducted both formally in the classroom as well as informally throughout the day over the course of many years.

The Tadoma method was used in the education of deaf–blind children (many as a result of meningitis) in various schools throughout the United States from the 1920s through the 1960s. Since that time, the use of Tadoma as a primary educational method for teaching speech and language has declined considerably due in large part to the changing characteristics of the deaf–blind population. As a result of advances in medicine leading to increased infant survival rate, there is now a large number of deaf–blind children who have a range of cognitive and sensorimotor problems in addition to severe impairments of hearing and sight. A recent survey of the current use of Tadoma in programmes for the deaf–blind (Schultz et al., 1984) indicates that Tadoma is no longer used as a primary method for teaching speech and language. Tadoma is sometimes employed as a supplement to other educational methods including auditory training, sign language, fingerspelling, and visual speechreading (for students with some residual sight). The current educational trend appears to be the use of sign systems to develop communication skills appropriate to the child's cognitive and social level of functioning (Robbins et al., 1975; Wilbur, 1979: 263–4).

Despite the current limited use of the Tadoma method, there are a group of adults who were trained in its use as children and are now highly experienced users of the method. These adults are in a sense unique in that they are highly practised in the use of a method of communication that relies solely on tactual input. As such, they are a valuable source of information concerning the potential of the tactual sense for communication for several reasons. First, demonstration of successful speech reception through Tadoma provides the field of tactual research with an existence proof for the use of the skin for communication. In addition, study of this particular natural method of communication may lead to insights concerning the design of synthetic tactual devices and factors involved in learning to use tactual displays.

This chapter is organized around research that has been carried out on the Tadoma method. These topics include: (a) research on the Tadoma method with experienced deaf–blind subjects; (b) research on the Tadoma method with naive laboratory subjects; and (c) development of an artificial Tadoma system. The final section of the chapter discusses the implications of research on the Tadoma method in the development of tactual devices for the deaf.

Research on the Tadoma Method with Experienced Deaf–Blind Subjects

Studies of experienced deaf–blind users of the Tadoma method have been concerned with the speech-reception (Norton *et al.*, 1977; Reed *et al.*, 1982c, 1985, 1989a), speech-production (Tamir, 1989), and linguistic (Norton *et al.*, 1977; Reed *et al.*, 1985; Chomsky, 1986) abilities of these individuals. The studies which will be summarized here were conducted with a group of deaf–blind adults who received training in the Tadoma method as children and who currently use Tadoma as a means of communication. Information on the history of these subjects is available in Reed *et al.*, 1985: Table 1. The most common etiology of deaf/blindness among this group is childhood meningitis (in seven of the nine subjects) with occurrence before the age of 2 (again, for seven of the nine subjects). Of the nine subjects who took part in the studies, three participated in an in-depth series of analytic testing, while the remaining six were tested on a smaller battery of probe tests. Results from both groups of subjects will be drawn on to provide a picture of the abilities of Tadoma users.

Speech-reception ability

The speech-reception abilities of experienced Tadoma users have been studied for a variety of test materials, including nonsense syllables, isolated monosyllabic words, words in sentences with varying degrees of context, and connected discourse. A summary of performance on these tasks (reported by Reed *et al.*, 1985) indicates a range of abilities across individual subjects. At the segmental level, greater inter-subject variability was observed for vowel identification compared to consonant identification. Scores ranged from 18 to 60% for the identification of 16 medial vowels in /h/-V-/d/ syllables and from 52 to 69% correct for the identification of 24 initial consonants in C-/ɑ/ syllables. For meaningful speech materials, larger inter-subject variability was observed on the W-22 word test (Hirsh *et al.*, 1952) and the SPIN test (Kalikow *et al.*, 1977) than on the CID 'Everyday' sentences (Davis and Silverman, 1970). Scores for open-set monosyllabic words presented in isolation ranged from 26 to 56% across subjects. Results from the SPIN test provide an indication of the role played by context in the ability to identify monosyllabic words. For the identification of the final word in sentences where little context is established for the word (low-predictability words), scores ranged from 20 to 54% correct, compared to a range of scores from 24 to 86% when the sentence provided a context for the final word (high-predictability words). Differences in scores between the high-predictability and low-predictability words on the SPIN test ranged from −4 to +56 percentage points. Four of the subjects indicated substantial ability to use contextual information to enhance word recognition (with difference scores ranging from 28 to 56) while the remaining five subjects evidenced no such ability (their difference scores ranged from −4 to +4). Results on the CID 'Everyday' sentences indicated that seven of the nine subjects scored in the range of 70–85% correct key words, with the remaining two subjects exhibiting scores below 50% correct.

Sentence-reception ability was dependent on speaking rate as well as on the difficulty of the materials. Of the three in-depth subjects who were tested on CID sentences as a function of speaking rate, scores for two of the subjects dropped rapidly at rates above 3 syllables/second, while the third was able to maintain good performance up to roughly 6 syllables/second (normal speaking rate is in the range of 4–5 syllables/second). The Harvard or IEEE (1969) sentences proved to be more difficult in that scores for the three in-depth subjects ranged from 45 to 60% correct at slower-than-normal speaking rates compared to their CID scores of 80-85% correct at similar speaking rates. Some indication of the ability to process connected discourse through Tadoma is provided by results from the three in-depth subjects using the tracking paradigm of De Filippo and Scott (1978). Tracking scores ranged from 30 to 40 words/minute across the three subjects compared with tracking scores for the normal auditory/visual reception of speech of roughly 100 words/minute.

Taken together, the results from different speech materials suggest that the performance of Tadoma users may be compared to that of listeners in adverse speech-to-noise ratios or to lipreaders: that is, less-than-perfect segmental information appears to be combined with contextual cues to achieve reasonably good reception of conversational speech. Reed *et al.* (1992c) suggest that the reception of speech through Tadoma may be comparable to that of normal-hearing listeners under speech-to-noise ratios in the range of 0–6 dB.

Insight into the basic cues used to receive speech through Tadoma is provided through analyses of segmental-reception data obtained in consonant and vowel identification tests. For consonants, feature analyses of confusion data indicate that voicing and manner of production are generally better perceived than features related to place of production. For vowels, features related to lip-rounding, tenseness, and jaw lowering are better received than features such as low and back which describe the location of the tongue within the mouth. The reception of segmental speech cues through Tadoma appears to be related to four basic types of actions available on the face and neck during speech production: laryngeal vibration, lip movements, jaw movements, and airflow at the lips. The effects of systematic removal of these cues on the reception of small sets of consonants and vowels are described by Reed *et al.* (1989a). Different patterns of performance were observed for different features as a function of hand position. For example, removal of the hand from the neck resulted in reduced reception of consonant voicing while having little effect on manner or place reception, while removal of thumb contact with the lips strongly reduced the reception of place, had a moderate effect on manner reception, and no effect on voicing. At the same time, the results also suggest that the cues are not totally independent of each other in that certain types of information were conveyed redundantly among the cues. For example, information concerning manner of production is transmitted both through airflow at the lips and through lip movements and voicing information is present on both the jaw and neck.

Speech-production ability

Characteristics of the speech produced by the three in-depth Tadoma subjects have been assessed through measurements of intelligibility as well as objective acoustic properties. The basic trends observed in these measurements were similar across the three Tadoma users despite the fact that two of the subjects can be classified as prelingually deaf (with onsets around the age of 1.5) while the third subject was postlingually deafened at the age of 7.

The intelligibility of productions of Clarke sentences (Magner, 1972) recorded by the three Tadoma users was evaluated using a panel of three listeners who had little, if any, previous experience listening to deaf speech. Percentage-correct syllable reception averaged across the three listeners ranged from 63 to 70%. The listeners were also asked to assign intelligibility ratings to the speech of the Tadoma users on a scale from 1 to 5 (where 1 represents 'easily understood' and 5 represents 'completely unintelligible'). The ratings averaged roughly 3 ('only partially understood') across listeners for each talker, and were thus consistent with the intelligibility scores obtained on these materials. These speech intelligibility measures compare favourably to average results on intelligibility of deaf speech reported in the literature (e.g., Smith, 1975).

Various objective measurements of segmental and suprasegmental properties were obtained on the Clarke sentences recorded by the Tadoma users (Tamir, 1989). Measurements of vowels produced in sentence context indicated reduced F1–F2 space, relatively normal fundamental frequency, longer-than-normal intrinsic vowel durations but fairly normal patterns of relative vowel durations, and little change in formant values throughout the duration of diphthongs. Measures of consonants indicated fairly normal patterns of VOT and spectral characteristics of plosives and fricatives. Suprasegmental measures indicated that speaking rate was slower than normal by roughly a factor of two and that, for two of the three speakers, the ratio of pause-to-vocalization time was extremely high. Fundamental-frequency contours indicated very little movement in F0 over the course of a sentence. Generally, these trends are similar to those described for sighted deaf speakers (e.g. Monsen, 1978).

Linguistic ability

A variety of tests of linguistic competence have been conducted with the Tadoma subjects, including standardized language tests as well as special-purpose tests derived from the research literature on linguistics. This testing addresses the question of the extent to which the learning of language can stimulated and/or extended through Tadoma input following the onset of deafness and blindness. The nine Tadoma subjects were administered (in Braille) the Test of Syntactic Ability (TSA) developed by Quigley *et al.* (1978) for evaluating the English skills of deaf and hearing-impaired students. Scores on the TSA, which samples performance on a set of nine grammatical features in multiple-choice format, ranged from 48 to 100% correct across the nine subjects. Six subjects (including the four who made substantial use of context in the SPIN test) scored higher than the normative score of 68% for a population of 500 students with mild to profound hearing loss. Of the three subjects who performed below the normative value, two are believed to have been deaf and blind from birth.

Further evaluations of the linguistic competence of the three in-depth subjects are reported by Chomsky (1986). Of these three subjects, two suffered onset of deaf/blindness in the second year of life, while the onset for the third occurred at age 7. Chomsky's tests included extensive probes of the subjects' knowledge of various grammatical and semantic distinctions and of their abilities to provide objective accounts of a variety of linguistic phenomena. For the two subjects with early onset, Chomsky reports vocabulary development and oral and written language abilities that compare favourably to the normal-hearing population and syntactic abilities that are excellent relative to the deaf population. For both subjects, some deficits were noted in their ability to interpret special types of syntactic constructions (structural ambiguity in sentences and tag questions). The testing of the subject with later onset of deaf/blindness indicates that she has developed full and normal linguistic competence that undoubtedly goes beyond the competence she would have achieved at the age of 7. Based on her extensive evaluations, Chomsky concludes that 'our observations reveal a relatively minor effect on language achievement of severe restriction on amount and range of language exposure' (page 344) and clearly indicate that linguistic competence may be acquired and extended through Tadoma input.

Research on the Tadoma Method with Naive Subjects

Research on Tadoma with laboratory subjects includes studies of discrimination and identification of speech segments (Reed *et al.*, 1978, 1982a; Snyder *et al.*, 1982), long-term studies of the reception of speech, including connected discourse, through Tadoma (Reed *et al.*, 1982a), and a series of studies concerned with improving segmental reception through Tadoma by means of supplementary tactual displays (Reed *et al.*, 1992c). These studies have typically employed normal-hearing and sighted subjects and used masking noise and blindfolds to eliminate auditory and visual cues.

Segmental performance

The ability of naive subjects to discriminate pairs of speech segments was studied for a variety of speech materials using an ABX discrimination paradigm (Reed *et al.*, 1978). Although the subjects had no previous experience using Tadoma and were unable to identify the materials presented, they were asked to attend only to differences between the stimuli and to decide whether the third item in an experimental trial was a repetition of the first or second item (which were always different from each other). Thus, the ability to perform the task relied only on the ability to attend to differences in sequentially presented stimuli and did not require the type of higher-order cognitive processing involved in interpreting connected speech. Discrimination scores for the two naive subjects ranged from roughly 70 to 90% correct across the different types of materials and compared quite favourably to performance of an experienced Tadoma user on the same task.

Snyder *et al.* (1982) compared the ability of naive subjects to discriminate a set of 32 consonant pairs through Tadoma and through an artificial tactile display of the speech spectrum. Common subjects, test materials, and procedures were employed for the two methods. Results indicated superior performance through Tadoma for contrasts of voicing (90% vs 55%) and place (82% vs 57%) and similar performance for the two methods for manner constrasts (roughly 78%). The poor results obtained with the tactile display may have been related to the specific device employed in the study, which was a 24 × 6 finger-sized array of vibrators which encoded frequency and amplitude, respectively.

The ability of naive subjects to identify speech segments through Tadoma was studied for a set of 24 consonants and for a set of 15 vowels and diphthongs in fixed monosyllabic context (Reed *et al.*, 1982a). Following roughly 100 hours of training, identification scores averaged roughly 75% correct for the set of 24 consonants and 82% correct for the set of 15 vowels and diphthongs. These scores, which were obtained with the speaker used in the training sessions, exceed the range of scores observed on these tasks for experienced deaf–blind Tadoma users (see Reed *et al.*, 1985). When the naive subjects were tested with unfamiliar speakers, their scores dropped to levels of 40–60% correct but were within the range of scores obtained by the experienced Tadoma users. Analyses of the identification results showed similar patterns of confusion for the naive and experienced subjects, suggesting that both groups of subjects monitored the same types of information in performing the segmental identification task.

The results of the discrimination and identification tests are useful (a) in establishing that there are no inherent differences in basic tactile sensitivity between experienced deaf–blind subjects and normal subjects, (b) in providing further insight into the cues available through Tadoma, and (c) in serving as a reference point for evaluating the performance of laboratory subjects on artificial tactual displays of speech.

Long-term training in the use of Tadoma

Long-term studies of the acquisition of speech-reception abilities through Tadoma by naive subjects have been undertaken as a first step in understanding the process involved in learning to use Tadoma. The use of normal-hearing and sighted subjects with simulated sensory impairment eliminates the need to learn language and thus focuses the learning problem on the use of the Tadoma display itself (as would be the case with any other tactual display of speech). In one study (Reed *et al.*, 1982a), two naive subjects, who first were given some preliminary training at the segmental level, received roughly 40 hours training on the acquisition of a 43-word vocabulary and on the identification of sentences constructed from the vocabulary. Post-training tests of the ability to receive sentences constructed from this limited vocabulary indicated scores of roughly 30% correct for the initial presentation and an average of roughly four presentations required for a correct repetition of the entire sentence.

In a follow-on study, a group of three new subjects each received roughly 500–600 hours training on identification of speech segments, isolated words, and sentences formed from a fixed vocabulary that reached 250 words. Final tests performed with the 250-word vocabulary indicated a range of performance across the three subjects: identification of isolated words drawn from the complete vocabulary ranged from 30 to 52%; identification of words on the first presentation of sentences (averaging eight words in length) ranged from 28 to 57%; and the average number of presentations required for complete identification of a sentence ranged from 2 to 7. Overall, these results suggest that the difficulty of learning Tadoma in subjects who have acquired language through the normal route may be roughly comparable to the difficulty of learning a 'difficult' foreign language. Of course, this problem is much simpler than that posed for the deaf–blind child whose ultimate task is the acquisition of both speech and language through Tadoma.

Augmented Tadoma

Reed *et al.* (1992c) report on a series of studies examining the possibility of improving the reception of speech segments through Tadoma through the addition of supplementary tactual information. A knowledge of the structure of segmental confusions through Tadoma (see section above on speech-reception ability of experienced deaf–blind subjects) leads to speculation that many of these errors might be eliminated by introducing additional information concerning the location of the tongue within the oral cavity. Ultimately, the goal of this research was to establish a 'super-Tadoma' system that (a) relied solely on tactual input, (b) led to near-perfect segmental reception, and (c) provided a new standard of performance through the tactual sense.

Experiments were conducted with three types of supplementary tactual displays: (1) a tactile display of tongue contact with the palate; (2) a tactile display of the short-term speech spectrum; and (3) tactual reception of the manual cues associated with Cornett's (1967) Cued Speech system. The discriminability of pairs of consonants and vowels that were highly confused under Tadoma was studied for conditions that included Tadoma alone, the supplemental tactual display alone, and Tadoma combined with a particular supplementary display.

Supplementary information on tongue position was measured by detection of tongue contact with the hard palate (using the Rion

Electro Palatograph) and presented through a finger-sized vibrotactile array. Consonant discrimination scores indicated that performance for either the tactile display alone (82%) or for Tadoma augmented by this display (81%) was substantially greater than that obtained for Tadoma alone (65% correct). For vowels, on the other hand, performance for Tadoma alone and for augmented Tadoma were similar (roughly 65%) and superior to that obtained with the tactile display of tongue contact presented by itself (56%). Thus, the display of tongue contact with the hard palate proved to be more effective in improving consonant than vowel discriminability.

In an effort to improve vowel discriminability, Tadoma was supplemented with a spectral display of the acoustic waveform based on results suggesting that vowel identification using multichannel displays of the short-term spectrum may be superior to that obtained through Tadoma (see Reed et al., 1982b). The supplementary display of the speech spectrum was a laboratory version of the 16-channel Queen's University tactile vocoder (Brooks and Frost, 1983) in which speech is filtered into 16 bandpass channels and presented through a linear array of solenoid vibrators worn along the forearm. Average vowel discriminability for Tadoma augmented by this display (80%) was slightly better than that obtained for either the tactile vocoder alone (75%) or Tadoma alone (73%). Thus, the supplementary spectral display proved to be more effective than the tongue–palate-contact display in improving the discriminability of vowels through Tadoma.

Finally, experiments were conducted using tactual reception of the manual cues associated with Cued Speech as a supplement to Tadoma ('Cued Tadoma'). Based on near-perfect levels of performance on the consonant and vowel discrimination task, testing was extended to include identification of sets of consonants and vowels. Improvements of 25 percentage points for Cued Tadoma (roughly 85% correct) over Tadoma alone (roughly 60%) were obtained for both consonants and vowels. The results obtained with Cued Tadoma indicate (a) that the hand actions used in visual cueing can be well perceived tactually, (b) that subjects can integrate tactual cueing with Tadoma, and (c) that the cues are effective in disambiguating speech segments that are confused through Tadoma. Thus, Cued Tadoma provides an effective demonstration of the possibility of a tactual system for speech communication that results in higher performance than that obtained through natural Tadoma.

Development of an Artificial Tadoma System

Research has been conducted on the development and evaluation of a synthetic Tadoma system (Skarda, 1983; Leotta, 1985; Leotta et al., 1988; Reed et al., 1985; Henderson, 1989; Tan et al., 1989). The goal of this research was to develop an accurate simulation of Tadoma and to use this simulation as a research tool to explore various hypotheses concerning the properties of Tadoma that are responsible for its success.

Construction of synthetic face

The basis of the synthetic Tadoma system is an anatomical-model skull that was adapted to produce movements corresponding to those that occur in the articulation of speech (Reed *et al.*, 1985; Leotta, 1985). In particular, these movements were chosen to be those that previous research suggested were most important for speech reception through Tadoma. Among this previous research (in addition to segmental studies of speech reception through Tadoma on both experienced and naive subjects – see above) was an early study conducted by Hansen (1964) on the relationship between facial actions during speech production and Tadoma performance. The actions that were incorporated into the anatomical-model skull included: jaw movements, up–down and in–out movements of the lower lip, up–down movements of the upper lip (all through the use of position-controlled actuators), airflow at the lips (through valving actions on a tank of compressed air), and vibration in the laryngeal area (through a bone-conduction vibrator). Each of these actions was controlled by a digital signal derived from physical measurements of a talker's face while producing a set of test materials (Skarda, 1983). For example, strain gauges were used to record lip and jaw movements and a microphone to record laryngeal vibrations.

Speech performance with synthetic Tadoma system

In a preliminary evaluation of the performance of this synthetic Tadoma system, Leotta *et al.* (1988) conducted experiments on the discriminability of pairs of speech segments using naive laboratory subjects. The discriminability of 11 vowel contrasts and 38 consonant contrasts using the synthetic display was compared to results reported by Reed *et al.* (1978) for natural Tadoma. Overall vowel discriminability was similar for natural (70%) and synthetic (71%) Tadoma, while average consonant scores were better for natural (roughly 83%) than for synthetic (roughly 65%) Tadoma. The most striking difference between artificial and natural Tadoma was on the discrimination of consonant voicing contrasts (56% for synthetic compared to 70% for natural Tadoma). When the synthetic system was modified to display the voicing signal over a larger region of the face, the score was improved to a level comparable to that obtained with natural Tadoma.

Following a set of further modifications to the synthetic face to improve the specification and control of airflow signals and lip closure, Henderson (1989) conducted a series of evaluations of speech reception using the modified system. Normal laboratory subjects received training on the identification of sets of consonants and vowels presented through the artificial face. Post-training scores averaged roughly 65% for identification of a set of 24 consonants or for a set of 15 vowels and compared favourably to performance through natural Tadoma. Furthermore, error analyses indicated that confusion patterns were qualitatively similar for natural and synthetic Tadoma. The subjects were also tested in a study of the effects of the removal of each of the facial actions on reception of a set of 12 consonants. Results showed decreased performance with the elimination of any one cue, and different error patterns depending on the specific cue that was removed. Testing was also conducted with one experienced deaf–blind Tadoma user on the identification of various sets of consonants and vowels and on sentence reception. On the segmental tests, this subject's performance was inferior to his scores on natural Tadoma but similar to that of the laboratory-trained subjects after an equivalent amount of experience (in terms of number of trials on a given task) with the synthetic display. For CID sentences presented through the synthetic face, the experienced Tadoma user scored 20% on recognition of key words, compared to his score of 85% on natural Tadoma. The results from the laboratory subjects and the experienced Tadoma user suggest that although the synthetic Tadoma system does not provide a perfect simulation of natural Tadoma, it is capable of transmitting roughly the same amount of information, at least at the segmental level.

Basic studies with synthetic Tadoma system

The information-transmission properties of the synthetic Tadoma display were studied further in an investigation that focused on the four separate lip and jaw movements that occur on the artificial face (Tan et al., 1989). Measurements of the just-noticeable-difference (JND) for displacement of each of these movements indicated a Weber fraction of roughly 9% across a range of reference displacements when the values of the remaining channels were held fixed. When random variations were introduced into the displacement values of the non-relevant channels, the Weber fraction increased by a factor of roughly 2–6 depending on the particular movement channel being measured. Identification of displacement values was studied for one-dimensional stimuli (using both fixed and randomly selected values along the non-relevant dimensions) and for four-dimensional stimuli. Information transfer along each of the single dimensions was roughly 1.5 bits for fixed backgrounds and decreased by a factor of roughly 2 when random variations were introduced into the non-relevant dimensions. Information transfer for the four-dimensional stimuli (roughly 3.3 bits) was similar to the sum of the information transfer across the single dimensions with roving background. This study did not include measurements of the airflow and vibration channels of the synthetic Tadoma system; however, if one assumes similar information-transmission properties for these channels as for the movement channels, then total information transfer along the six dimensions of the synthetic system may be estimated at roughly 5–6 bits. This estimate of information transfer for a synthetic Tadoma system suggests (a) that the system carries roughly the amount of information necessary for identification of the set of segmentals used in English and (b) that the synthetic Tadoma system is not exceptional in its information-bearing capacity.

Implications of Tadoma Research in the Development of Tactual Aids for the Deaf

Studies with experienced deaf–blind users of the Tadoma method have demonstrated the capability of the tactual sense for speech communication, thereby providing an impetus for continued efforts in the development of sensory-substitution devices. Research on Tadoma has begun to examine the particular properties of this method that account for its success as a basis for improving the design of artificial tactual devices. These characteristics (discussed previously by Reed *et al.*, 1985, 1989b, 1992a) include the use of the hand for sensory input, the use of an articulatory-based display, the multi-dimensional aspects of the Tadoma display, and, finally, the extensive training in and long-term use of Tadoma by its practitioners. Although preliminary insight into these issues has been provided through studies of the acquisition of Tadoma by naive subjects and of augmented Tadoma, as well as through work on a synthetic Tadoma system, our understanding of these issues is still incomplete. In particular, a more comprehensive understanding of the properties that govern information transfer in the tactual sense is necessary for advancements in the development of practical tactual speech-communication devices.

Studies of other natural methods of tactual communication also provide support for the potential of the tactual sense for communication. For example, data obtained on a natural tactual supplement to speechreading used by an expert subject (Plant and Spens, 1984; Öhngren, 1992) offer an existence proof for the successful integration of speechreading with supplementary information presented tactually. More generally, research on methods of tactual communication used by members of the deaf–blind community (including the tactual reception of fingerspelling and sign language as well as Tadoma) suggest that the tactual sense is capable of receiving information encoded in a variety of different ways at rates and performance levels that allow for efficient communication (e.g., see Reed *et al.*, 1989b, 1990, 1992a, 1992b; Working Group on Communication Aids for the Hearing-Impaired, 1991). The natural methods of tactual communication provide a baseline of performance against which artificial devices may be compared and help suggest guidelines which may be followed in the design of future tactual aids. But perhaps most importantly, these methods serve as an inspiration for continued research in the area of tactual communication.

Acknowledgement

This research was supported by a grant from the National Institutes of Health (NIH Grant No. 5-R01-DC00126).

References

Alcorn, S. (1932) The Tadoma method. Volta Review 34: 195–8.

Brooks, P.L. and Frost, B.J. (1983) Evaluation of a tactile vocoder for word recognition. Journal of the Acoustical Society of America 74: 34–9.

Chomsky, C. (1986) Analytic study of the Tadoma method: Language abilities of three deaf–blind subjects. Journal of Speech and Hearing Research 29: 332–47.

Cornett, O. (1967) Cued Speech. American Annals of the Deaf 112: 3–13.

Davis, H. and Silverman, S.R. (1970) Hearing and Deafness. New York: Holt, Rinehart, and Winston.

De Filippo, C.L. and Scott, B.L. (1978) A method for training and evaluating the reception of ongoing speech. Journal of the Acoustical Society of America 63: 1186–92.

Hansen, A. (1930) The first case in the world: Miss Petra Heiberg's report. Volta Review 32: 223.

Hansen, R.J. (1964) Characterization of Speech by External Articulatory Cues as the Basis for a Speech-to-Tactile Communication System for Use by the Deaf–blind. M.S. Thesis, Massachusetts Institute of Technology, Cambridge, MA.

Henderson, D.R. (1989) Tactile Speech Reception: Development and Evaluation of an Improved Synthetic Tadoma System. M.S. Thesis, Massachusetts Institute of Technology, Cambridge, MA.

Hirsh, I., Davis, H., Silverman, S.R., Reynolds, E., Eldert, E. and Benson, R.W. (1952) Development of materials for speech audiometry. Journal of Speech and Hearing Disorders 17: 321–37.

IEEE (1969). Recommended practice for speech quality measurements. IEEE Transactions on Audio Electroacoustics 17: 225–46.

Kalikow, D.N., Stevens, K.N and Elliott, L.L. (1977) Development of test of speech intelligibility in noise using sentence materials with controlled word predictability. Journal of the Acoustical Society of America 61: 1337–51.

Leotta, D.F. (1985) Synthetic Tadoma: Tactile Speech Reception from a Computer-Controlled Artificial Face. M.S. Thesis, Massachusetts Institute of Technology, Cambridge, MA.

Leotta, D.F., Rabinowitz, W.M., Reed, C.M. and Durlach, N.I. (1988) Preliminary results of speech-reception tests obtained with the synthetic Tadoma system.

Journal of Rehabilitation Research 25: 45–52.

Magner, M.E. (1972) A Speech Intelligibility Test for Deaf Children. Clarke School for the Deaf, Northampton, Massachusetts.

Monsen, R.B. (1978) Toward measuring how well hearing-impaired children speak. Journal of Speech and Hearing Research 21: 197–219.

Norton, S.J., Schultz, M.C., Reed, C.M., Braida, L.D., Durlach, N.I., Rabinowitz, W.M. and Chomsky, C. (1977) Analytic study of the Tadoma method: background and preliminary results. Journal of Speech and Hearing Research 20: 574–95.

Öhngren, G. (1992) Touching Voices: Components of Direct Tactually Supported Speechreading. Doctoral Dissertation, Uppsala University, Uppsala, Sweden.

Plant, G. and Spens, K.E. (1986) An experienced user of tactile information as a supplement to lipreading. STL-QPSR 1: 87–110.

Quigley, S.P., Steinkamp, M.W., Power, D.J. and Jones, B.W. (1978) Test of Syntactic Abilities. Beaverton, Oregon: Dormac.

Reed, C.M., Delhorne, L.A., Durlach, N.I. and Fischer, S.D. (1990) A study of the tactual and visual reception of fingerspelling. Journal of Speech and Hearing Research 33: 786–97.

Reed, C.M., Doherty, M.J., Braida, L.D. and Durlach, N.I. (1982a) Analytic study of the Tadoma method: further experiments with inexperienced observers. Journal of Speech and Hearing Research 25: 216–23.

Reed, C.M., Durlach, N.I. and Braida, L.D. (1982b) Research on tactile communication of speech: a review. ASHA Monographs, Number 20.

Reed, C.M., Durlach, N.I., Braida, L.D. and Schultz, M.C. (1982c) Analytic study of the Tadoma method: identification of consonants and vowels by an experienced Tadoma user. Journal of Speech and Hearing Research 25: 108–116.

Reed, C.M., Durlach, N.I., Braida, L.D. and Schultz, M.C. (1989a) Analytic study of the Tadoma method: effects of hand position on segmental speech perception. Journal of Speech and Hearing Research 32: 921–9.

Reed, C.M., Durlach, N.I. and Delhorne, L.A. (1992a) Natural methods of tactual communication. In Summers, I.R. (Ed) Tactile Aids for the Hearing Impaired. London: Whurr Publishers.

Reed, C.M., Durlach, N.I. and Delhorne, L.A. (1992b) The tactual reception of speech, fingerspelling, and sign language by the deaf–blind. SID 92 Digest, 102–5.

Reed, C.M., Durlach, N.I., Delhorne, L.A., Rabinowitz, W.M. and Grant, K. W. (1989b) Research on tactual communication of speech: ideas, issues, and findings. Volta Review (Monograph) 91: 65–78.

Reed, C.M., Rabinowitz, W.M., Durlach, N.I., Braida, L.D., Conway-Fithian, S. and Schultz, M.C. (1985) Research on the Tadoma method of speech communication. Journal of the Acoustical Society of America 77: 247–57.

Reed, C.M., Rabinowitz, W.M., Durlach, N.I., Delhorne, L.A., Braida, L.D., Pemberton, J.C., Mulcahey, B.D. and Washington, D.L. (1992c) Analytic study of the Tadoma method: improving performance through the use of supplementary tactual displays. Journal of Speech and Hearing Research 35: 450–65.

Reed, C.M., Rubin, S.I., Braida, L.D. and Durlach, N.I. (1978) Analytic study of the Tadoma method: discrimination ability of untrained observers. Journal of Speech and Hearing Research 21: 625–37.

Robbins, N., Cagan, J., Johnson, C., Kelleher, H., Record, J. and Vernacchia, J. (1975) Perkins Sign Language Dictionary. Perkins School for the Blind. Watertown, Massachusetts.

Schultz, M.C., Norton, S.J., Conway-Fithian, S. and Reed, C.M. (1984) A survey of the use of the Tadoma method in the United States and Canada. Volta Review 86: 282–92.

Skarda, G.M. (1983) An Analysis of Facial Action Signals during Speech Production Appropriate for a Synthetic Tadoma System. M.S. Thesis, Massachusetts Institute of Technology, Cambridge, MA.

Smith, C.R. (1975) Residual hearing and speech production in deaf children. Journal of Speech and Hearing Research 18: 795–811.

Snyder, J.C., Clements, M.A., Reed, C.M., Durlach, N.I. and Braida, L.D. (1982) Tactile communication of speech. I. Comparison of Tadoma and a frequency-amplitude spectral display in a consonant discrimination task. Journal of the Acoustical Society of America 71: 1249–54.

Stenquist, G. (1974) The Story of Leonard Dowdy: Deaf–blindness Acquired in Infancy. Perkins School for the Blind, Watertown, Massachusetts.

Tamir, T.J. (1989) Characterization of the Speech of Tadoma Users. B.S. Thesis, Massachusetts Institute of Technology, Cambridge, MA.

Tan, H.Z., Rabinowitz, W.M. and Durlach, N.I. (1989) Analysis of a synthetic Tadoma system as a multidimensional tactile display. Journal of the Acoustical Society of America 86: 981–8.

Vivian, R. (1966) The Tadoma method: a tactual approach to speech and speech reading. Volta Review 68: 733–7.

Wilbur, R. B. (1979) American Sign Language and Sign Systems. Baltimore: University Park Press.

Working Group on Communication Aids for the Hearing-Impaired (1991) Speech perception aids for hearing-impaired people: current status and needed research. Journal of the Acoustical Society of America 90: 637–83.

5

Design Fundamentals for Electrotactile Devices The Tickle Talker Case Study

ROBERT S.C. COWAN, KARYN L. GALVIN,
PETER J. BLAMEY and JULIA Z. SARANT

Introduction

Since the work of Gault in the 1920s, the literature has chronicled the development of numerous tactile devices for use by the hearing-impaired in improving communication. Devices have been developed to target improvements in both speech perception and speech production. In each development, the inventors have attempted to encode speech information through stimulation of the intact kinaesthetic system of the individual, as a supplement or replacement for speech input available from the damaged auditory pathway.

Use of the tactile modality for encoding speech has mainly been approached through either vibratory stimulation, relying on pressure deformation of receptors in the skin or underlying tissue, or through direct electrical stimulation of nerve endings in the skin surface or nerve bundles in the underlying tissue. Piezo-electric stimulation has also been employed. In these designs, electric currents are employed, resulting in deformation of either a mechanical rod or foil material which produces a vibratory stimulus for the user (Ifukube, 1989; Leysieffer, 1986). A myriad of transducer designs and body sites for placement of both vibrotactile and electrotactile transducers have been trialed with varying degrees of success. A wide range of speech encoding schemes have also been employed, in both single-channel and multiple-channel approaches to transducer design and tactile encoding schemes. Encoding schemes have included tactile transforms of the entire speech waveform, cues to single speech features such as fundamental frequency or speech amplitude, or cues to multiple spectral and amplitude features. These developments have been well-reviewed by Levitt, Pickett and Houde (1980), Pickett (1986) and McGarr (1989).

Despite these concerted efforts, tactile devices have not achieved the same level of acceptance nor impact on rehabilitation of hearing impairment as use of the various forms of manual communication, the development of the modern hearing aid or the development of multi-channel cochlear implants. More recently, the development of the auditory brainstem implant, an admittedly surgically-invasive approach to providing speech information, threatens to overtake tactile devices as the habilitation approach of choice for profoundly hearing-impaired individuals unable to proceed with cochlear implantation.

This raises the obvious question – what evidence leads us to believe that the tactile modality can in fact be employed as a communication avenue for the hearing-impaired? The prima facie evidence for tactile perception of speech, cited by those working in the field, has been the success of deaf–blind users of the Tadoma method (Alcorn, 1932; Reed *et al.*, 1982) or the natural tactiling method developed by Söderlund (1990). In addition, evidence from studies of Braille have suggested that the tactual perception abilities of adults and children can be developed to high levels with consistent long-term training. However, in each of these cases, the innate perceptual ability of the human hand to sense shape, movement or pressure is exploited to the fullest. In a sense, the human hand is employed as the tactile 'device', allowed to explore the speech source in a fluid and investigative manner, searching for the richest stream of information. In contrast, most tactile devices have a fixed display which cannot tap into this innate perceptual ability.

If we for the moment accept the evidence supporting tactile perception of speech, a further obvious question then arises – what factors might be responsible for limiting the acceptance and use of tactile devices by hearing-impaired adults and children? The effects of a number of factors should be considered:

- cosmetics and ease of use,
- safety for acute or long-term use,
- efficacy of the device including:
  - ability of users to perceive information presented, and
  - ability of users to integrate information presented to assist communication,
- training required for optimum performance, and
- cost of the device relative to potential benefits.

There are obvious interrelationships between these factors, and in making a decision as to acceptance of any particular tactile device, the user may well accept trade-offs between them. For example, cochlear implant users accept a higher cost and the cosmetic presence of the microphone and transmitter coil and associated cables in return for the established safety and reliability of implants and the significant speech information provided to most users. Hearing aid users accept the lower power of the in-the-ear (ITE) hearing aid over the behind-the-ear (BTE) or body aid in return for the reduced cosmetic 'presence' of the ITE. Similarly, Tadoma users accept the need for close interpersonal contact and the extensive long-term training required in return for the speech information provided, particularly given that there is no alternative source of speech information available.

Scope of the Chapter

To explore the question of why tactile devices have achieved only limited acceptance and use in the wider hearing-impaired population to date, it is appropriate to evaluate how the potential impact of these factors has been considered in the development programme for particular tactile devices. In this chapter, we will use the development of the Tickle Talker™ to illustrate and evaluate the influence of the factors we have identified on implementation, acceptance and use of the device. This case study may help to identify design fundamentals which are critical to achieving broader acceptance and use of tactile devices in the hearing-impaired community.

The Tickle Talker™ – A Case Study

The Tickle Talker, or electrotactile speech processor, was developed at the University of Melbourne (Blamey and Clark, 1985) to provide a non-invasive alternative for adults and children who did not receive significant speech perception assistance from hearing aids, and who were unable to proceed with cochlear implantation. The Tickle Talker, shown in Figure 1, consists of an ear-level or lapel microphone, a speech processor/stimulator unit and an electrode handset with associated cabling. Speech sounds received through the input microphone are passed to the speech processor, which is similar to that used in the 22-channel cochlear implant developed by the University of Melbourne and Cochlear Pty Limited (Clark et al., 1984). Several generations of Tickle Talker (UM1, UM2, UM3, UM4) have been developed during the programme, incorporating redesigns of the electrode handset and speech processor/stimulator hardware and improvements in the signal processing scheme employed. Each of the factors which we have identified have been considered in the research and development programme and their potential impact addressed through sequential prototype redesigns. The impact of factors and subsequent redesign strategies have been assessed and confirmed in laboratory studies with normally-hearing subjects and in clinical field trials with hearing-impaired adults and children.

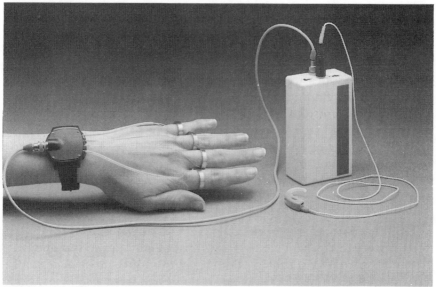

Figure 1. University of Melbourne Tickle Talker, version UM3, showing integrated speech processor/stimulator, wide-band directional microphone and redesigned electrode handset.

Cosmetics and Ease of Use

The electrode handset

The first step in the development is design of the means through which the user will perceive the signal. This involves both the mode of and the site of stimulation. The early fundamental decision to explore the use of electrical means of stimulation in the Tickle Talker was made for a number of reasons. First, our intention was to develop a small portable multichannel tactile device which could employ the speech processor developed for the 22-channel cochlear implant, saving the need for a separate costly and time-intensive speech processor development. Due to the power consumption of the speech processor itself and size restrictions, the maximum possible space and power allocation was for two AA cells or a single PP33 battery. Vibrotactile transducers available at the time were considered too large and had too great a power consumption for these requirements. Initial experiments with electrical stimulation of the skin surface, however, had not identified an acceptable stimulus site, due to involvement of pain receptors in the skin surface rendering the stimulation unpleasant (McLeod *et al.*, 1983). A breakthrough occurred with the discovery that stimulation by electrodes overlying the digital nerve bundles in the fingers resulted in a more pleasant stimulus with larger dynamic ranges than had been found with stimulation at other body sites (Blamey and Clark, 1985).

The resulting design for the electrode handset consisted of eight electrodes, two in each of four rings worn on the fingers of the non-dominant hand. The electrodes were positioned on the sides of the rings to overlie the position of the digital nerve bundles in each of the four fingers. The electrodes were numbered sequentially from 1 on the outside of the index finger through 8 on the distal side of the little finger.

In the UM1 and UM2 designs, eight 50 mm² electrodes were constructed of folded stainless steel, supported in pairs in plastic or plastic-coated metal rings positioned on the skin surface. A 9 cm² common electrode fabricated from rubber was located on the underside of the wrist. Only one electrode was activated at a time and the stimulus current passed between the active finger electrode and the wrist electrode.

Detailed studies were undertaken to identify the optimum electrode surface area, shape and electrical paradigm required to minimize power requirements and to render the stimulus most acceptable. Radical changes in handset and electrode design were also investigated in the UM3 design, where the use of platinum, titanium and stainless steel, shaped into flat or raised electrodes, and mounted in rings or in a continuous flexible printed-circuit board (PCB) carrier, were evaluated. Additional studies explored the use of an alternative ground circuitry, as some subjects had noted occasional electrical sensations at the wrist electrode. The subsequent design of the UM4 processor overcame this problem by employing the non-active finger electrodes as a ground, eliminating the need for the wrist electrode.

Figure 2 shows results of these electrode studies, designed to identify the optimum size and shape of electrodes and to evaluate the effects of changes in ground strategy. Users were asked to subjectively set their threshold and comfortable pulse widths (described as the highest level of stimulus acceptable for continuous application over a 2 minute period) for different ground strategies (wrist electrode circuit versus finger electrode circuit), different electrode surface areas (5 mm × 5 mm – 8 mm × 8 mm), different electrode shapes (flat versus raised) and for different carriers (rings versus PCB carrier). The evaluation of the newly-designed PCB carrier was necessary as it altered the pressure holding the electrode in position over the digital nerve bundle.

Results showed that the optimum threshold (T) and comfortable (C) pulse widths (a measure of the tactile dynamic range and power requirements for the device) were achieved with 7 mm (49 mm²) flat electrodes, mounted in rings, and using the finger ground paradigm. Subjects also subjectively rated the 7 mm ring electrodes as producing the most pleasant sensation. As shown, electrical charge required for T and C levels was also much higher for the raised versus the flat electrodes. The PCB carrier was found to be less effective in maintaining adequate pressure and position of the electrodes, resulting in higher T

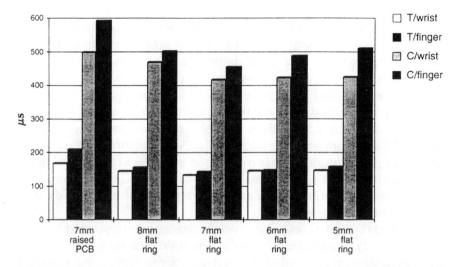

Figure 2. Comparison of mean subjective threshold (T) and most comfortable (C) pulse widths for 12 subjects with different electrode surface areas, shapes, carriers and grounding strategies.

and C pulse widths and resultant power consumption. This factor, coupled with the high cost of production and the observed fragility of the PCB design in field trials, resulted in abandonment of this concept and a return to a redesigned ring handset.

In summary, the electrode studies identified the following design requirements:

- the optimum electrode surface area should be 49 mm²,
- the optimum electrode shape is flat, with a raised contact area on the support ring,
- electrode material must be biocompatible, with stainless steel the choice due to ease of machining, cost and current-carrying capacity,
- the two electrodes must be electrically isolated from each other on the support ring,
- the degree of separation in the support ring must be 210°ᵒᴾ to position the electrode over the digital nerve bundles, and there must be adequate pressure from the support ring to maintain good contact,
- the use of the non-active finger electrodes in the ground circuit was more effective than a large surface area wrist-ground paradigm and avoids the potential for inadvertent wrist stimulation,
- at least 10 different size graduations of ring are required to fit the population range of children aged 6 through to adults (additional sizes required for children aged 2–6)
- colour is not an important factor for children or adults, but function and robustness are critical to long-term use and acceptance.

The speech processor/stimulator

The UM1 and UM2 device employed the WSPIII cochlear implant speech processor. RF output from the speech processor was hard-wired into a separately-powered stimulator unit. This unit was compact, weighing 435 grams. It was powered by a rechargeable 9 volt NiCd PP33 battery. The two units were carried in a single pouch worn on a strap over the shoulder or on the belt using an attached belt loop. Input was through a Sony ECM 16T electret condenser lapel microphone. This design was clinically trialed with normally-hearing and hearing-impaired adults and proved to be effective in transmitting the tactile signal to the users, resulting in significant improvements in speech feature discrimination and in the perception of words, sentences and running speech.

In the UM1 and UM2 speech processor, estimates of second formant frequency (F2), speech amplitude (A) and fundamental frequency (F0) were extracted and encoded as electrical parameters. The electrical parameters as selected were presented through the electrode handset and were perceived by the user as a changing pattern of tactual sensation on the fingers of the non-dominant hand. The UM3 processor was a significant development, integrating the new MSP cochlear prosthesis speech processor and stimulator into one combined unit, reducing the size and weight of the device to 200 grams and reducing the power supply required for both devices to a single 1.5 volt AA cell. In addition, the microphone was replaced with a Knowles ear-level EB1843 wide-band receiver and a 4000–10 000 Hz high frequency band-pass filter was incorporated. These two latter changes allowed additional spectral information to be encoded. Specifically, the presence/absence of high frequency energy (HF) was presented as stimulus output to electrode 8 on the outside of the little finger. In the UM4 processor, further evolution of the speech processor circuitry reduced the number and costs of components and redesign of the power supply reduced power consumption resulting in improved battery life. The option of a wide-band lapel microphone and RF compatibility was added. The UM4 version also incorporated an additional speech feature cue to the presence/absence of voicing (UV) in the speech processing/encoding scheme. Table 1 shows a summary of the speech processing scheme employed in the Tickle Talker prototype developments.

As shown, second formant frequency (F2) was encoded as electrode selected and sensed by the user as the position of stimulation. Sounds with low F2 values such as the vowel in the monosyllable 'hoard' would result in stimulation on electrode 1 (or electrode 2 in UM4), whereas high frequency consonants would be sensed on electrode 8. Frequency boundaries between electrodes were individually adjustable and were programmed into the speech processor memory through a computer interface. Speech waveform amplitude (A) was encoded as pulse width of 1.5 mA constant current biphasic pulses and sensed by the user as the stimulus strength. Fundamental frequency (F0) was encoded as variations in the pulse rate and sensed by users as the quality of stimulus – from rough through smooth

Table 1. Speech processing/encoding schemes employed in Tickle Talker prototypes

	Speech feature	Electrical parameter	Electrical sensation
UM1/UM2			
	F2	electrode selected	stimulus position
	A	pulse width	stimulus strength
	F0	pulse rate	stimulus quality
UM3 (added)	HF	pulse width (electrode 8)	stimulus strength (electrode 8)
UM4 (added)	UV	pulse width (electrode 1)	paired stimulus (electrode 1)

The speech processor hardware and encoding schemes have been continually improved, with the inclusion of additional spectral and speech feature cues, for example presence/absence of high frequency and a cue to initial voicing. These developments have resulted from laboratory studies with normally-hearing subjects. Resultant redesigns have been evaluated in field trials with hearing-impaired adults and children using the device to ensure robustness and function.

Safety

Although no obvious surgical risks are associated with use of tactile devices, the potential exists for biomedical problems which might arise after prolonged use of any particular transducer or electrical stimulus paradigm. The aim of the safety studies incorporated into the research programme were to assess:

– the possibility of risks inherent in the electrical stimulus or the device, and
– the possibility of long-term contraindications to use resulting from irreversible changes in physiological function.

Electrical safety assessments focused on the electrical parameters selected for use in the electrical stimulus waveform, the design of the electrode circuit in the handset and the electrical circuitry employed in the speech processor/stimulator and programming interface.

Physiological studies were both acute and chronic and included evaluation of potential effects on local tissue, peripheral nervous system, or central nervous system function.

Electrical safety

To enable safe and painless stimulation, it is vital that the electrical stimulus should not cause electrolytic processes at the skin/electrode interface, dielectric breakdown of current channels across the skin, or result in large conversion of energy to heat (Brummer and Turner, 1977; Mason and MacKay, 1976; Rugerri and Beck, 1985). The most direct means of controlling the charge applied to the skin is to use rectangular constant current pulses, with the charge being a function of a fixed current applied over a variable pulse width. Rectangular pulses have the advantage that the charge per pulse does not vary with repetition frequency as is the case with sine wave stimuli (Butikofer and Lawrence, 1979). Several studies have demonstrated the safety of such pulses for biomedical applications (Lilly, 1955).

For this reason, the stimulus waveform selected for the Tickle Talker was a biphasic constant current waveform, with equal charge in each phase and no net current flow. By limiting the current applied in each phase to 1.5 mA the possibility of skin breakdown due to electrical stimulation is also reduced, as is the remote possibility of electrical interference effects on cardiac tissue (Cabanes, 1985; Green and Ross, 1985). For a 1.5 mA constant current, the range of pulse widths used in the device (10–1000 μs) would result in a potential range in charge between 15 and 1500 nC/phase, representing a maximum current density of 3.06 μC/cm^2 geometric/phase. Studies of neural tissue survival following prolonged electrical stimulation through implanted platinum electrodes with similar electrical stimuli have shown no damage to tissue from charge densities ranging from 20 to 40 μC/cm^2 geometric /phase (Shepherd *et al.*, 1983). Although these studies have primarily been aimed at establishing the safety of subcutaneous stimulation, the charge densities employed in the Tickle Talker for cutaneous stimulation would appear to be well below recommended safety limits.

The choice of electrode material for use in the Tickle Talker focused on the needs for mechanical strength, ease of machining, biocompatibility, cost and the ability to pass adequate charge without electrolysing tissue components. Although the electrodes are mounted on the skin surface and no electrolyte material is introduced to reduce skin electrical impedance, studies with dry electrodes have shown that a small amount of sweat rapidly accumulates on the surface of the skin under the electrode, and that in fact a weak saline fluid interface results (Bergey *et al.*, 1971; Lewes, 1965). While stainless steel is an ideal electrode material from the perspective of strength, it may not be completely corrosion-resistant. Platinum is a more stable electrolytic material, but is also more costly. The use of biphasic current pulses, already stressed as important in limiting potential electrolysis (Pfeiffer, 1968) is also important in limiting potential corrosion problems with stainless steel electrodes. The electrodes must also be capable of delivering high current densities and the current-carrying capacities of stainless steel and platinum are intermediate, being greater than for copper or aluminium, but less than rhodium (Ragheb and Geddes, 1981).

As mentioned already, the UM1 and UM2 Tickle Talker designs incorporated a rubber ground electrode worn on the underside of the wrist. While this design inherently spread current over a larger circuit (i.e. finger to wrist), some subjects noted a wrist stimulation, which may have resulted from a breakdown in the high resistance of the rubber electrode which normally allows the current to be spread over multiple pathways under large surface electrodes. This could result in a large portion of the current being shunted through a single skin pathway in which the higher resistance was broken down, causing the current densities under both the ground and active electrode to become similar, thereby producing a sensation at the wrist. To overcome this problem, the long-term solution selected was elimination of the wrist electrode. In the UM4 design, the seven 'inactive' finger electrodes have been used as the reference.

A final consideration at the interface between skin and electrode is production of locally-generated heat due to electrical stimulation, particularly when electrodes are applied to dry skin (Burton and Maurer, 1974). Studies have indicated that this could be reduced or eliminated through use of relatively short separation between the positive and negative phases of biphasic pulses, since the energy stored in the skin capacitance by the first phase is removed by the second instead of being discharged through skin resistance creating heat (Butikofer and Lawrence, 1979). The relatively short interstimulus gap of $100\,\mu s$ used in the Tickle Talker should be effective in reducing the potential for local heat generation, and in fact local heat generation has not been noted as a limiting problem by any user.

Additional electrical safety assessments of the stimulator circuitry and the system programming interface were made to ensure compliance with relevant Australian and international standards for biomedical devices. Independent biomedical engineering analysis excluded potential risks from accidental electric shock through breakdown of mains-powered equipment during programming, or for accidental overstimulation through breakdown of the speech processor circuitry. The device incorporated a number of specific design features to eliminate or reduce these potential risks and to ensure electrical isolation of the user. The speech processor and stimulator circuitry were electrically isolated through use of an opto-isolator. In addition, each of the electrodes was capacitively coupled, limiting the potential for DC current leaks between the user and programming equipment. The speech processor circuitry was also waterproofed and was designed so that a failure in any one component could not result in accidental overstimulation. The 1.5 mA output current was controlled by a field-effect transistor (FET) which functioned as a current-limiter. In addition, a constant current-limiting diode was fitted to the output of the stimulator unit.

Physiological safety

Systematic studies of long-term electrotactile stimulation using the specific electrical transducers and stimulus paradigm employed in the Tickle Talker were required to establish that the device was biomedically safe for long-term application in adults and children. Detailed safety studies (Cowan *et al.*, 1992) were undertaken with normally-hearing and hearing-impaired adults to evaluate the effects of electrotactile stimulation on:

– local tissue,
– peripheral nervous system function, and
– central nervous system function.

Local tissue studies

Local tissue evaluations included measurements of finger temperature, as well as hand and finger blood flow. Initial studies had shown that the fingers of some users cooled slightly (up to 3°C) following 30 minutes of stimulation (Blamey and Clark, 1987). A more detailed study with seven normally-hearing subjects evaluated the prevalence and degree of skin cooling. Large individual variations across subjects were present. However, comparison of mean pre- and post-stimulation finger temperatures did not show a significant cooling effect for either the stimulated or non-stimulated fingers in the group of subjects tested.

These results did suggest that some vasoconstriction in the fingers might occur as a result of the electrical stimulus. To evaluate the degree and to clarify causative factors for any observed vasoconstriction, a long-term vascular study was undertaken with five subjects. Analysis of vascular circulation in the hands and fingers of each subject was undertaken following 3 months of training with the Tickle Talker. A number of measures were performed including: hand blood flow (HBF) measured by water plethysmography at ambient hand temperatures of 20°C and 40°C, and following body heating to abolish cutaneous sympathetic activity; finger blood flow (FBF) measured by strain gauge plethysmography at similar temperatures; heart rate (HR) and mean arterial blood pressure (MAP). After measurement of each of the parameters in the pre-stimulus condition, the effects of electrical stimulation on the

Table 2. Mean results for hand blood flow (HBF), finger blood flow (FBF), mean arterial pressure (MAP) and heart rate (HR) measured at plethysmograph temperatures of 20°C and 40°C and following body heating, prior to and during electrotactile stimulation

Test	20°C		40°C		Body heating	
	Pre	Stim	Pre	Stim	Pre	Stim
HBF	2.22	2.04	12.84	11.78	33.78	32.14
FBF	4.16	4.0	22.6	20.6	38.4	35.1
MAP	81.4	81.8	80	81	77.4	77
HR	66.4	67.4	69.2	70.4	86	87

HBF and FBF in ml/100 ml/min, MAP in mmHg, HR in beats/min.

parameter were recorded. Table 2 shows the results of a number of these measurements.

Following application of electrotactile stimulation, there was a small reduction in mean HBF for all three temperature environments. Individual results varied across subjects. However, statistical analysis showed no significant difference between mean HBF in the pre-stimulation or stimulation conditions. Although there was a slight reduction in mean finger blood flow (FBF) at all three temperatures tested, again there was no significant difference in mean FBF for the two conditions tested. Similarly, no significant effect of stimulus condition on either mean arterial pressure or heart rate was found.

Although these studies did not demonstrate a significant group reduction in HBF or FBF, some individuals did show evidence of vasoconstriction. Analysis of potential causative factors showed that sympathetic efferent and pathological causes for the observed cooling and vasoconstriction noted could be eliminated. The most likely causative effect was baseline alteration in conditions in the arterio-venous anastomoses, resulting in a changed ratio between blood flow to these structures and to nutritive capillary beds. No contraindication to long-term use was evident in the results. The degree of cooling was minimal for any individual, being of a similar order of magnitude to normal variations in everyday temperature or to that associated with intense mental concentration (approximately 3°C).

Peripheral nervous system studies

To assess potential changes which might occur to tactual sensitivity following prolonged electrotactile stimulation, evaluations of tactual acuity for sharp–dull, hot–cold and two-point difference limen discrimination were made in a group of six subjects following electrotactile stimulation.

Measurements of both the stimulated and non-stimulated fingers were made to evaluate changes which might have occurred as a direct consequence of prolonged electrotactile stimulation with the selected electrodes and stimulus paradigm. Prior to measurement, each of the subjects had 6 months experience with the Tickle Talker. For each test, stimuli were presented immediately before and immediately following 50 minutes of continuous electrotactile stimulation. Two different measures were conducted on different days for each of the six subjects and mean results are shown as Table 3.

No differences were evident between mean scores for the stimulated and non-stimulated index finger for the six normally-hearing subjects over 10 trials each on identification of sharp vs dull, or of hot vs cold stimuli. Results for two-point discrimination limens show a reduction in mean scores for both the stimulated and non-stimulated fingers following the 50 minute electrotactile stimulation period, consistent with an improvement in tactual sensitivity. However, results of paired t-tests indicated that these differences were not significant for either the stimulated or non-stimulated hands. While admittedly these measures are of a gross nature, it would be expected that any marked decrement in tactual sensitivity resulting from electrotactile stimulation would be manifest following either acute or chronic long-term stimulation.

Table 3. Mean results for measures of sharp–dull discrimination, hot–cold discrimination, and two-point discrimination limens measured for six normally-hearing subjects prior to (pre) and following (post) electrotactile stimulation for both the stimulated (St) and unstimulated (NSt) index fingers

	Pre-stim		*Post-stim*		*Pre/Post diff*	
Test	St	NSt	St	NSt	St	NSt
Sharp/dull	10	10	10	10	0	0
Hot/cold	10	10	10	10	0	0
Two-point	1.64	1.6	1.43	1.37	–0.21	–0.23

Sharp–dull and hot–cold discriminations are from a total of 10 trials in each condition averaged across two test sessions, two-point discrimination limens are in millimetres.

Further investigation of chronic stimulation was undertaken with normally-hearing subjects and with hearing-impaired adults who were consistent long-term users of the device. The main aim of the evaluation was to establish that there was no change in the last factor, the sensitivity of the nerve bundles to electrical current. To evaluate this, mean T and C pulse widths were recorded over a 6 month training period for the normally-hearing subjects and with five hearing-impaired adults who had between 6 and 36 months experience with the device. It was assumed that changes in sensitivity would be manifested as either temporary or irreversible increases in C and particularly T thresholds. Results showed that after prolonged experience, little change was noted in T widths, but that significant increases in mean C pulse widths were present for most subjects.

Although the long-term measurements showed an increase in mean C pulse widths, no significant increase was noted in T widths, suggesting that no physiological effect on sensitivity was present. To confirm this, a more direct measure of change in sensitivity was to compare the mean T and C pulse widths across a group of experienced subjects in both the stimulated and non-stimulated hands. If in fact a change in physiology were present, one would anticipate that this change would be evidenced in a recordable difference between the two hands. Comparison of mean T and C pulse widths in a group of five hearing-impaired subjects (Figure 3) showed no significant differences between the stimulated and non-stimulated hands for experienced long-term users of the device.

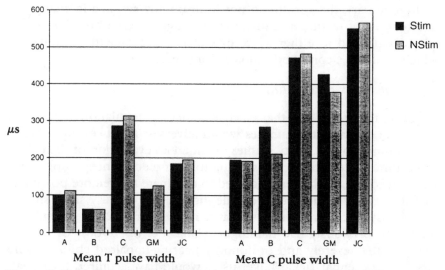

Figure 3. Mean T and C pulse widths measured in μ for eight electrodes in stimulated and non-stimulated hands for five adults following extensive electrotactile experience. (The letters A,B,C,GM and JC refer to individual subjects.)

These results, coupled with the fact that T widths showed little increase over time, suggest that the observed increase in C pulse widths shown for users of the device were not due to physiological changes in sensitivity of the digital nerve bundles of the stimulated hand. A more feasible rationale for the changes in C levels would be readjustment of the subjective criterion used by subjects to set C pulse widths. A number of factors may contribute to the subjective setting of T and C pulse widths including:

– the geometry of the electrode/skin interface;
– the electrode position relative to the nerve bundles;

- the subjective criteria used to establish T and C levels by each individual user; and,
- the sensitivity of the nerve bundles to electrical current.

The first two factors were beyond experimental control, since exact positioning of electrode rings varied between recording sessions and different electrode shapes, sizes and materials incorporated as part of the continuing design programme were included in the long-term measurements. Subjective criteria may also have varied across sessions, particularly as the users became aware of the potential speech perception benefits available through use of the device and accepted higher C levels to increase their useable tactile dynamic range. It would appear reasonable to suggest that the observed increase in C levels was primarily due to subjects accepting stronger sensations as they become more familiar with both the sensation and the potential speech perception benefits.

In summary, the results do not indicate any systematic change or habituation of tactual sensitivity in the digital nerve bundles of the stimulated hand in either acute or chronic electrotactile stimulation which could be a contraindication to long-term use.

Central nervous system studies

While it is very unlikely that electrocutaneous stimulation of the skin surface or digital nerve bundles would adversely affect central nervous system function, the safety studies included an evaluation of the effects of continuous electrotactile stimulation on electroencephalographic (EEG) recordings. This was included to eliminate the remote possibility that the stimuli could produce epileptic foci, particularly since studies of epilepsy in children suggest that it may occur in 2–3% of children who have previously had meningitis (Jadavji *et al.*, 1986). Given that many of the severely and profoundly hearing-impaired children who would be potential Tickle Talker users would have acquired their hearing loss as a sequela to meningitis, it appeared prudent to eliminate this as a potential contraindication.

Seven normally-hearing and three hearing-impaired subjects had standard EEG recordings taken in three conditions: immediately prior to, during and immediately following cessation of electrotactile stimulation of the digital nerves through the Tickle Talker. Each of the subjects had three separate recording sessions, the first one prior to any exposure to electrotactile stimulation, the second session following approximately 35 hours of exposure and the last following 70 hours of exposure. No systematic difference in recordings during or subsequent to acute or long-term electrotactile stimulation were evident for any subject. No paroxysmal activity of an epileptic pattern or other abnormality were recorded during the periods of stimulation. These results do not suggest that the electrotactile stimulation could act to predispose users to epileptic episodes.

In summary, the combined electrical and physiological safety studies indicated that the Tickle Talker was safe for long-term use. Potential problems inherent in the use of electrotactile stimulation were evaluated and addressed through redesigns of the circuitry used in the device. No biomedical contraindication to long-term use was evident in any of the studies of tactual sensitivity, vascular or neurological evaluations of acute or chronic stimulation.

Efficacy of the Device

While the influence of electrical design and safety factors can be directly assessed and addressed, the efficacy of the device is a more complex amalgam of effects operating at several different levels including:

- the actual speech information selected for encoding,
- the efficiency of the transducers and speech encoding strategy in presenting this information in an accessible form,
- the psychophysical ability of the user to perceive the information,
- the ability of the user to convert the tactual percept to meaningful speech perception, and
- the interrelationship and redundancies between the speech information presented through the tactile device, with speech information available from other sources such as lipreading or aided residual hearing.

Psychophysical studies

Extensive psychophysical testing was undertaken to establish that the stimuli presented to the user could be recognized as distinct tactual sensations, to define the operating ranges for the electrical stimulus parameters, to measure the information transmission characteristics of the electrical parameters and to assess the feasibility of the proposed speech encoding strategy (Blamey and Clark, 1987; Blamey et al., 1990).

Pilot studies demonstrated that placement of electrodes over the digital nerve bundles resulted in a more comfortable sensation than electrical stimulation at other body sites. These findings were consistent with physiological studies showing nerve fibre stimulation to be characterized by different evoked sensations than stimulation of nerve end organs (Pfeiffer, 1968). A more important advantage of the electrode placement, however, was that the digital nerve bundles form a well-ordered spatially distinct series of stimulation sites. It has also been well-established that the tactual sensitivity of the fingers is maximal and that cerebral representational area is proportionately larger for the facial region and for the hands (Geldard, 1973).

Electrode identification was studied in seven subjects, using a single-interval electrode recognition task. Mean score for all eight electrodes was 98%, with all subjects scoring at 95% or greater. Identification of pulse width was also measured with a single-interval recognition task, using eight test stimuli with pulse widths equally spaced on a log scale between threshold and comfortable level. Mean scores for five subjects ranged from 43–69%. Identification of pulse rate was evaluated in seven subjects, who were asked to identify a set of seven stimuli presented on a single electrode for a fixed duration, ranging in pulse rate from 25 to 200 pps in a single-interval forced choice task. Subjects showed a wide variation in performance, with the range of performance being 28–76%. These results indicated that subjects would be able to recognize electrode site and pulse width efficiently, but that pulse rate identification would be poor above 250 pps. Based on these studies, these three stimulus parameters were employed in the first encoding scheme to convey the prosodic and spectral features F2, A and F0. Given the pulse rate findings, a scaled version of F0 was employed. Subsequent studies of pulse duration identification and discrimination, gap detection, and integration times for pulsatile electrical stimulation have confirmed that gross amplitude envelope variations should be well conveyed by the stimulus parameters used in the Tickle Talker (Blamey *et al.*, 1990).

Initially, the non-dominant hand was chosen as the preferred site for the electrode array in order to reduce the potential for use of the device to affect everyday function or activities. Subsequent psychophysical studies (Sarant *et al.*, 1993) evaluated differential performance of subjects using the Tickle Talker on the dominant versus the non-dominant hand. No significant differences were found between the right and left hands for measures of threshold pulse widths, dynamic range, multiple electrode identification tasks, or on a tactile discrimination battery. These results suggested that the tactual sensitivity of the hands for the electrotactile stimuli employed did not differ to a significant degree between the dominant and non-dominant hands.

Following the initial clinical trials of the Tickle Talker, it was suggested that the observed lower scores for transmission of initial consonant voicing cues shown by some subjects might be due to the inability of these subjects to perceive differences in pulse rate. Further psychophysical studies were undertaken to identify alternative means of providing cues to initial consonant voicing. Pilot studies (Cowan, 1991) with an extended linear involving 16 electrodes on both hands, or a two-dimensional array using two electrode rings on each finger (2 × 8 matrix), were undertaken. Although promising in terms of high electrode identification scores, the extended linear array was discarded due to the obstruction of everyday function that might result from use of both hands. Similarly, the two-dimensional array was ruled out as subjects found it difficult to differentiate between electrode positions on the same side of the fingers. The use of simultaneous multiple electrode stimulation delivered through the existing eight electrodes was subsequently evaluated as an alternative (Cowan, 1991). This approach had distinct advantages since it could be implemented without a redesign of the speech processor circuitry or electrode handset.

Table 4 shows both mean electrode identification scores and information transmission scores for four different sets of multiple electrode stimuli presented through the Tickle Talker (Cowan *et al.*, 1991b).

Table 4. Mean percentage electrode identification scores and information transmission scores for nine subjects on four stimulus sets presented through the Tickle Talker

Stimulus pattern	Identification score (%)	Stimulus information (bits)	Information transmitted (bits)	Information transmission (%)
Single electrodes	97.8	3.0	2.84	95.7
Pairs	61.9	4.74	2.99	62.1
Triplets	31.8	5.68	2.84	48.9
Pairs/singles	73.6	5.13	3.88	75.1

Absolute identification of electrode position was shown to decrease as the number of electrodes in the test stimulus increased. Although recognition of electrodes in paired stimuli was lower than for single stimuli, subjects were able to identify accurately whether the test stimulus was a pair of electrodes or single electrode with reasonable accuracy (74%). Information transmission for the paired/single stimuli also increased to 3.88 bits. While this was a lower percentage information transmission than for single electrodes, it represented a substantial increase over single electrodes (2.84 bits) or paired electrodes (2.99 bits) in actual information transmitted. This confirmed the possibility of using the additional stimulus parameter of presence/absence of paired stimuli to encode additional cues to speech features, particularly cues to initial consonant voicing. These findings were implemented in the speech processing strategy employed in the UM4 device, which used paired stimuli (i.e. electrode 1 plus one of electrodes 2–7 to encode F2 frequency) to signal the presence of an unvoiced initial consonant.

Speech feature discrimination studies

Given the psychophysical evaluations showing that users could in fact perceive differences in the electrical parameters used to encode cues to speech features, evaluation of efficacy next focused on the ability of users to access these tactually-encoded speech cues. Assessments were made at a number of linguistic levels including: sound/speech detection; discrimination of feature cues such as prosody; recognition of words and sentence level materials; and recognition and comprehension of running speech in connected discourse tracking.

Sound and speech detection threshold assessment is important to establish that users can detect cues from the Tickle Talker operating on speech input that is within normal conversational levels. Figure 4a shows mean sound detection thresholds for 14 profoundly hearing-impaired children using the Tickle Talker versus thresholds for aided residual hearing (Cowan *et al.*, 1990). At each frequency, mean tactile detection thresholds were at lower levels than for hearing aid thresholds, particularly in the high frequency region beyond 2000 Hz. In this region, mean hearing aid thresholds drop below the conversational speech spectrum limits. In contrast, the tactile detection thresholds remain within the speech spectrum limits, confirming that the Tickle Talker users would be able to detect higher-frequency cues to consonants encoded in the tactile signal which would be inaudible through their hearing aids.

Figure 4b shows mean speech reception thresholds for the Ling 5-Sound test for 14 profoundly hearing-impaired children using the Tickle Talker. Results confirm that the children are capable of detecting speech sounds across the frequency range at normal conversational levels using only tactual cues presented through the Tickle Talker.

Given the ability to detect cues to speech features, the next focus is to establish that users can distinguish between tactually-encoded words with varying speech cues. A number of studies have assessed efficacy of

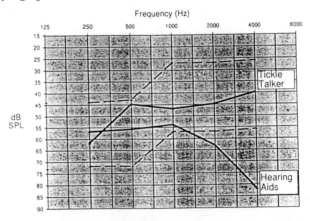

Figure 4a. Mean sound detection thresholds for 14 profoundly hearing-impaired children using hearing aids (lower solid line) or Tickle Talker (upper solid line). (Solid lines show thresholds for short duration pure tones presented free-field measured in dB SPL for either device, dashed lines show upper and lower threshold values for average 70dB speech spectrum.)

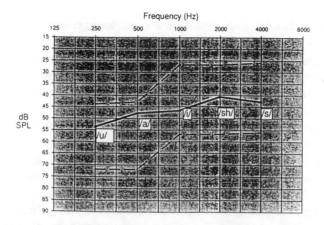

Figure 4b. Mean speech reception thresholds measured for the Ling 5-Sound Test in 14 profoundly hearing-impaired children using the Tickle Talker alone without hearing aids. (Solid lines show thresholds for each phoneme presented free-field and measured in dB SPL, dashed lines show upper and lower threshold values for average 70dB speech spectrum.)

the Tickle Talker at this linguistic level (Cowan *et al.*, 1989a, 1989b). In the first study, the ability of eight subjects to use tactile input only to differentiate between sets of suprasegmental and segmental speech feature contrasts using an ABx task devised by Plant (1989) was assessed. Table 5 shows results of the ABx test battery evaluations. In each case, both the mean percentage correct responses for all subjects on each subtest and the number of subjects out of a total of eight who achieved significant levels of feature discrimination are shown.

Table 5. Tactile-alone feature contrast scores for eight subjects

Speech feature	*Specific speech feature contrast*	*No.*[1] subjects	*%*[2] correct
syllable number/stress	monosyllables/spondees/trochees /b/	8	78
syllable number/stress	monosyllables/spondees/trochees /m/	6	76
vowel length	vowel length with final stop	8	84
vowel length	vowel length with final nasal	8	80
vowel formant	F1 frequency contrasts	7	77
vowel formant	F2 frequency contrasts	7	75
consonant voicing	initial consonant voicing	3	60
consonant manner	initial manner (nasal/stop)	4	70
consonant manner	initial manner (fricative/stop)	7	74
consonant manner	initial manner (stops/affricates)	4	64
consonant manner	initial manner (nasal/fricative)	6	75
consonant manner	initial manner (s/t/st)	8	89

[1]Number of subjects scoring significantly above chance for each subtest (p<0.05).
[2]Percentage correct responses for eight subjects on each subtest.

Results show that subjects could detect prosodic contrasts with high accuracy. In addition, vowel formant frequency contrasts were well-discriminated. Results for the various consonant contrasts were more variable, with lowest performance on initial consonant voicing and highest performance on discrimination of high frequency consonant manner cues. Results for the prosodic tests indicate efficient encoding of time/intensity cues in the tactual signal. Subjects were able to perceive contrasting vowel length and syllable number through cues of changing stimulus strength and electrode position. Scores for vowel formant cues suggest that the tactual cue of electrode position used to encode spectral cues is also well-perceived. Scores for initial consonant voicing show that cues to this feature were not as well-perceived as for other features, consistent with psychophysical results which showed variable perception of pulse rate differences, the main tactual cue encoding initial voicing contrasts. To overcome this limitation, a new speech processing scheme was introduced in the UM4 device to provide a specific cue to this speech feature. Results for the high frequency contrasts of the unvoiced fricative /s/, unvoiced stop /t/ and blend /st/ showed efficient encoding of high frequency consonant fricative information through the tactual display, suggesting that the high frequency filter and wide-band microphone incorporated in the UM3 and UM4 devices was effective in improving transmission of high frequency spectral information.

Additional studies (Cowan *et al.*, 1987; 1989b; 1991a) have evaluated the ability of normally-hearing and hearing-impaired adults to use tactile cues provided through the Tickle Talker to improve discrimination on speech feature discrimination tasks including the Minimum Auditory Capabilities Battery (Owens *et al.*, 1985), SPAC Battery (Boothroyd, 1984) and discrimination of closed-set of vowels and consonants. Results for each of these evaluations are consistent with the ABx results, showing good discrimination of time/intensity and spectral formant cues and suggesting the need for additional cues to initial consonant voicing contrasts. Following 70 hours of systematic training, normally-hearing adults reached tactile-alone mean scores of 75% on vowel discrimination and 47% on consonant discrimination. Similar testing with hearing-impaired adults following 40 hours of training showed tactile-alone discrimination scores of 56% on vowels and 43% on consonants.

Speech perception studies

Psychophysical and tactile-alone speech feature discrimination testing established that prosodic and segmental speech feature information were accurately presented through the encoding scheme of the Tickle Talker and that users were able to detect and to discriminate speech feature contrasts as variations in the parameters of the tactile stimuli.

While good tactile-alone detection thresholds and feature discrimination are vital to the successful design of the Tickle Talker and choice of speech processing strategy, in few instances would the hearing-impaired user be cut-off from other sources of speech cues. A more likely scenario would be use of the tactually-encoded speech information in combination with cues from either lipreading or aided residual hearing. Given that features such as consonant voicing and manner are not easily distinguished by lipreading and the likelihood that high frequency consonant cues would be inaudible through hearing aids for most severely or profoundly hearing-impaired people, the additional tactile information may be very valuable to the user in a combined modality approach. Table 6 summarizes data which confirm that tactile input provided through the Tickle Talker can effectively supplement lipreading and/or aided residual hearing in identification of vowels and consonants (Cowan *et al.*, 1988, 1989a).

Table 6. Mean vowel and consonant identification scores for three hearing-impaired adults using three models of Tickle Talker

Prototype model	Vowel identification (%)						Consonant identification (%)					
	TLA	LA	TL	L	TA	A	TLA	LA	TL	L	TA	A
UM2	99	96	98	87	99	90	86	68	86	53	66	57
UM3	100	97					91	61			71	65
UM4	100	93					91	64			79	50

As shown, the tactile input can be used to supplement lipreading (L), aided residual hearing (A), or the combination of aided residual hearing and lipreading (LA) to improve perception of both vowels and consonants.

Benefits to speech feature discrimination from tactile input used as a supplement to aided residual hearing have also been assessed in hearing-impaired children using the Tickle Talker (Cowan *et al.*, 1990). Mean scores for 14 profoundly hearing-impaired children on subtests of the PLOTT feature contrast test (Plant, 1983) were recorded with hearing aids alone (A) and with the Tickle Talker combined with hearing aids (TA). Statistical analysis showed significant increases in mean scores on vowel length, vowel formant and initial consonant manner resulting from the addition of tactually-encoded speech feature cues. Scores in the tactually-aided condition also showed a significantly reduced range (82–100%) as compared with the hearing aid alone condition (40–92%).

Again, while these results are important in trialing design changes and choice of speech processing strategy, the primary focus of the evaluation of device efficacy must not be on discrimination of features, vowels or consonants. To establish real benefit to communication from use of the Tickle Talker or any other tactile device, tactually-encoded speech cues must be integrated at conversational level. The most critical evaluation of efficacy is the ability of users to improve their perception of open-set words, sentences and running speech, as this is a true measure of the benefits to everyday communication. Involvement of hearing-impaired adults and children in field evaluations is vital, since their ability to lipread or to use residual audition will differ from the abilities of normally-hearing subjects with an intact auditory system listening to degraded or filtered speech.

Speech perception studies with hearing-impaired adults

The benefits from use of supplemental tactile cues would be expected to vary between individual hearing-impaired adults, as a function of their hearing thresholds and ability to use their aided residual hearing, since this would determine what tactile cues presented by the Tickle Talker would be redundant with input from hearing aids. The aetiology and age at onset of the hearing loss will also have an effect, with congenitally deaf adults having in general more experience with lipreading, but perhaps poorer linguistic skills and less auditory experience than postlingually deafened adults. Benefits of the tactually-encoded speech feature information to both lipreading and lipreading plus aided residual hearing have been assessed and Figure 5 shows results of open-set word and sentence discrimination evaluations with four hearing-impaired adults using the Tickle Talker. The four adults have a range of residual hearing, age at onset and presence of other disabilities.

Patient 1 was an 82-year-old profoundly deaf male. He had suffered a step-wise progressive hearing loss due to otosclerosis and had been totally deaf for 15 years. He had previously been implanted with a Nucleus 22-channel cochlear implant, which was explanted after 4 years due to the presence of an undetected acoustic neuroma on the implanted side. Overall, perception scores for this patient were low, in part due to residual visual problems from the acoustic neuroma which affected his lipreading. However, after one year of experience with the Tickle Talker small improvements in words and sentences were evident. Without the tactile input, he was unable to perceive any words or sentences and subjectively felt isolated from the environment.

Patient 2 was a 31-year-old profoundly hearing-impaired male. He acquired his hearing loss at age 4 as a sequela to meningitis. He did not

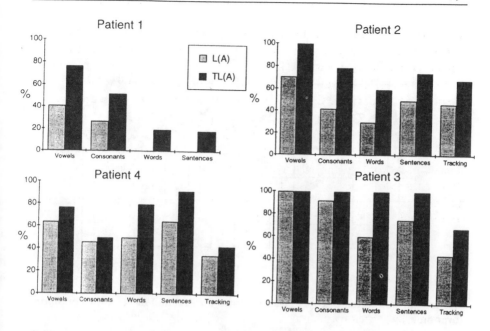

Figure 5. Speech perception scores for four hearing-impaired adults.

wear hearing aids and had previously decided against cochlear implantation as a communication option. Results after 2 years of experience with the Tickle Talker show Patient 2 was able to combine speech cues from the tactile input and from lipreading to improve significantly his perception of words and sentences. His perception of running speech in connected discourse tracking also improved by an average 21 words-per-minute. Tracking scores continued to show an increase over an 18 month period following initial tactile device fitting, as shown in Figure 6a, indicating that the patient was learning to incorporate more of the tactile information with additional experience with the device as an everyday communication aid.

Patient 3 was a 27-year-old profoundly hearing-impaired male. He had a congenital hearing loss and wore a single postauricular hearing aid on his left ear. Results after 3 years experience with the Tickle Talker show Patient 3 was able to combine tactually-encoded speech cues with those available from both aided residual hearing and lipreading. It is of note that Patient 3 scored 100% correct on perception of open-set words and sentences in the TLA condition, suggesting that the added tactile input had provided the additional cues missing in both lipreading and aided residual hearing. Patient 3 also showed a mean increase in perception of running speech in connected discourse tracking of 23 words per minute. Figure 6b shows that tracking rates increased over a 24-month period of tactile training and experience.

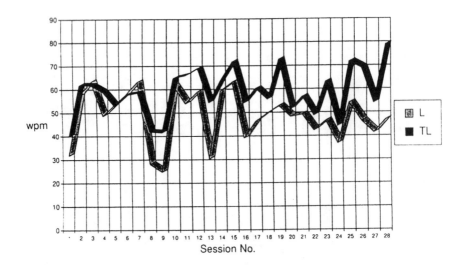

Figure 6a. Connected discourse tracking rates for Patient 2 in TL and L conditions over time.

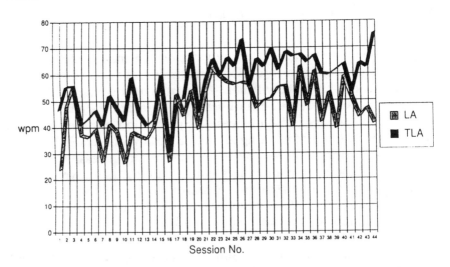

Figure 6b. Connected discourse tracking rates for Patient 3 in TLA and LA conditions over time.

Patient 4 was a 53-year-old profoundly hearing-impaired female. She had an acquired hearing loss as a result of head injuries. She used a single postauricular hearing aid on the right ear. Following 40 hours of training with the Tickle Talker, she showed significant benefits on words, sentences and speechtracking from the additional tactile information. Improvements on speechtracking were more modest, consistent with her level of experience with the device.

In summary, these results demonstrate that the Tickle Talker can effec-tively provide speech cues which are not available through either lipreading and/or aided residual hearing. These tactually-encoded speech cues could be integrated by all four adults with cues from lipreading and/or aided residual hearing to improve perception of words, sentences and running speech in connected discourse tracking. Benefits were shown for hearing-impaired adults with a range of hear-ing impairment, with both congenital and acquired hearing loss and for both non-users and users of hearing aids.

Speech perception studies with children

Hearing-impaired children are, in general, a more heterogeneous group than adults, with a wide range of hearing-impairment, aetiology, age at onset, years of severe and profound deafness, ability to use aided residual hearing, auditory experience, receptive and expressive vocabu-lary, knowledge of language, communication method (e.g. total com-munication or oral), educational placement, and familial and social support for habilitation.

Studies with the Tickle Talker have focused primarily on a group of eight children enrolled in oral education environments. Clinical field trials have also been conducted with an additional seven children in a total communication setting (Galvin *et al.*, 1991). Figure 7 shows mean percentage scores on speech feature discrimination and on perception of open-set words and sentences for these eight children, measured in both the tactually-aided (TLA and TA) and unaided (LA and A) condi-tions. The children were all using the UM3 prototype Tickle Talker for the evaluations and had experience ranging from 6 months to 4 years with the tactile input.

As shown, the children showed a significant improvement on percep-tion of open-set monosyllabic Phonetically-Balanced Kindergarten (PBK) words and key words in Bamford-Kowal-Bench (BKB) sentences when using the Tickle Talker. Although our focus is on open-set word and sen-tence perception, it is of interest to note that the children were able to access tactual cues to a variety of speech features which were not as read-ily available through their hearing aids. The results for words and sen-tences confirm that additional tactually-encoded cues were integrated into higher level perceptual tasks and that they could be effectively combined with information available from aided residual hearing and lipreading.

In summary, there is significant evidence for the following:

– that the Tickle Talker provides significant cues to speech features which are not available through either lipreading or aided residual hearing,
– that both hearing-impaired adults and children can detect and dis-criminate this tactually-encoded information,

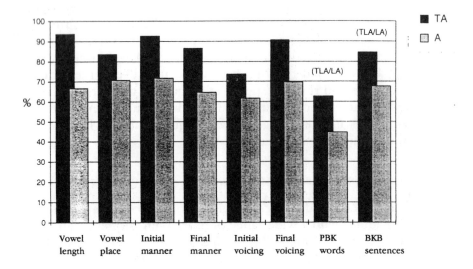

Figure 7. Speech test results for profoundly hearing-impaired children in tactually-aided (TLA and TA) and unaided (LA and A) conditions.

- that the tactually-encoded speech feature cues can be readily integrated with input from lipreading or aided residual hearing,
- that the added tactile input results in significant improvements in perception of words, sentences and running speech in connected discourse tracking, and
- that speech perception benefits continue to increase with additional experience.

Speech production studies

While our discussion has concentrated on assessing and establishing device efficacy by measuring benefits to speech detection, discrimination and perception, it is also interesting to assess the use of the Tickle Talker as a means of improving speech production skills, which are often poorly developed in congenitally hearing-impaired children. A pilot study has assessed the impact of the Tickle Talker on articulation when used as an on-line speech self-monitoring device by hearing-impaired children (Galvin *et al.*, in press). Figure 8 shows partial results of the pilot study, evaluating mean articulation of one child in both the Tickle Talker on and Tickle Talker off conditions.

As shown, the numbers of vowels, consonants, clusters and total phonemes correctly articulated was increased with the presence of on-line tactile self-monitoring. More detailed analysis of speech production improvements over time for a larger group of children are being made to assess the impact of the device on long-term speech production.

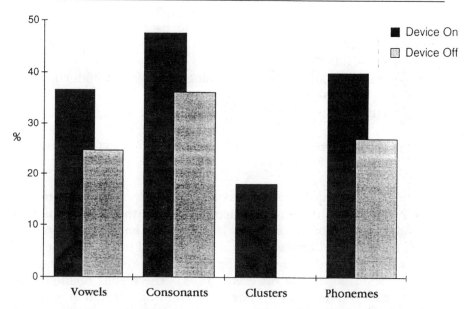

Figure 8. Articulation accuracy for one child using on-line tactile self-monitoring.

Training

It has been well-established that the training provided with any sensory device is a critical component in achieving maximum benefits from use of the device and of eventual user acceptance. This is particularly true for use of tactile devices, which require the user not only to learn to detect and discriminate a novel sensory signal, but also to learn to interpret the encoded information as meaningful speech messages and to integrate tactually-encoded signals with input from other sensory modalities such as vision and aided residual hearing. This is a formidable task as evidenced by studies of Tadoma training.

It is vital that tactile device development programmes include consideration and production of training programmes suitable and optimized for their particular device. While there will, of course, be generality in application of materials, the training must be suited to the content and saliency of the speech cues which are tactually encoded. In addition, thought must be given to the modalities to be employed in training. While significant progress in feature discrimination can be made with concerted closed-set training, this will not ensure that tactually-discriminable cues can be effective in improving perception of running speech (Alcantara *et al.*, 1990).

Important factors which have been identified as critical in design of tactile training programmes include:

- type of training task (analytic versus synthetic),
- amount of training (both total training required and frequency),

- motivation and consistency of device use, user characteristics (needs of individuals for supplementary cues based on residual hearing or presence of other disabilities),
- response formats employed in training (inclusion of both conversation and closed-set tasks),
- information encoded by the tactile device (the most critical factor), and
- evaluation procedures employed to monitor subject progress and identify training targets.

A full discussion of these factors and their relevance to optimizing benefits from use of tactile devices including the Tickle Talker is beyond the scope of this chapter. However, the impact of these individual factors have been assessed in a number of training studies and results incorporated in the development of the training programme for the Tickle Talker (Galvin *et al.*, 1993). The results highlight the need to concentrate training efforts on achieving integration of tactile input for perception of words, sentences and running speech through use of conversational materials. The results also confirm the importance of a knowledge of the saliency of the tactually-encoded speech cues provided by the particular tactile device in the development of training materials. Lastly, the need for long-term field trials of both tactile device use and training programmes with hearing-impaired adults and children is mandatory. While laboratory studies of training in normally-hearing subjects can shed light on underlying mechanisms of perceptual learning, only studies of real tactile device use and benefits can optimize the training programmes required for particular devices.

Cost

Cost of the Tickle Talker reflects not only the particular hardware and software to be implemented in the commercial-model device, but also the development costs incurred over the lengthy laboratory and field trials required to demonstrate efficacy. In addition, licensing costs for intellectual property and costs associated with the extensive patent protection required for marketing of biomedical devices must be considered. These costs must obviously be considered in light of and with knowledge of the potential intended market of users for the device. The concept of trade-offs again becomes important at the commercialization and marketing stage of the development. While it would be ideal to include a fully-programmable series of front-end speech encoding strategies or interchangeable vibratory or electrotactile transducers to provide the individual with the greatest flexibility, this would be reflected in much higher costs both in hardware and software developments.

It is vital that these eventual cost factors be considered at all stages of the development programme. For example, the potential advantages in use of platinum as the electrode material were outweighed in favour of stainless steel by the cost differential, difficulty in machining and less stringent requirements of the cutaneous electrode position in contrast to a subcutaneous environment. Similarly, the Tickle Talker uses the commercially-available speech processing hardware developed for the 22-channel cochlear implant. While development of a speech processor specifically tailored for use in the Tickle Talker might have achieved superior speech perception, the aim of producing an effective tactile device as a supplementary aid has been achieved and the additional costs for such a development would have been prohibitive. In addition, given the supplemental nature of the speech information provided, it is unlikely that users would accept the resultant higher price tag necessary with device developments such as the cochlear implant. This last consideration may of course be overcome by a breakthrough in speech processing which allows sufficient information to be presented through the tactile modality to allow open-set tactile-alone perception of running speech.

Summary

Our discussion has focused on identifying critical factors in the development of the Tickle Talker which have been addressed in order to achieve greater user acceptance by hearing-impaired adults and children. While we have been encouraged by the benefits available to users of this device, release of a commercial model is of paramount importance. If we draw on the example of the 22-channel cochlear implant produced by the University of Melbourne and Cochlear Pty Limited, there can be little argument as to the significant speech perception benefits being provided to thousands of hearing-impaired adults and children world-wide. The development of the successful initial cochlear implant required extensive preliminary psychophysical and biomedical safety studies. Following release of the first commercial multichannel implant, a continuing series of hardware development and speech processing studies have seen an evolution and steady increase in benefits available to users, culminating in release of the current SPECTRA-22 cochlear implant speech processor.

A good example of the validity of this approach is the development programme of the Tactaid devices, which are currently the most-used commercial tactile device in Australia and the United States. Tactile device programmes, including the Tickle Talker, must learn from and use this successful model of achieving user acceptance. Development must not be focused only on laboratory studies aimed at achieving the optimum speech processor, but must incorporate field use trials where the actual use of the device with hearing-impaired adults and children can be observed and assessed. Our studies must also incorporate evaluations of the impact of improved speech perception on development of language if we are to achieve real benefits for young children, who must use their sensory devices to acquire language. We must listen and learn from results and feedback from users to continually improve our hardware, speech processing strategies and training programmes. Only in this way will be able to achieve our ultimate aim of providing communication assistance to the hearing-impaired through widespread use and acceptance of tactile devices such as the Tickle Talker.

Acknowledgements

In closing, we wish to acknowledge the leadership of Professor Graeme Clark and the support and collaboration of colleagues in the development of the Tickle Talker. We are also grateful to the Commonwealth of Australia, Cochlear Pty Limited, the National Health and Medical Research Council, and several trusts and benefactors who have generously supported the research and development programme.

Finally, we would like to pay tribute to Arne Risberg for his pioneering efforts in the field of tactile and auditory research, which continue to inspire his many colleagues to pursue better communication for the hearing-impaired.

References

Alcantara, J.I., Cowan, R.S.C., Blamey, P.J. and Clark, G.M. (1990) A comparison of two training strategies for speech recognition with an electrotactile speech processor. Journal of Speech and Hearing Research 33: 195–204.

Alcorn, S. (1932) The Tadoma Method. Volta Review 34: 195–8.

Bergey, G.E., Squires, R.D. and Simple, R.W. (1971) Electrocardiogram recording with pasteless electrodes. IEEE Trans. Biomed. Eng., BME-18, 206–11.

Blamey, P.J. and Clark, G.M. (1985) A wearable mutiple-electrode electrotactile speech processor for the profoundly deaf. Journal of the Acoustical Society of America 77: 1619–20.

Blamey, P.J. and Clark, G.M. (1987) Psychophysical studies relevant to the design of a digital electrotactile speech processor. Journal of the Acoustical Society of America 82: 116–25.

Blamey, P.J., Alcantara, J.I., Cowan, R.S.C., Galvin, K.L., Sarant, J.Z. and Clark, G.M. (1990) Perception of amplitude envelope variations of pulsatile electrotactile stimuli. Journal of the Acoustical Society of America 88: 1765–72.

Boothroyd, A. (1984) Auditory perception of speech contrasts by subjects with sensorineural hearing loss. Journal of Speech and Hearing Research 27: 133–44.

Brummer, S.B. and Turner, M.J. (1977) Electrochemical considerations for safe electrical stimulation of the nervous system with platinum electrodes. IEEE Trans Biomed. Eng. BME-21, 81–8.

Burton, C. and Maurer, D.D. (1974) Pain suppression by transcutaneous electrical stimulation. IEEE Trans. Biomed. Eng. BME-21, 81–8.

Butikofer, R. and Lawrence, P.D. (1979) Electrocutaneous stimulation II: Stimulus waveform selection. IEEE Trans Biomed Eng. BME-26, 69–75.

Cabanes, J. (1985) Physiological effects of electric currents on living organisms, more particularly humans. In: Bridges, J.E. *et al.*, (Eds) Proceedings of the First International Symposium on Electric Shock Safety Criteria. Toronto: Pergamon Press.

Clark, G.M., Tong, Y.C., Patrick, J.F., Seligman, P.M., Crosby, P.A., Kuzma, J.A. and Money, D.K. (1984) A multi-channel hearing prosthesis for profound-to-total hearing loss. Journal of Medical Engineering and Technology 8(1): 3–8.

Cowan, R.S.C., Alcantara, J.I., Blamey, P.J. and Clark, G.M. (1987) Interim results of open-set speech discrimination with a wearable multichannel electrotactile speech processor. Journal of the Acoustical Society of America 82: 1456–7.

Cowan, R.S.C., Alcantara, J.I., Blamey, P.J. and Clark, G.M. (1988) Preliminary evaluation of a multichannel speech processor. Journal of the Acoustical Society of America 83: 2328–38.

Cowan, R.S.C., Alcantara, J.I., Whitford, L.A., Blamey, P.J. and Clark, G.M. (1989a) Speech perception studies using a multi-channel electrotactile speech processor, residual hearing, and lip reading. Journal of the Acoustical Society of America 85: 2593–607.

Cowan, R.S.C., Blamey, P.J., Alcantara, J.I., Whitford, L.A. and Clark, G.M. (1989b) Speech feature recognition with an electrotactile speech processor. Australian Journal of Audiology 11: 57–75.

Cowan, R.S.C., Blamey, P.J., Galvin, K.L., Sarant, J.Z., Alcantara, J.I. and Clark, G.M. (1990) Perception of sentences, words and speech features by profoundly hearing-impaired children using a multichannel electrotactile speech processor. Journal of the Acoustical Society of America 87: 1374–84.

Cowan, R.S.C. (1991) Speech Feature Encoding Through an Electrotactile Speech Processor. PhD. Dissertation. University of Melbourne.

Cowan, R.S.C., Blamey, P.J., Sarant, J.Z., Galvin, K.L. and Clark, G.M. (1991a) Perception of multiple electrode stimulus patterns: Implications for design of an electrotactile speech processor. Journal of the Acoustical Society of America 89: 360–8.

Cowan, R.S.C., Blamey, P.J., Sarant, J.Z., Galvin, K.L., Alcantara, J.I., Whitford, L.A. and Clark, G.M. (1991b) Role of a multichannel electrotactile speech processor in a cochlear implant program for profoundly-totally deaf adults. Ear and Hearing 12: 39–46.

Cowan, R.S.C., Blamey, P.J., Alcantara, J.I., Blombery, P.A., Hopkins, I.J. Whitford, L.A. and Clark, G.M. (1992) Safety studies with the University of Melbourne multichannel electrotactile speech processor. Journal of Rehabilitation Research and Development 29: 35–52.

Galvin, K.L., Cowan, R.S.C., Sarant, J.Z., Blamey, P.J. and Clark, G.M. (1991) Use of multichannel electrotactile speech processor by profoundly hearing-impaired children in a total communication environment. Journal of the American Academy of Audiology 2: 214–25.

Galvin, K.L., Cowan, R.S.C., Sarant, J.Z., Tobey, E.A., Blamey, P.J. and Clark, G.M. (in press) Articulation self-monitoring using electrotactile speech processor. Ear and Hearing.

Galvin, K.L., Cowan, R.S.C., Sarant, J.Z., Blamey, P.J. and Clark, G.M. (1993) 'Factors in the development of a training programme for use with tactile devices'. Ear and Hearing 14: 118–27.

Geldard, F.A. (1973) The Human Senses. New York: Wiley.

Green, H.L. and Ross J. (1985) Danger levels of short electric shocks from 50Hz supply. In: Bridges, J.E. *et al.*, (Eds) Proceedings of the First International

Symposium on Electrical Shock Safety Criteria.

Ifukube, T. (1989) Discrimination of synthetic vowels by using tactile vocoder and a comparison to that of an eight-channel cochlear implant. IEEE Trans. Biomed. Eng. BME-36(11), 1085–91.

Jadavji, T., Biggar, W.D., Gold, R. and Proben, C.G. (1986) Sequel of acute bacterial meningitis in children treated for seven days. Pediatrics 78: 21–5.

Leysieffer, H. (1986) A wearable multi-channel auditory prosthesis with vibrotactile skin stimulation. Audiological Acoustics 25: 230–51.

Levitt, H., Pickett, J.M. and Houde, R.A. (Eds) (1980) Sensory aids for the hearing impaired. New York: IEEE Press.

Lewes, D. (1965) Multipoint electrocardiography without skin preparation. Lancet ii: 17–18.

Lilly, J.C. (1955) Brief non-injurious electric waveform for stimulation of the brain. Science 121: 468–9.

Mason, J.L. and MacKay, N.A.M. (1976) Pain sensations associated with electrocutaneous stimulation. IEEE Trans Biomed. Eng. BME-23, 405–9.

McGarr, N.S. (Ed) (1989) Research on the use of sensory aids for hearing-impaired people. Volta Review 91: 1–138.

McLeod, G.A., Clarke, G.M. and Pengellerey, C.J. (1983) A speech processing strategy for an electrotactile vocoder: Preliminary psychological study. University of Melbourne Research Progress Report.

Owens, E., Kessler, D.K., Raggio, M.W. and Schubert, E.O. (1985) Analysis and revision of minimum auditory capabilities battery. Ear and Hearing 6: 280–7.

Pfeiffer, E.A. (1968) Electrical stimulation of sensory nerves with skin electrodes for research, diagnosis, communication and behavioral conditioning: a survey. Medical Biological Engineering 6: 637–51.

Pickett, J.M. (1986) Speech communication for the deaf: visual, tactile and cochlear implant. Journal of Rehabilitation Research and Development 23: 95-9.

Plant, G.L. (1983) The Plott Test (Stage Two). National Acoustic Laboratories: Sydney.

Plant, G.L. (1989) A comparison of five commercially-available tactile devices. Australian Journal of Audiology 11(1): 11–19.

Reed C.M., Rabinowitz, W.M., Durlach, N.I., Braida, L.D., Conway-Fithian, S. and Schultz, M.C. (1982) Research on the Tadoma method of speech communication. Journal of the Acoustical Society of America 77: 247–57.

Ragheb, T. and Geddes, L.A. (1981) Electrical properties of metallic electrodes. IEEE Med. biol. Eng. Comp. BMEC-28, 182–6.

Rugerri, R.T. and Beck, T.R. (1985) Calculations of temperature rise produced in body tissue by a spherical electrode. Annals of Biomedical Engineering 13: 177–94.

Sarant, J.Z., Cowan, R.S.C., Blamey, P.J., Galvin, K.L. and Clark, G.M. (1993) The effect of handedness in tactile speech perception. Journal of Rehabilitation Research and Development 30: 423–35.

Shepherd, R.K., Clark G.M. and Black R. C. (1983) Chronic electrical stimulation of the auditory nerve in cats. Acta Otolaryngologica (Stockh) 399: 19–31.

Söderlund, G. (1990). 'Natural tactiling: A personal account'. Paper presented at International Conference on Tactile Aids, Hearing Aids and Cochlear Implants, Sydney NSW, May 1-3.

6

Education of Deaf Children with Tactual Aids: the Miami Experience

D. KIMBROUGH OLLER, KATHLEEN VERGARA and
REBECCA E. EILERS

Introduction: The Miami Program

The study of speech perception through tactual artificial hearing devices raised hope in the mid-1970s that deaf children would soon profit from educational approaches incorporating advances supported by high technology. That hope inspired the development of a programme of training and research at the University of Miami. The effort includes device development, psychophysical testing of tactual vocoders, as well as training in tactual speech perception of both deaf and hearing subjects. The linguistic and academic accomplishments of deaf users constitute the bottom line of practical benefits from the research. Training begins with profoundly deaf children when they are 2 years of age or younger and includes full-time education within a laboratory school at the University for a period of usually 4 to 6 years. Thereafter children graduate into satellite programs where they are mainstreamed in the public schools of Dade County. The academic training the children receive in the satellites and their continued utilization of artificial hearing devices is supervised by a committee composed of University faculty and staff of the public school system.

The success of the model program has been notable. Deaf children have performed much better in speech production, speech comprehension, language use, reading, and other academic subjects than would have been expected in traditional programs. Recent comparisons, outlined below, suggest that outcomes for children in the model program are in many respects similar to those for congenitally deaf children with cochlear implants. The primary focus of the model educational program has been to evaluate and develop methods of training for deaf children based on high technology aids. It appears that the content and intensity of training are critical predictors of the success of education using tactual aids. The present report is intended to provide an update on the role that tactual aids can be expected to play in effective education of deaf children in the coming decades. The chapter outlines educational methods designed to optimize outcomes for children whose access to the world of sound can be augmented by tactual aids, and provides a summary of results obtained with children in the program.

Definition: the Family of Tactual Vocoders

The term 'tactual vocoder' is used here to refer to a family of devices that (1) receive sound through a microphone, (2) divide the sound into bands of information based on acoustic frequency, and (3) use the information in each band to drive one of a linear array of stimulators (vibrotactile or electrotactile) worn on the skin, where each stimulator reacts proportionally to the energy in its corresponding band. Historically, the number of bands or 'channels' in tactual vocoders has varied widely, and the devices used in the Miami programme have included systems with two, four, seven, eight, sixteen, twenty-four and thirty-two channels. In addition, both vibrotactile and electrotactile stimulators have been used. The vibrotactile stimulators have been of the 'plunger' variety (operating at a fixed frequency) as found in the designs of Engelmann and Rosov (1975) and Brooks and Frost (1983), and of the resonance-tuned variety as found in the Tactaid systems designed by Franklin (1986). The electrotactile stimulators of the Tacticon 1600 were designed by Saunders (1985).

The signal processing systems in the devices used in the Miami program have mostly been based on either analogue or digital filtering systems. However, in recent years the program has made use of a system called the Digivoc, which employs fast Fourier transforms (FFT) to determine energy levels at each selected frequency and consequent input to each stimulator. The system was developed through collaboration of engineers from Intelligent Hearing Systems in cooperation with the research team at the University of Miami (see Ozdamar *et al.*, 1992). The FFT tactual vocoder is now in miniaturization, and the signal processing approach has been augmented to include formant tracking algorithms based on linear predictive coding (Oller, *et al.*, in press).

The tactual vocoders that have been available for use in the Miami programme have varied substantially in where they are worn on the body, and whether or not they are sufficiently miniaturized to be worn full-time. The devices that have proven most effective in transmitting speech information have not been miniaturized, and as a result have been used only in speech training within special periods (of from 20 minutes to 1 hour daily), while more wearable devices such as the Tacticon 1600, Tactaid II+, and the Tactaid 7 are utilized by the children during the entire school day.

In miniaturized systems the processor box varies from the size of a beeper to the size of a paperback book, and can be worn on the children's belts. In non-miniature tactual vocoders, the processors are hard-wired systems housed in a table-top unit, or digital systems incorporated into a computer. Each type of tactual aid is connected to microphones and an array of stimulators. The stimulator arrays have been worn on the arm or leg (the Engelmann and Rosov system for example), on the abdomen (the Tacticon 1600, the Tactaid 7 and the Digivoc), or on the forehead (the Tactaid devices). The preferred location for miniaturized systems is often the abdomen (because the stimulator belt can then be hidden under clothing, and mobility is unimpaired) even though tactual sensitivity of other locations (especially the forehead) appears to be superior to that of the abdomen. The children themselves sometimes make the choice about where to place the stimulator arrays depending on cosmetic preferences and personal opinions regarding relative transmission capabilities of stimulators in varying locations.

Background Research

The inspiration to begin the Miami program came from training studies that showed tactual vocoders could transmit a substantial portion of the speech code in real time (Engelmann and Rosov, 1975; Richardson and Frost, 1977; Brooks and Frost, 1983). The encouraging results reversed an earlier pessimism that had emerged when short-term experience with tactual vocoders had produced good perception of isolated speech features, but little ability on the part of wearers to perceive running speech (see review by Kirman, 1973). In particular, the new hope was inspired by results of Engelmann and Rosov (1975) indicating that, with sufficient systematic training, both deaf and hearing subjects using a 24-channel tactual vocoder, could learn to recognize substantial vocabularies of words, as well as sentences composed over the learned vocabulary through the tactual sense alone. Perhaps even more important, subjects showed consistent learning and continuous acquisition of new tactual vocabulary even after months of training. Their learning curves did not level off, and they demonstrated the ability to recognize new words that differed in phonetically limited ways from previously learned vocabulary. These results indicated that the subjects were learning to recognize the phonetic system of English, and to utilize that knowledge creatively rather than simply to process each new word as an independent gestalt. This pattern of open-ended learning was a key ingredient that stoked the dormant fires of hope that sensory substitution could play a major role in speech reception for deaf learners. In addition, research indicated that a wide variety of tactual vocoders were capable of transmitting substantial speech information (Spens, 1980).

At the University of Miami, we began artificial hearing research with studies designed to confirm the validity of the Engelmann and Rosov results. After encouraging outcomes (reported in Oller, Payne and Gavin, 1980 and Oller and Eilers, 1988a) the research team proceeded to device development and psychophysical testing where tactual speech signals were presented to hearing subjects (Mandalia *et al.*, 1983; Eilers, Bull and Oller, 1984; Bull *et al.*, 1985; Ozdamar, Eilers and Oller, 1987; Eilers *et al.*, 1988a). At the same time we initiated a program of training for deaf children that quickly expanded from individual therapy to speech training with five youngsters every weekday afternoon. By the early 1980s we had established a full-day educational program wherein deaf children at the preschool and early elementary levels studied a full range of subjects and used tactual vocoders and hearing aids in an eclectic approach to speech and speech reception training. Presently more than 50 children are involved in the model program and its satellites.

Design of the Miami Program

An eclectic approach

A fundamental assumption of the Miami program is that severe to profound hearing impairment does not imply inferior cognitive abilities. The majority of deaf children have the ability to function normally in cognition given normal input of information (Quigley and Paul, 1984). The hitch in this reasoning concerns the notion 'normal input'. By adopting an eclectic approach to education, the Miami program provides the opportunity for children to receive maximal input. To insure that speech and speech reception are developed optimally, children are presented with a wide array of systematically designed speech tasks where the input is multimodal – children read lips, use auditory information through hearing aids (or cochlear implants in the cases of an increasing number of the children), and utilize tactual vocoders to provide additional acoustic information. In addition, sign language plays an important role in children's cognitive and communicative development within the program (see below). Language and speech are taught in this eclectic setting in a systematic pattern designated in the Miami CHATS curriculum (Vergara *et al.*, 1993a), the formal guide to speech and speech reception training within the program.

Multimodal and unimodal training

The Miami program focuses on both unimodal and multimodal training. Our early work focused on training all three modalities (visual, auditory, tactual) simultaneously, in the hope that deaf children would learn to integrate information across modalities. However, these initial attempts yielded mixed results, and the cross-modal integration outcome was deemed unsatisfactory given expectations based on previous laboratory work with adult subjects trained in recognition of words and sentences through tactual aids, and then tested for cross-modal integration in reception tasks that involved information presented through lipreading and the tactual sense simultaneously (Brooks *et al.*, 1986; Weisenberger and Miller, 1987; Weisenberger, 1988; Lynch, Oller and Eilers, 1989).

Consequently, we instituted a new training effort with the intention of enhancing cross-modal integration. The new method begins with multimodal (auditory-tactual-visual) training within particular tasks, and then moves on to unimodal versions of the same or similar tasks, in an attempt to focus the child's attention on each modality individually. Thereafter, training in combinations of modalities (auditory–tactual, auditory–visual, tactual–visual and auditory–tactual–visual) is used to encourage integration of information across modalities. This procedure is now routine within the training program. To exemplify, a child might be taught to recognize a class of words (say, numbers from one to five) first multimodally to some criterion level of success (say 60% correct). Thereafter the same task would be conducted with tactual signal only, and then with auditory signal only. After some criterion level of success in each modality, the child might be trained to recognize the same class of words with a combination of auditory and tactual information, then with auditory and visual information, and so on.

Research within the program has indicated effective integration of tactual, auditory and visual information as a result of this training approach. Children recognize syllables and words better in multimodal presentation than in presentation of tactual alone, auditory alone, or visual alone conditions (Lynch *et al.*, 1989a). It is notable that the generalization across modalities is still not found in every circumstance. On occasions of high task complexity or low task familiarity (as sometimes occurs with presentation of a novel evaluation protocol) children sometimes appear to revert to reliance upon one or two modalities and do not show the expected advantages of sensory integration found in other circumstances (Eilers *et al.*, 1993). A primary goal of current training efforts in the Miami project is to refine methods in order to instill integration abilities that are resistant to such limitations.

Teacher awareness of pattern perception on the skin and the function of auditory aids including cochlear implants

In training children within specific modalities it has proven important to ensure that teachers have specific and practical knowledge of the function of the devices that deliver acoustic information to the deaf child. Consequently, the curriculum encourages teachers as often as possible to wear the same kinds of tactual vocoders that their students wear, and to focus on the patterns of stimulation they feel in order to facilitate their description of patterns to the child. Teachers are also encouraged to study charts provided in the curriculum indicating ways in which particular sounds produce particular patterns of stimulation on the skin. Such charts provide a schematic representation of how the signal processing systems of the tactual vocoders control the delivery of acoustic information. Similarly, teachers are encouraged to study the signal processing characteristics of auditory amplification units and cochlear implants used by the children, in order to make clear what kinds of acoustic information may be available to the child.

The modular training approach: The role of Activities in the Miami CHATS curriculum

Speech and language training according to the Miami CHATS curriculum is built around Activities that are designed to provide the teacher with sample formats for the implementation of goals and objectives. The Activities have the flavour of games, and in general, the academic objectives of the training are opaque to the child. Each Activity is a recipe with criteria for success indicated and procedures fully specified. The intent of the curriculum as a whole is to focus the child's attention on speech through all modalities, to help the child recognize sounds, words and sentences, and to foster speech production development through systematic attention to feedback provided through tactual and auditory signals.

Goals, activities and cycling

There is a hierarchy of organization and a suggested procedure within the curriculum for selection of Activities day by day. The procedure is patterned after the phonological training system of 'cycling' (Hodson and Paden, 1991). Selection of Activities is based in part on the child's success in prior Activities, but is also decided on the basis of a pattern of recurrence of different goal types (for example, suprasegmental, segmental, vocabulary, etc.), different modalities, and different task levels. Cycling encourages the teacher to cover the field of learnable skills at a pace that maximizes the child's progress across the whole scope of speech and speech reception needs that are reflected in the curriculum's structure. Obsessive concern over reaching criterion level performance on any particular Activity is discouraged. The central aim is to maintain a pattern of training that engages the child's interest and balances the content objectives across a variety of domains.

While the curriculum specifies Activities as examples, the teacher is encouraged to create additional Activities using the published ones as models. Furthermore, while the curriculum indicates a possible order for presentation of the goals and objectives, flexibility is emphasized, and the teacher is expected to monitor child progress in each domain of training and to seek a day-to-day pattern of training that maximizes learning rate and maintains the child's interest through fun and a sense of success.

Receptive task levels

A hierarchy of task levels is specified in the curriculum to assist the teacher in the daily selection of Activities of an appropriate level of complexity. Higher level tasks require the abilities implied by the lower level tasks, and consequently, it is sometimes necessary to follow the order specified by the hierarchy in order to maintain progress. At the same time, if a child can succeed in a particular content domain without going through Activities at the lower levels of the hierarchy, the teacher is encouraged to skip or move quickly through the lower levels.

At the first receptive task level, children are taught to give evidence of detection or *awareness* of sounds within each modality. The goal of the awareness activities (often framed in the form of psychophysical vigilance tasks) is to focus the child's attention on information being presented in a particular modality. The Activities focused on detection prove especially important to make children aware of tactual and auditory signals at low sensation levels.

At the second receptive task level, children are taught to give indications of *discrimination* between differing sounds or words, first with pairs that are maximally distinct from an acoustic standpoint, and later with pairs that are minimally distinct. Discrimination Activities can be based on various responses of the child, for example, raising of a hand when a change occurs in a repeating background, saying or signing 'same' or 'different', or selecting one of two possible choices discriminatively. Discrimination tasks heighten the child's sensitivity to speech sounds and focus attention on properties of the sounds that have significance.

At the third receptive level, children are taught *recognition*, or the ability to identify sounds and associate them with meaningful symbols. For example, in a recognition Activity the teacher may name an object and the child may be asked to point to the appropriate picture from an array. Simple recognition tasks are based on two-choice identification with words that are maximally distinct phonetically, while more complex recognition tasks are based on multiple-choice identification with words that are minimally distinct.

At the fourth level, *comprehension* of meaningful speech, children are asked to respond meaningfully to words and eventually to sentences. Comprehension Activities require the child to generalize from knowledge developed systematically in simpler Activities and to respond to speech in contexts of potential educational significance as well as of real life experience.

Expressive task levels

Expressive tasks occur at one of two levels, *imitative* and *initiative*. Imitative tasks are designed to elicit systematically distinct pronunciations of sounds and sound sequences. Teachers are encouraged to facilitate imitation through explicitly directing the child's attention to any of the modalities. For example, in training a child to imitate the syllable [sa] as opposed to the syllable [ta], the teacher may produce the sounds and indicate to the child through verbal or signed description coupled with pointing to particular stimulators on the tactual array that the [s] is 'longer' than the [t], although both occur in the same location on the skin. Following successful imitation by the child, the training sequence may move on to elicitation of the target through a direct request (but not modelling), and finally to unprompted production in a meaningful linguistic exchange.

Goal categories

The content of the training provided within each task level is sequenced systematically to maximize learning rate and to ensure a firm foundation for further progress. Considerable effort in speech and speech reception training for the very young deaf child is directed toward the establishment of *phonological foundations*. Deaf children are often greatly delayed in the production of speech-like vocalizations and babbling (Stoel-Gammon and Otomo, 1986; Oller and Eilers, 1988b). Consequently, expressive training focuses at early stages on eliciting categories of vocalizations that progressively approximate well-formed syllables. The categories of vocalizations that are elicited are tailored to the child's current vocal stage, based on a model of normal vocal development that is by now well-documented (Oller, 1978; Stark, 1980; Holmgren *et al.*, 1986; Roug, Langberg and Lundberg, 1989). At the same early developmental point, receptive training is focused on establishment of phonological foundations by efforts to focus the child's attention on sound presented in each modality. Special effort is made to teach the child to recognize a variety of tactual patterns that bear a specific relationship with phonemic units or features and consequently are referred to as 'tactemes' or 'tactual phonetic features'.

As children progress, it becomes possible to move toward more traditional phonological training in all three modalities. From the standpoint of traditional speech and language categories, the training focuses on *suprasegmental* features such as duration, rate, intensity, pitch, and voice quality. Suprasegmental training in individual features encourages the child to recognize variations along significant speech parameters and to practice the productive control of the same parameters. *Segmental* training focuses on consonants, vowels, and diphthongs, and children are taught to discriminate contrasts in each modality, as well as to recognize and contrastively produce the segmental sounds of speech. In both the segmental and suprasegmental realms, a developmental model is used to determine the order in which sounds and contrasts are taught (Ingram, 1976; Oller and Eilers, 1981; Locke, 1983).

Both expressive and receptive training Activities are directed toward the learning of *vocabulary*, and in many cases the teaching of segmentals and suprasegmentals is conducted in the context of vocabulary learning. Similarly, as words become available to the child in expression and reception, *phrases and sentences* are systematically targeted.

As children gain facility with the reception and production of words and phrases in the limited circumstances of closed set training, the curriculum focuses on goals of *generalization*. At this level of goals, the Activities specified by the curriculum are integrative, incorporating all modalities, both expressive and receptive skills, and recruiting children's knowledge of all the vocabulary and syntax at their disposal. The systematic progression of objectives incorporated in the curriculum has much in common with other training manuals and training models written to guide teachers in the use of tactual aids (Plant, 1991; Hesketh and Osberger, 1990; Youdelman, Behrman, and Franklin, 1989).

The role of non-simultaneous total communication

By the time children are participating in generalization Activities, they are capable of meaningful, pragmatically significant use of speech. However, the Miami CHATS curriculum leaves room for a major role to be played by sign language. It should be noted at the outset that in the Miami program to date, the vast majority of the deaf children who have participated have had profound losses, most have been from homes where Spanish is a primary language (although English is the language of instruction at school), many are from conditions of low socioeconomic status and about one-third have additional secondary handicaps such as learning disabilities and mild motoric disorders.

These children would have extremely low prognosis for speech development in traditional programs, and in the absence of special programming, virtually all of them would be assigned to Total Communication (TC) classes based on the expectation that if they were in traditional oral programs, they would fail.

Given these conditions of prognosis, we have chosen to have sign language play an integral role in the Miami programme to date, but it is important to emphasize the uniqueness of the approach. In traditional TC, signing and speech are presented simultaneously at all times, and the results with regard to speech outcome have not been encouraging (Geers, Moog and Schick, 1984; Ling, 1984; Geers and Moog, 1992). In non-simultaneous TC, teachers present activities modularly, with considerable emphasis on natural, rapid communication through sign language during designated portions of the school day, and with emphasis on speech production and speech reception during other portions. This division is intended to foster 'bilingualism' in speech and sign, and to ensure success in both modalities of communication. Speech success is spurred on by a rapid growth of sign language knowledge, and hinges on a curriculum designed accurately to predict the sequence of progress that can be expected for deaf children through various speech communication skills. By consistently targeting speech skills at appropriate levels of difficulty, and by building on the foundations of previously acquired speech and sign skills, children are able to experience consistent effective speech communication and to acquire confidence in their vocal capacities. All the while, they gain new vocabulary, new syntactic structures, and new discourse skills that have already been established within the sign language domain.

Sign language skills consistently outpace speech skills in deaf children who are exposed to fluent signing, and in the Miami program sign language skills are intended not only to constitute a basic mode of interchange but also to pave the way for rich speech communication by providing a linguistic structure and conceptual frame within which speech training can be directed. To achieve the speech goals, it is critical to maintain a daily, intensive speech training program in order to establish confidence and build momentum in the use of vocal communication.

Advocates of traditional TC are sometimes sceptical of the Miami program's non-simultaneous approach, assuming that it may be a thinly veiled form of traditional oralism, where sign language is discouraged or prohibited. Similarly, advocates of traditional oralism have sometimes criticized the non-simultaneous approach as a thinly veiled manualism, where speech is presented along with sign but is not explicitly taught, and deaf children are tacitly encouraged to abandon the goal of active participation in speaking communities. These criticisms are inconsistent with the facts of the implementation in the Miami program classrooms, where both speech and sign are aggressively taught. At the same time, the arguments about appropriate methods should not, and perhaps cannot, be resolved without evaluation of outcomes. The proof of the pudding is in comparative speech and sign language skills of the children who have studied in the non-simultaneous environment of the Miami program as opposed to children who have experienced traditional educational methods.

Outcomes for Children in the Miami Program

Studies on tactual reception of acoustic information on the skin

A series of studies have been conducted within the project to illustrate that tactual vocoders can and do provide substantial information to deaf users. For example, Eilers, Widen and Oller (1988b) provided data on detection levels for tactual aids and amplified hearing in individual deaf children from 200 to 8000 Hz. The data indicated that while amplified auditory sensitivity thresholds dropped off precipitously above 500 Hz, tactual thresholds were roughly even out to 8000 Hz (at 40–55 dB). The data suggested that tactual detection of information across the spectrum necessary for speech is possible, and that tactual aids can provide substantial acoustic information not available through lipreading. Detection levels with tactual aids were found to be comparable to those of children with cochlear implants. Phoneme identification studies with the same deaf children indicated that speech sound contrasts that are difficult to hear (with amplification) and difficult to see (by lipreading) are sometimes easy to recognize tactually. Other studies in our laboratories (Oller *et al.*, 1980; Lynch, Eilers, Oller and LaVoie, 1988) also provided empirical data indicating that deaf children could use tactual information to advantage, especially since acoustic information provided through tactual vocoders is substantially different from that provided through lipreading and auditory amplification. The complementarity of acoustic information provided by tactual vocoders and lipreading has been verified in studies from other laboratories as well (e.g. Sparks *et al.*, 1978; Brooks and Frost, 1983; Plant and Spens, 1986).

Deaf children's speech progress in the Miami programme

In order to evaluate the speech progress of children in the Miami programme, it is useful to consider a variety of comparative perspectives. The problem of obtaining the requisite information is not trivial because outcomes are influenced by many variables, including the devices used by the children, the training procedures employed, the enthusiasm levels of the teachers, the prognostic levels of the children before entering the program, etc. It is not practically possible to control all such variables, and consequently, it becomes necessary to consider outcomes from a variety of studies in order to acquire information that may converge upon a reasonable conclusion regarding the role that tactual vocoders, in conjunction with specialized curricula, can play in educational outcomes.

The first systematic study to assess speech progress of deaf children in the Miami program considered speech gains across a year (Oller *et al.*, 1986). All the 13 children (mean age 5 years) who at the time of the report had been trained in speech therapy using tactual vocoders, showed substantial gains in speech sound inventory. Each child at least doubled the number of consonants produced in a syllable imitation task. Increases in vowel imitation were also found in every child. In addition, 10 of 13 children showed discernible gains in production of fricative/stop contrasts, indicating progress in a domain that is commonly difficult for deaf children. It has been suggested that the gain in fricative/stop production may have been supported by the high frequency information supplied effectively through the tactual vocoders, information that is hard to lipread and hard to transmit through auditory amplification to deaf students. All the children also showed discernible gains across the year in speech sounds produced contrastively in real words elicited in a naming task.

In order to evaluate the gains found in the children working with tactual vocoders in the context of gains that might be expected for children in other, more traditional training programmes, Eilers, Oller and Vergara (1989) compared outcomes for two groups, one composed of 11 of the children from the previous study, and one composed of 15 socioeducationally similar children educated in a traditional program. The groups were selected to be similar in socioeconomic status, ethnicity, hearing loss level, and secondary handicapping conditions. Across a year of study, the children in the tactually aided group showed a 17% gain in the number of contrastive speech sounds produced in a meaningful speech task, while the comparison group gained 1%. In addition, syllable inventory gains of the tactually aided group exceeded those of the comparison group by a factor of six.

A subsequent evaluation considered improvements in speech for eight tactually aided children over a three-year period, by comparison with those of another group of nine socioeducationally matched deaf children (Eilers *et al.*, in press). Again, children in both groups were evaluated in terms of their production of speech sounds in an elicitation task, although the test was a different one from that employed in the prior study, Eilers *et al.* (1989). The analysis of results considered the proportion of the speech code of English that was accurately produced by each child both at the beginning of the study and at the end. This analysis evaluated the pronunciations of the child in terms of the overall accuracy of each word attempted, calculating the degree of accuracy through a software implemented formula that assigned differential weights to errors of production that tend to have differential effects on intelligibility. For example, a segment substitution was penalized less in the formula than a segment deletion, and common, developmentally predictable segment substitutions were penalized less than uncommon substitutions, of a sort not often found in child speech. With this method, implemented in LIPP (Logical International Phonetics Programs, Oller, 1991), it was possible to obtain a global measure of the accuracy of children's speech production expressed as a proportion of the total speech code of English.

The two groups were closely matched in the baseline evaluations of year one, with the tactually aided group showing 21% correct production and the comparison group 23% correct production as determined by the LIPP-implemented correctness formula. Three years later, however, the tactually aided group had improved to 39%, while the comparison group's final score was 27%. While both groups showed discernible progress, the tactually aided group improved by a statistically greater amount. Furthermore, the eight tactually aided children gained 10% to 30% over the three years, while the most improved comparison child showed an improvement score of 12%.

The Eilers *et al.* (in press) study provided additional empirical support for previous findings of improvement in speech production by tactually aided children in the Miami program, and showed such gains across a longer period of time than prior studies. In addition, through use of the new formula for evaluation, the results provided a perspective that appears to correspond better with intuitive impressions of educators than previous traditional evaluations wherein all errors, regardless of seriousness, are treated equivalently. Further, the reliability of the transcriptionally-based results of the study was confirmed through a check in which transcribers who were blinded to the identity of the children whom they evaluated, revealed a pattern of gains that matched that of the original evaluation.

Comparisons of spoken language for children in the Miami program against national norms

Another way to consider the gains of children in the program is to evaluate their speech and language knowledge in the perspective of national norms. The GAEL (Grammatical Analysis of Elicited Language, Moog and Geers, 1985) provides evaluations for various ages that are normed for deaf children nationwide, in some cases for both TC programs and exclusively oral programs. Eilers *et al.* (1989) provided an initial comparison of growth in GAEL scores both in speech production and comprehension across a 5-month period by seven preschool deaf children in the Miami program. While all seven were below the 50th percentile for the comprehension section of the GAEL-P (preschool level) at the beginning of the study, and the mean ranking was 19th percentile (reflecting the low initial speech prognosis of children who have typically been admitted to the programme), the rankings after 5 months of training were at a mean level of the 39th percentile, and three of the students were above the 50th. In production, the gains were less over the 5-month period, with an initial mean ranking of 26th percentile and a 30th percentile mean at the end of the period. This pattern of more rapid growth in reception than in production has come to be an expected characteristic of outcomes for children with artificial hearing (Osberger, 1990). The Eilers *et al.* (1989) study also reported on three children who were 6–8 years of age. The GAEL-S (simple sentence level, appropriate for elementary-school-aged deaf children) percentile rankings for these three deaf children were over the 80th percentile for both production and comprehension based on the TC norms. The children had by that time graduated from the University-based model program into a public school follow-up program where they were partially mainstreamed into daily classes with hearing children, although they continued in a tactually aided, TC program for the hearing-impaired for regular portions of each school day. The high scores in both comprehension and production suggest that with long-term training the expressive/receptive gap seen in early training with artificial hearing can be narrowed.

A more recent evaluation by Vergara *et al.* (1993) followed up outcomes at ages 6 to 7 for 27 of the Miami program's deaf children who had graduated into follow-up programs with partial mainstreaming. The mean GAEL-S percentile rankings in the prompted section of the tests improved from the 60th to the 70th percentiles across the year, and in the imitative section they improved from the 65th to the 75th. Thirteen additional children who had graduated from the Miami program's model into the tactually aided follow-up programs, were 8–10 years of age, and able to be evaluated with the highest level GAEL test, the GAEL-C (Complex Sentence Level). The mean outcomes for these children at the last interval of testing were near the 90th percentile for both prompted and imitative productions based on the TC norms. The percentile rankings provide a benchmark of the levels of speech and language function that the children in the program attain, and they indicate that with aggressive treatment and eclectic usage of artificial hearing, children with initially low prognosis can move from low percentile rankings in preschool to very high ones by late elementary or junior high school.

Outcomes in sign language

One might imagine that the Miami program's efforts are successful in producing children who perform well in speech because there is such extraordinary effort devoted to speech training. Sign language outcomes might be expected to suffer. However, sign language training is pursued within the program by teachers who are highly skilled and who present important segments of the academic curriculum in sign language every day. The results of the Vergara *et al.* (1993) study include additional data from the GAEL on the children for both prompted and imitative signing as well as speech. The children proved to be excellent signers, ranking on the average at the 75–80th percentile by age 7, and above the 90th percentile for the total group of children older than age 7. Consequently, it is clear that sign language growth in the tactually aided children was rapid and exceeded that to be expected in traditional (simultaneous) TC programmes.

Comparative outcomes with cochlear implant users

The Miami program has recently initiated studies on the gains made by children in the tactually aided program compared with children who are users of cochlear implants. Only a few children within the Miami program have cochlear implants to date (though the number is now growing rapidly), but it has been possible to make preliminary comparisons of performance among tactually aided children and implanted children from other programmes for which results have been published.

It is important to emphasize that there are many differences between the experiences of the implanted children who have been reported on in published studies and the tactually aided children in the Miami programme. For example, the tactually aided children do not take their tactual devices home, and they use them only for portions of the school day, with a year-round average of about two hours per day of artificial hearing experience. This is an unfortunate practical fact, imposed upon the program by availability of equipment and financial constraints. Implanted children, on the other hand, tend to have access to artificial hearing on a more regular basis, both at school and at home, with a year round average usage of 10 hours per day or more (R. Fifer, personal communication). It should also be noted that intervention begins in the Miami program usually when children are 2 years old or younger, while cochlear implantation is done at a variety of ages, and consequently implanted children do not always experience early intervention to the degree that tactually aided children do. Eilers *et al.* (1993) reported results for 27 children from the Miami program, compared with results on a variety of implanted children from studies of Osberger *et al.* (1991). Judging from the children's ages and the ages of implantation, it appears that the implanted children had more total artificial hearing experience than the tactually aided children, though during a shorter period of time, and generally starting at more advanced ages.

The tests administered to children from both groups included the SCIPS (Screening inventory of Perception Skills), the MPT (Minimal Pairs Test), the Change/No Change Test, and the MTS (Monosyllable, Trochee, Spondee) Test. Children in the tactually aided group showed discernible gains on all tests across a one year period, and when compared with implanted children of similar age, showed scores that were generally comparable, or lower by relatively small amounts. For example on the SCIPS, the average score for tactually aided children was 82% across the four parts of the test (chance performance = 50%), while the average score for implanted children was 88%. On the Change/No Change Test the average score for tactual children was 75% across seven subtests while the average score for implanted children was 81%. On the MPT tactual children showed an average score of 63% while implanted children had an average score of 69%. Finally on the MTS, the tactually aided group had an average score of 50% (chance performance = 8%) while the implanted group's score was 54%. These outcomes suggest that with aggressive training using tactual aids (even when they are not available full-time), it is reasonable to expect speech reception growth not unlike that occurring in children with cochlear implants. Other results suggesting similarity of outcome for deaf children with tactual vocoders and cochlear implants have been reported by Cowan *et al.* (1992) and Plant (1992). Less encouraging results for users of tactual aids were reported by Robbins, Todd and Osberger (1992). The better outcomes appear to have depended on more intense, longer-term educational treatment focused on the use of the tactual aids.

Independent evaluation of the Miami programme

The studies thus far reviewed regarding tactually aided children were conducted by scientists and educators within the Miami program. It is worthwhile to consider results produced by an independent evaluation. Such a study was conducted over a 2-year period by the Division of Program Evaluation of the Dade County Public Schools. The study was intended to assist the School Board in determining whether or not to continue subcontracting education of deaf children to the University of Miami at substantial expense, during a period in which budget cuts were being implemented throughout the system and in subcontractual programs.

All testers were public school personnel unconnected to the program and to the University, and the designers of the evaluation as well as the writers of the final report were officials of the Division of Program Evaluation that had no connection with and knew nothing of the program prior to the study. Thirty-five children at various ages who were in the Miami program or were follow-up graduates of the program were compared with 24 children in traditional programs with similar hearing losses and socioeducational characteristics.

The outcomes for the two groups on the two sections of the standardized SAT (Stanford Achievement Test) provide a perspective on academic growth in the two groups. The average scores for the tactually aided group were more than 100 points higher than the comparison scores for reading, and more than 60 points higher in mathematics, differences that were in both cases highly statistically reliable.

In the independent study, the outcomes of the tactually aided and comparison groups in speech and language were compared using the GAEL battery. However, the scores were not reported because few children in the comparison group were able to complete any level of the test. All the 35 tactually aided children completed at least the GAEL-P (preschool level) the first year and the majority moved up a level the second year, but only 11 of 24 comparison children were able to complete any level the first year, and by the second year there were 'insufficient scores ... to warrant an analysis'. Similarly, 86% of the children from the tactually aided group completed the Carolina Picture Vocabulary Test and showed significant growth in scores across the year of study, while only 36% of the comparison group completed the test and their gains across the year were far less. Results on the SPINE (Speech Intelligibility Test) proved hard to interpret because the test was too advanced for the groups as a whole. Only 20% of the tactually aided group and only 13% of the comparison group were able to complete the test.

Of the 13 children who had graduated into the tactually-aided follow-up, all were mainstreamed partially and the average was 3.8 classes per day. Of the 15 children from the comparison group who were similarly eligible for mainstreaming, the average was 0.6 classes per day.

The authors of the study were cautious in their interpretations, taking note of methodological flaws of the work, but, on the basis of the results, recommended that the school district should 'continue to support' the project. The key concerns about methodological flaws were related to matching of the two groups of children. The authors noted that the two groups, which they had attempted to match to the extent possible on relevant socioeducational variables, differed in IQ at the time of the evaluation. Overall, the tactually aided group had a mean IQ of 103 while the comparison group's IQ was 96. However, by breaking the groups down into younger (through first grade) and older (after first grade) subgroups, it can be determined that the tactually aided group had lower IQs at the younger ages (95 to 103), while among the older children, the tactually aided group's IQs substantially exceeded those of the comparison group (117 to 92). This difference across age suggests, consistent with observations of teachers, that the IQs of children admitted to the Miami program grow discernibly and consistently as a function of intensive education and artificial hearing training.

Consequently, in assessing the outcome of the educational treatment, it is not appropriate to match groups on IQ. On the contrary, IQ is a legitimate dependent measure in and of itself, and has been used as such in much educational and intervention outcome research (Zigler *et al.*, 1982; Ramey *et al.*, 1985; Ramey and Campbell, 1987). Further, it is well-known that achievement test scores such as those of the SAT (one of the primary dependent measures in the study) are highly correlated with IQ. The concern about matching appears to have been based upon the ill-founded assumption that educational training procedures might affect language and academic outcomes without affecting IQ. If the authors had managed to match the groups for IQ, it is likely they would have masked many of the primary effects of the intensive education and training with tactual aids. A research approach that results in obscuring of real effects through matching of groups on variables correlated with dependent measures is referred to as 'overmatching' and is an increasing concern in the design of educational research where successful treatments can affect a variety of variables (Rothman, 1986).

Conclusions

The study of speech and speech reception improvement in children utilizing tactual aids within the Miami program shows a consistent pattern of growth, and outcomes that are far better than could be expected with traditional training methods. In addition, the outcomes in speech reception appear nearly comparable to those for children with cochlear implants even though the tactually aided children receive less experience with artificial hearing than their implanted counterparts. When compared with socioeducationally similar children based on national norms, the children from the Miami program reach levels of both speech and sign language performance that are commonly near or above the 90th percentile. Perhaps equally important, tactually aided children, by the late elementary and junior high school years, perform academically at excellent levels, substantially outperforming their deaf peers from traditional training programmes.

It is not the contention of the present authors that the success of children in the Miami program is due to the use of tactual vocoders alone. The comparisons with other programs and other studies involve many variables that may play a role in the outcomes. Our experience suggests that a complex combination of aggressive treatment with both unimodal and multimodal training (tactual, auditory, visual) as well as sign language, as well as enthusiastic teaching and a carefully tailored curriculum designed to exploit the advantages of artificial hearing in an eclectic training approach, accounts for the growth of speech, language and academic skills.

Acknowledgement

The authors would like to thank Austin and Marta Weeks, Jerome and Rita Cohen, Amelia and Donald Farquhar and many others who have contributed to support of the research reported here. The role of the Dade County Public Schools in supporting the training programme is also gratefully acknowledged.

References

Brooks, P.L. and Frost, B.J. (1983) Evaluation of a tactual vocoder for word recognition. Journal of the Acoustical Society of America 74: 34–9.

Brooks, P.L., Frost, B.J., Mason, J.L. and Gibson, D.M. (1986) Continuing evaluation of the Queen's University tactile vocoder. I: Identification of open set words. Journal of Rehabilitation Research and Development 23(1): 119–28.

Bull, D., Eilers, R.E., Oller, D.K. and Mandalia, B. (1985) The effect of frequency change on discrimination of pulse bursts in an electrocutaneous tactual vocoder. Journal of the Acoustical Society of America 77: 1192–8.

Cowan, R.S.C., Sarant, J.Z., Dettman, S.J., Galvin, K.L., Blamey, P.J. and Clark, G.M. (1992) Comparative performance of children using the Cochlear 22-channel implant and the 8-channel 'Tickle Talker'. Presented at the Tactile Aids Conference '92, June, Stockholm, Sweden.

Eilers, R.E., Bull, D.H. and Oller, D.K. (1984) Tactual perception of speech-like stimuli withan electrocutaneous vocoder. Artificial Organs 8: 494-497.

Eilers, R.E., Oller, D.K. and Vergara, K. (1989) Speech and language progress of hearing-impaired children in a systematic training program using tactual vocoders. Volta Review 91: 127–38.

Eilers, R.E., Vergara, K.C., Miskiel, L.W. and Friedman, K. (1993) Comparing cochlear implants and tactile vocoders in a model educational program for the hearing impaired. Poster presentation at the American Academy of Audiology annual convention, April, Phoenix, AZ.

Eilers, R.E., Fishman, L.M., Oller, D.K. and Steffens, M.L. (in press). Tactile vocoders as aids to speech production in young hearing-impaired children. Volta Review.

Eilers, R., Ozdamar, O., Oller, D., Miskiel, E. and Urbano, R. (1988a) Similarities between tactual and auditory speech perception. Journal of Speech and Hearing Research 31: 124–31.

Eilers, R.E., Widen, J. and Oller, D.K. (1988b) Assessment techniques to evaluate tactual aids for hearing-impaired subjects. Journal of Rehabilitation Research and Development 25(2): 33–46.

Engelmann, S. and Rosov, R.J. (1975) Tactual hearing experiment with deaf and hearing subjects. Journal of Exceptional Children 41: 243–53.

Franklin, D. (1986) Tactaid II. Audiological Engineering, Somerville, MA.

Geers, A.E. and Moog, J.S. (1992) Speech perception and production skills of students with impaired hearing for oral and total communication education settings. Journal of Speech and Hearing Disorders 35: 1384–93.

Geers, A., Moog, J. and Schick, B. (1984) Acquisition of spoken and signed English by profoundly deaf children. Journal of Speech and Hearing Disorders 49: 378–88.

Hesketh, L. and Osberger, M.J. (1990) Training strategies for profoundly hearing-impaired children using the Tactaid II+. Volta Review 92: 265–73.

Hodson, B.N. and Paden, E.P. (1991) Targeting intelligible speech: A phonological approach to remediation, 2nd edition. Austin, TX: Pro-ed.

Holmgren, K., Lindblom, B., Aurelius, G., Jalling, B. and Zetterstrom, R. (1986) On the phonetics of infant vocalization. In Lindblom, B. and Zetterstrom, R. (Eds), Precursors of Early Speech. New York: Stockton Press. pp 51–63.

Ingram, D. (1976) Phonological disability in children. New York: Elsevier.

Kirman, J.H. (1973) Tactile communication of speech: A review and an analysis. Psychological Bulletin 80: 54–74.

Ling, D. (1984) Early Intervention For Hearing Impaired Children: Total Communication Options. San Diego: College Hill Press.

Locke, J.L. (1983) Phonological Acquisition and Change. New York: Academic Press.

Lynch, M.P., Eilers, R.E., Oller, D.K. and Cobo-Lewis, A.B. (1989a) Multisensory speech perception by profoundly hearing impaired children. Journal of Speech and Hearing Disorders 54: 57–67.

Lynch, M. P., Oller, D. K. and Eilers, R. E. (1989b) Portable tactile aids for speech perception. Volta Review 91: 113–26.

Lynch, M., Eilers, R., Oller, D. and LaVoie, L. (1988) Speech perception by congenitally deaf subjects using an electrocutaneous vocoder. Journal of Rehabilitation Research and Development 25(3): 41–50.

Mandalia, B.D., Tapia, M.A., Oller, D.K., Bull, D.H. and Eilers, R.E. (1983) A non-real time software vocoder for tactual communication. In Proceedings of the Fifteenth Southeastern Symposium on System Theory, 249–52.

Moog, J. and Geers, A. (1985) Grammatical Analysis of Elicited Language (GAEL). St. Louis, MO: Central Institute for the Deaf.

Oller, D.K. (1978) Infant vocalization and the development of speech. Allied Health and Behavioral Sciences 1: 523–49.

Oller, D.K. (1991) Computational approaches to transcription and analysis in child phonology. Journal for Computer Users in Speech and Hearing 7: 44–59.

Oller, D.K. and Eilers, R.E. (1981) A pragmatic approach to phonological systems of deaf speakers. In Lass, N. (Ed), Speech and Language: Advances in Basic Research and Practice, Vol. 6. New York: Academic Press.(pp. 103–141.

Oller, D.K. and Eilers, R.E. (1988a) Tactual artificial hearing for the deaf. In Bess, F. (Ed) Hearing Impairment in Children. Parkton, MD: York Press. pp 310–28.

Oller, D.K. and Eilers, R.E. (1988b) The role of audition in infant babbling. Child Development 59: 441–9.

Oller, D.K., Eilers, R.E., Vergara, K. and LaVoie, E.F. (1986) Tactual vocoders in a multisensory program training speech production and reception. Volta Review 88: 21–36.

Oller, D.K., Miskiel, E., Eilers, R. and Ozdamar, O (in press) Formant tracking for tactual vocoders. Proc. 2nd International Conference on Tactile Aids, Hearing Aids, and Cochlear Implants.

Oller, D.K., Payne, S. and Gavin, W.J. (1980) Tactual speech perception by minimally trained deaf subjects. Journal of Speech and Hearing Research 23: 769–78.

Osberger, M.J. (1990) Speech perception abilities of children with tactile aids and cochlear implants. Keynote address at Tactile Aids, Hearing Aids and Cochlear Implants International Conference, May. National Acoustic Laboratories Central Laboratory, Sydney.

Osberger, M.J., Miyamoto, R.T., Zimmerman-Phillips, S., Kemink, J., Stroer, B., Firszt, J. and Novak, M. (1991) Independent evaluation of speech perception abilities of children with the Nucleus 22 channel cochlear implant system. Ear and Hearing 12(Suppl.): 66S-80S.

Ozdamar, O, Delgado, R.E. and Lopez, C. (1987) FFT-based digital vocoder for artificial hearing. IEEE Proceedings EMBS, 1892-3.

Ozdamar, O, Eilers, R.E. and Oller, D.K. (1987) Tactile vocoders for the deaf. IEEE Engineering in Medicine and Biology Magazine, September, 37-42.

Ozdamar, O., Lopez, C.N., Oller, D.K., Eilers, R.E., Miskiel, E. and O Lynch, M.P. (1992). FFT-based digital tactile vocoder system for real-time use. Medical and Biological Engineering and Computing, March, 213-18.

Plant, G. (1991) Tactaid II Training Program. New South Wales, Australia: National Acoustic Laboratories.

Plant, G. (1992) Development of speech in an acochlea child. Presented at the Tactile Aids Conference '92, June, Stockholm, Sweden.

Plant, G. and Spens, K.E. (1986) An experienced user of tactile information as a supplement to lipreading. An evaluative study. Speech Transmission Laboratories-Quarterly Progress Status Report 1: 87-110.

Quigley, S. P. and Paul, P. V. (1984) Language and Deafness. San Diego, CA: College Hill Press.

Robbins, A.M., Todd, S.L. and Osberger, M.J. (1992) Speech perception performance of pediatric multichannel tactile aid or cochlear implant users. Presented at the Tactile Aids Conference '92, June, Stockholm, Sweden.

Ramey, C.T., Bryant, D.M., Sparling, J.J. and Wasik, B.H. (1985) Educational interventions to enhance intellectual development: Comprehensive daycare versus family education. In Harel, S. and Anastasiow, N. (Eds) The 'At-risk' Infant: Psycho/socio/medical Aspects Baltimore, MD: P.H. Brookes Publishing. pp 75-85.

Ramey, C.T. and Campbell, F.A. (1987) The Carolina Abecedarian Project: An educational experiment concerning human malleability. In Gallagher, J.J. and Ramey, C.T. (Eds) The Malleability of Children. Baltimore, MD: P. H. Brookes Publishing. pp 127-39.

Richardson, B.L. and Frost, B.J. (1977) Sensory substitution and the design of an artificial ear. Journal of Psychology 96: 259-85.

Rothman, K.J. (1986) Modern Epidemiology. Boston: Little Brown and Co.

Roug, L., Landberg, I. and Lundberg, L. J. (1989) Phonetic development in early infancy: A study of 4 Swedish children during the first 18 months of life. Journal of Child Language 16: 19-40.

Saunders F.A. (1985) Wearable multichannel electrotactile sensory aids. Presented at the Tactual Communications Conference, Wichita, KS.

Sparks, D.W., Kuhl, P.K., Edmonds, A.A. and Gray, G.P. (1978) Investigating the MESA (Multipoint Electrotactile Speech Aid): The transmission of segmental features of speech. Journal of the Acoustical Society of America 63: 246-57.

Spens, K. E. (1980) Tactile speech communication aids for the deaf: A comparison. Speech Transmission Laboratories Quarterly Progress Status Report 4: 23-39.

Stark, R.E. (1980) Stages of speech development in the first year of life. In. Yeni-Komshian, G , Kavanagh, J. and Ferguson, C. (Eds) Child Phonology. New York: Academic Press. pp 73-90.

Stoel-Gammon, C. and Otomo, D. (1986) Babbling development of hearing-impaired and normally-hearing subjects. Journal of Speech and Hearing Disorders 51: 33–41.

Vergara, K.C., Miskiel, L.W., Lewis, B.J., Chiarello, K.A., Chojnicki, M., Donovan, P.A. and Punch, T.A. (1993a) A comprehensive cochlear implant, auditory and tactile skills curriculum. Miniseminar presented at American Speech, Language and Hearing Association annual convention, November, Anaheim, CA.

Vergara, K.C., Miskiel, L.W., Lewis, B.J., Eilers, R.E., Oller, D.K., Pero, P. and Hoffman, D. (1993b) Curricula used in a nonsimultaneous total communication program. Presented at CAID/CEASD Convention, June, Baltimore, MD.

Weisenberger, J.M. (1988) Effects of number of channels on speech perception with tactile aids. Journal of the Acoustical Society of America 84(Suppl. 1): S46.

Weisenberger, J.M. and Miller, J.D. (1987) The role of tactile aids in providing information about acoustic stimuli. Journal of the Acoustical Society of America 82: 906–16.

Youdelman, D., Behrman, A.M. and Franklin, D. (1989) Tactaid II+ Teachers Manual M-1. Somerville, MA: Audiological Engineering Corporation.

Zigler, E., Abelson, W.D., Trickett, P.K. and Seitz, V. (1982). Is an intervention program necessary in order to improve economically disadvantaged children's IQ scores? Child Development 53: 340–8.

7

Tactile Aid Usage in Young Deaf Children

ADELE PROCTOR

Significant Historical Background

As early as 1819, Arrowsmith discussed the advantages of providing tactile stimulation to teach lipreading and speech to young deaf children. Subsequently, educators devised different ways to use the sense of touch, independently and in coordination with vision, to augment the deaf child's loss of hearing. For example, young deaf children were taught to feel the sound patterns of language and the rhythm of speech when the teacher stroked the child's arm or back of the hand to the beat of a sentence being produced. At the same time the teacher held the child's hand, the child was required to look at the teacher's face.

With technological advances, attempts were made to design instruments which replicated the type of language and speech information provided to the deaf child by the teacher. Tactual delivery of speech and language by use of specially designed instruments was viewed as a means of increasing educational effectiveness. With a vibrotactile device a large number of school children could simultaneously receive the same types of acoustic information. Theory holds that use of such a device would free the teacher from the time intensive, one-to-one speech teaching paradigm.

To enhance the rate of acquisition of lipreading skills and to encourage intelligible speech production, R.H. Gault and his associates (1926a, 1926b, 1934) used a 'high quality' microphone, an amplifier, and a receiver or vibrator unit to develop the 'Teletactor', which was later called the 'Phonotactor' (Gault and Goodfellow, 1937; Goodfellow, 1934). The Teletactor user placed a finger or fingers on the vibrator to feel the rhythm, stress, duration and relative intensity of the speaker's voice.

In addition to testing the Teletactor with adults, one study systematically evaluated device usage in a classroom of deaf children (Carhart, 1935). A group of eight hearing-impaired children between the ages of 5 and 7 years were followed for 3 years while using the Teletactor. Results revealed that the children: (a) improved their lipreading ability; (b) became more aware of different types of sound; (c) were able to monitor their own voices; and (d) improved in many aspects of speech production (Cloud, 1933; Plouer, 1934). Additional tactile aid training was found to result in even further improvements in lipreading abilities. Lipreading is defined here as the perception of speech and the comprehension of oral language via the visual modality.

Gault's pioneering work is of significance today for several reasons. He demonstrated that deaf adults and children who used a vibrotactile device improved their lipreading, voice quality, and the intelligibility of selected aspects of speech production. Most importantly, Gault's experiments revealed that tactual delivery of the speech waveform envelope supplements the ability to lipread (cf. Gault, 1928).

The speech waveform provides temporal acoustic cues such as duration and rise–fall timing which signal consonant manner and voicing information about consonants and vowel durational information. The envelope also supplies acoustic information which assists with syllabic distinctions and prosodic cues such as emphatic stress. In recent years, other investigators (Erber, 1972a, 1972b, 1979; Van Tasell *et al.*, 1987, 1992) substantiated Gault's claim that the speech waveform envelope provides important acoustic information which supplements lipreading. Understanding the potential of the type of information that can be provided by transmitting the speech waveform envelope is meaningful since the design of many of the tactile devices currently used with children capitalize on presenting envelope information.

Since Gault's initial work, a relatively large body of literature has evolved regarding different types of tactile aids for children. Tactile aid evaluations have been carried out in English and non-English speaking countries (c.f. Ifukube, 1982; Kringlebotn, 1968; Ling and Sophin, 1974; Perier and Boorsma, 1982; Schulte, 1978; Spens, 1980, 1983; Traunmuller, 1977). Available data suggest that tactile aids, as presently designed, are effective cross-linguistically.

The cross-linguistic value of tactile aids suggests that the devices capture at least some universal features of human speech. When speech features are tactually delivered and coordinated with vision, deaf children can be trained to receive and to interpret oral language whether it is English, French, German, Japanese, Swedish or some other language. It appears that the ability to present the deaf user with some of the acoustic cues in the speech waveform envelope has been integral to achieving this cross-linguistic success.

Research Results: Selected Evaluation Studies

There were several basic questions which evaluation studies have attempted to answer: (1) can the tactile device be worn/used without deleterious effects; (2) can the device be worn/used with hearing aids and; (3) what are the benefits of a deaf child using or wearing a vibrotactile aid or an electrocutaneous device? To illustrate the variability among devices studied and the range of methodological approaches used to measure device efficacy, Table 1 summarizes selected studies exploring tactile aid use among children who learned some variation of English as a first language. The first column of Table 1 shows the investigator(s) and the date of the publication. A complete citation is given in the reference list.

The second to sixth columns of Table 1 display: the purpose of the research; the characteristics of the children in the study such as the total number (N) participating in the study, the subjects' degree of hearing loss and their chronological ages (CA); the type of device used; how device efficacy was measured and; the significant findings of the study. Direct application of some type of tactile device with children who ranged in chronological age (CA) from infancy to 19-years-old were among the primary criteria used to select studies for review.

Table 2 summarizes the results of the studies cited in Table 1. The relative speech and language benefits reported for the children who used tactile aids have been organized by five different categories in Table 2: (1) sound perception; (2) sound discrimination; (3) lipreading (speechreading); (4) speech production (articulation) and; (5) communication.

Candidacy for Tactile Aids and Other Frequently Asked Questions

In previous years, the primary factors considered in determining that a child is a candidate for a vibrotactile aid included: (1) the presence of a profound bilateral sensorineural hearing loss; (2) the child had not demonstrated any change in his/her response to sound after a trial period with personal amplification and/or FM trainer and; (3) the results of pure tone and speech audiometry suggested that his/her response to sound may be vibrotactile in nature. However, these criteria were established when the typical age of identification of hearing loss ranged from 1 to 3 years old. With technological advances and changes in our ability to detect hearing loss below the age of 1 year, the criteria for tactile aid use must be modified to manage successfully the increased numbers of profoundly deaf children who will be identified during infancy. Tactile aid usage in infancy will be addressed when

Table 1. Selected studies of tactile aid usage with hearing-impaired and deaf children: from birth (0) to late adolescence (19 years)

Reference	Purpose	Child characteristics Total(N)/Degree loss Chronological age(s)
Alcantara *et al.* (1990) (See also Galvin *et al.* 1993)	• To determine if children who were known to achieve partial benefit from personal amplification could learn to employ tactually delivered phonetic information to improve speech perception above the levels achieved with hearing aids only • To determine if training in one speech feature might be generalized to related but untrained contexts; measured (1) effects of direct training on subject performance; and (2) performance levels before, during and after training	7 – Profound loss/ 7 to 11 years
Bond. and Scott (1982)	• To devise a set of procedures for evaluating effects of the Speech Reception Aid (SRA) on speech reception of pre-lingual profoundly deaf children	4 – Profound loss/ 3.7–4.3 years
Boothroyd (1972)	• Programme consisted of testing different types of visual and tactile sensory aids. Designed to determine: a. capacity of different sensory modalities in receiving information b. methods for assessing benefits of aids c. most appropriate means of incorporating device into school curriculum when aid found to have educational benefit;	• Profound losses- • Exploratory report, mainly descriptive of device; device developed at the Clarke School for the Deaf; Specific ages for tactile study were no given, but ages in related visual aids project included the following: Lower School 5.1–7.0 years Middle School 11.7–14.0 year Upper School 14.9–17.6 year

Type aid/Placement of aid on body	Measures	Findings
Tickle Talker – 8 finger electrodes worn as bands around fingers and 1 common electrode worn at wrist level ** Investigators note that two different versions of this multichannel electrotactile device were used during the course of the study	• Training involved three phases, pre-training, training and post-training; multiple baselines taken in pre-training phase and compared to performance on similar speech test material when tested in the post-training phase • Subjects received phonetic feature level training on vowel (V) duration, V place, /s/ detection in word initial position of monosyllables, /s/ detection in word final position of monosyllables, identification of /m/ versus /b/ in word initial and word final positions of monosyllables and identification of /s/ versus /t/ in word initial and word final positions of monosyllables • Subjects also received conversational-level training with closed sets of sentences that varied in length and complexity and connected discourse training • Subjects training under three different conditions, tactile plus hearing aid (TA), tactile only (T) and aided hearing (A)	• In all conditions, higher test scores found for TA and T conditions than for A alone • Higher test scores found in the training and post-training phases relative to pre-training scores • Statistically significant interaction found for phase of training under TA and T conditions, suggesting tactile aid facilitated feature perception • Speech perception skills learned during training were retained and generalized to untrained contexts • Training did not improve perception in A only condition
RA 10 multichannel vibrotactile aid with stimulation at abdomen	• Detection task to assess sound awareness • Tested ability to perceive and reproduce syllable structure of short utterances • Used animal sounds to assess ability to receive and produce phonemes of English	• Significant difference found in rate of learning with tactile aid as compared with no tactile aid
Bone conduction (BC) oscillator with extended low frequency response attached to mitt worn on the hand High powered hearing aid with Y cord – BC oscillator on one end and air conduction (AC) receiver on the other end; AC receiver fit in ear and BC oscillator in mitt worn on the hand	• Response to pure tones in free field • Experimenter and teacher observational reports	• Awareness for pure tones increased by 25 dB when using vibrator and AC receiver versus using only AC receiver • With vibrator, able to distinguish syllabic patterns and voicing • When using tactile device, teachers reported improved voice control

Table 1. Cont.

Reference	Purpose	Child characteristics
Brooks *et al.* (1987) (See Scilley, 1980)	• To replicate results from Scilley (1980) with a larger number of subjects, i.e., to determine if the Queen's University Vocoder would be beneficial in supplementing lipreading and in improving speech intelligibility	2 – Profound loss/ 18 years old
Carhart(1935)	• To assess effects of Gault-Teletactor on speech perception and speech production	2 – Profound loss/ 1 at 16 years 1 at 18 years
Cloud(1933) (See also Plouer, 1934)	• To assess educational and practical value of the Teletactor in a classroom for deaf children; Teletactor room	8 Hearing-impaired (HI)/ (Degree of hearing loss reported as percentage of hearing loss – percentage loss for subjects from 43 to 82% as measured by the 2-A Audiometer] 5.5 to 7.7 years
Eilers, Oller and Vergara (1989) (See also Eilers, Widen and Oller, 1988)	Study 1: To determine comparative effectiveness of intensive tactual training programme Study 2: To compare speech and oral language abilities of deaf children in a tactual training programme and a matched group of deaf children not enrolled in a tactual training programme	Study 1: Tactual group – 15 – Profound loss/ Average age: 5.3 years Comparison group / Average Age: 7.3 years Study 2: Tactual group – 7 – Profound loss/ 3- to 6-year-olds selected from Study 1 to compare their

Type aid/Placement of aid on body	Measures	Findings
Queen's University Vocoder with 16 solenoids spaced 3 cm apart on a piece of plexiglass and worn on the right ventromedial forearm	• Word learning task with a 50 word vocabulary; vocabulary contained words with a range of frequency and intensity levels for phonemes • Feature identification tasks; required subjects to place 16 consonant–vowel (CV) combinations into five phonemic categories and 12 vowel–consonant (VC) combinations into four phonemic categories	• Subjects 1 and 2 achieved 80% correct criterion for a 50 word vocabulary after 28.5 hours and 24.0 hours of training, respectively • For feature identification of CVs, the average for both subjects was 84.5% correct and 89.6% correct for VCs • Although subjects' learning rates were similar, the subject with more knowledge of English learned at a slightly faster rate
Gault-Teletactor Subjects placed fingers on the device	• Teachers observations and reports	• Teletactor aided in developing the concept of poetic rhythms • Device useful in teaching rhythmic patterns, stress and speech inflection
Teletactor system with 'high quality' microphone at teacher's desk; teacher's desk similar to a switchboard Powerful amplifier and electromagnetic, low impedance vibrator, at each student's desk Each student also fitted with pair of earphones	• Teachers observations and reports	• Although multisensory approach, using tactile, visual and auditory, teachers' observation credits Teletactor for assisting deaf children in the following ways: – Able to feel their own voices – Able to monitor their own voices – Able to recognize rhymes by tempo – Improved tone production – Able to differentiate long–short vowels, voiced–unvoiced elements of words, number of syllables of words – Stimulated interest in oral communication – Able to produce 'smoother' speech patterns
Study 1: 3 Subjects used a Teletactor 32 channel electrocutaneous device worn around abdomen subjects used the Oregon vibrotactile aid – 24 channels worn on ventral surfaces of thighs Study 2: Same as Study 1	Study 1: • All subjects evaluated at beginning of training and 5 months later, at the end of training • Speech samples from all subjects audio-taped before and after training; one group received tactual training programme over the course of the school year and the matched comparison group received no tactual training for the same time frame	Study 1: • Intelligibility ratings revealed that Subjects in tactual training programme showed greater gains in speech production • Overall speech intelligibility ratings were considerably better for children who experienced tactual training versus those who did not receive tactual training

Table 1. Cont.

Reference	Purpose	Child characteristics
		language performance with US national normative data for hearing-impaired children; Subject sample for Study 2 included some children who had multiple handicaps
Englemann and Rosov(1978)	• To determine if an increased amount of training on a vibro-tactile device would improve speech perception of pro-foundly deaf children	4 normal hearing/ adult instructors 4 – profound Loss/ 8 to 14 years old
Franklin and Saunders (1981)	• To determine effects of mul-tichannel electrotactile display on deaf and deaf–blind chil-dren's speech production	3 – Profound loss/ 1 Subject 10 years 2 Subjects 8 years old

Type aid/Placement of aid on body	Measures	Findings
	• Recorded speech samples were analysed for misarticulations and overall speech intelligibility; data adjusted to consider bilingual and bidialectal language differences for both groups Study 2: • A psychometric language measure, the Grammatical Analysis of Elicited Language – Pre-sentence (GAEL-P) (Moog and Geers, 1985) was administered to deaf subjects • Results of tactile aid users compared to national norms for GAEL-P; US norms established for 150 hearing-impaired students who were between the ages of 3 and 6 years • Comprehension and production test results of tactile aid users were analysed for rate of progress, determined by amount of change in percentile points of the psychometric instrument (GAEL-P)	Study 2: • Tactile aid users scored 19 percentile points for comprehension and 4 percentile points for production at the beginning of training • At the end of training, 5 months later, tactile aid users scored 38 percentile points for comprehension and 30 percentile points for production • Data suggest a rapid rate of progress in understanding language and in improving speech production, even in presence of secondary handicaps
• Tactual vocoder with 200 Hz to 4000 Hz spread over 15 channels; four low frequency channels extended frequency range down to 85 Hz and four high frequency channels extended upper limits to 10,000 Hz Vibrators located on subjects' thighs	• Subjects' training time ranged from 20 to 80 hours • Normal-hearing subjects trained on isolated words, words in sentences and voice pitch patterns while wearing vocoder • Hearing-impaired subjects trained on articulation (speech production), words and sentences, isolated sounds and rhyming and language action tasks	• Deaf subjects were able to achieve fine speech discrimination by tactual only modality • Increased performance on tactual only mode is related to practice and training • Both normal-hearing and deaf subjects can learn to attend to prosodic elements of speech via the tactual only mode
Tacticon – Electrotactile belt with 16 channels	• Each child received training with the device two times a week for 30 minutes each session • Training consisted of imitation of single syllables, repetition of syllables, isolated words and words in context	• Increase in intelligibility of speech noted for each child at the end of the training programme • 2 subjects improved suprasegmental features • 2 subjects improved in tongue control • Overall voice quality became less nasal for all subjects and improved production of /m/ and /n/ observed

Table 1. Cont.

Reference	Purpose	Child characteristics
Friel-Patti and Roeser (1983).	• To assess effectiveness of the SRA 10 in improving speech, language and communication • To develop an effective procedure for evaluating tactile aids on young deaf children	4 – Profound loss/ 3.10 to 4.6 years
Gault(1926a)	• To determine if tactile device would aid in recognition and discrimination of speech patterns • To determine if tactile device would affect voice control	15 HI / Age range from 17 to 31 years old • Separated into groups of 6, 5 and 4 members each
Geers (1986)	• To determine effects of a wearable, single-channel vibrotactile aid on speech, language and communication performance	1 Profound loss/ 2.5 years. to 3.8 years. (longitudinal)
Goldstein, Jr. *et al.* (1983)	• To develop a wearable, single-channel vibrotactile aid for deaf infants • To measure effects of tactile device on lipreading and oral communication	1 – Profound loss/ 32 months to 42 months (longitudinal)

Type aid/Placement of aid on body	Measures	Findings
• SRA 10 multichannel vibro-tactile aid with three vibrators worn on abdomen	• Used subjects as own control; Tactile aid worn in Phase I versus tactile aid not worn by same subject in Phase II • Total Communication Index used to calculate amount and quality of changes in vocalization only, sign language only and vocalization plus sign language • Five expressive language measures taken; total number of utterances, multiword utterances, explicit verbs, basal sentences and mean length of signed utterances	• With tactile aid worn (Phase I) versus tactile aid not worn (Phase II), all subjects showed improvement in perception of conversational skills, syntax, semantics and improved productive use of language, both oral and sign • Decrement of language performance when tactile aid was removed (Phase II)
• Teletactor; Hand-held receiver (vibrator) Teletactor consisted of a powerful amplifier and electromagnetic, low impedance vibrator on which students could place their hands or hold in their hands	• Employed 58 words in a story • After subjects familiarized with words and sentences introduced in story, tested child's ability to identify vowel and diphthong elements • Scored ratios of word identification to number of presentations • Vowels and diphthongs scored in ratio of percentage correct	• Teletactor is a feasible means of interpreting speech • Teletactor assisted deaf speakers in improving pitch, accent and number of syllables in a word • All subjects improved in response to auditory stimuli, speech perception and speech production after tactile aid usage initiated
• Tactaid 1, single-channel, wearable vibrotactile aid with vibrator at sternum • Radioear B72 BC oscillator (See Goldstein et al., 1983)	• Vocabulary counts to determine progress in understanding single words • Formal speech-language pathology tests administered before tactile aid usage and during periodic intervals of tactile aid usage	• Improved in oral language comprehension (lipreading) for single words • Developed awareness to own speech and speech of others • Improved imitation of speech • Improved voice quality, prosody and segmentation of speech
• Single-channel, wearable vibrotactile aid with components in a vest and vibrator worn at the sternum • Power from rechargeable batteries and electronics designed to interact and to drive Radioear B72 BC oscillator	• Vocabulary count of number of single words subject could lipread • Administration of frequently used psychometric tests that are frequently used by speech-language pathologists to assess communication, language and speech	• Child progressed in understanding (lipreading only) five words presented orally to understanding over 500 words by lipreading only in a 10 month period • Impressive gains made in lipreading including ability to lipread familiar people from their profiles; • Rapid rate of lexical (vocabulary) acquisition found • Rate of acquisition combined with later diagnosis that child has limited peripheral vision suggests that tactile aid contributed to child's performance

Table 1. Cont.

Reference	Purpose	Child characteristics
Goldstein, Jr. and Proctor (1985)	• To reduce size of vibrotactile aid reported in the 1983 study; to determine if other profoundly deaf children would derive similar benefits as found with one child in the 1983 study	2 – Profound loss/ 1 Subject followed longitudinally from 42 to 53 months and the other Subject followed longitudinally from 70 to 81 months
Goldstein, Jr. and Stark (1976)	• To determine if profoundly deaf children will use a vibrotactile aid to monitor own speech production as hearing children are believed to use auditory feedback • To determine if a vibrotactile aid will improve speech production of young deaf children	12 – Profound loss/ 2 – 4 years
Kozma-Spytek and Weisenberger (1988) (See also Weisenberger and Kozma-Spytek, 1991)	• To assess device effectiveness as a speech reception aid	1 – Profound loss/ 12 years old (longitudinal)
Lynch et al. (1989)	• To determine effects of unimodal (tactile only) versus multimodal (tactile aid and hearing aid) on speech perception training of deaf subjects' ability to generalize novel speech stimuli	Study 1: 4 – Profound loss 5 to 7 years old Study 2: 4 – Profound loss 9 to 11 years old

Type aid/Placement of aid on body	Measures	Findings
• Wearable device using a Radioear B72 vibrator mounted gently against sternum; and electronics consisted of Knowles BT-1759 microphone, amplitude modulation (AM) of a 250 Hz sinusoid and automatic gain control (AGC) fit into a leather pouch that children could wear	• Psychometric language tests including the Test for Auditory Comprehension of Language (TACL) standardized on normal-hearing children	• Both deaf subjects exhibited a rapid rate of oral language comprehension (lipreading) as measured by the TACL • Improved rate and trend of language acquisition achieved by way of lipreading supported with vibrotactile input found to be consistent with subjects' performance reported in Geers (1986) and Proctor and Goldstein, Jr (1983)
Multichannel vocoder with fingertips placed on stimulators	• Three groups with 4 children in each group; all trained on consonant vowel syllables • measured amount of vocalization output as related to visual only, tactile only and control group • measured increase in CV combination and how closely children approximated target CV combinations	• Tactile aid users and visual aid users showed a significant increase in amount of vocalization as compared with the control group that used no special aids
Tacticon – 16 channel electrocutaneous vocoder with electrodes on a belt worn around the abdomen	• Device worn one hour per day for 8 months • Speech reception training and testing conducted first 30 minutes of each session • Tasks included Minimal Pairs Phoneme Discrimination; closed set word learning; Probe testing for word learning at four month intervals to determine ability to retain a 20 word vocabulary; syllable and number stress task; syllable identification task and; Connected Discourse Tracking	• Improvement found across all tasks • Data suggest device can provide a supplement to lipreading in reception of isolated words and connected discourse
Study 1: Tacticon 1600 Electrocutaneous vocoder and Tactaid II vibrotactile device	Study 1: Training Phase – Subjects trained to recognize 15 words presented via live voice to one of the two tactile devices; Testing Phase: Recognition paradigm used to test subjects in three conditions: (1) tactual aid only; (2) hearing aid only and; (3) combine tactile and hearing aid	Study 1: Subjects performed at statistically significant higher levels when using a tactile device and hearing aids
Study 2: Tacticon 1600 Electrocutaneous vocoder and Tactaid II vibrotactile device	Study 2: Training Phase – Similar to Study 1 with exception of adjustment to	Study 2: Subjects performed at statistically significant higher levels when using the tactile device and hearing aids

Table 1. Cont.

Reference	Purpose	Child characteristics
Miyamoto *et al.* (1989) (See also Miyamoto *et al.*, 1987)	• To compare speech perception abilities of children who used different types of sensory devices	42 Profound loss/ Age range of onset of hearing loss: 3 – 13.2 years
Neate (1972)	• To determine effects of tactile stimulation on improving speech production and voice quality	• Specific number and ages not given; Sample derived from the Whitebrook School for the Deaf, Manchester, UK
Osberger, Maso and Sam (1993) (See also Osberger *et al.*, 1990; Robbins *et al.*, 1988, 1992)	• To determine if productive speech intelligibility improves after sensory devices are provided • To determine the characteristics of speech if improvement found • To determine the comparative nature of speech production of three different types of sensory aid users relative to a control group of non-device users	N = 45 Profound loss/Age range device fit 7 months – 13.2 years • Experimental and control group subjects were subcategorized based on age of onset of hearing loss (early onset defined as hearing loss before age 4 years old and late onset, after 4 years old) • Experimental Group N = 31 – 12 with 3M House single-channel cochlear implant –

Type aid/Placement of aid on body	Measures	Findings
	vocabulary due to older ages of subjects in Study 2; Testing Phase – Similar procedures used as supplied in Study 1	Summary of results for Study 1 and Study 2: • Deaf children from 5 to 11 years old learned to recognize tactual patterns that corresponded to words • No significant difference was found in tactual word recognition with the two different tactile aids, although the electrocutaneous had 16 channels and the vibrotactile had 2 channels • Word recognition abilities were significantly better when children used a tactile aid and hearing aids simultaneously
• Tactaid II vibrotactile aid, House 3M cochlear implant and Nucleus 22-channel cochlear implant	• Speech discrimination test, Change/No Change Test – considered an alternative to word recognition tasks, includes nine subtests and measures detection of an acoustic change in a suprasegmental or segmental feature of speech • Recognition Test, The Minimal Pairs Test – a 20 item forced choice test that assesses ability to differentiate phonetic feature differences • Speech Tracking – requires verbatim repetition of connected discourse	• Considerable improvement observed with all three devices • Slightly higher performance for cochlear implants and tactile aids than for conventional hearing aids
• Bone conduction oscillator held in hand • Vibrator paired with hearing aids during speech training	• Teachers' and speech therapists' descriptive observational reports of changes in children's communication, language and speech abilities at school	• Increased vocalization observed • Improved rhythmic quality of speech noted • Aid assisted children in controlling vocal output
• Device types included a single-channel cochlear implant, a 22 channel cochlear implant and two-channel Tactaid II+ vibrotactile aid	• Speech perception tasks included two closed-set word recognition tests obtained on the last day of data collection for speech production; speech perception tests administered were the Minimal Pairs Test and Monosyllable Trochee Spondee Test (MTS) • Speech production tasks included 10 sentences drawn from three separate lists of 10 sentences containing 42 words per list	• No apparent difference in speech intelligibility scores among subjects who had implant or those who wore tactile aid • Subjects with implants and tactile aids and who had early onset of hearing loss produced speech intelligibility similar to hearing aid users with hearing levels (HL) between 100 to 110 Hz and limited high frequency hearing • For subjects who experienced

Table 1. Cont.

Reference	Purpose	Child characteristics

		• 15 with Nucleus 22 channel cochlear implant
		– 4 with two-channel Tactaid II+ vibrotactile aid
		• Control Group N = 14
		  – 12 with conventional hearing aids
		  – 2 used no sensory aid
		• Control group subdivided into two separate groups, gold and silver hearing aid users
		• Gold users had slightly better thresholds than silver users, determined by results of audiological testing

Oller *et al.* (1986)	• Progress report of 6 deaf subjects who participated as part of a larger study designed to develop improved tactual prostheses for deaf children	6 – Profound loss/ 3–6 years 1 at 3 years 4 at 4 years
Plant(1979)	• To determine if a single bone conduction oscillator would improve lipreading and subject's awareness to auditory environment	1 – Profound loss/ Adventitiously deafened at 17 years old

Type aid/Placement of aid on body	Measures	Findings
	• Speech production material controlled for syllabicity, syntactic complexity and articulatory characteristics of speech	late onset of hearing loss, a marked deterioration observed in speech intelligibility after onset of hearing loss followed by relatively large improvements after being fit with some type of sensory device • The single subject with late onset and tactile aid user did not show improvement in speech intelligibility
• Twenty-four channel vibrotactile aid with stimulation on thigh (see Gavin and Rosov, 1984) • Thirty-two-channel electrotactile aid with stimulation on abdomen (see Saunders, 1974)	1. Compared pre- and post-test measures for one academic year; 2. Transcribed and analysed tape-recorded speech sample for changes in subjects' elicited imitations of 64 nonsense syllables, 6 isolated vowels, spontaneous and imitative naming of 34 common pictures; imitation of correct number of syllables in nonsense words and imitation of loudness and pitch levels 3. Speech perception measures included two choice identification tasks and differentiation of number of syllables per utterance 4. Adults trained in phonetics served as listener judges and rated tapes	• Children made impressive gains in all areas measured for speech perception and speech production • Improved in number of vowels and consonants produced • Improved in production of speech contrasts • Improved in production of new vocabulary words • Words produced were judged to be more intelligible after tactile aid usage • Improved in ability to control pitch and loudness • Improved in perceptual ability to differentiate two and three choice items by tactual modality only

• Wearable, vibrotactile system driven by high powered body aid with bone conduction (BC) vibrator held in hand – BC oscillator – Radioear B-70-A	• Pre- and post-training measures taken
	• Training time 15 hours per week for 1 month
	Pre–Post-training measures:
	  I. Two formal lipreading (speechreading) tests administered to assess
	    a. Speechreading with tactile aid
	    b. Speechreading with no tactile aid
	  II. Fingerspelling
	  III. Tactile perception assesses with subtests of the Pittsburgh Auditory Test
	    a. Subtest 1- Duration of Gross Sounds
		• Improvements observed when sentence material presented on the formal lipreading tests and the Pittsburgh Auditory Test
		• No improvements observed when tests required frequency discrimination
		• Tactile supplement with lipreading showed significant improvement over lipreading alone

Table 1. Cont.

Reference	Purpose	Child characteristics
Plant(1983)	• To determine if deaf children would derive similar benefits from vibrotactile aids as found for deaf adults (Plant, 1982)	3 – Profound loss/ 7–11 years old
Proctor(1990)	• To measure effects of a single-channel vibrotactile aid, worn in conjunction with hearing aids, on oral language comprehension (lipreading) of young deaf children	3 – Profound loss/ Longitudinal study Subjects ranged in age from 3.5 years to 5.8 years at start of study and from 4.4 to 6.7 years at end of study
Proctor and Goldstein, Jr (1983)	• To determine effects of a wearable, single-channel vibrotactile aid on communication, language and speech of a profoundly deaf toddler	1 – Profound loss/ 33 to 43 months

Type aid/Placement of aid on body	Measures	Findings
	b. Subtest 2- Duration of Words and Phrases c. Subtest 5 – Sentence Discrimination	
• Single-channel vibrotactile devices with hand-held bone conduction vibrator (Radioear B70A) • Power source – high powered body type hearing aid; with a high frequency detector supplied by the Sentiphone	• Subjects followed longitudinally over a three year time frame with each child receiving 15 minutes of tactile training per week • Pre- and post-training measures taken for segmental and suprasegmental features • Segmental Features included: Vowel length Final voicing Initial /s/ Final /s/ Initial/Final /s/ Suprasegmental (Prosodic) Features included: Word identification Word classification Syllables in words Number of sentence patterns Nonsense patterns Sentences (i) Personal sentences Sentences (ii) Complex sentences	• Scores for all measures revealed that children performed well above chance • Data suggest that tactile aids are useful in providing information about both segmental and suprasegmental aspects of speech
• Single-channel, wearable vibrotactile aid with components mounted in a leather pouch and vibrator worn at sternum; tactile aid and hearing aids worn concurrently on a daily basis	To assess oral language comprehension, administered two different psychometric language tests, Scales for Early Communication Skills for Hearing-Impaired Children (SECS) and Test for Auditory Comprehension of Language (TACL)	• Subjects exhibited a faster than average rate in learning to understand oral language, as determined by psychometric measures • Comparison of test items on TACL from first to last test administration showed greatest improvement in vocabulary; improved comprehension also found for morphology and syntax
• Vibrotactile circuitry mounted in a vest that the child wore • Radioear B-72 vibrator fit into vest and designed to press gently against child's sternum	• Device worn during speech and language therapy at home and at school • General aspects of therapy consisted of developing awareness to sound, increasing amount and type of age appropriate vocalization and child learning strategies for coordinating visual and (See Proctor, 1983 for details of training programme)	• Rapid rate of oral language comprehension (lipreading) found; child moved from understanding only five single words via lipreading to comprehension of more than 500 words via lipreading in a 10 month period • Some portion of this rapid rate of lexical comprehension attributed to tactile aid • Rate and pattern of lexical comprehension similar to younger, normal-hearing children

Table 1. Cont.

Reference	Purpose	Child characteristics
Scilley (1980)	• To measure effectiveness of Queen's University Vocoder	1 – Profound loss/ 13 years old
Sheehy and Hansen (1983)	• To determine effects of vibrotactile stimulation on speech production of deaf children	3 – Profound loss/ 4.6 years
Sparks (1977)	• To determine if information can be communicated effectively to hearing-impaired who use a remotely activated tactual device	5 – Normal-hearing 17 and 21 years old 5 – Profound loss 8 to 14 years old
Stratton (1974)	• To determine if immediate and continuous corrective tactile feedback will improve intonation patterns of hearing-impaired children	12 – Severe to profound losses Age range from 12 to 16 years old

Type aid/Placement of aid on body	Measures	Findings
• Queen's University Tactile Aid – 16 channel solenoid array with solenoids fitted to contour of subject's right arm	• Discrimination tasks involved differentiation of environmental sounds, phonemes, word pairs and lipreading tests with and without wearing vocoder • Listener judges rated recorded speech samples; speech intelligibility measured by percentage of words in sentences understood by normal-hearing listeners	• After 12 hours of training, subject achieved 80% correct on test requiring differentiation of 50 environmental sounds; data suggest rapid rate for ability to discriminate environmental sounds • After 12 hours of training and while using device, subject improved to 88% on Utley Test of Lipreading as contrasted with 39% with no device • Rating of speech samples revealed 104% improvement in speech intelligibility • When wearing device, subject's phrasing, stress when speaking improved
• Siemens' Fonator with vibrator worn on wrist	• Effectiveness of device determined by using a rating scale with 11 separate categories for judging speech production, response to sound, voice quality and suprasegmentals; parents and teachers served as observers and judged changes in children's speech, voice and prosodic productions	• Increased awareness to sounds • Improved awareness to non-segmented aspects of speech and discrimination of vowels • Improved rhythm and intensity of production imitation, bisyllabic words
• System composed of a radio frequency (RF) transmitter, an RF receiver and an electrotactile stimulator • Remotely activated tactual system to be used by a sender and a hearing-impaired receiver within a 500 yard radius • Stimulator-receiver mounted on belt and the electrode adhered to skin of abdomen	• Subjects learned Morse codes delivered tactually • In laboratory setting, normal-hearing Subjects obtained 100% correct on third session • In same laboratory setting, hearing-impaired subjects obtained 100% correct on fourth session	- Field results: (1) Normal-hearing tested while running and obtained 92% correct responses to commands (2) Hearing-impaired tested while running scored 86% correct and while skating, hearing-impaired subjects scored 100% correct
• Portable vibrotactile display with 10 miniature solenoids; solenoids activated by subjects' voice pitch; subjects' palm held on device and can feel own fundamental frequency contours	• Subjects separated into two groups: (1) received tactile feedback and pitch transcription during training and; (2) received only pitch transcription feedback during training; all subjects asked to practice imitation of frequently produced short phrases and sentences • Speech samples were tape recorded from all subjects	• Subjects acquired awareness of voice pitch at a rapid rate • Statistically significant improvement was found in ability to control intonation

Table 1. Cont.

Reference	Purpose	Child characteristics
Zeiser and Erber (1977).	• To compare abilities of profoundly hearing-impaired children and normal-hearing adults to perceive syllabic patterns both acoustically and vibrotactually	20 Normal-hearing adults with an age range of 22 to 31 years 20 – Profound loss 8 to 15 years old

Table 2. Benefits reported for tactile aids

Sound perception

- develops awareness to presence or absence of sound
- increases awareness to the presence of speech
- increases awareness to different types of environmental sounds
- assists in getting and maintaining the child's attention
- improves hearing aid use by emphasizing aspects of the speech signal that the hearing aid cannot provide

Sound discrimination

- improves ability to differentiate loud–soft sounds
- improves ability to differentiate long–short sounds
- improves ability to differentiate continuous versus interrupted sounds
- improves ability to distinguish the number of sounds in a word, phrase or sentence
- improves ability to distinguish number of syllables in words and sentences
- improves ability to distinguish different types of sounds in the environment

Lipreading (speechreading)

improves ability to lipread; supplements lipreading cues and lipreading improvement has been reported for isolated phonemes, single words and sentences

Speech production (articulation)

- increases amount of vocalization and willingness to use speech
- improves stress patterns and syllabification

Type aid/Placement of aid on body	Measures	Findings
	before and after a training phase with the device • A group of 20 adult listeners were asked to judge the taped pre- and post-training taped samples	
• Laboratory vibrotactile device designed to present spectral shape of speech to users' fingers • Auditory comparison presented through earphones	• A list of 180 syllable names with 60 monosyllabic, 60 disyllabic and 60 trisyllabic names were randomly amplified and presented to both groups of subjects, in a tactual and an auditory condition • Normal-hearing adults were artificially deafened with masking noise during the tactual presentations	• Normal-hearing listeners reported similar numbers for syllabification in both the tactual and auditory condition • Number of syllabic patterns perceived by deaf children differed from those reported by normal-hearing adults • Number of syllable shapes identified by deaf children was more consistent with what was felt than what was heard

Table 2. Cont.

– improves ability to articulate commonly used words and phrases such as family
– names and greeting routines
– reduces and often eliminates of bilabial clicks (lip smacking sounds that deaf children
– often produce)
– improves production of vowel duration and fewer neutralized vowels are heard
– reduces frequency of occurrence of the intrusive schwa [ə], a sound that deaf
– children often insert between adjacent consonants
– consonant production is closer to target
– the above cited improvements in articulation result in increased intelligibility

Communication

– assists the individual in becoming more responsive to the auditory and verbal environment, therefore, oral communication is improved with hearing parents, siblings and other family members and friends

Laura's case is presented in the case studies section of this paper.

There is consensus, internationally, that a tactile device can improve lipreading and speech perception as well as improve voice quality and selected features of speech production for profoundly deaf children. Yet, many parents, educators and others interested in the welfare of deaf children ask questions that can be answered most effectively by interpreting the research literature. Several of these frequently asked questions can be answered by reviewing Tables 1 and 2. Some of the frequently asked questions are:

1. What is the purpose of the device?
2. What can a tactile aid do?
   (Answer contingent on number of channels.)
3. Is the device easy to operate?
   (A manufacturer's manual for the device should be available to the family.)
4. How much does the device cost? Who will pay for it?
5. When should the child use it? Optimum times? Least effective times?
6. Can the device be worn in conjunction with hearing aids?
7. At what age can a tactile aid be used?
8. How do tactile aid wearers fare over time?
9. How much wearing time is required of the child?
10. Should adjustments be made for home versus school environments?

Case Studies

Rate of change and amount of gain or progress in some aspect(s) of language relative to a reference group have often been used in evaluation studies of children's performance with tactile aids. Case studies of two sisters, Erin and Laura, have been selected to elaborate on the interactive relationship between tactile aid usage and language development. Both sisters used a single-channel vibrotactile aid. Both children were trained with the Tactaid 1 for the first two years of tactile aid usage and later wore the Minivib 3. Non-verbal tests of cognition revealed that both sisters are well within a normal range of functioning.

Erin began to wear a tactile aid at 24 months while Laura began tactile aid usage at the age of 8 weeks. Each of the children wore binaural amplification and their individual tactile aids at the same time. Erin was identified as having a profound, bilateral sensorineural hearing loss when she was 18 months old. From age 24 months, she wore a single-channel vibrotactile aid for an average of 5 hours per day at home and at school and her school curriculum was a Total Communication (TC) approach with signed English.

Erin's auditory brainstem response (ABR) results and pure tone audiograms in Figure 1 and show that she has a profound bilateral sensorineural hearing loss. Her early audiological test results are shown for ages 18 months, 38 months and 43 months. This child's unaided response to sound did not change after the 43 month audiogram. The 'A' in Figure 1 represents her response to sound in the soundfield with hearing aids while 'T' represents her response to sound with the tactile aid. Although the tactile responses to sound (T) are displayed on the audiogram, this does not mean that she heard sound at the same level at which she felt the presence of sound.

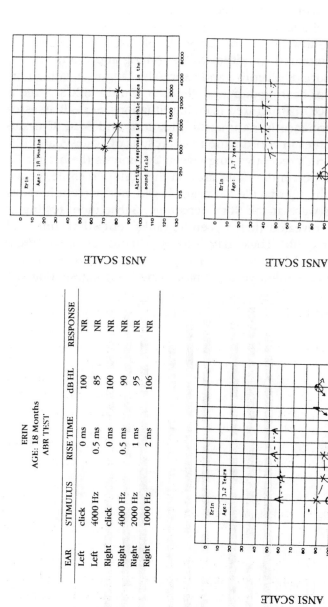

EAR	STIMULUS	RISE TIME	dB HL	RESPONSE
Left	click	0 ms	100	NR
Left	4000 Hz	0.5 ms	85	NR
Right	click	0 ms	100	NR
Right	4000 Hz	0.5 ms	90	NR
Right	2000 Hz	1 ms	95	NR
Right	1000 Hz	2 ms	106	NR

ERIN
AGE: 18 Months
ABR TEST

Figure 1. Erin's audiological picture: 18 months, 3.2 years and 3.7 years. A = response to sounds with tactile aids. T = response to sounds with hearing aids.

ANSI - American National Standards Institute

Rate of progress in receptive and expressive language after a tactile aid fitting has been used as one method of determining device effectiveness in very young children who are in the process of learning their first language. A developmental 'rule of thumb' that is often employed in assessment is that we can expect one month's progress in one month's time. Erin's progress in receptive and expressive language is shown in Figures 2, 3 and 4.

Figures 2 and 3 show results for the Scales of Early Communication Skills for Hearing-Impaired Children (SECS) (Moog and Geers, 1975). The SECS is a measure of receptive and expressive language with a normative population of hearing-impaired children. On the SECS, Scale A assesses performance in structured teaching situations, Scale B assesses spontaneous performance in naturalistic situations and Scale C evaluates non-verbal abilities in coordination with results of Scales A and B.

Pre-testing for Erin's receptive language at 24 months (before tactile aid fitting) revealed percentile ranks around the 10th percentile. At age 31 months, 7 months after tactile aid usage began, her percentile ranks for all three scores were at the 90th percentile. Subsequent testing at 42 and 47 months revealed that percentile ranks centred around and above the 90th percentile. These data suggest a rapid rate of progress for understanding oral language. Her ability to maintain percentile ranks at the 90th percentile over a 16-month period suggests that she

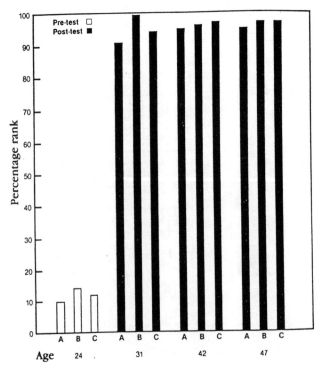

Figure 2. Erin: SECS – receptive language. See text for A, B, C.

continued to acquire and understand new concepts since the SECS is adjusted for increasing language complexity as a function of age.

For expressive language, Erin's percentile ranks before the tactile aid was fitted were below the 25th percentile on all three scales. She consistently performed above the 50th percentile 7 months later. By age 42 months, she consistently performed above the 75th percentile on all three SECS scales. By 47 months, she achieved the 100 percentile, a rating that would not have been attained by oral deaf children in the sample population. The rapid change in percentile ranks provide evidence that Erin progressed at an unusually rapid rate during the 16 month period of tactile aid usage.

For evaluation studies of tactile aids, it has been difficult to demonstrate that all of the child's rapid rate of progress can be attributed to the tactile aid. Young tactile aid users consistently demonstrate that they retain and expand on the language concepts that they learned while wearing the device. Erin's continued language progress reflects this behaviour. She wore the tactile aid until she was about 5 years old and then indicated a preference for hearing aids only. Figure 4 shows the results of our continued evaluation of Erin's receptive language progress at 51, 57 and 63 months.

The Test for Auditory Comprehension of Language – Revised (TACL-R) (Carrow-Woolfolk, 1985), a test with a normative population of

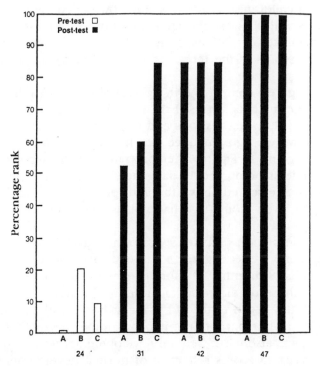

Figure 3. Erin: SECS – expressive language.

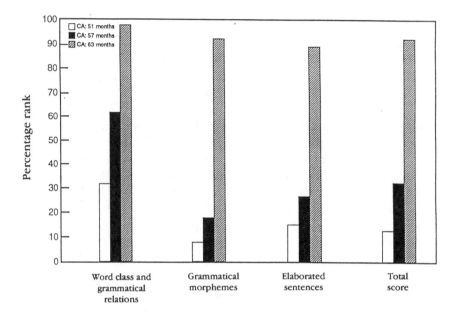

Figure 4. Erin: TACL-R.

normal-hearing children, was administered. TACL-R contains three different subtests which assess the child's ability to understand single words and grammatical relations, grammatical markers and elaborated sentences. The scores of the three subtests are combined to derive a total score.

Recall that Figure 4 compares Erin's percentile rank with that of normal-hearing, age matched peers. Erin wore her hearing aids during each of the TACL-R testing sessions and was allowed to see the examiner's face. However, sign language was not used in the testing sessions. The histograms in Figure 4 demonstrate that she showed steady progress in understanding spoken language over a 2 year period. By age 63 months, she scored above the 90th percentile on each of the TACL-R subtests, even though she had not used a tactile aid for more than a year.

Laura was identified as having a profound bilateral sensorineural loss at the age of 5 weeks. Figures 5 and 6 show her audiological history at 2 months, 8 months, 13 months, 3 years and 4 years of age. These confirm the early diagnosis of profound bilateral sensorineural hearing loss. Laura began tactile aid usage at home and continued to use the device in her parent–infant programme in which TC with signed English was also used. General developmental testing for Laura consistently revealed scores reflective of normal development since infancy.

LAURA   Age: 5 Weeks
Auditory Brainstem Response (ABR)

Ear	1000Hz	2000Hz	4000Hz	Click
R	NR 90	NR 95	NR 95	NR 100
L	NR 90	NR 95	NR 95	NR 100

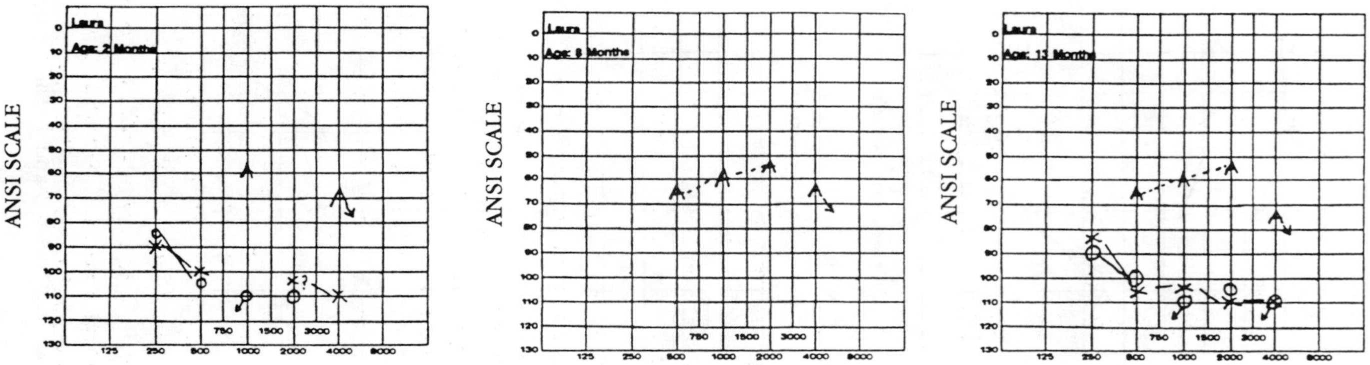

Sound Detection Threshold
(SDT)
R – 95 dB HL O
L – 85 dB HL ×

A – Aided
(Phonic Ear HC461)

Sound Detection Threshold
(SDT)
R – 95 dB HL
L – 95 dB HL

A – Aided
(Voice – 60 dB HL)
(Music – 60 dB HL)

Tested with Warble Tones Under Earphones
and with Warble Tones in Sound Field

Figure 5. Laura's audiological history: 5 weeks, 2 months, 8 months and 13 months.

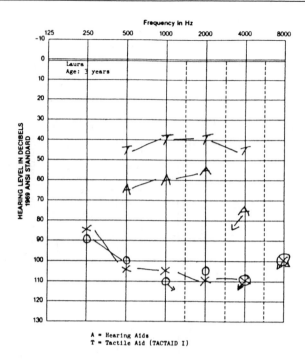

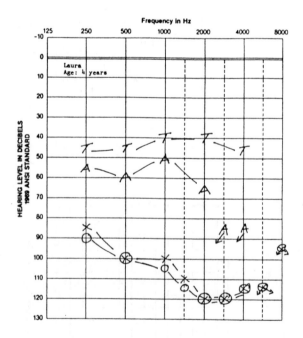

Figure 6. Laura's audiograms at 3 and 4 years of age. A = hearing aids. T = tactile aid (Tactaid I).

The single-channel tactile aid assists the child in developing a sense of awareness of the presence or absence of sound and develops other aspects of sound perception (see Table 2). It appears that our ability to record pure tone audiograms for both Erin and Laura at such early ages is related to the use of a tactile aid, worn in conjunction with their hearing aids.

During her first 36 months, Laura consistently wore the tactile aid and her hearing aids. By age 3 years 8 months, Laura's scores on the Grammatical Analysis of Elicited Language – Pre-sentence (GAEL-P) (Moog, Kozak and Geers, 1983) certainly compare favourably with those of Megan at the same age. Megan was a profoundly deaf, tactile aid user whom Geers (1986) discussed. For comparative purposes, cases reported in the literature such as Megan were selected since no other reports of children who began tactile-aid usage in infancy have been identified.

Table 3 shows comparative language results for Megan and Laura at the same ages. Laura's data suggest that there may be even greater long-term linguistic benefits when a tactile aid is provided in infancy and training occurs in the context of a total communication home and school. Laura wore her hearing aids and could see the Examiner's face, but sign language was not used when administering the GAEL-P.

Table 3. Percentile ranks on the GAEL-P

Scale	Megan (CA = 3.8 years)	Laura (CA = 3.8 years)
Comprehension	65	100
Production	50	100
Imitation	35	100

Between 3 years, 6 months and 4 years, 6 months, Laura inconsistently wore the tactile aid because she expressed a preference for hearing aids only. At age 4.6 years, the Grammatical Analysis of Elicited Language – Sentence level (GAEL-S) could be administered to Laura. The GAEL-S is syntactically more advanced than the GAEL-P and has 5-year-old hearing-impaired children as the youngest reference group.

Table 4 shows Laura's results of the GAEL-S for prompted and imitated performance as compared to profoundly deaf 5-year-olds and profoundly deaf 5-year-olds who use Total Communication (TC). Sign language was used with Laura in the administration of the GAEL-S. Although Laura was not 5 years old, her scores compare favourably with other profoundly deaf 5-year-olds in the US who use TC. For three of the areas assessed, Laura scores in the 75 percentile for 5-year-olds and achieves the 80th percentile in another area on the GAEL-S.

Table 4. GAEL-S prompted and imitated percentile ranks

Reference Group	Laura's Percentile Rank	
	Prompted	Imitated
Profoundly deaf 5-year-olds	75	75
Total Communication (TC): 5-year-olds	75	80

Again, Laura's results of the GAEL-S are impressive. This 4.6-year-old's language performance is nearing the upper limits of children who are chronologically 6 months older.

Summary and Discussion

Based on Gault's thesis, tactually providing information about the speech waveform envelope enhances the quality of the acoustic signal that the deaf child receives. Subsequent single-channel tactile aid studies that processed the speech waveform envelope in some manner supported Gault's notion. Others have further extended the concept of tactually supplementing hearing loss by developing multichannel tactile devices.

Our first subject, Tabitha, who used the Hopkins wearable vibrotactile aid (Proctor and Goldstein, 1983) as a toddler, is now a college freshman. Although she has not worn a vibrotactile aid for many years, neither she nor her parents report any negative side effects from device usage. Similarly, Erin and Laura's parents have not reported negative side effects for either child and we have no other reports of negative side effects for single-channel and two-channel vibrotactile devices which we have used with 30 different children ranging in age from 8 weeks old to 5 years old at onset of tactile aid usage. In summary, no safety risks have been reported for single-channel or multichannel vibrotactile aids after 15 years of observing paediatric tactile aid users.

Erin and Laura join the cases of other children who were early tactile aid users. The data for these two sisters, in conjunction with other cases reported (cf. Goldstein et al., 1983; Goldstein and Proctor, 1985; Proctor and Goldstein, 1983; Proctor, 1990), continue to provide evidence that a single-channel vibrotactile aid assists in developing auditory awareness and thereby facilitating the audiologist's ability to obtain an accurate pure tone audiogram at younger ages than in the past. It is unclear if the use of more than one channel at younger ages will change the rate at which deaf infants and toddlers will respond to sound. This is clearly an area that requires further investigation.

The tactile aid provides deaf children an entrée to the hearing world by feeling sound and developing a conceptual basis for understanding the complexity of sound. In today's society, the hearing world and Deaf culture are viewed as holding unique, and often mutually exclusive, characteristics. In one way or another, deaf children are expected to be bilingual and bicultural. The tactile aid increases lipreading (oral language comprehension) at a relatively rapid rate and enables children to improve their ability to negotiate those home and school settings which require interaction with hearing people who do not sign or who do not sign well. Sign language increases the child's ability to make felt sound meaningful in many different and subtle ways. Sign language also puts deaf children in touch with others who share their Deaf culture.

Acknowledgement

I am deeply grateful to Erin, Laura and Theresa and their parents Jean and Dan McManus of Whitman, Massachusetts. I also express sincere appreciation to Madeline Feldman, and all other teachers, parents and students at the former Boston School. As family and as educators, your model has enriched my life and positively touched the lives of many others.

References

Alcantara, J.I., Whitford, L.A., Blamey, P.J., Cowan, R.S.C. and Clark, G.M.(1990) Speech feature recognition by profoundly hearing impaired children using a multiple-channel electrotactile speech processor and aid residual hearing. Journal of Acoustical Society of America 88: 1260–73.

Arrowsmith, J.D. (1819) The Art of Instructing the Deaf and Dumb. London: Taylor and Hessey.

Bond, S.L. and Scott, B. L. (1982) Evaluating a tactile aid on four-year-old profoundly deaf children. Journal of Acoustical Society of America 71: S59.

Boothroyd, A. (1972) Sensory aids research project at the Clarke School for the Deaf. In Fant, G. (Ed) Speech Communication Ability and Profound Deafness. Washington, DC: A.G. Bell Association. pp 367–77.

Brooks, P.L., Frost, B.J., Mason, J.L. and Gibson, D.G. (1987) Word and feature identification by profoundly deaf teenagers using the Queen's University tactile vocoder. Journal of Speech and Hearing Research 30: 137–41.

Carhart, R. (1935) A method of using the Gault-Teletactor. American Annals of the Deaf 80: 260–3.

Carrow-Woolfolk, E. (1985) Test for Auditory Comprehension of Language – Revised. Hingham, MA: Teaching Resources.

Cloud, D.T. (1933) Some results from the use of the Gault-Teletactor. American Annals of the Deaf 78: 200–4.

Eilers, R.E., Oller, D.K. and Vergara, K. (1989) Speech and language progress of hearing-impaired children in a systematic training program using tactual vocoders. In McGarr, N.S. (Ed) Research on the Use of Sensory Aids for Hearing-Impaired People. Volta Review 91: 127–38.

Eilers, R.E., Widen, J.E. and Oller, D.K. (1988) Assessment techniques to evaluate tactual aids for hearing-impaired subjects. Journal of Rehabilitation Research and Development 25: 33–46.

Englemann, S. and Rosov, R. (1975) Tactual hearing experiments with deaf and hearing subjects. Exceptional Child 41: 243–53.

Erber, N.P. (1972a) Speech envelope cues as an acoustic aid to lipreading for profoundly deaf children. Journal of Acoustical Society of America 51: 1224–7.

Erber, N.P. (1972b) Auditory, visual and auditory-visual recognition of consonants by children with normal and impaired hearing. Journal of Speech and Hearing Research 15: 413–22.

Erber, N.P. (1979) Speech perception by profoundly hearing-impaired children. Journal of Speech and Hearing Disorders 44: 255–70.

Franklin, B. and Saunders, F.A.. (1981) The use of tactile aids with the deaf. Presented at the American Speech- Language-Hearing Association, Nov. 20–23, Los Angeles, CA.

Friel-Patti, S. and Roeser, R. J. (1983) Evaluating changes in the communication skills of deaf children using vibrotactile stimulation. Ear and Hearing 4: 31–40.

Galvin, K.L., Cowan, R.S.C., Sarant, J.Z., Blamey, P.J. and Clark, G.M. (1993) Factors in the development of a training program for the use with tactile devices. Ear and Hearing 14: 118–27.

Gault, R.H. (1926a) Touch as a substitute for hearing in the interpretations and control of speech. Archives Otolaryngology 3: 121–35.

Gault, R. H. (1926b) Extension of the uses of touch for the deaf. School and Society 23: 368–70.

Gault, R. H. (1928) Interpretation of spoken language when the feel of speech supplements vision of the speaking face. Volta Review 30: 379–86.

Gault, R. H. (1934) An interpretation of vibrotactile phenomena. Journal of Acoustical Society of America 5: 252–4.

Gault, R.H. and Goodfellow, L.D. (1937) Experimental evidence for a basic theory of vibrotactile interpretation of speech. Archives of Otolaryngology 25: 190–5.

Geers, A. E. (1986) Vibrotactile stimulation: Case study with a profoundly deaf child. Journal of Rehabilitation Research and Development 1: 111–17.

Goldstein, M.H., Jr and Proctor, A. (1985) Tactile aids for profoundly deaf children. Journal of Acoustical Society of America 77: 258–65.

Goldstein, M.H., Jr., Proctor, A., Bulle, L. and Shimizu, H. (1983) Tactile stimulation in speech reception: Experience with a non-auditory child. In Hochberg, L. N., Levitt, H. and Osberger, M.J. (Eds) Speech of the Hearing Impaired. Baltimore, MD: University Park Press. pp 147–66.

Goldstein, M.H., Jr and Stark, R.E. (1976) Modifications of vocalizations of preschool deaf children by vibrotactile and visual displays. Journal of Acoustical Society of America 59: 282–6.

Goodfellow, L.D. (1934) Experiments on senses of touch and vibration. Journal of Acoustical Society of America 6: 45–50.

Henoch, A. and Hunt, S.L. (1981) Application of a vibrotactile aid in improvement of speech production in deaf children. Journal of Academy of Rehabilitation Audiology XIV: 125–40.

Ifukube, T. (1982) A cued tactual vocoder. In Raviv, J. (Ed) Uses of Computers in Aiding the Disabled. NY: North-Holland. pp 197–215.

Kozma-Spytek, L. and Weisenberger, J.M. (1987) Evaluation of a multichannel electrotactile aid for the hearing impaired: A case study. Paper presented at the Meeting of the Acoustical Society of America, November, Miami, FL. Published in Journal of Acoustical Society of America 82: 523.

Kringlebotn, M. (1968) Experiments with some visual and vibrotactile aids for the deaf. American Annals of the Deaf 113: 311–17.

Ling, D. and Sofin, B. (1975) Discrimination of fricatives by hearing impaired children using a vibrotactile cue. British Journal of Audiology 9: 14–18.

Lynch, M.P., Eilers, R.E., Oller, K.D. and Cobo-Lewis, A. (1989) Multisensory speech perception by profoundly hearing-impaired children. Journal of Speech and Hearing Disorders 54: 57–67.

Miyamoto, R.T., Osberger, M.J., Robbins, A.J., Renshaw, J., Myres, W.A., Kessler, K. and Pope, M.L. (1989) Comparison of sensory aids in deaf children. Annals of Otology, Rhinology and Laryngology 98: Part 2, Supplement 142, 2–7.

Miyamoto, R.T., Myres, W.A., Wagner, M. and Punch, J.L. (1987) Vibrotactile devices as sensory aids for the deaf. Otolaryngology Head Neck Surgery 97: 57–63.

Moog, J. and Geers, A. (1985) Grammatical Analysis of Elicited Language – Presentence level. St. Louis, MO: Central Institute for the Deaf.

Neate, D. M. (1972) The use of tactile vibration in the teaching of speech to severely and profoundly deaf children. The Teacher of the Deaf 70: 137–46.

Oller, D.K., Eilers, R.E., Vergara, K. and LaVoie, E. (1986) Tactual vocoders in a multisensory program training speech production and reception. Volta Review 88: 21–36.

Oller, D.K., Payne, S.L. and Gavin, W.J. (1980) Tactual speech perception by minimally trained deaf subjects. Journal of Speech and Hearing Research 23: 760-78.

Osberger, M.J., Maso, M. and Sam, L.K. (1993) Speech intelligibility of children with cochlear implants, tactile aids or hearing aids. Journal of Speech and Hearing Research 36: 186–203.

Osberger, M.J., Miyamoto, R.T., Robbins, A.M., Renshaw, J.J., Berry, S.W., Myres, W.A., Kessler, K. and Pope, M.L. (1990) Performance of deaf children with cochlear implants and vibrotactile aids. Journal of American Academy of Audiology 1: 7–10.

Perier, O. and Boorsma, A. (1982) A prosthetic device utilizing vibrotactile perception of profoundly deaf children. British Journal of Audiology 16: 277–9.

Plant, G.L. (1979) The use of tactile supplements in the rehabilitation of the deafened: A case study. Australian Journal of Audiology 1: 76–82.

Plant, G. L. (1982) Tactile perception by the profoundly deaf. British Journal of Audiology, 16: 233–44.

Plant, G. L. (1983) The use of vibrotactile aids with profoundly deaf children. STL-Quarterly Progress and Status Report (QPSR) 1: 36-51.

Plouer, A.N. (1934) The Gault-Teletactor at the Illinois School. Volta Review 36: 83–4, 116.

Proctor, A. (1990) Oral language comprehension using hearing aids and tactile aids: Three case studies. Language, Speech, and Hearing Services in Schools 21: 37–48.

Proctor, A. (1983) Early home intervention for hearing-impaired infants and their parents. Volta Review, 85, 150-166.

Proctor, A. and Goldstein, M.H., Jr (1983) Development of lexical comprehension in a profoundly deaf child using a wearable vibrotactile communication aid. Language, Speech, and Hearing Services in Schools 14: 138–49.

Robbins, A.M., Osberger, M.J., Miyamoto, R.T., Renshaw, J.J. and Carney, A.E. (1988) Longitudinal study of speech perception by children with cochlear implants and tactile aids: Progress report. Journal of Academy of Rehabilitation Audiology 21: 11–28.

Robbins, A.M., Todd, S.L. and Osberger, M.J. (1992) Speech perception performance of pediatric multichannel tactile aid or cochlear implant users. Paper presented at the Second International Conference on Tactile Aids, Hearing Aids, and Cochlear Implants. Stockholm, Sweden.

Schulte, K. (1978) The use of supplementary speech information in verbal communication. Volta Review 80: 12–20.

Scilley, P.L. (1980) Evaluation of a vibrotactile auditory prosthetic device for the profoundly deaf. Unpublished master's thesis, Queen's University, Kingston, Canada

Sheehy, P. and Hansen, S.A. (1983) The use of vibrotactile aids with preschool hearing impaired children: Case studies. Volta Review 85, 14–26.

Sparks, D.W. (1977) A remotely activated tactual communication aid for the hearing impaired. Journal of Speech and Hearing Disorders 42: 412–21.

Spens, K-E. (1980) Tactile speech communication aids for the deaf: A comparison. Speech Transmission Laboratory: Quarterly Progress and Status Report 4: 23–39.

Spens, K-E. (1983) A tactual 'hearing aid' for the deaf. Paper presented at the IX World Conference of the Deaf, July 1–6. Palermo, Italy.

Stratton, W.D. (1974) Intonation feedback for the deaf through a tactile display. Volta Review 76: 26–35.

Traunmuller, H. (1977) The sentiphone, a tactual speech communication aid. Paper presented at the Research conference on Speech Processing Aids for the Deaf, Gallaudet College, Washington, D.C.

Van Tasell, D.J., Soli, S.D., Kirby, V.M. and Widin, G.P. (1987) Speech waveform envelope cues for consonant recognition. Journal of Acoustical Society of America 82: 1152–61.

Van Tasell, D.J., Greenfield, D.G., Logemann, J.J. and Nelson, D.A. (1992) Temporal cues for consonant recognition: Training, talker generalization, and use in the evaluation of cochlear implants. Journal of Acoustical Society of America 92: 1247–57.

Weisenberger, J.M. and Kozma-Spytek, L. (1991). Evaluating tactile aids for speech perception and production by hearing-impaired adults and children. American Journal of Otology 12: 188–20 (Supplement).

Zeiser, M.L. and Erber, N.P. (1977) Auditory/vibratory perception of syllabic structure in words by profoundly hearing impaired children. Journal of Speech and Hearing Research 20: 430–6.

8

Toward Future Tactile Aids

LYNNE E. BERNSTEIN

Arne Risberg was an early player on the tactile aid stage, as Pickett's ·chapter documents. Although I argue below that progress in the area has been relatively limited, the argument does not diminish the vision exhibited by Arne Risberg in undertaking research for which there was scant precedent and even theoretically opposing arguments.

Levitt (1988) characterized tactile aid research as cyclic, with waves of enthusiasm followed by troughs of disappointment and disinterest. The first wave began with Gault (1926), followed by loss of interest in the 1930s and 1940s. This wave probably reached its peak with the installation of vibrators on the desks of each pupil in oral schools for deaf children (Pickett, 1993). Arguably, too little was known about tactile psychophysics and speech perception during Gault's time to achieve success. 1949–1965 marked a second wave that ended with few gains beyond those of the first cycle (Levitt, 1988). Tactile aids drew attention again in the 1970s, continuing through to the present, as a non-invasive alternative to cochlear implants. Also, new technologies and scientific knowledge had suggested new approaches to be tried. Some gains have been made in this recent cycle (see Summers, 1992, for detailed reviews of work in the past decade or so): several wearable devices have been tested and marketed; several device designs have been tested in the laboratory (for example, Bernstein et al., 1991; Blamey et al., 1988; Boothroyd and Hnath, 1986; De Filippo, 1984; Eberhardt et al., 1990; Lynch et al., 1989; Weisenberger et al., 1989); knowledge has improved in the area of training and testing; and a small body of programmatic research has been conducted to obtain basic knowledge about the encoding of speech signals for the tactile system (for example, Bernstein, et al., 1989, 1993a; Hnath-Chisolm and Medwetsky, 1988; Cowan, et al., 1991; Green et al., 1983; Hanin et al., 1988; Rothenberg et al., 1977; Rothenberg and Molitor, 1979). But the goal of a highly effective tactile aid has not been achieved.[1]

One thing that has been learned in the history of tactile aids is that small-to-moderate benefits can be achieved with a variety of different schemes for tactual encoding of speech information. Perhaps, because these gains can be made within the current framework of knowledge, tactile aid research is frequently conducted as a strictly applied science. Experiments are comparisons between commercial devices or between tactile aids and cochlear implants. Of course, a main rationalization for applied studies is to obtain data that may be clinically useful. The factors in an applied tactile aids experiment are typically defined in terms of the linguistic levels of the stimuli (for example, nonsense syllables, words, sentences, texts), the receptive conditions (speechreading alone, speechreading with the aid, and occasionally the aid alone and/or speechreading with a tactile aid and a hearing aid), and the experience afforded the subject (for example, in the laboratory versus outside). The measures obtained in the experiment are almost invariably related to stimulus identification accuracy on the part of the subject, although discrimination procedures are also employed. This scenario contrasts with that in basic research in tactile and speech perception for which answers are sought to questions like: What is the stimulus (in psychophysical, acoustic-phonetic, linguistic, or functional terms) (see, for example, Fowler, 1986; Remez et al., 1993)? What is the basic unit of speech perception? What is the nature of multi-modality speech perception (for example, Summerfield, 1991; Massaro, 1987)? What are the levels of processing that are traversed between the sensory periphery and the recognition of a word (for example, Nygaard and Pisoni, 1992; Melara and Marks, 1990)? A thesis of this chapter is that major advances in tactile aids require a greater emphasis on basic science.

It is not difficult to point out issues in the tactile aid literature that support the notion that lack of basic knowledge may be severely restricting the possibility for making significant improvements over current levels of enhancement with tactile aids. For example, it is frequently supposed that arrays of vibrators can deliver more information than a single vibrator. Yet, scant evidence is available to demonstrate an advantage for multichannel configurations as aids to lipreading (Bernstein et al., 1993a; Hanin et al., 1988; cf. Cowan et al., 1991). Likewise, it is frequently supposed that tactile aids should deliver phonetic cues. But it is questionable what if any phonetic information is delivered during connected speech by any tactile aids studied to date. A plausible alternative hypothesis is that tactile aids mainly deliver prosodic information (possibly rhythm and duration) that contributes to discovering word boundaries (Cutler and Butterfield, 1992). The question alluded to by the channels example is how best to use the skin surface to encode speech information. The question alluded to by the prosody example is what speech information should be delivered.

If future tactile aids are to achieve large significant improvements over current levels of benefit, it is likely that the knowledge base available for the work needs to be increased commensurately.

Theories of Speech Perception

If tactile aid research were only an applied branch of speech science, a reasonable expectation would be that literature on speech perception would provide a theoretical basis for tactile aid research. Unfortunately, speech scientists do not even agree on how to describe the speech stimulus. The contemporary discussion of this issue has been couched in terms of the question: What is the object of speech perception (Fowler, 1986; Remez et al., 1993)? The current lack of certainty is a particularly inconvenient state of affairs for the development of tactile aids, since the availability of knowledge might introduce some constraints on what should be presented to the skin.

Motor theory

One major theory, motor theory (Liberman et al., 1968), initially argued that speech perception is accomplished by an innately specified analysis-by-synthesis mechanism that refers perception of articulatory gestures to production. Liberman et al. (1968) posited that a specialized phonetic decoder is needed to recover phonemes from a speech signal. Furthermore, that decoder was said to be specialized for acoustic signals: '...that decoder can be made to work only from an auditory input' (p. 128). Research in this tradition has been concerned with showing that auditory speech perception reveals implicit knowledge of articulatory gestures.

What does motor theory offer to tactile aid research? Kirman (1973) essentially suggested that it is irrelevant since its exclusive reliance on an auditory mechanism for speech perception was not justified by the available data. In their revised motor theory, Liberman and Mattingly (1985) relax the assumption that speech information requires auditory processing and acknowledge that viewing a talker may also afford speech information. In the revised version of the motor theory, both auditory and optical speech information is processed by an innately given module specialized for speech.

Recently, Fowler and Dekle (1991) have argued that an innate decoding mechanism is unlikely to be specialized for haptic speech perception, as occurs with the haptic method of speech perception known as 'Tadoma'. Tadoma is a method used by some people who are deaf and blind to perceive speech by placing a hand on the face and neck of the talker (Reed et al., 1985; Schultz et al., 1984). The argument that the innate speech mechanism should not be able to decode arcane stimuli such as Tadoma could also be made with regard to artificial stimulation via tactile aids. However, the issue here may be one of stimulus information versus stimulus modality. That is, irrespective of the sensory source of the speech information, the theoretical speech module may be capable of decoding that information. However that debate is resolved, that the effective speech stimulus is the articulatory behaviour of the talker is supported by the Tadoma example. A consequence of this observation is the suggestion that the source of speech information for transformation to the tactile sense ought to be of articulatory origin, for example, electroglottograph signals, nasal accelerometer signals, or perhaps more practically (and in the future), signals derived from models that predict speech physiology from speech acoustics. This is a suggestion that has resulted in relatively little research to date other than studies of artificial Tadoma, that is Tadoma involving a mechanical face (Reed *et al.*, 1985; Tan *et al.*, 1989; an exception is De Filippo, 1984). In current research we are now beginning to examine implications of this suggestion (see below).

Auditory theories

Auditory theories have been the traditional countervailing force against motor theory as an explanation for speech perception. Two types of auditory theories can be distinguished. One views speech perception as a mapping between proximal auditory stimulation patterns (acoustic-phonetic cues) and phonetic perception, and within this category there are a variety of specific positions (see, for example, Pisoni and Luce, 1987; Stevens *et al.*, 1986). Acoustic cues are characteristics such as release bursts, formant frequencies, spectral shapes, and the myriad other characteristics that have been the subject of much speech research (see Lisker, 1978, for a discussion of cues). The research programme from this perspective is to describe the speech stimulus in terms of its linguistically relevant acoustic characteristics. The second type of auditory theory explains speech perception in terms of auditory impressions, or psychoacoustic processes (Diehl *et al.*, 1990; Kuhl *et al.*, 1991).

Theories that account for speech perception in terms of auditory mechanisms or acoustic-phonetic stimulus characteristics per se cannot account for visual or tactile-visual speech perception. However, most tactile aid research has implicitly or explicitly adopted an auditory view of speech perception. That is, all tactile devices that use microphone signals as their input extract signal characteristics that can/could (presumably) be shown to contain acoustic-phonetic cues. Tactile vocoders are an example of this approach; a wideband of speech frequencies is filtered by a set of adjacent narrowband filters, and the speech energy passed by each band is used to modulate a corresponding tactile vibrator in a

linear or two-dimensional array. Were the same signals presented to the
ear as acoustic stimuli, highly intelligible speech would be produced
(see, for example, Bernstein *et al.*, 1993b).

Acoustic-phonetics is extremely valuable to tactile aid development.
It provides information about sufficient conditions for auditory speech
perception. But it would be a mistake to confuse the analytic properties of acoustic-phonetic stimuli for what is perceived in speech perception. (In this regard, the theoretical thrust of motor theory is
well-taken.) Similarly, it would be a mistake to confuse proximal tactile
stimulation patterns (for example, tactile vocoder signals) with what is
actually perceived by the user of a tactile aid. Keeping these caveats in
mind, knowledge from acoustic-phonetics can be mined to provide
sources of acoustic-to-tactile transformations. But the onus is on the
tactile aid researcher to show that those transformations induce the
same perceptual effects in the tactile domain that they do in the auditory one.

One particularly relevant counter case to auditory theories

Auditory theories fail to account for demonstrations of speech perception without natural acoustic-phonetic characteristics. Remez *et al.*
(1993) have shown that some very unspeechlike acoustic signals can
induce speech perception. Remez *et al.* employ digitally synthesized
sinewave replicas of speech stimuli. What stands for speech here are
three or four time-varying sinusoids, each of which is specified by the
centre frequency and amplitude of a vocal resonance in a natural utterance. Sinewave speech lacks the fine-grained properties of speech signals that are the stuff of acoustic-phonetics. Sinewave speech has
characteristics that preclude its having been produced by a natural
vocal tract, lacking comodulation by a fundamental frequency, aperiod-
icities (associated with frication and aspiration), and broadband formants. Sinewave replicas do not sound like speech, nor do they convey
speech information to naive subjects. Naive subjects describe sinewave
replicas as modern music, radio interference, or other non-speech
sounds. Nevertheless, after being told that the stimulus is speech, subjects can perceive its linguistic content at reasonably high levels of
accuracy. What sinewave speech appears to preserve is critical dynamic
speech properties that are invariant across the extreme transformation
that is involved in generating sinewave speech.

The challenge that sinewave speech sends to auditory theories is to
explain speech perception in the absence of auditory impressions that
are similar to those induced by natural speech and in the absence of
proximal auditory stimulation patterns that contain the usual acoustic-
phonetic characteristics. A benefit this work offers to tactile aids is that it
demonstrates a case of apparently severe transformation that preserves

speech intelligibility at the expense of natural acoustic-phonetic characteristics. It supports the notion that speech perception can be induced with arcane stimuli. It also suggests that a theory of speech perception is required to explain how both natural and arcane speech stimuli can induce speech perception. Similarly, an adequate theory of speech perception needs to comprise an account of tactile and visual speech perception. A theory of speech perception that explained how speech perception is accomplished on the basis of multiple modality inputs and a variety of stimulus types would likely contribute greatly to development of future tactile aids.

One Approach to the Selection of Tactile Speech Cues

Presently lacking a proven theoretical basis for designing tactile speech stimuli, the approach of selecting acoustic speech signals that may be matched to tactile psychophysical characteristics continues to be a potentially fruitful approach. Research on the use of voice fundamental frequency (F0) exemplifies this approach. Signals derived from voice F0 have been studied by several groups of investigators who sought to obtain significant enhancements to lipreading. Several experiments have demonstrated that auditory signals designed to convey voice F0 can result in large enhancements to lipreading (Boothroyd et al., 1988; Breeuwer and Plomp, 1986; Grant et al., 1985; Rosen et al., 1981). The typical effect-size for combining F0 information with lipreading was reported by Breeuwer and Plomp (1986), who showed that experienced normal-hearing subjects improved their syllable identification scores on an open-set sentence identification task from 33% lipreading alone to 73% with the auditory F0 signal.

Several groups have attempted to obtain equally favourable results with tactile indication of F0 (Bernstein et al., 1989, 1993a; Eberhardt et al., 1990; Boothroyd and Hnath, 1986; Hanin et al., 1988; Grant et al., 1986; Plant, 1987; Plant and Risberg, 1983). Among the reasons for predicting that F0 will be effective tactually are the following: (1) voice F0 rates are fairly well matched to the skin's best frequencies or can be relatively easily transposed in that region (Rothenberg and Molitor, 1979); and (2) prosodic characteristics of speech conveyed in part by voice F0 change fairly slowly, on a syllabic scale, and may not greatly challenge the temporal processing characteristics of the skin (Rothenberg et al., 1977; Weisenberger, 1986).

In tactile aid experiments, investigators have reported that subjects can identify prosodic characteristics such as intonation and stress (Bernstein et al., 1989; Hnath-Chisolm and Kishon-Rabin, 1988; Rothenberg and Molitor, 1979) with the tactile aid alone. But the size of the enhancement to lipreading of connected speech has been more modest compared with results obtained with auditory F0 signals. Among the most successful experiments, one by Hanin *et al.* (1988) employed three adults with postlingual severe or profound hearing loss. The difference between lipreading with and without a multichannel tactile aid that presented F0 in terms of rate as well as position of the active vibrator in a linear array was between 11% and 20% words correct in sentences. At Gallaudet University, we recently completed testing a group of postlingually deafened adults with a wearable F0 tactile aid. At this stage in the analysis of results (Auer *et al.*, 1994; Bernstein *et al.*, 1994), it appears that the aid provides similar enhancement to that reported by Hanin *et al.* (1988).

It is important to explain why a signal that seems so well suited for a tactile aid has not been as effective as its auditory counterpart. To their credit, Boothroyd and his colleagues asked this question directly in a study of the effects of F0 extraction and quantization on enhancement with auditory stimuli (Hnath-Chisolm and Boothroyd, 1992). In their study, a filtered electroglottograph signal that measured voice fundamental frequency directly was compared with a sinusoid whose frequency was based on the electroglottograph signal but was restricted by frequency quantization of from one to twelve steps. Results of this study showed that quantization had a significant detrimental effect. For example, there was a significant decrement in subjects' performance with eight levels of F0 quantization versus twelve (50% words correct versus 54% words correct). This result was interpreted as suggesting the need for an increased number of vibrators in the Boothroyd F0 tactile aid, which employs both rate and spatial coding. Thus the lesson here is that the tactile aid signal should putatively provide at least the information that appears critical for the audiovisual enhancement effect; otherwise, the expectation of equivalent levels of performance is ill-founded. This type of careful research to isolate critical factors contributing to aid performance is essential to the future success of tactile aids.

A potentially important class of auditory speech signals that deliver surprisingly high levels of benefit to speechreading are speech envelope signals obtained from input analysis filters of an octave or narrower in width. The energy passed by the analysis signal is used to amplitude modulate a fixed frequency carrier signal. An early study by Risberg (1974) appears to be the first to consider use of these auditory signals to supplement lipreading. Breeuwer and Plomp (1984) demonstrated their effects in an experiment in which speech energy in either one or two bands of speech was used to modulate a corresponding fixed-frequency tone. For example, energy in a 1/3-octave band at 500 Hz was used to modulate a 500-Hz sinusoid. Among a set of single-band or dual-band signals, the most effective for enhancing lipreading were a 500-Hz sinusoid with energy from an octave band at 500 Hz, and a combination of 500- and 3160-Hz sinusoids again modulated by energy from corresponding octave bands. Lipreading alone in this study was at approximately 23% syllables correct. The single isolated 500-Hz signal resulted in a 43% enhancement to syllables correct in sentences (66% correct performance level), and the dual-sinusoid signal resulted in a 64% enhancement (87% correct performance level). A single amplitude-modulated sinusoid would be expected to convey virtually no speech information by itself. The dual 500-Hz and 3160-Hz signal resulted in 22.9% syllables correct in sentences without lipreading.

Grant et al. (1991) tested lipreading with a large set of different single-band amplitude signals based on appropriate combinations of analysis filters (wideband, or octave band at 500, 1600 or 3150 Hz), smoothing filters (from 12.5 to 1600 Hz), and carriers (wideband noise, or sinusoid at 200, 500, 1600 or 3150 Hz). Not every combination of signal processing was effective in enhancing lipreading. The most effective, a 500-Hz analysis filter with carrier at 200 Hz, resulted in lipreading scores approximately 40 percentage points above the level obtained for lipreading alone. Audiovisual performance was at approximately 80% words correct for relatively easy sentences and approximately 60% words correct for relatively difficult sentences. Notably, a wideband prefilter combined with a 200-Hz carrier resulted in only a 10–15% gain. It appears that the overall amplitude envelope is less informative than the amplitudes of fixed narrow bands.

We can compare the auditory signals above with the tactile stimulus obtained with the Tactaid II (Franklin, 1988). The Tactaid II uses one low-pass prefilter up to 2000 Hz and one high-pass prefilter from 2000–8000 Hz. The energy from each analysis filter is used to modulate a fixed rate pulse train activating a single vibrotactile channel. Although there are no identical experiments on the Tactaid to compare with the audiovisual experiments discussed above, it appears that none of the results with the Tactaid II indicate the level of enhancement reported with the auditory signals. For example, in Lynch et al. (1989), a subject with congenital profound hearing impairment was tested with the Tactaid II using a connected discourse tracking (De Filippo and Scott, 1978) procedure. At the conclusion of the experiment, the subject's tracking with the device was approximately 5 words per minute faster than by lipreading alone (Lynch et al., 1989 Figure 3), a small although significant enhancement.

In attempting to explain results such as the Lynch et al. (1989) study, there has been some tendency among tactile aid researchers to focus on gross characteristics of the vibrotactile psychophysical display such as number of channels and on duration of training. However, Grant et al.'s (1991) results suggest that a major limitation with the tactile aid may have been the choice of wideband prefilters, which for auditory signals are less effective than narrowband filters. Grant *et al.* also suggest that careful attention should be paid to not only the overall amplitude characteristics of the signal but also the short-term details of the amplitude envelope. Some of these characteristics have been categorized by Rosen (1992) as envelope, periodicity, and fine-structure. Rosen considers envelope characteristics to be those fluctuations in overall amplitude between 2 and 50 Hz. Properties in the envelope that are related to the distinction between periodic and aperiodic vocal tract excitation and to the rate of periodicity fall under the category of periodicity. Fine-structure characteristics refer to variation in waveform shape over single periods.

In theory, for a tactile aid to be as effective as an auditory signal, not only must the signal processing preserve the critical speech information, but the tactile psychophysical display must be designed to convey this information to the skin. To date, research on the tactile perception of the envelope, periodicity, and fine-structure characteristics of narrowband speech envelopes is extremely sparse but encouraging (cf. Rabinowitz *et al.*, 1994; Weisenberger, 1989; Formby *et al.*, 1992).

The Nature of the Psychophysical Display

Tadoma has been held up repeatedly as an existence proof for tactile speech perception, because without speechreading it has been shown effective for learning language as well as for communication at slow to moderate rates (Reed *et al.*, 1992). This level of success has yet to be demonstrated for any tactile aid. However, the use of the term 'tactile' to describe the Tadoma method ignores a potentially important distinction between perception of cutaneous stimuli and haptic perception. Tactile perception usually refers to cutaneous stimulation, not to proprioception or kinaesthesia. Tactile stimulation includes skin deformation and vibration. Haptic perception has received diverse definitions involving both the type of information available to the observer and the observer's involvement as an active or passive agent in obtaining information (Loomis and Lederman, 1986). However, all definitions assign both cutaneous and kinaesthetic stimulation to haptic perception. Kinaesthesia defined in the broadest manner includes awareness of positions and movements of limbs and other body parts independent of the nature of the participation (active or passive) of the observer (Clark and Horch, 1986). According to the distinctions being drawn here, Tadoma is an example of haptic not tactile perception. What is important to note here is that the more impressive results that have been reported for Tadoma may be due to the qualitatively different stimulation received by the Tadoma user. Haptic perception hypothetically can provide more information than stimulation to cutaneous receptors alone.

Although Tadoma demonstrates the efficacy of a natural haptic stimulus, the demonstration itself does not disclose the effective stimulus. Research on haptic perception, although it has a distinguished history (Gibson, 1966), has focused on spatial and object perception rather than dynamic stimulation available from the face of a talker. One thing that study of haptic perception has shown is that it is fast and accurate for recognizing complex three-dimensional objects (Klatzky, *et al.*, 1985).

Reed and her colleagues at MIT (Reed *et al.*, 1985) have investigated Tadoma over the past 15 years. Their research has involved two primary components: (1) evaluation of practised and novice users of natural Tadoma, and (2) development and testing of a synthetic Tadoma system based on a mechanical face that gives indication of laryngeal vibration, oral airflow, jaw height, lower lip height and protrusion, and upper lip protrusion. The artificial system comprises sampling of physiological signals from talkers and representation of those signals by an artificial skull with movement, vibration, and air-jet sources. The research on natural Tadoma has made a significant contribution to our knowledge of what can be achieved by practised subjects and has suggested which speech articulatory features may be perceived via Tadoma. The synthetic Tadoma system has been less studied, but one study by Tan *et al.* (1989) was not encouraging regarding haptic speech perception.

Tan *et al.* (1989) examined information transmitted by four of the synthetic facial movement dimensions and concluded that 'reception of facial movement information by itself does not appear to account for the extraordinary success of the Tadoma method' (p. 981). Possible inadequacies of the synthetic system were acknowledged. As an alternative to the richness of the display as the explanation for Tadoma's success, extensive long-term training was suggested. However, extensive training could not result in accurate performance in the absence of an adequate stimulus and effective perceptual processing.

Because of its generally negative conclusions regarding haptic perception, the Tan *et al.* study requires examination. In the study, three subjects with normal hearing and vision participated first in making discrimination judgements for estimates of just-noticeable-differences (jnds) of displacement for the upper lip protrusion, lower lip protrusion, lower lip displacement, and jaw displacement on the synthetic display. Then they identified either one-dimensional stimuli composed of displacement from 0 to 24 mm along a continuum of either 16 or 14 steps, or four-dimensional stimuli at one of four displacements per dimension. The duration of movement to and from each target was held at 150 ms regardless of extent of displacement. The target position was held for 300 ms.

The results of discrimination trials in which only one channel was activated were Weber fractions of approximately 8–10%, with reference values between 0.1 and 21.3 mm. When irrelevant channels were randomly activated at the same time, Weber fractions increased three-fold. These results are not particularly troublesome. The results from identification trials are of more concern.

In one-dimensional identification trials, subjects assigned numerical labels to absolute displacements for the jaw and for lower lip vertical and horizontal displacement. Information transmitted in the one-dimensional condition varied between 1.3 and 2.0 bits out of the possible 3.8 or 4 bits (34% and 50% transmitted information, respectively). Movement of the irrelevant channels reduced one-dimensional identification accuracy to between 0.2 and 1.4 bits transmitted information. Four-dimensional identifications were made by subjects who were required to give numerical labels to four simultaneous displacements. The total number of alternative stimuli was 256, corresponding to 8 bits of information. Results showed approximately 3.3 bits (41%) transmitted information across the entire stimulus–response matrix. These results support the notion that haptic perception is deficient.

Several factors could explain the Tan *et al.* results. Subjects may have been unable to use the brief intervals (300 ms) that the fingers were in static positions to identify their absolute locations. The experimental task also required use of memory to encode the four independent movement channels. Errors could therefore arise in either the encoding or retrieval process. In addition, subjects had only 5000 trials of training.

Bernstein (1992) calculated the percentage transmitted information for natural nonsense syllable stimuli identified by subjects who are deaf–blind using Tadoma in Reed *et al.* (1982). Transmitted information was 49% (2.27 bits transmitted of 4.58, corresponding to 100% accurate transmission of 24 consonants). Two normal-hearing subjects achieved 3.67 bits transmitted information (80%) when trained on identification of 24 naturally-produced consonants, a level higher than that reported in the Tan *et al.* study. A difference between the two studies was that in the Tadoma study, subjects identified an assembly of haptic stimulation as a single phoneme, while in the Tan *et al.* study, the subjects made absolute judgements for each of the component movements. A plausible hypothesis is that the haptic system works by detecting information across stimulation sites in relation to each other (see Gibson, 1966) rather than by absolute measurements at each site. If so, the conclusions of the Tan *et al.* study were based on an incorrect notion of haptic perception.

In my laboratory, we are initiating basic studies of haptic perception using a new hand stimulator (Eberhardt *et al.*, 1993) that does not attempt to mimic the natural face. It is hypothesized that natural face geometry is likely not required in order to convey speech haptically. This position is supported by other examples of speech transformations, such as sinewave speech (Remez *et al.*, 1993), that preserve the critical information while destroying natural characteristics of the stimulus. Our haptic stimulator comprises independent channels for delivering low-amplitude high-frequency cutaneous stimulation and high-amplitude low-frequency kinaesthetic stimulation to the fingers. Each movement/vibration channel is independently controlled by a microprocessor, and the ensemble of channels is orchestrated by a personal computer. Stimuli composed of multiple channels of data can be computed either in realtime or in advance. Stimulus properties can be derived from physiologic measures obtained during speech articulation or from acoustic measures obtained from microphone signals. With this new system, we hope to discover: (1) the extent to which the success of Tadoma versus vibrotactile aids depends on the nature of the psychophysical display (haptic versus cutaneous only stimulation); (2) whether the source of the stimulus parameters (acoustic or articulatory) affects haptic speech perception; and (3) whether there are differential training effects with cutaneous only versus haptic stimuli.

Conclusions

Much remains to be done in the area of tactile aids. Research of the past decade or so suggests that the effort is worthwhile, but that the goal of an extremely effective tactile aid is likely not to evolve from ad hoc or atheoretical efforts. On the contrary, research in tactile aids needs to vigorously enter into discussions about basic science in speech perception and haptic perception. Tactile aid research needs to regard itself as an area of both basic and applied science. The need for a basic science approach will remain as long as many of the fundamental principles required for an applied science are yet to be discovered. As an application of science, tactile aid research can put to direct test implications of basic studies and theories.

Acknowledgements

This paper benefited from discussions with Philip F. Seitz, Edward T. Auer, J. Mac Pickett, Marilyn E. Demorest, Robert E. Remez, Ken W. Grant and David C. Coulter. The work was supported by grants from NIH, DC01577 and DC00695. The author is now at House Ear Institute, 2100 West Third Street, Los Angeles, CA 90057.

Note

1. Within the field itself, criteria for tactile aid success during the past decade or so have been defined informally as providing significant enhancement to speechreading and to signaling environmental events. *De facto* standards for success are evolving in relation to success with cochlear implants. The magnitude of benefit with implants varies widely across individuals. Five to ten per cent of implant users can perceive speech effectively without speechreading

(CHABA, 1991), but for many others the implant functions as a speechreading aid. Among the latter group, however, levels of enhancement for postlingually deafened adults frequently exceed levels reported in tactile aid studies (see for example, Blamey and Cowan, 1992). Rabinowitz *et al.*, (1992) report enhancements to reading sentences of 40 to 50 percentage points (audiovisual minus visual alone) among adult implant users who receive benefit.

References

Auer, E.T. Jr., Bernstein, L.E. and Coulter, D.C. (1994) Examining the effects of long-term experience using tactile supplements to speechreading. Journal of the Acoustical Society of America 95, 2, 987.

Bernstein, L.E. (1992) Evaluation of tactile aids. In Summers, I.R. (Ed) Tactile Aids for the Hearing Impaired. London: Whurr.

Bernstein, L.E., Auer, E.T., Jr. and Tucker, P.E. (1994) Spoken word recognition with tactile stimuli. Manuscript submitted for publication.

Bernstein, L.E., Auer, E.T., Coulter, D.C., Tucker, P.E. and Demorest, M.E. (1993a) Single- versus multichannel vibrotactile supplements to intonation and stress by normal-hearing and hearing-impaired adults. Journal of the Acoustical Society of America 93: 2336.

Bernstein, L.E., Coulter, D.C., O'Connell, M.P., Eberhardt, S.P. and Demorest, M.E. (1993b) Vibrotactile and haptic speech codes. In Risberg, A., Felicetti, S., Plant, G. and Spens, K-E.(Eds) Proceedings of the Second International Conference on Tactile Aids, Hearing Aids, and Cochlear Implants, Stockholm, June 7-11, 1992.

Bernstein, L.E., Demorest, M.E., Coulter, D.C. and O'Connell, M.P. (1991) Lipreading with vibrotactile vocoders: Performance of normal-hearing and hearing-impaired subjects. Journal of the Acoustical Society of America 90: 2971–84.

Bernstein, L.E., Eberhardt, S.P. and Demorest, M.E. (1989) Single- channel vibrotactile supplements to visual perception of intonation and stress. Journal of the Acoustical Society of America 85: 397–405.

Blamey, P. J. and Cowan, R. S. C. (1992).The potential benefit and cost-effectiveness of tactile devices in comparison with cochlear implants. In Summers, I.R. (Ed) Tactile Aids for the Hearing Impaired. London: Whurr.

Blamey, P.J., Cowan, R.S.C., Alcantara, J.I., Whitford, L.A. and Clark, G.M. (1988) Phonemic information transmitted by a multichannel electrotactile speech processor. Journal of Speech and Hearing Research 31: 620–9.

Boothroyd, A. and Hnath, T. (1986) Tactile supplements to lipreading. Journal of Rehabilitation Research and Development 23: 139–46.

Boothroyd, A., Hnath-Chisolm, T., Hanin, L. and Kishon-Rabin, L. (1988) Voice fundamental frequency as an auditory supplement to the speechreading of sentences. Ear and Hearing 9: 306–12.

Breeuwer, M. and Plomp, R. (1984) Speechreading supplemented with frequency-selective sound-pressure information. Journal of the Acoustical Society of America 76: 686–91.

Breeuwer, M. and Plomp, R. (1986) Speechreading supplemented with auditorily presented speech parameters. Journal of the Acoustical Society of America 79: 481–99.

CHABA (1991) Speech-perception aids for hearing-impaired people: Current status and needed research. Journal of the Acoustical Society of America 90: 637-585.

Clark, F.J. and Horch, K.W. (1986) Kinesthesia. In Boff, L.R., Kaufman, L. and Thomas, J.P. (Eds) Handbook of Perception and Human Performance, Vol. 1. NY: Wiley.

Cowan, R.S.C., Blamey, P.J., Sarant, J.Z., Galvin, K.L. and Clark, G.M. (1991) Perception of multiple electrode stimulus patterns: Implications for design of an electrotactile speech processor. Journal of the Acoustical Society of America 89: 360–8.

Cutler, A. and Butterfield, S. (1992) Rhythmic cues to speech segmentation: Evidence from juncture misperception. Journal of Memory and Language 31: 218–36.

De Filippo, C.L. (1984) Laboratory projects in tactile aids to lipreading. Ear and Hearing 5: 211–27.

De Filippo, C.L. and Scott, B.L. (1978) A method for training and evaluating the reception of ongoing speech. Journal of the Acoustical Society of America 63: 1186–92.

Diehl, R.L., Kluender, K.R. and Walsh, M.A. (1990) Some auditory bases of speech perception and production. Advances in Speech, Hearing and Language Processing 1: 243–67.

Eberhardt, S.P., Bernstein, L.E., Demorest, M.E. and Goldstein, M.H. (1990) Lipreading sentences with single-channel vibrotactile transformations of voice fundamental frequency. Journal of the Acoustical Society of America, 88, 1274–85.

Eberhardt, S.P., Bernstein, L.E., Coulter, D.C. and Hunckler, L. (1993) OMAR – A Haptic display of speech for speech perception by deaf and deaf–blind individuals. Proceedings Virtual Reality Annual International Symposium, The IEEE Neural Networks Council, September 18–22, 1993.

Formby, C., Morgan, L.N., Forrest, T.G. and Raney, J.J. (1992) The role of frequency selectivity in measures of auditory and vibrotactile temporal resolution. Journal of the Acoustical Society of America 91: 293–305.

Fowler, C.A. (1986) An event approach to the study of speech perception from a direct-realist perspective. Journal of Phonetics 14: 3–28.

Fowler, C.A. and Dekle, D.J. (1991) Listening with eye and hand: Cross-modal contributions to speech perception. Journal of Experimental Psychology: Human Perception and Performance 17: 816–28.

Franklin, D. (1988) Tactaid II+ users manual. Somerville, MA: Audiological Engineering Corp.

Gault, R. H. (1926). Touch as a substitute for hearing in the interpretation and control of speech. In Levitt, H., Pickett, J. M. and Houde, V. (Eds) Sensory Aids for the Hearing Impaired. New York: IEEE (1980). [Reprinted from Archives of Otolaryngology 3: 121–35.]

Gibson, J.J. (1966) The Senses Considered as Perceptual Systems. NY: Houghton Mifflin.

Grant, K.W., Ardell, L., Kuhl, P. and Sparks, D. (1985) The contribution of fundamental frequency, amplitude envelope, and voicing duration cues to speechreading in normal-hearing subjects. Journal of the Acoustical Society of America 77: 671–7.

Grant, K., Ardell, L., Kuhl, P. and Sparks, D. (1986) The transmission of prosodic information via an electrotactile speechreading aid. Ear and Hearing 7: 328–35.

Grant, K.W., Braida, L.D. and Renn, R.J. (1991) Single-band amplitude envelope cues as an aid to speechreading. Quarterly Journal of Experimental Psychology 43A: 621–45.

Green, B. G., Craig, J. C., Wilson, A. M., Pisoni, D. B. and Rhodes, R. P. (1983) Vibrotactile identification of vowels. Journal of the Acoustical Society of America 73: 1766–78.

Hanin, L., Boothroyd, A. and Hnath-Chisolm, T. (1988) Tactile presentation of voice fundamental frequency as an aid to the speechreading of sentences. Ear and Hearing 9: 329–34.

Hnath-Chisolm, T. and Boothroyd, A. (1992) Speechreading enhancement by voice fundamental frequency: The effects of F0 contour distortions. Journal of Speech and Hearing Research 35: 1160–8.

Hnath-Chisolm, T. and Kishon-Rabin, L. (1988) Tactile presentation of voice fundamental frequency as an aid to the perception of speech pattern contrasts. Ear and Hearing 9: 329–34.

Hnath-Chisolm, T. and Medwetsky, L. (1988) Perception of frequency contours via temporal and spatial tactile transforms. Ear and Hearing 9: 322–8.

Kirman, J.H. (1973) Tactile communication of speech: A review and an analysis. Psychological Bulletin, 80, 54-74.

Klatzky, E.L., Lederman, S.J. and Metzger, V.A. (1985) Identifying objects by touch: An 'expert system'. Perception and Psychophysics 37: 299–302.

Kuhl, P.K., Williams, K.A. and Meltzoff, A.N. (1991) Cross-modal speech perception in adults and infants using nonspeech auditory stimuli. Journal of Experimental Psychology: Human Perception and Performance 17: 829–40.

Levitt, H. (1988) Recurrent issues underlying the development of tactile sensory aids. Ear and Hearing 9: 301–5.

Liberman, A.M., Cooper, F.S., Shankweiler, D.P. and Studdert-Kennedy, M. (1968) Why are speech spectrograms hard to read? American Annals of the Deaf 113: 127–33.

Liberman, A.M. and Mattingly, I.G. (1985) The Motor Theory of Speech Perception Revised. Cognition 21: 1–36.

Lisker, L. (1978). Rabid vs. rapid: A catalog of acoustic features that may cue the distinction. Haskins Laboratories Status Report on Speech Research, SR-54, 127–32.

Loomis, J.M. and Lederman, S.J. (1986) Tactual perception. In Boff, L.R., Kaufman, L. and Thomas, J.P. (Eds) Handbook of Perception and Human Performance (Vol. 1). NY: Wiley.

Lynch, M.P., Eilers, R.E., Oller, D.K., Urbano, R.C. and Pero, P.J. (1989) Multisensory narrative tracking by a profoundly deaf subject using an electrocutaneous vocoder and a vibrotactile aid. Journal of Speech and Hearing Research 32: 331–8.

Massaro, D.W. (1987) Speech Perception by Ear and by Eye: a Paradigm for Psychological Inquiry. Hillsdale, NJ: Erlbaum.

Melara, R.D. and Marks, L.E. (1990) Dimensional interactions in language processing: Investigating directions and levels of crosstalk. Journal of Experimental Psychology: Learning, Memory, and Cognition 16: 539–54.

Nygaard, L.C. and Pisoni, D.B. (in press) Speech perception: New directions in research and theory. In Miller, J.L. and Eimas, P.D. (Eds) Handbook of Perception and Cognition. Vol. 11: Speech, Language, and Communication. New York: Academic Press.

Pickett, J.M. (1993) Personal communication.

Pisoni, D. B. and Luce, P. A. (1987) Acoustic-phonetic representations in word recognition. In Frauenfelder, U.H. and Tyler L.K. (Eds) Spoken Word Recognition. Cambridge, MA: MIT Press.

Plant, G. (1987) A single-transducer vibrotactile aid to lipreading. Speech Communication 6: 335–42.

Plant, G. and Risberg, A. (1983) The transmission of fundamental frequency variations via a single channel vibrotactile aid. Speech Transmission Laboratory. Quarterly Progress and Status Report, 2-3, 61–84.

Rabinowitz, W.M., Eddington, L.A., Delhorne, L.A. and Cuneao, P.A. (1992). Relations among different measures of speech reception in subjects using a cochlear implant. Journal of the Acoustical Society of America 92: 1869–81.

Rabinowitz, W.M., Reed, C.M., Delhorne, L.A. and Besing, J.M. (1994) Tactile and auditory measures of modulation resolution. Journal of the Acoustical Society of America 95: 2987.

Reed, C.M., Doherty, M J., Braida, L.D. and Durlach, NI. (1982). Analytic study of the Tadoma method: Further experiments with inexperienced observers. Journal of Speech and Hearing Research 25: 216–23.

Reed, C.M., Durlach, N.I. and Delhorne, L.A. (1992) Natural methods of tactual communication. Summers, I. (Ed) Tactile Aids for the Hearing Impaired. London: Whurr.

Reed, C.M., Rabinowitz, W.M., Durlach, N.I. and Braida, L.D. (1985) Research on the Tadoma method of speech communication. Journal of the Acoustical Society of America 77: 247–57.

Remez, R.E., Rubin, P.E., Berns, S.M., Pardon, J.S. and Lang, J.M. (1993, submitted). On the perceptual organization of speech.

Risberg, A. (1974) The importance of prosodic speech elements for the lipreader. Scandinavian Audiology 153–64.

Risberg, A. and Lubker, J. (1978) Prosody and speechreading. Speech Transmission Laboratory. Quarterly Progress and Status Report 4: 1–29.

Rosen, S. (1992).Temporal information in speech: Acoustic, auditory and linguistic aspects. Philosophical Transactions of the Royal Society, London B 336: 367–73.

Rosen, S., Fourcin, A.J. and Moore, B.C.J. (1981). Voice pitch as an aid to lipreading. Nature 291: 150–2.

Rothenberg, M., Verrillo, R. T., Zahorian, S.A., Brachman, M.L. and Bolanowski, S.J. (1977) Vibrotactile frequency for encoding a speech parameter. Journal of the Acoustical Society of America 62: 1003–12.

Rothenberg, M. and Molitor, R. (1979) Encoding voice fundamental frequency into vibrotactile frequency. Journal of the Acoustical Society of America 66: 1029–38.

Schultz, M.C., Norton, S.J., Conway-Fithian, S. and Reed, C.M. (1984) A survey of the use of the Tadoma method in the United States and Canada. Volta Review 86: 282–92.

Stevens, K.N., Keyser, S.J. and Kawasaki, H. (1986) Toward a phonetic and phonological theory of redundant features. In Perkell, J.S. and Klatt, D.H. (Eds) Invariance and Variability in Speech Processes. Hillsdale, NJ: Erlbaum.

Summers, I. (1992). Tactile Aids for the Hearing Impaired. London: Whurr.

Summerfield, Q. (1991). Visual perception of phonetic gestures. In Mattingly, I.G. and Studdert-Kennedy V. (Eds) Modularity and the Motor Theory of Speech Perception. Hillsdale, NJ: Erlbaum.

Tan, H.Z., Rabinowitz, W.M. and Durlach, N. (1989) Analysis of a synthetic Tadoma system as a multidimensional tactile display. Journal of the Acoustical Society of America 86: 981–7.

Weisenberger, J.M. (1986) Sensitivity to amplitude-modulated vibrotactile signals. Journal of the Acoustical Society of America 80: 1707–15.

Weisenberger, J.M., Broadstone, S.M. and Saunders, F.A. (1989) Evaluation of two multichannel aids for the hearing impaired. Journal of the Acoustical Society of America 86: 1764–75.

Part II
Cochlear Implants

9

Cochlear Implants: Historical Perspectives

GRAEME M. CLARK

These historical perspectives are seen from a personal point of view, and date back to the author's first involvement with cochlear implant research at the beginning of 1967. The perspectives are aimed at presenting the questions asked, the difficulties faced and the solutions achieved in the development of our multichannel cochlear prosthesis. Work in other centres is discussed when relevant, to set our research in context. Space does not permit a detailed presentation of our research or the contributions of others. It is hoped, however, that by presenting personal perspectives on the cut and thrust of human endeavour, and its interface with technology, a contribution will be made to the overall goal of understanding the origins of cochlear implants.

Cochlear implants arose, firstly, as a result of initial demonstrations in the nineteenth century that electrical stimulation of the ear produced hearing sensations, and, secondly, from the development of electronics in the twentieth century, enabling speech information to be presented electrically to the auditory nerve in a controlled way.

Count Alessandro Volta (1745–1827) was the first to report hearing with electrical stimulation of the ear, following an experiment on himself in which he inserted metal rods in his two ears and connected them to a battery compound of 30 or 40 zinc/silver couples. He reported his results to the president of the Royal Society of London, the Right Honourable Sir Joseph Banks, Bart, K.B.P.R.S., and the report was read before the Royal Society in 1800. This was published in French in the Philosophical Transactions of the Royal Society of London for the year 1800, part I, pages 403–31. An English translation of a section of this report is as follows:

> It only remains for me to say a word about hearing. I had tried without success to excite this sense with two single metallic plates, although they were the most active among all the movers of electricity, namely, one of silver or gold and the other zinc, but I finally managed to effect it with my new

apparatus, made up of 30 or 40 pairs of these metals. I introduced right into both ears two probes or rods of metal with rounded ends; I linked them up immediately to the two extremities of the apparatus. The moment when the circuit was completed in this way, I received a jolt in the head; and a few moments later (the circuit operating continuously without any interruptions), I began to feel a sound, or rather a noise, in my ears which I cannot define clearly; it was a kind of jerky crackling or bubbling, as though some paste or tenacious matter was boiling. This noise continued without stopping and without increasing all the time the circuit was complete, etc. The disagreeable sensation of the jolt in the brain, which I feared might be dangerous, was such that I did not repeat this experiment several times (translated by E.C. Forsyth).

In spite of the unpleasant sensation experienced by Volta, sporadic attempts to investigate the phenomenon were carried out over the next 50 years, but the sensation was always momentary and lacked tonal quality.

Hearing Due to Electrical Stimulation of the Ear: 1850 to the 1950s

More detailed investigations of the phenomenon of hearing with electrical stimulation began in the middle of the nineteenth century. These were possible due to a knowledge of electromagnetism and electric circuit design, and are summarized in the Doctorate of Philosophy thesis (Clark, 1969a) a book chapter (Clark et al., 1990) and a review paper (Clark, 1992).

The first report of stimulating the ear with an alternating current was by Duchenne of Boulogne who in 1855 (cited by Simmons, 1966) achieved this by inserting a vibrator into a circuit containing a condenser and induction coil. A sound which resembled 'the beating of a fly's wings between a pane of glass and a curtain' was experienced. This phenomenon was studied more extensively by Brenner in 1868 (cited by Simmons, 1966), and he showed that hearing was better with an electrical stimulus which produced a negative polarity in the ear.

More thorough investigations were made possible by the introduction of the thermonic valve which allowed the auditory system to be stimulated with greater precision. An important question that needed to be answered, which is still relevant today, was what caused the phenomenon. The Russian investigators Gersuni and Volokhov (1936) showed that hearing could be produced even after the removal of the ossicles, suggesting that the cochlea was the site of stimulation. Stevens and Jones (1939) and Jones et al., (1940) showed there were three mechanisms which produced hearing when the cochlea was stimulated electrically. Firstly, the middle ear could act as a transducer which obeys the 'square law', and convert alterations in the strength of an electrical field into the mechanical vibrations that produce sound. Secondly, electrical energy could be transduced by a linear mechanism into sound by a direct effect on the basilar membrane, which would then vibrate maximally at a point determined by the frequency, and these vibrations would stimulate the hair cells. Thirdly, a crude hearing sensation could be produced in patients with minimal or absent hearing, and this was probably due to direct stimulation of the auditory nerve.

Initial Studies on Speech Perception when Electrically Stimulating the Cochlea and Auditory Nerve: the 1950s and 1960s

The above reports summarize work from 1850 to the 1950s carried out primarily to study the phenomenon of hearing induced by electrical stimulation. Initial studies on patients were carried out in the 1950s and 1960s to see if speech perception could be achieved in profoundly deaf people using electrical stimulation. In these studies although the patients could recognize some stimuli as speech-like, they were basically not able to understand what was said. These studies were reviewed in my Doctorate of Philosophy thesis (Clark, 1969a).

One of the first recorded attempts to stimulate the auditory nerve was by Lundberg in 1950 (cited by Gisselsson, 1950), who did so with a sinusoidal current during a neurosurgical operation. The patient, however, could only hear noise.

A more detailed study was performed by Djourno and Eyries (1957), and the stimulus parameters appear to have been well controlled. In their patient, the electrodes were placed on the auditory nerve, which was exposed during an operation for cholesteatoma. The patient was able to appreciate differences in pitch in increments of 100 pulses per second (pulses/s) up to a frequency of 1000 pulses/s. He was able to distinguish certain words such as 'papa', 'maman', and 'allo'.

Another investigation was carried out by Simmons et al., (1964) who were able to stimulate the auditory nerve and inferior colliculus in a patient undergoing a craniectomy for a cerebellar ependymoma. The stimuli were varied in frequency from 1 to 1000 pulses/s, in pulse duration from 0.1 to 1.0 milliseconds (ms), and in amplitude from 0.01 to 2.0 V. The patient was able to differentiate different frequencies from 20–3500 pulses/s, and at 850 pulses/s had a difference limen of 5 pulses/s. Electrode placement was found to be critical, and hearing could not be experienced unless the two electrodes were aligned parallel to the fibres of the auditory nerve. In this study, the patient had satisfactory cochlear function, and thus his ability to detect a frequency of 3500 pulses/s was probably due to the fact that hearing was electrophonic in origin. Stimulation of the inferior colliculus, however, produced no hearing sensation.

At about the same time a study was performed by Doyle *et al.*, (1964). They superimposed speech signals on a train of square waves using an active electrode placed extracochlearly on or near the round window. The patients were able to perceive the rhythm of speech and music, to differentiate high from low tones, and to distinguish an occasional word. Similar results were obtained with a single active electrode inserted directly into the cochlea. In one patient four electrodes were introduced at four locations in the cochlea. These electrodes were stimulated sequentially with square waves upon which were superimposed speech signals. There was, however, no filtering of the speech, but nevertheless the patient was reported to be able to repeat phrases. It is not clear whether these phrases were from an open or closed set.

A more extensive study was reported by Simmons *et al.*, (1965), and Simmons (1966) who described the results of implanting six electrodes into the modiolus of the cochlea in a patient with complete perceptive deafness. The electrodes were implanted along the modiolus so that nerve fibres representing different frequencies could be stimulated. The patient was then tested to determine the effect of alterations in the frequency and intensity of the signal. Monopolar and bipolar stimulation were compared, speech and pulse-encoded speech were given, and the waveform of the stimulus was also varied.

The results indicated that the patient could detect a change in pitch up to a frequency of 300 pulses/s. Single stimuli produced a pitch sensation, and this varied according to the position of the stimulating electrode. There was also correlation between the position of the electrode and the pitch elicited with stimulation, so that a rough frequency scale was apparent. This is evidence in support of the place theory of hearing.

When speech signals were used as electrical stimuli, the patient could not understand their meaning, but could recognize them as speech, possibly from the rhythm. An attempt was made to separate the speech spectrum into frequency bands, and to process each band to produce pulse stimuli which would make more efficient use of the characteristic 'pitches' of the various electrodes, but this also failed to produce speech intelligibility.

Work was also carried out by W.F. House and associates during this period, but was not published till later (House *et al.*, 1976). Some of Dr House's initial studies were undertaken with J.M. Doyle and J.B. Doyle whose independent work is referred to above. In 1961 the promontory of a deaf patient was electrically stimulated for a period of several weeks and 'his best responses were within the range 40–200 pulses/s'. Electrodes were subsequently implanted in the scala tympani of this and another patient. Hearing sensations were induced but special tests were not available at the time to determine specific responses. The intracochlear electrodes were removed from both patients after a few weeks because of adverse effects thought to be due to infection and allergy (Clark *et al.*, 1990).

Basic Research in the 1960s

In the 1950s and 1960s the above attempts to help deaf people understand speech, although unsuccessful, led to the hope that eventually this would be possible. Furthermore, in the 1960s there was excitement in the medical profession as a whole that there were two frontiers in medicine that remained to be enlarged. These were firstly genetic engineering, and secondly the restoration of central nervous and sensory function, of which the alleviation of sensorineural deafness was an example. The initial spirit of optimism, in the latter case, however, was tempered by reservations from scientists involved in hearing research.

These reservations were voiced as early as 1964 by M. Lawrence (1964) who said that 'direct stimulation of the auditory nerve fibres with resultant perception of speech is not feasible'. He came to this conclusion on a number of grounds. Firstly, previous studies had shown that there was only a 10 dB dynamic range for electrical stimulation which would be too small to be practicable when considering the 120 dB range of the normal ear. Secondly, the innervation patterns of dendrites in the cochlea were complex, and no one-to-one relation existed between the dendrites of the ganglion cells and a position on the basilar membrane. It was assumed that the discrimination of frequency and intensity depended on these innervation patterns, and it would therefore be difficult for electrical stimulation to simulate the results of acoustic stimulation. Thirdly, there was evidence that if hair cells were lost, the fibres eventually degenerated back through the cell bodies in Rosenthal's canal. Furthermore, it was conceivable that entering the inner ear fluids with an electrode would eventually lead to degeneration of any remaining nerve fibres.

To help answer some of these questions I firstly commenced a physiological study in 1967 to compare the unit responses in the brainstem for acoustical and electrical stimulation using different stimulus parameters. This was done to see how well electrical stimulation could simulate the temporal responses to acoustical stimulation.

The study showed that the main differences between the responses to electrical square wave and acoustical stimulation were that neurons fired more synchronously or deterministically to electrical stimulation, and more asynchronously or stochastically to acoustical stimulation (Clark, 1969a, 1969b). In view of these findings it was hoped that by stimulating electrically with a sine rather than square wave it would be possible to induce more stochastic firing as occurs with sound. Unfortunately no differences were seen between these two modes of electrical stimulation. The above study also showed sustained firing did not occur for most neurons above 200 pulses/s. A small number responded up to 500 pulses/s and even then as shown in the perstimulus time histogram in Figure 1 there was loss of the normal onset response, and suppression of firing after the stimulus.

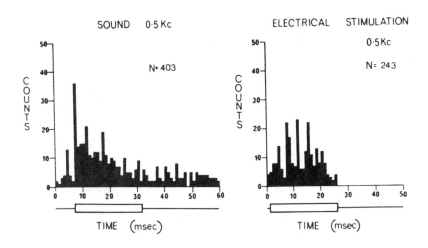

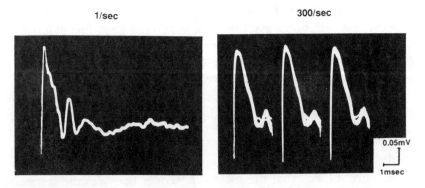

Figure 1. Top left: perstimulus (poststimulus) time histogram of unit responses from the superior olivary complex of the cat to a 500 Hz tone burst (Clark, 1969a, 1992). Top right: perstimulus time histogram for a 500 pulses/s burst of electrical square wave pulses. Bottom left: field potentials from the superior olivary complex of the cat in response to electrical pulses at 1 pulse/s. Bottom right: field potentials as above for pulses at 300 pulses/s (Clark, 1970, 1992).

To overcome the problem of sampling responses from a limited number of neurons in an auditory brainstem nucleus, the changes in the amplitudes of field potentials were also determined for different rates of stimulation. This was carried out since field potentials are the result of unit activity in a number of neurons. The results (Figure 1) showed marked reduction in field potential amplitudes at various sites within the superior olive for stimulus rates of 300 pulses/s and above (Clark, 1970). The field potential studies confirmed the perstimulus time data that there were limitations in maintaining unit responses to electrical stimulation above about 200–300 pulses/s.

The neurophysiological research, summarized above, showing the limitations of coding frequency on a rate coding basis, suggested that in order to adequately understand speech, the frequencies would need to be represented by place of stimulation.

In the 1960s the physiological effects of electrical stimulation of the auditory nerve were also studied by Moxon (1967, 1968). The prime aim of this research was to determine whether the maximum firing rate of auditory nerve fibres to acoustical stimuli (approximately 200 spikes/s) was a result of the refractoriness of the nerve fibres or to more peripheral mechanisms in the cochlea. Electrical stimulation was used as it would bypass the cochlea and determine whether the refractory properties of the auditory nerve were similar to those of other nerves, and whether or not they would account for the maximum response rate to acoustical stimulation. The refractory period of the auditory nerve fibres was determined by presenting pairs of electrical stimuli. It was shown that the absolute refractory period could be as short as 0.5 ms. While the refractory period recorded this way indicates the maximum possible instantaneous discharge rate, it does not necessarily mean the fibre is able to fire continuously at this rate. In a further study it was shown that with bursts of electrical stimuli the initial maximum rate of stimulation was 900 pulses/s, but this fell to 500 pulses/s over two minutes. The maximum rate of stimulation possible with electrical stimulation was dependent on the stimulus intensity, being greater with a higher current level. The study also showed that the dynamic range from threshold to a 100% response rate was much narrower with electrical compared to acoustical stimulation.

Subsequently, Moxon (1971) carried out research to find out if there was a physiological basis for electrophonic hearing, previously studied by Stevens and Jones (1939) and the others referred to above. The research showed that with electrical stimulation there were two types of auditory nerve responses. Firstly, there were responses due to direct electrical stimulation of the auditory nerve. These responses were more deterministic than for clicks. Secondly, there were responses due to electromechanical stimulation of the cochlea. These were similar to those induced by acoustical stimuli.

In the 1960s there were strong reservations that implanting electrodes into the cochlea could lead to degeneration of the nerve fibres it was hoped to stimulate. This reservation was one of those voiced by Lawrence (1964), and it persisted well into the 1970s and even into the 1980s. It arose from basic experimental studies which had shown that cochlear pathology could lead to degeneration of auditory nerve fibres (Schuknecht, 1953). It was also thought by others that electrode insertion itself would result in a similar marked loss of neural elements. This view received support from clinical observations by otologists that the cochlea was very sensitive to trauma during a stapedectomy. As a result otologists treated the cochlea with great respect and avoided inserting anything into it if at all possible.

The possibility of implanting electrodes into the cochlea without significant loss of nerve fibres was initially investigated in the experimental animal by Simmons (1967). This research showed that the round window membrane could be incised, perilymph aspirated and a metallic electrode inserted for weeks to months without widespread cochlear degeneration.

At this time concern was also expressed that a majority of profoundly deaf people would not have sufficient residual spiral ganglion cells or auditory nerve fibres to stimulate electrically and produce speech comprehension. This was based on data from Kerr and Schuknecht (1968) that only 25% of the cochleas they examined histologically had two-thirds or more of a normal spiral ganglion cell population remaining, and their hypothesis was that a two-thirds proportion was required for speech comprehension.

So in summary, by the end of the 1960s there had been, as discussed above, a few preliminary studies on patients to see what percepts were experienced when varying electrical stimulus parameters. It had not been possible, however, to present speech by electrical stimulation in a way that enabled subjects to comprehend words or sentences. The mid to late 1960s also saw the start of the physiological research aimed at specifically studying the coding of frequency by electrical stimulation (Clark, 1969a, 1969b). Furthermore, there had been a preliminary study to see if it was feasible to implant electrodes into the cochlea without an inevitable loss of nerve fibres or ganglion cells (Simmons, 1967).

Research Directions for the Future: Proposed in 1969

As a result of the above reported studies it was my personal view, at the time, that progress would be best achieved by a more basic and detailed scientific study of the different aspects of the problem. This is outlined in the introduction to my Doctorate of Philosophy thesis quoted below (Clark, 1969a).

> In the case reports described above, experience with direct electrical stimulation of the auditory nerve and its terminal fibres indicates that the surgical treatment of perceptive deafness is possible. A number of problems will have to be solved, however, before satisfactory speech intelligibility can be achieved.
>
> Electrical stimulation of the auditory nerve could not be expected to produce hearing in patients with damage to the higher auditory centres. Many children and some adults with perceptive deafness, however, have a lesion involving the cochlea and not the higher centres (Ormorod, 1960), and could be helped when their deafness is severe. A number of patients with presbycusis also have a lesion involving the cochlea (Schuknecht, 1964), but their hearing loss is usually not severe enough to warrant this form of treatment.
>
> It would also be desirable to have clinical tests which enable patients to be selected into those most likely to benefit from the operation. Tests of speech intelligibility and the presence of recruitment are satisfactory when some residual hearing remains, but in the patients where severe or total deafness is present these methods would not be adequate. It is possible that an objective test of hearing using preliminary electrical stimulation of the cochlea could be devised.
>
> The type of electrodes used, and their method of implantation will also have to receive careful consideration. Simmons (1967) has shown that when electrodes are chronically implanted their resistance increases, and this could lead to unreliable stimulation. He has also demonstrated that when electrodes are chronically implanted in the scala tympani of cats through an incision in the round window, the surgical trauma need not cause permanent cochlear damage. The factors responsible for degeneration of the organ of Corti and auditory nerve fibres were unpredictable, however, infection was found to consistently produce widespread destruction of tissue.
>
> Consequently, the site and method of implantation are important as the neural pathways can be damaged, and this would prevent the electrical signals being transmitted to the higher centres. Destruction of the cochlea can lead to transneuronal degeneration in the cochlear and superior olivary nuclei up to a year after the production of the lesions (Powell and Erulkar, 1962). If the hair cells can be preserved, however, this degeneration would probably not occur, as Schuknecht (1953) has shown that experimental damage of hair cells does not cause secondary nerve degeneration. This only occurs when the changes in the organ of Corti become so severe that they involve the supporting cells.
>
> Not only do these technical problems require solution, but a greater understanding of the encoding of sound is desirable. As emphasized by Lawrence (1964), the terminal auditory nerve fibres are connected to the hair cells in a complex manner, which could make it difficult for electrical stimulation to simulate sound.
>
> The relative importance of the volley and place theories in frequency coding is also relevant to the problem. If the volley theory is of great importance in coding frequency, would it be possible for different nerve fibres, conducting the same frequency information, to be stimulated in such a way

that they fired in phase at stimulus rates greater than 1000 pulse/s. If this was possible, it would then have to be decided whether this could be done by stimulating the auditory nerve as a whole, or whether local stimulation of different groups of nerve fibres in the cochlea would be sufficient. On the other hand, if the place theory is of great importance in coding frequency, would it matter whether the electrical stimulus caused excitation of nerve fibres at the same rate as an auditory stimulus, or could the nerve fibres passing to a particular portion of the basilar membrane be stimulated without their need to fire in phase with the stimulus?

If the answers to these questions indicate that stimulation of the auditory nerve fibres near their terminations in the cochlea is important, then it will be necessary to know more about the internal resistances and lines of current flow in the cochlea, and whether the electrical responses normally recorded are a reflection of the transduction of sound into nerve discharges, or directly responsible for stimulating the nerve endings.

The final criterion of success will be whether the patient can hear, and understand speech. If pure tone reproduction is not perfect, meaningful speech may still be perceived if speech can be analysed into its important components, and these used for electrical stimulation. More work is required, however, to decide which signals are of greatest importance in speech perception (Clark, 1969a).

Research in the 1970s

The beginning of the 1970s saw a change in goals from the preliminary human and experimental animal studies to the pursuit in earnest of speech understanding, using electrical stimulation of the auditory nerve.

In my own case I decided in 1970, on the basis of the initial animal experimental study discussed above, to develop a multiple-channel implant. As there were limitations to the coding of sound by using temporal information via a single stimulus channel it was reasoned that multiple-channel stimulation could provide the necessary additional information. I also considered that it would not be appropriate to use a percutaneous plug and socket for the investigation of speech processing strategies in initial patients, as my experience with plugs and sockets in experimental animals had been that they frequently became infected. This meant, however, that a difficult and prolonged engineering design task was required to produce an implantable package that had the necessary electronics to permit speech processing strategies to be evaluated that would help profoundly deaf people understand speech. As the task was going to require years of work and there were many design problems to overcome, it was very important to make a correct decision on the circuit design, so that not only could the correct stimulus parameters be tested, but the power consumption of a speech processor would be low enough to reduce the number of batteries, and hence overall size, to convenient proportions. Although it would have been a lot easier to investigate different speech processing strategies with the flexibility of a plug and socket it was considered inappropriate to subject the initial patients to the greater risk of infection.

The development of an implantable receiver-stimulator also required research to determine the best method of: transmitting data and power through the skin; packaging the electronics so that signals could pass to and from the device without the ingress of corrosive body fluids; and designing and fabricating a multiple-electrode array to allow stimulation of discrete groups of nerve fibres.

Experimental animal behavioural research

When our work to develop an implantable multiple-channel receiver-stimulator commenced, research on experimental animals was continued to confirm the previous physiological findings showing the limitations of using single-channel stimulation to convey temporal information. This was also carried out so we could be sure the large investment in time, money and effort to produce a prototype multiple-channel implant was needed.

As it was considered that the firing patterns of cells to acoustic and electric stimulation seen with the physiological research (Clark 1969a, 1969b), did not necessarily correlate with percepts experienced by the alert animal, behavioural studies were carried out on experimental animals to examine the limitation of using stimulus rate by determining rate difference limens.

The first study (Clark *et al.*, 1972) showed that cats had only a very limited ability to discriminate changes in rate of stimulation above 200 pulses/s in spite of the fact that loudness differences associated with rate of stimulation were not controlled for. Even at rates of 100 and 200 pulses/s the difference limens for rate of stimulation were considerably poorer than for sounds of the same frequency. Furthermore, at the conclusion of the experiments the temporal bones were sectioned and the cochleas examined to ensure that there were no residual hair cells that could have led to false results from electrophonic hearing. The results of this study therefore indicated that there would be serious limitations in using single-channel electrical stimulation to code the high frequencies required for speech intelligibility.

A second behavioural study on cats (Clark *et al.*, 1973) was carried out to help confirm the results of the first study, and to compare the responses for varying the rate of electrical stimulation over time with those for comparable acoustic stimuli. This was done as a great deal of information in speech is conveyed by variations in frequency over time, and it was considered important to see how well a rate or time-period code could also convey this information along a single stimulus channel.

The two parts of the study were undertaken by conditioning cats to respond to sound and electrical stimuli that were frequency-modulated. Electrodes were implanted in the basal turn of the cochlea and responses compared for changing rates of electrical stimulation. The measurements were also repeated after any residual hair cells were destroyed using an ultra-high frequency electron beam to exclude electrophonic hearing. The destruction of hair cells was determined by failure to record cochlear microphonics, and by the absence of hair cells in the cochleas subsequently examined under light microscopy.

The results from the first part of this study showed that changes in rate of stimulation could be detected for electrophonic hearing at 2400 pulses/s in cat 1 and 1600 pulses/s in cat 2, but for direct electrical stimulation of the auditory nerve only at 600 pulses/s in cat 1 and 800 pulses/s in cat 2. This indicated that hair cell function could be preserved for frequencies below 2400 Hz when an electrode was inserted through the round window into the scala tympani of the basal turn of the cochlea. This also meant that care would need to be taken when interpreting results from deaf implant patients as residual hair cells and electrophonic hearing could lead to better speech perception scores than when auditory nerve fibres alone were stimulated. On the other hand, they also suggested that electrical stimulation in patients with some residual hearing may be beneficial.

The second part of the above behavioural study on cats was undertaken to measure more accurately the ability of cats to detect a changing stimulus rate, as this is an important cue in speech comprehension and was relevant to the design of a cochlear implant that would help patients understand running speech. The study was carried out by varying the slope or rate of change in stimulus rate or frequency for electrical stimuli of 200 pulses/s and 2000 pulses/s, and sound at 200 Hz and 2000 Hz. The carrier frequencies were modulated by triangular waves to produce graded changes in frequency over a duration of 500 ms. The results for sound at 200 Hz and electrical stimuli at 200 pulses/s were similar. The ability of cats to detect changes in rate of stimulation at high stimulus rates (2000 pulses/s) was poor compared to that for sound at the same frequency.

A third study was undertaken to help confirm the findings on rate of stimulation in the above two cat behavioural studies (Williams et al., 1976). The effect of rate of stimulation was evaluated by requiring the cats to make comparative judgements of whether a stimulus was higher or lower than a reference rather than requiring 'same' or 'different' judgements as in the first two studies. With this experimental design it was considered that the cats were more likely to respond to the psychophysical correlate of pitch. The intensity variations that occur with changes in stimulus rate were controlled for. In this series of experiments signal detection theory was the basis for determining thresholds for different combinations of stimuli. The thresholds were obtained by scoring responses as hits, misses, false alarms and correct rejections, and plotting a receiver-operating curve. The thresholds recorded by this method were independent of decision criterion levels. In this study electrophonic hearing was controlled for by administering neomycin in dose levels needed to destroy hair cells. The destruction of hair cells was subsequently confirmed by serially sectioning the cochleas and examining the sections under light microscopy.

The results of the study showed that, when electrophonic hearing was excluded by the destruction of hair cells, the cats could at least discriminate stimulus rates which varied from 348 to 490 pulses/s, but not at higher rates. These stimulus rates could be discriminated with electrodes placed in either the apical or basal turns of the cochlea.

The three behavioural studies on experimental animals described above were carried out in parallel with the engineering development of a prototype multiple-channel cochlear implant. They helped confirm the limitation of using rate information on a single channel alone, and further emphasized the need for the development of the multiple-channel implant.

The engineering development of the implantable receiver-stimulator for multiple-channel stimulation of the auditory nerve

The physiological and behavioural studies on the experimental animal discussed above provided data for the design (Forster, 1978) of The University of Melbourne's prototype receiver-stimulator first implanted on 1 August 1978.

The information showed, firstly, that as there were limitations in coding pitch by rate or timing of stimulation it would be necessary to code pitch on a place basis as well, in order to maximize speech understanding. To do this would require implanting a number of electrodes in the cochlea so that discrete groups of auditory nerve fibres could be stimulated. This would require either transmitting speech information to the multiple-electrode arrays by direct link through the skin (percutaneous plug) or by implanting a receiver-stimulator unit and sending the information transcutaneously through the intact skin.

The engineering development of the receiver-stimulator is summarized in Table 1.

Transcutaneous vs percutaneous link

It was decided back in 1971 to use transcutaneous stimulation. This decision was made for a number of reasons. Firstly, my experience with the long-term use of percutaneous plugs in animals had shown that there was a tendency for the skin to become macerated at its junction

Table 1. The engineering of the receiver-stimulator

Receiver-stimulator

Transutaneous vs percutaneous link
Type of transcutaneous link
Analogue vs digital circuits
Data and power transfer
Electronic design
Packaging
Connector
Lead wire assembly
Biocompatibility
Reliability

---

with the plug, and for a sinus to occur beside the plug. The sinus provided a nidus for infection which could track around the foreign body and become chronic. Eradicating the infection became difficult and it had to be controlled with the topical application of antibiotics or the removal of the foreign material. Secondly, the percutaneous plugs could be easily damaged and the electrodes dislodged or fractured. Thirdly, it was considered that percutaneous plugs would not be aesthetically acceptable, especially in children.

Transcutaneous link

The next decision was how to transmit the coded speech information through intact skin to an implanted receiver-stimulator. Should this be carried out by an electromagnetic link, by optical signals, or ultrasonically? After consideration it was decided to use electromagnetic induction as the most efficient and reliable method. Electromagnetic induction is based on the principle that a magnetic flux produced by passing a current through a coil (external) will induce a current in a second coil (internal).

In addition, it was necessary that adequate power be transferred from the external to internal coils over a distance that would vary depending on the thickness of a patient's skin and underlying tissues. It was desirable that some lateral misalignment be possible between the two coils. The engineering studies showed that there would be adequate power transfer over a distance of up to 10 mm when the coils were coaxial, with some degree of misalignment possible at a shorter distance.

Analogue vs digital circuits

For transmitting coded speech signals and power another important decision was whether to use analogue or digital circuitry or a combination of both in the design of the receiver-stimulator unit.

Analogue circuits are those where continuously varying physical parameters such as voltages can be altered or combined. With analogue circuitry the instantaneous amplitude of speech could be converted into a voltage proportional to the amplitude. The voltage could then be transmitted to the receiver-stimulator where the induced voltages (or currents) would be used to stimulate nerve fibres. On the other hand, with digital circuitry the frequency and instantaneous amplitude of speech would be transmitted and extracted as a digital code. The digital code would be represented by discrete pulses, and could be quantified as a series of digits or numbers which could then be manipulated mathematically.

There were, and still are, a number of advantages in using a digital system. Firstly, it is straightforward to combine the control information for each electrode pair into a single signal, and to recover this information in the receiver-stimulator. A single transmission path or pair of induction coils can then be used for a multiple-electrode implant. On the other hand, with a multiple-electrode analogue system, separate coils would be needed for each electrode pair in order to minimize power consumption. This would mean a bulky receiver-stimulator system which would be awkward to implant, especially in children. Secondly, digitally controlled current sources are more reliable with high noise immunity and would therefore deliver well-defined stimuli. The speech processor could be precisely adjusted to suit individual patients.

In view of the above advantages and the ready availability of digital designs in integrated circuit silicon chip technology, a digital receiver-stimulator system was realized.

Data and power transfer

Data and power were transmitted by modulating a carrier wave. The modulated wave was decoded by the implanted receiver-stimulator electronics, and the power and coded speech signals extracted. In the case of the prototype receiver-stimulator power was transmitted at a carrier frequency of 112 kHz, and speech data at 10.752 MHz (Clark *et al.*, 1977a, 1977b).

Electronic design

The design of the prototype receiver-stimulator (Clark *et al.*, 1977a, 1977b) needed to allow for as much flexibility as possible in the use of stimulus parameters as we were not sure how to produce a speech-processing strategy that would enable patients to understand running speech, or the range of parameters required. It was designed so that intensity could be varied from a minimum of 80 μA to a maximum of approximately 1 mA in 70-μA steps. The rate of stimulation could be varied in 125-μs steps up to 1 kHz on each of ten stimulus channels, and the phase relations between pulses could be varied in eight 126-μs periods (Clark *et al.*, 1977a, 1977b).

The design of the prototype receiver-stimulator was realized using a hybrid circuit in which various commercially available components as well as a custom-made integrated circuit were interconnected on three substrates using thick film technology.

Packaging

The packaging of the receiver-stimulator electronics was considered to be very important, and this was carried out using an hermetically sealed Kovar container impervious to body fluids. The sealing needed to be validated using helium leak testing. Helium was used as it can be detected in very small concentrations, and has a fast diffusion rate. The Kovar containers had metal-to-glass feedthroughs and the two sections were sealed by soldering. Although these containers were satisfactory for space flights, the body is a more hostile environment. There was therefore still concern that the body tissues and fluids could erode the glass insulation around the wires, or surface tension forces could enlarge small cracks in the glass so they became fluid entry paths. Furthermore, with time, the metals in the solder could migrate or produce corrosion from an electrolytic reaction, and thus lead to weaknesses in the seal. Nevertheless, this was the best packaging option at the time.

Connector

The initial receiver-stimulator needed a connector so that it could be replaced if there was an electronic failure. It should be added, however, that with pacemakers the least likely failure is an electronic one, and the same situation was envisaged with cochlear implants. Furthermore, it was shown with experimental animal work prior to our second implant in 1979 that as implantations and reinsertions could be carried out with ease using our smooth, free-fitting electrode array, a connector would not be necessary.

With a connector, pressure between contact points needed to be maintained for many years, and the same metals were required to avoid corrosion. Furthermore, the connector had to be designed so that body fluids could not enter and cause current leakage between the electrodes.

The connector used for the prototype receiver-stimulator consisted of a pair of substrates with conductor patterns printed on them, and layers of conducting and non-conducting elastomate material between the two substrates. The elastomate was compressed between the substrates thus connecting matching sections of the conductor patterns. It was found that the elastomate lost compression over time.

Research for the design and development of an electrode array

The design and development of an electrode array for a multiple-channel cochlear implant required answers to a number of questions. These were: where to locate an array within the cochlea to minimize trauma; where to place electrodes so they would lie close to the auditory nerves that normally convey the speech frequencies; how to localize the stimulus current to discrete groups of nerve fibres, to provide frequency coding on a place basis; which metals to use for the electrodes; and how to avoid corrosion with electrical stimulation? We commenced research in 1971 to help answer these questions.

Electrode placement to minimize trauma

To determine where to optimally locate electrodes within the cochlea to minimize trauma, we either placed electrodes in the scala vestibuli or scala tympani of the cat cochlea by drilling separate openings through the overlying bone or inserting an electrode carrier along the scalae. The cochleas were subsequently examined for histological evidence of trauma and loss of spiral ganglion cells. The results showed that considerable damage could occur (Figure 2) when separate electrodes were placed in the cochlea through individual openings in the overlying bone. In a separate study, other bones were implanted through openings drilled in the bone overlying the cochlea and the results are reported in detail by Clark et al. (1975a). Less trauma (Figure 3), however, was seen when a free-fitting electrode carrier was inserted along the scala tympani of the basal turn (Clark et al, 1975a). The histological sequelae of electrodes placed through separate drill holes in the cochlea were such (Figure 2) that this placement was not considered the best option for a multiple-electrode implant.

Electrode placement close to the auditory nerves in the speech frequency range

Having demonstrated that there would be less trauma if electrodes were passed along the scala tympani, the next problem to be faced was how to insert electrodes far enough around the scala tympani so that they could lie close to the nerve fibres normally transmitting the speech frequency range. Our preliminary attempts to insert electrodes along the scala tympani of the basal turn through the round window were not very successful, and the electrodes did not pass more than

Figure 2. A photomicrograph of the cat cochlea following the insertion of electrodes directly into the cochlea through openings drilled through the overlying bone.

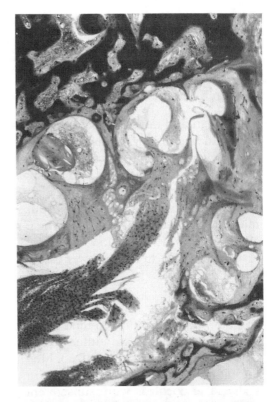

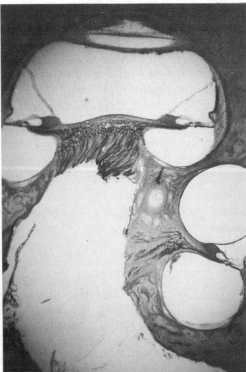

Figure 3. A photomicrograph of the cat cochlea following the insertion of a free-fitting electrode carrier through the round window and along the scala tympani of the basal turn.

about 15 mm. Indeed, the electrodes needed to be inserted 20 mm and preferably 25 mm to lie opposite the nerve fibres conducting the speech frequencies. To overcome this difficulty we experimented with alternatives which included drilling with care into the scala tympani at points around the cochlea so that electrode arrays could be threaded up the cochlea (anterograde insertion) along segments of both the basal and middle turns (Clark, 1975). With this technique the carrier could only be inserted a limited distance, and there was the problem of damage to underlying structures as a result of the fenestration. It was also difficult to expose the scala tympani of the middle turn due to its being overlapped by the scala vestibuli of the basal turn.

Another alternative was to pass an electrode array in a reverse direction (retrograde) along the scala tympani. In this case the electrode array was inserted through an opening drilled in the apical-to-middle turns and passed down to and along the basal turn. This method of insertion was studied in models of the human cochlea as well as in human temporal bones (Clark et al, 1975a). It was found that once the carrier was inserted into the scala tympani it moved freely along the scala as it passed into an expanding rather than a tightening spiral. However, a histopathological study on cats (Clark, 1977), in which the effects of inserting an array along the scala tympani through the round window were compared with those from a retrograde insertion through an opening in the apical-to-middle turns, showed that the latter method of insertion could cause more trauma than one through the round window. The increased trauma was due firstly to the fact that an opening drilled into the cochlea could damage underlying structures, and secondly, the array could enter the scala vestibuli and tear Reissner's membrane as it passed around the cochlea. In addition, the study established that if the electrode array was free-fitting and inserted through the round window it would cause minimal trauma.

Having shown with the studies referred to above that it was preferable to insert a smooth free-fitting electrode array via the round window along the scala tympani of the basal turn of the cochlea, the problem still remained how to insert it sufficiently far for it to lie opposite the nerves in the speech frequency range. To help answer this question we carried out a theoretical analysis of the strains within the array, and the effects of friction on the outer wall of the cochlea (Hallworth, 1976). The analysis demonstrated that a significant limitation to a deep insertion was friction between the electrode array and outer wall of the cochlea. Consequently, anything which would reduce this friction would result in a deeper insertion. The solution did not come, however, until it was realized that an electrode array could be inserted with reduced friction between it and the outer wall if it was made from a Silastic tube and had graded stiffness from the tip to the base. The latter was achieved with an electrode array by the sequential addition of wires along its length. As the wires were needed to provide electrical contact with the electrodes along the array, the solution was ultimately simple. Lubricants such as glycerine were also considered as a means of reducing the friction between the array and outer wall, but as they would have needed extensive biocompatibility studies the simplest solution of using a Silastic carrier with graded stiffness alone was finally adopted.

Current localization

Not only was it necessary to determine the optimal site for introducing electrodes into the cochlea to minimize trauma, but it was also necessary to determine the optimal sites for placing stimulating electrodes to achieve adequate current localization. To do this we developed a computer model of resistances within the cochlea using existing data (Black and Clark, 1977). This computer model plotted the voltage distributions for different electrode stimulus configurations: for example when stimulating between the scala vestibuli and scala tympani or between two electrodes in the scala tympani. The results showed that the best current localization could be expected from any array within the scala tympani.

The spread of current within the scala tympani of the cochlea was also studied using bipolar and monopolar electrodes. Using a technique developed by Merzenich (1974) it was possible to determine the spread of current along the cochlea by recording the thresholds of cells in the inferior colliculus to the electrical stimulus. The inferior colliculus receives a binaural input so that the frequency of best response for an acoustic stimulus from the contralateral ear indicates the site of stimulation along the cochlea of the implanted ear. In this way the thresholds for electrical stimulation can be plotted at different points along the cochlea. The results showed that for bipolar stimulation the voltage attenuation was 3–4 dB/mm, and for monopolar stimulation it was less than 1 dB/mm (Black and Clark, 1977; Black, 1978). These results were in agreement with those recorded by Merzenich (1974) who showed attenuation which ranged between 3.3 and 8 dB/mm. In his study, however, the results were only obtained with a moulded array which filled a large proportion of the scala tympani and restricted the flow of current around it.

The results from our study described above were obtained with a pair of bared wire electrodes lying radially across the scala tympani and freely within it (Black, 1978; Black and Clark, 1977).

Electrode metal

In developing an electrode array one of the issues was the metal to be used for the electrodes. Candidate materials included gold, platinum, stainless steel and tungsten. Gold electrodes were initially preferred by some (Michelson, 1971). We decided, however, to use platinum even though it was not a reversible electrode, and required an overvoltage before current flowed (Clark, 1973). It was also necessary to determine whether to use platinum black or polished platinum. The advantage of platinum black (a granular deposit of platinum produced by electrolysis) was that it increased the surface area, but this was significantly reduced in the presence of protein. We chose polished platinum, however, as being less likely to have impedance variations, and more likely to be reliable for the long-term interface with the nervous system.

Electrode corrosion

In designing an electrode array it was also necessary to ensure that the electrical stimulus parameters would not lead to corrosion and ultimately the complete loss of the electrodes. Furthermore, the release of heavy metal ions into the tissues could cause degeneration of auditory neurons. We also feared that heavy metals such as platinum could be taken up systemically from the cochlea and affect vital organs.

Studies to determine the effect of different stimulus parameters on the corrosion of platinum electrodes are outlined in the Doctorate of Philosophy thesis by Black (1978). The electrical stimuli investigated were either direct current or sinusoidal waves and pulses. The effect of current density on all these stimuli was determined, as well as rate of stimulation for the sinusoidal and pulsatile stimuli. The pulsatile stimuli were either monophasic or biphasic. In the latter case they were presented as either anode or cathode first, and were either charge-balanced or unbalanced.

The results showed a very high dissolution rate with d.c. currents especially when using a cathodic current. Monophasic stimulation produced dissolution one order of magnitude greater than biphasic stimulation. With biphasic stimuli the dissolution decreased as both current densities and pulse widths were reduced. With sinusoidal stimulation dissolution decreased with increasing frequency.

In summary, the study showed that for both biphasic pulsatile and sinusoidal stimulation a range of parameters existed where dissolution was very small. For biphasic stimulation this occurred for pulse widths of 5 ms or less, and current densities of 2.5 mA/geom. mm^2 or less. The information gained from this series of studies was very important in setting safe limits for presenting current to the stimulating electrodes. It established the use of biphasic, charge-balanced pulses with each phase being 180 μs in duration. In addition, the dissolution studies influenced the design of the electrode array where it was considered important to have electrodes with a large surface area to keep the charge density small and hence corrosion at a very low level.

To ensure also that if corrosion occurred it would not lead to systemic effects, we carried out a study in 1976 in which high concentrations of platinum chloride were injected into the cat cochlea and platinum levels determined spectrophotometrically in other structures and viscera (Shepherd, 1977). The results showed platinum in the subarachnoid space presumably via the cochlear aqueduct, but it was not detected elsewhere. It was assumed that if corrosion occurred it would be released in much smaller concentrations than with the cochlear injection in this study, and surrounding fibrous tissue would also restrict any spread via the cochlear aqueduct. Furthermore, as platinum was not detected elsewhere, systemic effects from corrosion, if they occurred, were not considered a problem.

Electrode design

As demonstrated above our research showed the preferred electrode site, the materials to be used, and the importance of having a large surface area for the electrodes in order to reduce corrosion, provided this did not significantly affect our ability to restrict current to a number of discrete groups of auditory nerve fibres. It remained to decide on the geometry and construction of the electrodes themselves.

In 1975 one line of investigation was the development of a multiple-electrode array by sputtering platinum onto a thin ribbon of Teflon so that a large number of electrode tracks and electrode pads could be condensed into a small space (Clark and Hallworth, 1976). The work was carried out in collaboration with the Weapons Research Laboratory, Salisbury; the Ammunition Factory, Maribyrnong; and the Royal Melbourne Institute of Technology. A number of variations to the thin film fabrication and etching techniques were explored, but it proved difficult to achieve an array that would bend sufficiently well to pass around the cochlea without cracks developing in the electrode tracks or pads. Furthermore, when the Teflon strips were inserted into the cats' cochleas their edges cut the basilar membrane as shown (Clark *et al.*, 1987 page 39: Fig. 16). As a result of the above findings this electrode array was not used with the first prototype receiver-stimulator.

While this work was being undertaken, research also commenced to see if it would be possible to make an appropriate array by more conventional procedures.

Initially, we decided to wrap the bared ends of 20 individual electrodes around a Silastic carrier as illustrated in Figure 4. This would have provided a large surface area. However, not long before the first operation was scheduled it was considered important to implant these arrays in human temporal bones to see if significant trauma would occur especially if removed for replacement with another. Alarmingly, removal of the electrode resulted in it cutting through the bone as though it were a Gigli saw. To avoid this problem a banded electrode was conceived and used for the first and subsequent patients (Figure 5). It provided the required large area to minimize the current density. Being circumferential it also had the advantage that it could be rotated to facilitate insertion, and still make good contact with the auditory neurons.

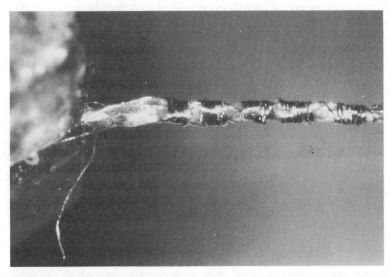

Figure 4. A multiple-electrode array with the bared ends of individual wires wrapped around a Silastic tube.

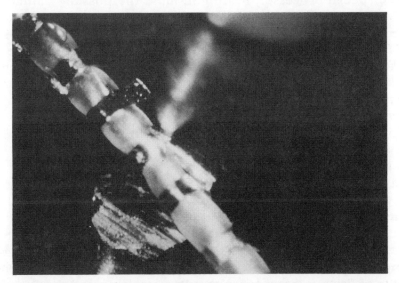

Figure 5. The banded multiple-electrode array being constructed in the Department of Otolaryngology, The University of Melbourne (improved manufacturing techniques are now being used by Cochlear Pty Limited for its fabrication).

Preliminary speech processing research

My initial speech research, aimed at developing a speech processing strategy for a multiple-channel cochlear implant, commenced in 1976 in collaboration with Dr William Ainsworth, Keele University, UK. This research was carried out to specify in a parallel speech synthesizer the formant frequencies of fricatives, plosives and nasals for optimal comprehension. This work was supplemented by a visit to the Department of Speech Communication and Music Acoustics, Royal Institute of Technology, Stockholm, where I met Gunnar Fant, Arne Risberg, Karl-Erik Spens and other members of the group, and saw some of the speech research being undertaken. I continued further work on the perception of speech formants in the Department of Otolaryngology, The University of Melbourne later in 1976. In this latter research, synthesized speech was presented to deaf children to determine what speech cues or formants they used in successfully understanding speech, when the more usual ones could not be heard because of their hearing loss (Clark *et al.*, 1976). The results of the initial study suggested that children were relying on the perception of the formant frequency transitions seen with coarticulation in consonant-vowel syllables, rather than the high frequency spectral energy normally of importance in say the recognition of fricatives.

As the time approached for the completion of the prototype receiver-stimulator and its first implantation in a profoundly deaf patient, it was also considered important to develop a physiologically-based speech processor, bearing in mind the possible limitations shown previously in the physiological and animal behavioural results referred to above (Clark 1969a, 1969b, 1970; Clark *et al.*, 1972, 1973, 1976). At the time the whole question of whether it was possible for profoundly deaf people to understand connected or running speech by electrical stimulation was completely open, so we had to be prepared to try a number of strategies, including physiologically-based ones. The development of this speech processor commenced jointly in the Departments of Otolaryngology and Electrical Engineering, The University of Melbourne in February 1978, 6 months prior to the first implantation (Laird, 1979).

The physiologically-based speech processor was designed to model the population responses of auditory neurons. This was carried out by using bandpass filters to approximate the frequency selectivity of the neurons. A delay mechanism was introduced to mimic that of the basilar membrane. A system was also incorporated to allow the stochastic firing of nerves to be reproduced. It was also designed so that the probability of firing increased over the dynamic range and the fine time structure of the phase-locking of the stimuli was preserved.

Selection of patients

The initial selection of patients required careful consideration. The future success of the programme would depend on this. If the first patient could not be helped, this would produce doubt in the minds of those watching the development. Obviously children were not suitable, as it was too experimental, and they would not be able to cooperate with us over what could be a long period of testing. Prelinguistically deaf adults were considered, but it was decided it should be preferable to study only postlinguistically deaf adults, as they should have memory for the sounds previously heard, and be able to compare the sensations obtained from electrical stimulation with those previously experienced with sound.

Although there were statistics to show there were significant numbers of profoundly deaf people who could benefit from an implant, there were initially no satisfactory volunteers. I was particularly concerned at first to see people who had no hearing, or virtually none, so that any effects obtained from electrical stimulation could not be attributed to electrophonic hearing (electrically mediated stimulation of residual hair cells).

Fortunately at the appropriate time two volunteers came forward. One was a 46-year-old man who lost all hearing following a recent car accident. The other volunteer was a 63-year-old man who had a partial hearing loss in 1944 following a bomb blast, and whose hearing deteriorated to the point where he had obtained no help with hearing aids for the previous 13 years. Both were thoroughly evaluated audiologically, had X-rays of the skull and temporal bones, and electrical stimulation of the cochlea to establish if they were able to obtain some hearing percepts. The details of their evaluations are described in more detail elsewhere (Clark *et al.*, 1977c, 1981a, 1981b, 1981c, 1981d).

Finally, the 46-year-old man was selected to be the first to have the implant, as he had a more recent hearing loss, and it was hoped he would therefore be better able to remember how the individual percepts compared with sounds previously heard.

Prior to any implantation it was considered important to have ethics approval from the organization to which we were responsible. At this time ethics committees were not in operation at a number of public hospitals, and it was necessary to have one created for the Department of Otolaryngology, The University of Melbourne at the Royal Victorian Eye and Ear Hospital, specifically for the purpose of reviewing the patients.

Operative procedure

One main concern in planning the operative procedure was to do everything possible to minimize the risk of infection. This was necessary as implanting any foreign body is associated with an increased incidence of infection. Furthermore, as the electrode entered the inner ear through the middle ear cavity there was also the additional likelihood that infection extending up the Eustachian tube could result in labyrinthitis. As a result, we developed a protocol to minimize infection which is presented in detail in Clark *et al.* (1980). The nose, pharynx, and skin in the area of the proposed incision were swabbed prior to surgery, and appropriate treatment instituted if a pathogen was found. In addition, apart from taking care with asepsis we developed a technique for operating in a horizontal laminar flow of filtered air.

It was decided to expose the operative area using an invented U-incision. Our anatomical dissections confirmed that if the incision was first made in the postauricular sulcus then extended upwards and backwards for 5 cm before taking it downwards and backwards for 4 cm, the flap would provide adequate exposure and still have an arterial supply from the occipital and postauricular arteries. In addition, the downward venous drainage, assisted by gravity, would be preserved. Thus we considered it to be a flap which should have good viability in most circumstances because of its arterial supply and venous drainage, as well as having a large width/length ratio.

The round window was exposed through a posterior tympanotomy using the procedures described by Jansen (1968) for middle ear surgery. We found it was preferable to use this approach to the round window rather than one down the ear canal as we found it easier to insert the electrode array a satisfactory distance along the basal turn when pushing along the line of movement rather than at right angles to it. Claws that not only steered the electrode tip into the round window, but also applied a force to the array were developed by us as reported in Clark *et al.* (1979). It was also proposed that the electrode might be held by suction if the shaft of the claw was hollow.

In our initial plans for the development of an implantable receiver-stimulator, made in the early 1970s, it was proposed that the device should be placed in the bone behind the ear. One advantage was that the bone there was free of muscle attachments or could be made free by stripping up the fascial attachment of the occipito-frontalis muscle. Furthermore, only a short electrode lead would be needed to reach the inner ear. Our behavioural studies on the cat in 1971 had demonstrated that muscle movements from the temporalis could fracture single-stranded electrode wires within a period as short as 3 weeks. Consequently, a site where muscle movements would not be transmitted to the electrode, and also where the electrode lead wire could be buried, for example in the mastoid cavity, was seen as important. In addition, a site behind the ear would be an appropriate place to locate a transmitting coil so that the device would look similar to a conventional hearing aid, and indicate to observers the person had a hearing defect.

In deciding on the dimensions of the implantable device a conflict occurred between surgeons and engineers. The surgeons naturally wanted it as small as possible and the engineers as large as possible! A compromise was reached and it had the dimensions: length 42 mm; width 32 mm; height of anterior connector section 8.5 mm; and height of posterior receiver-stimulator section 13 mm. Although a round package would have been preferred as it would have been a little easier to drill a bed to retain it in place, it was necessary to accept a square box as that was the shape of the Kovar container. A significant problem, however, was its height (13 mm) as this could result in it protruding too far above the surface of the skull if a shallow bed was made in the bone. There is, however, considerable variation in the thickness of the skull at the proposed site, and fortunately in the patient concerned it was possible to drill down approximately 6 mm and not expose dura mater widely, and so not have the package protrude to an extent where it was unsightly or prone to get bumped. (Following the considerable experience now obtained in implanting the Cochlear Pty. Limited device, there would appear to be no problems in exposing the dura mater at the bottom of the receiver-stimulator bed. Also the device should be designed with a flange or have a section of it resting on the outside of the skull, so that a blow to the head does not easily force the receiver-stimulator into the cranial cavity.)

With the implantation in the first patient a Silastic foam collar was pre-glued to the electrode bundle at a location that would allow it to fit snugly into the round window niche after implantation. The idea of using a Silastic foam collar was that fibrous tissue would grow into it, and help prevent the entry of infection into the inner ear. This meant, however, the need to make an initial insertion with a dummy electrode to gauge how far an array would pass along the scala tympani. There was also a need to have packages with collars glued at different lengths so that an appropriate one would be available for implantation. However, a collar was subsequently shown not to be necessary as it was no more effective than either an autograft around the electrode entry point or allowing a fibrous tissue sheath to form naturally around the shaft of the electrode carrier (Clark and Shepherd, 1984).

Stabilization of the implanted package in the first patient was thought to present special problems as it could tilt forwards into the mastoid cavity. Stabilization was accomplished by making a Silastic mould during surgery that would fit into the mastoid cavity and support the front end of the device. Subsequently, the connector was removed from the implant used for the second implant so that the above method of fixation was not necessary. The second package was secured by drilling a bed in the mastoid, parietal and occipital bones just posterior to the mastoid cavity and by suturing an inferiorly-based fascial flap over it. Initially we thought it would be necessary to remove as many air cells as possible to avoid leaving them as a focus for infection. This was impracticable and also not found necessary. Since that time, the technique has been modified to leave as much bone as possible around the posterior air cells to help support the package.

Finally, at the operation on the first patient the electrode array passed easily along the scala tympani of the basal turn for a distance of 25 mm. The lead wire which was malleable and more than adequate in length was tucked into the mastoid cavity. It was not fixed, as the importance of doing this was not appreciated at the time. Unfortunately, some weeks later it slipped out 10 mm, hampering our research studies. This incident then led to it becoming our standard policy to recommend that the lead wire should be fixed. This policy has subsequently been substantiated when electrodes have slipped even when the fixation ties have not been adequately tightened.

Preliminary psychophysics

Prior to surgery there had been considerable discussion on the tests to be carried out and our policy towards rehabilitation. As often happens with initial studies on patients, many more tests were proposed than the patient would have been able to do even when working 40 hours a week. These, of course, had to be streamlined. The main concerns were to determine whether our electrode system and placement could code pitch on a place basis, what were the limitations of coding pitch on a rate basis (time period code), and the thresholds and dynamic ranges for stimulus current levels on each electrode. Another important psychophysical test proposed was to determine the ability of the patient to detect a change in frequency either by rate or place of stimulation over durations that corresponded to those of consonants. These were foreshadowed in earlier animal behavioural studies (Clark et al., 1972, 1973).

Although the above psychophysical tests were considered the first tests needed, thought was also required to decide what type of speech testing could be carried out when we were able to develop speech processing strategies. The most obvious ones were closed-sets of consonants and vowels, but as some people's expectations for open-set speech recognition were not high (derived from the lack of any open-set speech recognition being obtained on single-channel patients) open-set speech testing was not considered a priority. Instead there was discussion about testing the patient's ability to recognize 'minimal auditory cues'. At the time 'minimal auditory cues' referred to the recognition of speech elements rather than speech itself (for example, being able to categorize a second formant transition).

It was anticipated we would have to carry out a number of psychophysical tests to develop appropriate speech processing strategies to evaluate on our patient. As no one had been able to help profoundly deaf people understand connected speech with electrical stimulation, it was likely we would have had to spend considerable time exploring a great range of stimuli in the hope that this might provide information leading to a successful speech processing strategy. Although it might take considerable time to find the best possible strategy, the patient required help as soon as possible, and for this reason we decided to spend half our time rehabilitating him when we had a speech processing strategy that seemed to provide even minimal help.

After surgery the first question to be answered was when we should commence electrical stimulation of the residual auditory nerves. If the surgery had caused trauma to and partial damage of nerve fibres, would electrical stimulation aggravate the situation, and how long should one wait for healing to occur? A period of 3 weeks was chosen as a compromise between usual clinical recovery periods from neuropraxia, and the need to commence helping the patient.

The initial psychophysical investigations (Tong *et al.*, 1980b) commenced by determining thresholds for common ground stimulation on each electrode, and this showed significant variations (common ground was the only stimulus mode available with the prototype receiver-stimulator). The growth of loudness as a function of current was plotted and found to be much steeper than for sound. Pitch was then scaled for rate of stimulation after balancing the loudness of the stimuli. With pulse rates below 200 pulses/s, the pitch produced by electrical stimulation increased with pulse rate. For example, on one electrode the pitch increased from 78 mels at 50 pulses/s to 3000 mels at 200 pulses/s. However, for pulse rates above 200 pulses/s there was little increase in pitch. Place pitch was clearly demonstrated and was scaled in an orderly fashion from low in the more apical to high in the more basal region. An exception to this was a low pitch sensation from the most basal electrode lying near the round window. The percept in this case was attributed to the extracochlear spread of current. The place pitch percepts were different from those perceived by varying the stimulus rate, and were described as dull for apical electrodes and sharp for more basal ones. There were thus two types of pitch percepts, one for rate and the other for place of stimulation. Understanding how these percepts arose was helped by reference to research reports in Plomp (1976). In one study (Plomp and Steeneken, 1971) it was demonstrated that timbre was determined by the absolute frequency position of the spectral envelope rather than by the position of the spectral envelope relative to the fundamental. In another study (von Bismarck, 1974) it was found that sharpness, as the major attribute of timbre, was primarily related to the position of the loudness centre on an absolute frequency scale rather than to a particular shape of the spectral envelope. It was shown that low-frequency tones do indeed sound dull and high-frequency tones sharp.

Another important discovery on our first patient (Tong *et al.*, 1980b), was that when he was asked to mimic the pitch perceived by stimulating various electrodes he did so by voicing different vowel sounds. These were /ɛ/,/ɪ/,/ʊ/. It was also noted that the vowel could be changed by varying the duration and rate of the stimulus. The /ʊ/ became /ɔ/, and /ɪ/ became /i/ if the duration was increased from 200 ms to 400 ms. Furthermore, /ɔ/ could become /a/ by increasing the stimulus current or pulse rate.

In seeking to understand why these particular vowel sounds were experienced, help was obtained by reference to a previous acoustic study (Delattre *et al.*, 1952). In this research the authors determined one-formant equivalents of synthetic two-formant vowels. They found that the single formant usually lay between the first and second formants. However, for two vowels /u/ and /ʊ/ it was close to the first formant, and for /i/ close to the second formant. In this study the single formants representing the vowels /ɔ/,/ɛ/, and /i/ experienced by our patient had frequencies of 720 Hz, 2160 Hz and 3000 Hz. These frequencies corresponded approximately to the electrode location where these frequencies would normally cause excitation of the basilar membrane. The fact that we were able to shift the vowel perceived from /ɔ/ to an /a/ by increasing the current level was attributed to a shift in the population of neurons stimulated, and an averaging process referred to by Plomp (1976) for spectral components of acoustic stimuli.

We also carried out psychophysical studies using two electrodes stimulated simultaneously and at the same rate. The vowel perceived was different from that for each one stimulated separately. When we stimulated one electrode resulting in /ʊ/ and combined this with another resulting in /ɪ/ the percept was /ʌ/ as in hut. This suggested that an averaging process was taking place in the brain when two populations of neurons were excited for spectral components in the two vowels.

Another important finding was that when two nearby electrodes were stimulated simultaneously with rates which differed by approximately 5–7% the patient perceived a consonant and following vowel. With the electrodes used this was /d/. Data from the study suggested that beating was occurring, and that amplitude changes from the stimuli moving in and out of the phase were responsible for the perception of the consonant in conjunction with the vowel. It was thought that the stimuli were representing some of the acoustic cues for the coarticulation of consonants and vowels.

The psychophysical studies carried out in September/October 1978 on our first implant patient gave valuable information on how electrical stimulation reproduced percepts obtained with acoustic stimuli, and helped in the development of our cue extraction or formant-based speech processing strategy in November/December 1978.

Evaluation of physiologically-based speech processor

The development of the physiologically-based speech processor commenced in February 1978 and was ready for evaluation on our first patient in September/October 1978 (Laird, 1979). The details of how this processor operated are outlined above.

With the physiologically-based speech processor it was found that when three or four channels of simultaneous stimulation were used a 'coarser' percept was obtained than when using one channel alone. Furthermore, with multiple-channel stimulation the percepts often exceeded pain thresholds even though individual channels had been set at comfortable levels. Preliminary testing with speech stimuli using more than two channels gave percepts of such complexity that it was beyond the patient to categorize them adequately. The patient described speech as a series of vowel-type sounds the length of which roughly corresponded to the stimulus word length and the vowel colour depended on the electrode stimulated. He was able to perceive rhythm and could recognize certain tunes. The processor was also shown to benefit him with lipreading. When tested with a closed-set of ten vowels he gave above chance responses, and the main cues appeared to be vowel duration and to some extent vowel colour. Limited testing with closed sets of consonants in a CVC context only gave results above chance for the voiced–unvoiced distinction. The processor was tested with stimuli presented in either a stochastic or deterministic mode, but there was no difference in results. The patient, however, described the deterministic mode of stimulation as less complex, smoother and to some degree more intelligible. In summary, the main limitation of this processor was the unpredictable variation in loudness produced with simultaneous stimulation.

Development and evaluation of formant-based or cue extraction speech processor

In view of the very limited success that was occurring with the physiologically-based speech processor we were forced to reappraise the situation. One of the questions needing to be reconsidered was whether pre-processing of speech would be better? Should we select appropriate speech elements and present these in a meaningful way to the auditory nervous system?

We had seen with our psychophysical studies that stimulating single electrodes resulted in the perception of vowels which corresponded quite well to those heard by normal hearing people when presented with single formants. Furthermore, it was known from research by Potter *et al.* (1947), Cooper *et al.* (1952), Liberman *et al.* (1954), Fant (1956) and others that the second formant conveyed considerable speech information. This led to the decision to pre-process the speech by extracting the second formant frequency. The amplitude of the filter at this frequency was then used to set the current level on the electrode that corresponded to this frequency on a place coding basis. By stimulating one of the 10 electrodes non-simultaneously we were then avoiding the problem of the unpredictable summation in loudness for simultaneous stimuli seen with the physiologically-based speech processor. The problem remained, however, how to code the voicing frequency which was known to be another important element in speech perception. This needed to be extracted and presented to the nervous system in an appropriate way. A decision was made to stimulate each electrode at a rate that corresponded with the voicing frequency. Consequently the voicing frequency would be conveyed by stimuli across the electrodes as the site of stimulation, with a plosive consonant for example, varied over time. This required integration by the brain of rate information across the electrodes. The speech processing strategy was implemented as a laboratory-based speech processor using a Hewlett-Packard 2100 series computer.

The method of operation of the inaugural formant-based speech processor (Tong *et al.*, 1980a) is summarized in Figure 6 for the word 'wit'. The first, second and third formant frequencies are shown. As can be seen, the second formant rises over a short time interval for the consonant /w/, remains steady for a longer period over the duration of the vowel /I/, and there is then a burst of high-frequency energy for the unvoiced phoneme /t/. The electrical stimuli produced by the cochlear implant in response to this word are represented by the vertical lines. For the /w/ sound the place of stimulation shifts from a low-to-high frequency area of the cochlea, and as it is a voiced sound the spacing between the pulses is proportional to the voicing frequency. The rate of stimulation remains steady for the vowel (I) and again the stimulus period is proportional to the voicing frequency. Finally, for the /t/ sound which is a short burst of high frequency noise, an electrode in the basal area is excited. As it is unvoiced a low randomized pulse rate is used as this was identified by the patient as noise-like.

When evaluating this speech processing strategy which extracted the second formant (F2) and fundamental frequency (F0), the testing was certainly not as routine as it is today. We did not know what the patient was hearing or how best to test it. At the time very little could be done to help profoundly deaf patients so there were few standard tests. It was not until the MAC battery (Owens and Telleen, 1981) was developed that appropriate tests became available.

Our initial testing was carried out with a small closed-set of vowels and then even smaller sets of consonants with contrasting features. This showed encouraging results and led to informal testing with closed sets of sentences. Eventually the audiological team members

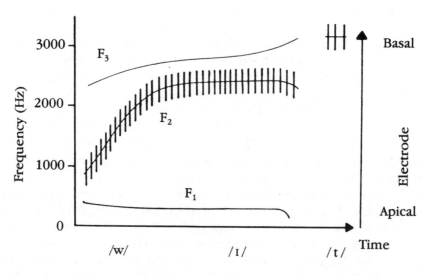

Figure 6 (Clark *et al.*, 1987). Implementation of the speech processing strategy as seen for the word 'wit' on its phonetic transcript /w/ /I/ /t/. The vertical bars represent the electrical pulses.

were encouraged to present open-sets of AB words (Boothroyd, 1968). This was the test we had commenced using and teaching in our new postgraduate course in Audiology, Department of Otolaryngology, The University of Melbourne. To our surprise and pleasure the patient was able to obtain significant open-set scores for these words scored phonemically, but also for words alone.

It was very significant that we had speech perception results which could register on a recognized audiological test. This test could also be used to make statements about how the multiple-channel cochlear implant would help with communication. Although single-channel devices were giving patients an awareness of sound and later shown to help in recognizing speech elements in closed sets and even as a lipreading aid, there was still considerable debate as to their benefits in communication and overall value. In achieving open-set speech recognition for both electrical stimulation alone and electrical stimulation combined with lipreading, we were on a measuring scale from which comparisons had been made of a person's ability to hear running speech (Davis and Silverman, 1970).

With the discovery that the patient could obtain some open-set speech understanding with electrical stimulation alone came the need to prove this to the scientific community. Fortunately this patient had been shown preoperatively to have had no hearing, and only gave vibration thresholds with bone conduction tests. Consequently, no improvements could be attributed to electrophonic hearing.

To establish the benefits of the implant required setting up a series of speech perception tests in standardized conditions. This involved making sure that the test material was prerecorded, not previously presented, and administered in controlled conditions. To show the benefits of the implant in understanding running speech not only did we use the phonetically-balanced AB word test (Boothroyd, 1968; Clark *et al.*, 1981c) but also the CID everyday sentence test (Davis and Silverman, 1970; Clark *et al.*, 1981a) and then later the Tracking test (De Filippo and Scott, 1978; Martin *et al.*, 1981). The testing was also carried out for electrical stimulation alone, lipreading alone and electrical stimulation combined with lipreading.

The results of the initial testing is reported in more detail elsewhere (Clark *et al.*, 1981 a, 1981b; Martin *et al.*, 1981). In summary, however, with AB words he obtained a score of 10% for words and 20% for phonemes using electrical stimulation alone. He also obtained scores of 40% (words) and 73% (phonemes) for electrical stimulation combined with lipreading, and scores of 10% and 53% for lipreading alone respectively. These represented improvements for electrical stimulation, combined with lipreading compared to lipreading alone, of 300% (words) and 38% (phonemes). With CID sentences he obtained scores of 14% for electrical stimulation alone 14% for lipreading alone and 68% for electrical stimulation combined with lipreading. The latter was a 386% improvement versus lipreading alone.

The initial testing was all carried out with the F0/F2 strategy implemented on the Department of Otolaryngology's free standing computer. To help the patient in his everyday life there was a need to build a portable unit that implemented the same speech processing strategy. The development of a portable speech processor commenced in March 1979, and by March 1980 a prototype was available for testing on this patient and a second patient operated on 13 July 1979.

While work was being undertaken to develop a wearable speech processor and plans were being made to operate on the second patient, it was considered essential to carry out further psychophysical studies on the first patient to better understand how the strategy worked, and to provide a good scientific basis for it. This involved, in particular, studying the perceptual limitations of varying the rate as well as place of stimulation for durations that corresponded to those of consonants (approximately 25 ms), or the minimum for vowels (approximately 100 ms). The results showed that for varying pulse rates discrimination deteriorated with a decrease in the duration of the stimulus burst from 100 ms to 25 ms. On the other hand the discrimination of stimuli which varied in their place of stimulation did not change as the duration became shorter (Tong *et al.*, 1982). These results were also seen in the second patient operated on 13 July 1979.

These studies helped establish that the coding of the second formant as place of stimulation was appropriate. The second formant is a most important cue in the perception of consonants, and as a change in the place of stimulation was well discriminated over a duration comparable to that of a consonant it could effectively represent a second formant transition. On the other hand, it was not so appropriate to use rate of stimulation due to its poor discrimination at short durations, but it was better used to code the voicing or fundamental frequency with its longer time course.

With the first patient getting encouraging results, further questions to be answered were:

Was this result achieved because we had found some way of coding sound that suited this particular individual?

How would other people find the coding strategy?

Did the strategy depend on someone being deaf only a short time?

Would this strategy benefit other people who had been deaf for a considerably longer period of time?

Would a person's memory for speech sounds be present after many years of deafness?

Would variations in disease and residual spiral ganglion cell populations affect the results?

Could we develop a portable speech processor?

To answer some of these questions it was necessary to carry out an implant on a second patient. This was done on 13 July 1979. The patient was older (63 years) and had been profoundly deaf for 13 years so it was of great interest to see if he could benefit as well. His first test session was carried out three weeks postoperatively and was largely taken up with setting thresholds and comfortable levels for his electrodes, and seeing if he too could scale pitch on a place coding basis. However, at the second test session to everyone's pleasant surprise it became apparent that he could understand running speech. Although not a standard test, our senior audiologist went and bought the morning paper, and we found that if he was read a news item first, he could have it read to him using electrical stimulation alone and he could understand most of it.

He too, like the first patient, underwent the series of standardized audiological tests, and although he had a more limited ability to understand speech using electrical stimulation alone, he obtained considerable help with the device as a lipreading aid.

In view of the encouraging findings on two postlinguistically deaf adults a third patient received an implant on 9 October 1979. This patient was a 43-year-old woman who had been profoundly deaf for more than 20 years due to an unknown aetiology.

Research in the 1980s

The demonstration in the late 1970s that our two postlinguistically deaf adults with profound-total hearing losses could understand some speech with electrical stimulation alone, and that they could obtain marked improvements in understanding speech when electrical stimulation was combined with lipreading, compared to lipreading alone, resulted in intensified activity not only to develop the multiple-channel device commercially, but also to undertake research to see how far speech processing could go in providing near normal speech understanding using electrical stimulation alone. Work was also directed towards using implants to help children.

In Melbourne the 1980s started with major problems. In January 1980 the receiver-stimulator implanted three months previously in a third patient started to fail. This was presumed to be due to fluid leaking into the receiver-stimulator and short circuits between the receiving coil and stimulating electrodes. Then later in January the second patient operated on on 13 July 1979 experienced an unexplained loud noise and the device went on and off intermittently, until it finally stopped completely in April 1980 one week after the wearable speech processor was developed. He had just one week to experience how beneficial the wearable unit could be.

We had to agonize over what had happened. No amount of checking could find a fault with the external system. The sudden failure suggested that it was not due to loss of nerve function and therefore we had to assume that the problem lay within the implanted receiver-stimulator. The whole programme had come to a halt. We could not implant any more people if we did not know the cause of the problem, and we could not find out the cause of the problem until we removed the package. We did not want to remove the system and replace it with another if the second system had the same problem. The matter was brought to a head, however, when we discovered the patient had developed a sinus over the front edge of the package. This occurred because he used to fall asleep at night wearing his glasses and the arm of the glasses eventually rubbed through the skin when he lay on that side. This led to an infection around the package requiring antibiotics. When this infection settled down we removed the foreign body, but cut the electrode just outside the round window.

The receiver-stimulator package was treated like a piece of moon rock. It had everyone looking at it. Finally, the fault was discovered and found to be due to a concentration of mechanical stress in the electrode wires at a point just after they emerged from the package. This had led to their breaking. This proved to be valuable information, and when Nucleus came to design their first commercial receiver-stimulator for clinical trial, this problem was avoided by the use of the helical wires—now standard for the present receiver-stimulator.

As a result of the above difficulties, we had, in 1980 and 1981, only one patient (our first) left to carry on with the research studies. The first of these was to show that he could obtain results with the wearable speech processor at least as good as those for the laboratory-based one. The results of the comparison are presented in Tong *et al.* (1981). For this evaluation a test battery was created. This consisted of AB words, CID sentences, closed sets of eight and 16 consonants, 16 spondees, a modified rhyme test, and the Craig lipreading inventory (Craig, 1964). This was the start of our using a battery of tests to assess communication skills which later continued with the use of the MAC battery (Owens and Telleen, 1981). (With improved speech processor performances in the late 1980s, however, the need for a battery of tests has diminished.)

In addition to the above difficulties with the prototype receiver-stimulator, considerable pressure was being created when people said that single-channel devices were as effective as multiple-channel ones, and it was questioned whether it would be worthwhile to go to the expense of developing a multiple-channel system.

To try and resolve this question we were able to carry out two comparative studies. It would have been best if we had our own patients with single- and multiple-channel implants tested under the same conditions. With the first study we compared the results obtained for closed-sets of spondaic words presented to our first two patients under similar conditions to those for nine patients at Los Angeles using their single-channel devices (Clark *et al.*, 1981b). When the second and third patients' devices failed and we were left with one patient, we compared his results when using the fundamental frequency (F0) alone on a single-channel, with those obtained when using our F0/F2 speech processor (Clark *et al.*, 1981d). The F0 strategy was similar to that used in London and enabled a comparison to be made (Fourcin *et al.*, 1979; Clark *et al.*, 1981d). The results of the comparison with the Los Angeles device showed significant advantages for multiple-channel stimulation as did the comparison with the London implant (Clark *et al.*, 1981d). In the latter case, as expected, the transmission of second formant information was significantly better but the transmission for F0 was similar. It was not until an independent comparison was made of the single-channel devices from Los Angeles (House and Urban, 1973) and Vienna (Hochmair-Desoyer *et al.*, 1980) and the multiple-channel devices from Utah (Eddington, 1983) and Melbourne (Clark *et al.*, 1978) by the clinic in Iowa (Gantz *et al.*, 1987; Tyler *et al.*, 1987) that it became more generally acknowledged that multiple-channel stimulation provided more information on speech than single-channel implants.

The industrial development of an implantable receiver-stimulator and wearable speech processor for clinical trial for the FDA

The failure of two of the prototype receiver-stimulators early in 1980 emphasized the need to produce an implant package and electrode array that was robust, reliable and well sealed. This led to renewed endeavours to obtain industrial participation, and the Sydney firm Telectronics was contracted to produce a new receiver-stimulator. Telectronics was a most appropriate choice as it had pioneered the sealing of pacemakers. Staff were the first to discover how to produce a ceramic-to-metal seal so that the electronics for pacemakers could be enclosed in a titanium package rather than embedded in Araldite as previously. Although they had succeeded in producing a larger package than the one required and with a single electrode feedthrough, the task of producing a package only about 30 mm in diameter with 22 electrode feedthroughs seemed daunting at the time.

During 1980/81 plans were made to design and fabricate a more reliable receiver-stimulator. Initial research was undertaken at The University of Melbourne in conjunction with the Commonwealth Industrial Research Organization's (CSIRO) Department of Materials Science and Technology, to determine the bonding between platinum and ceramics, and the shrinkage characteristics for different ceramic formulae. Other techniques for achieving hermetically-sealed feedthroughs for at least 20 electrodes were also investigated. When contract work with Telectronics commenced in mid-1981 further investigations of the ceramic-to-metal feedthrough problem were carried out, and finally a solution achieved which is still the most effective one. In addition, work to simplify the circuit design of The University of Melbourne's prototype, incorporate most of the circuitry on a single silicon chip, and use a single coil for the reception of data was undertaken. Developmental work was required to determine how best to seal the electronics into a titanium can. Experiences obtained in pacemaking were valuable in achieving reliable manufacturing methods for the task. The lead wire system had special stress relief incorporated into its design to avoid the problems that occurred in our second patient as discussed above, and the electrode array was similar to the prototype, only better construction methods were developed.

While the receiver-stimulator was being developed, work was also carried out by Nucleus Limited in conjunction with the Department of Otolaryngology, The University of Melbourne, to reduce The University of Melbourne's prototype speech processor in size to one that could be worn in a pocket. A number of engineering tasks were required, including the use of semi-custom made circuits and a more efficient data link to reduce the power consumption, so that the number and size of the batteries would be small. The speech processing strategy, however, was essentially the same as for The University of Melbourne's prototype device.

Biological safety studies for the FDA evaluation

While collaborating with industry in developing a new receiver-stimulator and wearable speech processor for clinical trial for the FDA, we had the task of carrying out research to ensure that the device was safe as well as effective. This required research to determine that: implanted materials to be used were biocompatible; that the electrical stimulus parameters would not result in the loss of spiral ganglion cells; and that inserting the banded multiple-electrode array into the cochlea would not cause significant trauma especially to spiral ganglion cells.

Initially a range of candidate materials were examined to determine tissue reactions. At the time there was little information in the literature on a number of suitable materials, and certainly not for those materials when implanted in the cochlea. These biocompatibility studies are reported in Clark *et al.*, (1987a), and were part of the more comprehensive safety data subsequently obtained by us and presented to the FDA, for approval of the Nucleus multiple-channel cochlear implant as being safe for postlinguistically deaf adults.

It was also necessary to be sure that the stimulus parameters to be used in the design of the new receiver-stimulator for clinical trial for the FDA did not lead to damage of spiral ganglion cells. For this reason we commenced a study on chronic stimulation of the cat cochlea. In the study (Shepherd *et al.*, 1983b) there were a number of electrode leadwire breakages that led to the need to modify its design. Data was obtained, nevertheless, on three cats for biphasic charge-balanced pulses at a rate of 200 pulses/s for up to 1000 hours of continuous stimulation, and showed no significant effects on the ganglion cells. The study led to a second one (Shepherd *et al.*, 1983a). This was a more extensive investigation on 10 cats using charge-balanced biphasic pulses at rates of 500 pulses/s for up to 2000 hours of continuous stimulation. Again there was no significant loss of spiral ganglion cells for charge densities up to $32 \ \mu C \ cm^{-2}$ geom. per phase.

Establishing that both the electrical stimulus parameters and the materials to be used in the new receiver-stimulator for clinical trial were safe was deemed important, and had been an essential part of the work leading up to the clinical trial. There remained, however, the need to establish with as much certainty as possible that the insertion of the electrode array would not result in significant trauma.

For this reason we embarked on a study in 1981/82 where electrode arrays prepared by the manufacturing process were inserted into the human temporal bones, and the bones subsequently sectioned and stained for evidence of trauma. The data was reported by Shepherd *et al.* (1985) and showed that the insertion of the banded scala tympani array resulted in minimal trauma. However, in five of nine cochleas there was a tear of the spiral ligament 7–11 mm from the round window; three of these tears were associated with tears of Reissner's membrane. Tears of the basilar membrane occurred in two of nine bones, and a fracture of the spiral lamina in one. The fracture and a tear of the basilar membrane was seen close to the round window and occurred when the electrode was pushed after resistance was felt, and it buckled just inside the scala tympani. The second tear of the basilar membrane occurred 15 mm from the round window, again after the insertion continued after resistance was felt.

The effect of electrode insertion on the cochlea was also studied by Clifford and Gibson (1987) who drilled away the overlying bone to expose the membranous cochlea and electrode array. They were then able to examine the cochlea macroscopically for evidence of trauma. Their results were similar to our own, and demonstrated that the most common form of trauma was a tear in the spiral ligament.

While carrying out our study on electrode insertion in human temporal bones, we also undertook further investigations on cat temporal bones that had been implanted to better determine how trauma to various structures might affect the loss of ganglion cells.

The above studies were carried out at a time when the debate over whether it was better to do single-channel or multiple-channel stimulation and extracochlear or intracochlear implantation intensified. There was also criticism that intracochlear electrodes inserted far enough to produce multiple-channel stimulation in the speech frequency range were unacceptably traumatic. This view arose partly because of an histopathological study by Johnsson *et al.* (1982) that a House single ball electrode inserted some distance into the cochlea had caused considerable trauma, and it was widely thought that a multiple-electrode array would cause even worse damage.

Although the human temporal bone studies (Shepherd *et al.*, 1985; Clifford and Gibson 1987) had shown that electrode insertions basically resulted in no significant trauma, critics were still concerned that tears of the basilar membrane had occurred in a small proportion of bones, that more serious trauma could occur if the electrode array was pushed too hard and that it might be difficult to feel initial resistance telling the surgeon when to stop. In addition, a high proportion of bones had tears of the spiral ligament at a point 10 mm inside the cochlea, and the effects of these tears on the cochlea were not known.

To help resolve the above questions the mechanical properties of the single electrode used by the Los Angeles device and our own multiple-electrode one were compared (Patrick and MacFarlane, 1987). The study showed that the maximum force transmitted to the tip of the single solid wire electrode was 25 times that transmitted to the tip of the multiple-electrode array, and the multiple-electrode array was ten times more flexible. Secondly, in our study in cats on the effects of trauma to cochlear structures, we found that a localized lesion of the spiral ligament did not lead to any loss of spiral ganglion cells, as illustrated in Clark et al. (1987, Figure 8). Thirdly, as a result of dissections in the temporal bone laboratory we discovered (Franz and

Clark, 1987) that if resistance is experienced during insertion then the electrode array should be withdrawn a little and rotated 90° before reinsertion (counterclockwise for the right ear and clockwise for the left ear). This manoeuvre then helped prevent the tip of the electrode being pushed through the basilar membrane.

The clinical trial of the receiver-stimulator and wearable speech processor

The new receiver-stimulator, having been thoroughly tested, was available in June/July 1982 for implantation. It was decided not to implant the first patient until the wearable speech processors were also ready so the patients would have a processor to use in their everyday life and we would not have a situation where they had undergone surgery and had to wait around expectantly for rehabilitation.

The speech processor became available in August 1982 and the first of six postlingually deaf patients had his operation on 14 September 1982. It was planned that we carry out surgery on a second patient after a short interval, and then review the two patients, to ensure that the new receiver-stimulator was performing according to expectations, before operating on further patients. After satisfying ourselves that this was the case, we operated on four more postlinguistically deaf adults, the last operation being 16 November 1982 (Clark *et al.*, 1984). The electrical stimulation alone, open-set AB word scores for the first four patients were: 10%, 0%, 37%, 33%. The AB phoneme scores were: 40%, 30%, 66%, 63% (Clark *et al.*, 1983).

In view of the successful initial trial of the receiver-stimulator at the Royal Victorian Eye and Ear Hospital negotiations took place to extend the clinical trial to Centres in the US, Canada, West Germany and Australia, so that the benefits of the implant could be determined on a greater number of people, and by more independent groups, so that the requirements of the FDA could be satisfied. The initial centres were: University of Iowa, DesMoines, Iowa; Baylor College of Medicine, Houston, Texas; Mason Clinic, Seattle, Washington; New York University, New York; Good Samaritan Hospital, Portland, Oregon; University of Toronto, Toronto, Canada; Louisiana State University, New Orleans, Louisiana; Medizinische Hochschule, Hannover, Germany; and University of Sydney, Sydney, Australia.

In following up the patients from these centres over time it was noted that their results continued to improve. This is demonstrated in Table 2 and Figure 7. This shows that for 23 patients their average post-operative open-set CID sentence score for electrical stimulation alone was 16% at 3 months, and this increased to 40% at 12 months (Dowell *et al.*, 1986) (further follow-up showed that performance continued to improve over 2 or more years).

Table 2. Open-set CID sentence scores : hearing alone preoperatively and F0/F2 electrical stimulation postoperatively

	Preoperative (%)	Postoperative (%)	
		3 months	12 months
Mean	0.1	16.2	39.7
Standard error	0.11	3.70	5.31
Range	0–4	0–58	0–86

(Dowell *et al.*, 1986; Clark *et al.*, 1987.)

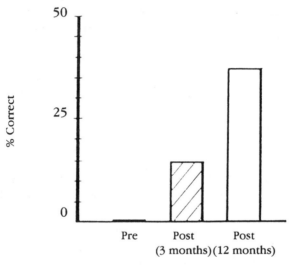

Figure 7 (Clark *et al.*, 1987). Mean CID sentence scores for hearing aid alone pre-operatively, and F0-F2 electrical stimulation alone 3 months postoperatively and 12 months postoperatively (n = 23).

While the FDA clinical trial of the F0/F2 multiple-channel system was being undertaken we were involved in additional streams of activity. The first was a commitment to patients who were now coming forward to receive help from the implant. This required organizing a clinical facility at the Royal Victorian Eye and Ear Hospital, and in 1983 a public hospital clinic came into being at the Hospital funded by the State Government of Victoria. The patients all had the battery of tests undertaken and were included in the trial for the FDA. A second stream of activity was to continue research to improve the formant-based or cue extraction strategy. Having been successful in extracting F2 and coding this on a place basis, the most logical improvement was to extract either the first formant (F1) or third formant (F3), and present one of these at the same time as F2. We could not carry out this research initially as we wanted to comply with the FDA requirements for the clinical trial of the F0/F2 strategy and follow up the patients for the required period of time. It was also reasoned that a comparison with the F0/F2 strategy would mean using the alternative strategy in the same everyday environment, and there was no indication that valuable engineering resources should be directed towards the necessary modification of the F0/F2 processor.

An F0/F1/F2 speech processor

To help establish that the extraction of an additional formant (preferably F1) would be of benefit, we first addressed the question could patients recognize two percepts when two separate sites in the cochlea were stimulated near simultaneously? It was assumed that the recognition of two percepts with these simple stimuli was a prerequisite for using two formants to represent vowels and consonants. With this study the dissimilarities in perception for two electrode stimulation was best represented in two-dimensional space (Tong *et al.*, 1984). This suggested that a two-formant speech processing strategy would be of benefit.

To provide additional information on the desirability of using a two-formant speech processing strategy, and in the absence of opportunities to investigate alternative strategies on patients, research effort was directed towards establishing an acoustic model for electrical stimulation, so that we could evaluate candidate strategies on normally-hearing volunteers.

With the model, a set of stimuli were generated from a pseudorandom white noise generator, the output of which was fed through separate bandpass filters corresponding to different electrode sites. The psychophysical tests showed similar results using the model on three normally-hearing subjects, compared to multichannel stimulation on two cochlear implant patients. The psychophysical tests were: pulse rate difference limens; pitch scaling and categorizations of stimuli differing in filter frequency or electrode position; and similarity judgements of stimuli differing in pulse rate as well as filter frequency or electrode position (Blamey *et al.*, 1984a; Clark *et al.*, 1987a). With speech perception tests the addition of F1 helped in the transmission of all speech features except place. In this study (Blamey *et al.*, 1984b) we also determined that the amplitude envelope was an important cue for consonant recognition, and the addition of F1 resulted in better amplitude detection.

Having shown with the acoustic model that an F0/F1/F2 speech processor gave better results than the F0/F2 processor, this strategy was implemented by The University of Melbourne and Cochlear Pty Limited in a bench-top laboratory-based speech processor. When the F0/F1/F2 strategy was initially tested in December 1983 in a pilot study on a small number of patients who had been using the F0/F2 processor, a conclusive improvement was not seen. It was discovered that the patients had some difficulties learning the new strategy and would need a wearable take home unit before a satisfactory comparison could be made. As a result, Cochlear proceeded to implement the F0/F1/F2 strategy as a wearable unit called WSPIII. When it was trialed in patients it was found to result in similar improvements to those obtained with the acoustic model (Clark, 1986; Dowell *et al.*, 1987). This result showed the predictive value of the acoustic model and, in doing so, indicated it was a good model for formant-based speech processors using multiple channel electrical stimulation.

The F0/F1/F2 speech processor not only provided better speech perception results in quiet than the F0/F2 processor, but also performed better in noise (Dowell *et al.*, 1987). Furthermore, the results in noise were as good as those obtained for the Symbion speech processor using the same test procedure described in Gantz *et al.*, (1987). This F0/F1/F2 (WSPIII) speech processor was approved by the FDA in May 1986 for postlinguistically deaf adults.

Cochlear implantation for prelinguistically deaf adults and children

While undertaking the further speech processing research on postlinguistically deaf patients, discussed above, we commenced studies in parallel to determine how to process speech for prelinguistically deaf people. The first prelinguistically deaf patient to receive the multiple channel implant was educated almost entirely by signing (signed English and sign language) and was operated on 20 September 1983 at age 25. A second patient, who had a similar educational history, had an implant on 15 November 1983 at age 24 (Clark *et al.*, 1987b, 1987c). Both were studied extensively and it was found from psychophysical research that although they performed well for current level identification and had satisfactory duration difference limens, their abilities for pulse rate and electrode position identification were poor (Tong *et al.*, 1986; Clark *et al.*, 1987b, 1987c; Tong *et al.*, 1988). This was also reflected in the poor speech perception scores they obtained using the formant-based speech processing strategy (Busby *et al.*, 1986; Clark *et al.*, 1987b, 1987c; Tong *et al.*, 1988). From this study it was concluded that the formant-based speech processing strategy used for postlinguistically deaf patients was probably not suitable for prelinguistically deaf people 20 years of age and over, and that the use of signing could have been a contributing detrimental factor. It certainly reduced their motivation to learn a new and auditory/oral based system. It was also felt that untreated deafness from an early age could lead to perceptual processing difficulties for frequency coding that could make speech processing using those cues unsatisfactory.

In view of the above findings it was decided to operate on younger people, and preferably those with an auditory/oral educational background. On 8 January 1985 a 14-year-old boy who had been taught with cued speech received a cochlear implant. His electrode place and pulse rate identifications were better than the two adult prelinguistically deaf patients, but not as good as those generally obtained for postlinguistically deaf people (Clark *et al.*, 1987b). His speech perception was also better than the prelinguistically deaf adults, and he obtained some help in understanding running speech when the implant was used in combination with lipreading.

Some months later (17 September 1985) we implanted a 22-year-old prelinguistically deaf woman who had received an auditory/oral education, and although born with a severe hearing loss, went profoundly-totally deaf over the first 18 years of her life. Interestingly, the speech perception results on the patient were more similar to those obtained with postlinguistically deaf people (Clark *et al.*, 1987b).

As the results on the third patient had suggested that it was desirable to operate on younger children, the decision was made to implant a 10-year-old. This child had a profound-total hearing loss at 3.5 years of age and was educated by Total Communication. The operation was only possible, however, with the development of the mini 22-electrode receiver-stimulator (Clark *et al.*, 1987c) which was more suitable for children because it was smaller and had a rare earth magnet embedded in it (Dormer *et al.*, 1980) so that an external transmitting coil, also with embedded magnet, could be held in place by bringing the magnets into close proximity. This new mini-22 prosthesis was implanted first in the 10-year-old on 20 August 1985. After establishing that it performed to specifications, a series of psychophysical and speech perception studies were undertaken, and these demonstrated an advantage for the perception of speech when the device was combined with lipreading, but little open-set speech recognition for electrical stimulation alone.

To evaluate the prosthesis on younger patients, a 5 year-old received a cochlear implant on 15 April 1986. This boy, who went deaf at 3 years of age from meningitis and was trained with cued speech, made excellent progress with the implant and after some months was able to get significant open-set speech identification scores from electrical stimulation alone.

Prior to implanting children, it was realized that the training and assessment would need to be quite different from that for postlinguistically deaf adults. It was considered important that we assess not only speech perception, but also speech production, as well as expressive and receptive language and communication skills (Nienhuys *et al.*, 1987). To this end a protocol was developed which has been used subsequently for the management of all our children.

The studies on children at The University of Melbourne and The Bionic Ear Institute have continued since that time, and congenitally deaf children as young as two years of age have been operated on. It has been found that congenitally and prelinguistically deaf children can benefit from the implant as well as postlinguistically deaf children, and a significant proportion can get open-set speech recognition for electrical stimulation alone (Dawson *et al.*, 1992). The prelinguistically deaf group, however, need a longer period of training and appear to do better if implanted at a young age.

The evaluation of children using the WSPIII (F0/F1/F2) speech processor was extended to centres in North America and Australia for the FDA study. The results in 80 children were presented to the FDA, and it was approved as safe and effective for children on 27 June 1990. Since that time the results on 142 children have been analysed (Staller *et al.*, 1991; Clark *et al.*, 1992) and they confirm the above findings from The University of Melbourne that pre and postlinguistically deaf children can receive significant improvements when the device is combined with lipreading, and approximately 40–50% can get significant open-set speech scores for electrical stimulation alone.

The second improvement in multiple-channel speech processing: extraction of formants and high frequency spectral peaks – Multipeak-MSP

While establishing that the F0/F1/F2 speech processing strategy (WSPIII) would help profoundly deaf children as well as adults understand running speech, research was also in progress to further improve the speech processing strategy. The motivation for this was that although there was significant improvement in the speech perception scores for the F0/F1/F2 compared to the F0/F2 processor, the results still fell short of the hoped for near normal findings for all patients. Furthermore, although there was a generally improved performance in noise, the consonant scores did not change markedly except for those in which the addition of F1 improved the transmission of voicing. To help overcome the information bottle-neck for electroneural stimulation that was particularly prominent for consonant perception, it was hypothesized that additional high frequency spectral information would help. The speech processor was accordingly modified so that in addition to the F0/F1/F2 processor, the amplitude of the three high frequency filters (ranges: 2000 Hz to 2800 Hz; 2800 Hz to 4000 Hz; and 4000 Hz to 6000 Hz) were determined. For voiced sounds, the outputs from the lower two frequency bands were used to stimulate the more apical two of three fixed electrodes in the high frequency end of the cochlea. For unvoiced sounds the amplitudes at the three high frequency filters were used to excite the three fixed electrodes and, in addition, the F2 but not F1 amplitude was used to stimulate a fourth electrode whose location was appropriate for the F2 frequency.

This strategy, which presented information from four spectral peaks for each glottal pulse, was named Multipeak and was implemented as a smaller wearable speech processor (MSP) by Cochlear Pty Limited. The initial comparison of the MSP with the WSPIII speech processor at The University of Melbourne showed there was significant improvement in the perception of speech both in quiet and in noise (Dowell *et al.*, 1990). A more detailed comparison of the two speech processors has also been made by Skinner *et al.*, (1991) in a controlled study on five patients and by Dowell (1991) also in a controlled study on five patients. These show significant improvements for most elements of speech perception in quiet and noise. The scores for closed sets of both vowels and consonants were better, and this applied to place The MSP-Multipeak speech processor was approved by the FDA in October 1989.

Research in the 1990s

We have continued our research to further improve monaural speech processing for cochlear implants. Recently, we have shown that if we select the outputs of 16 bandpass filters and present these as appropriate current levels to six electrodes on a tonotopic basis, using constant rate of stimulation, we can achieve better results than for the Multipeak-MSP processor (McKay *et al.*, 1991, 1992). The stimulus rate is typically 250 pulses/s, well below the highest rate (500 pulses/s) used in our safety studies (Shepherd *et al.*, 1983a). Further research is now needed to develop this and other strategies and to establish that they are safe.

We have also been undertaking research to determine if cochlear implants in each ear can help improve the total amount of information transmitted, and provide better speech understanding in noise. Initial results on our first patient are encouraging (van Hoesel *et al.*, 1990, 1993).

The monaural speech processing results for electrical stimulation are now better than those for some severely deaf people with residual hearing when using a hearing aid and we have therefore been able to offer implants to people with usable hearing in the opposite ear.

We have been carrying out research to determine how best to combine information through electrical stimulation of one ear, and acoustic stimulation of the other ear. Initial results are encouraging (Dooley *et al.*, 1993), but further research is needed to establish the possible benefits.

Finally, as our clinical results on children are showing better results when they receive their implant at an early age, and as our safety studies for operating under two years are showing no impediments to this

(NIH Contract 'Studies on Pediatric Auditory Prostheses Implants' N01-NS-7-2342), we should see research and clinical work on children as young as one year this decade.

Acknowledgements

I wish to acknowledge the stimulating and helpful collaboration I have had with my scientific and clinical colleagues over the last 29 years. Our research has of necessity been a team effort, and all members have played an important part in the overall development.

Funding the research has always been difficult, but at each stage of the work sources have become available when others have terminated. There has usually been enough, but not an abundance. To all those people who as individuals or as part of organizations or granting bodies have supported our work I say 'thank you'.

Finally, I would like to wish Arne Risberg, in whose honour this chapter is written, a very fruitful retirement and to congratulate him on his scientific achievements.

References

Bismark, G. von (1974) Sharpness as an attribute of the timbre of steady sounds, Acoustica 30:159–72.

Black, R.C. (1978) The Cochlear Prosthesis: Electromechanical and Electrophysiological Studies, Doctor of Philosophy Thesis, University of Melbourne.

Black, R.C. and Clark, G.M. (1977) Electrical transmission line properties in the cat cochlea. Proceedings Australian Physiological and Pharmacalogical Society 8: 137.

Blamey, P.J., Dowell, R.C., Tong, Y.C. and Clark, G.M. (1984a) An acoustic model of a multiple-channel cochlear implant. Journal of the Acoustical Society of America 76: 97–103.

Blamey, P.J., Dowell, R.C., Tong, Y.C., Brown, A.M., Luscombe, S.M. and Clark, G.M. (1984b) Speech processing studies using an acoustic model of a multiple-channel cochlear implant. Journal of the Acoustical Society of America 76: 104–110.

Boothroyd, A. (1968) Developments in speech audiometry. Sound (now British Journal of Audiology) 2: 3–10.

Busby, P.A., Tong, Y.C. and Clark, G.M. (1986) Speech perception studies in the first year of usage of a multiple-electrode cochlear implant by prelingual patients. Journal of the Acoustical Society of America 80 (Suppl 1): 530.

Clark, G.M. (1969a) Middle Ear and Neural Mechanisms in Hearing and in the Management of Deafness. Doctor of Philosophy Thesis, University of Sydney.

Clark, G.M. (1969b) Responses of cells in the superior olivary complex of the cat to electrical stimulation of the auditory nerve. Experimental Neurology 24:124–36.

Clark, G.M. (1970) A neurophysiological assessment of the surgical treatment of perceptive deafness. International Audiology 9:103–9.

Clark, G.M. (1973) A Hearing prosthesis for severe perceptive deafness – experimental studies. Journal of Laryngology and Otology 87:929–45.

Clark, G.M. (1975). A surgical approach for a cochlear implant in anatomical study. Journal of Laryngology and Otology 89: 9–15.

Clark, G.M. (1977) An evaluation of per-scalar cochlear electrode implantation techniques: an histopathological study in cats. Journal of Laryngology and Otology 91,185–99.

Clark, G.M. (1986) The University of Melbourne/Cochlear Corporation (Nucleus) Program; in Balkany, T. The Cochlear implant. Otolaryngologic Clinics. North America 19: 329–54.

Clark, G.M. (1992) The Development of speech processing strategies for The University of Melbourne/Cochlear multiple channel implantable hearing prostheses, JSLPA/ROA 16:1–13.

Clark, G.M. and Hallworth, R.J. (1976) A multiple-electrode array for a cochlear implant. Journal of Otology 90: 623–7.

Clark, G.M., and Shepherd, R.K. (1984) Cochlear implant round window sealing procedures in the cat: an investigation of autograft and heterograft materials. Acta Otolaryngologica (Stockh) Suppl, 410: 5–15.

Clark, G.M., Hallworth, R.J. and Zdanius, K. (1975a) A cochlear implant electrode. Journal of Laryngology and Otology 89: 787–92.

Clark G.M., Pyman, B.C. and Bailey, Q.R. (1979) The surgery for multiple-electrode cochlear implantations. Journal of Laryngology and Otology 93: 215–23.

Clark, G.M., Pyman, B.C. and Pavillard, R.E. (1980) A protocol for the prevention of infection in cochlear implant surgery. Journal of Laryngology and Otology 94:1377–86.

Clark, G.M., Tong, Y.C. and Gwyther, J. (1976) Speech perception and the development of language in deaf children. Proceedings of the 2nd Conference of Audioogical Society of Australia. 1–3.

Clark, G.M., Tong, Y.C., and Martin, L.F.A. (1981a) A multiple-channel cochlear implant: an evaluation using open-set CID sentences. Laryngoscope 91: 628–34.

Clark, G.M., Tong, Y.C. and Martin, L.F.A. (1981b) A multiple-channel cochlear implant: an evaluation using closed-set words. Journal of Laryngology and Otology 95: 461–4.

Clark, G.M., Tong, Y.C. and Patrick, J.F. (1990) Cochlear Prostheses. Edinburgh: Churchill Livingstone. pp 1–5.

Clark, G.M., Nathar, J.M., Kranz, H.G. and Maritz, J.B. (1972) A behavioral study on electrical stimulation of the cochlea and central auditory pathways of the cat. Experimental Neurology 36: 350–61.

Clark, G.M., Tong, Y.C., Martin, L.F.A. and Busby, P.A. (1981c) A multiple-channel cochlear implant: an evolution using an open-set word test. Acta Otolaryngologica 91: 173–5.

Clark, G.M., Kranz, H.G. and Minas, H. (1973) Behavioral thresholds in the cat to frequency modulated sound and electrical stimulation of the auditory nerve. Experimental Neurology 41:190–200.

Clark, G.M., Kranz, H.G., Minas, H. and Nathar, J.M. (1975b) Histopathological findings in cochlear implants in cats. Journal of Laryngology and Otology 89:495–504.

Clark, G.M., O'Loughlin, B.J., Rickards, F.W., Tong, Y.C. and Williams, A.J. (1977b) The clinical assessment of cochlear implant patients. Journal of Laryngology and Otology 91: 697–708.

Clark, G.M., Black, R.C., Dewhurst, D.J., Forster, I.C., Patrick, J.F. and Tong, Y.C. (1977a) A multiple-electrode hearing prosthesis for cochlear implantation in deaf patients. Medical Progress in Technology 5: 127–40.

Clark, G.M., Busby, P.A., Dowell, R.C., Dawson, P.W., Pyman, B.C. and Webb, R.L. (1992).The development of the Melbourne/Cochlear multiple-channel cochlear implant for profoundly deaf children. Australian Journal of Otolaryngology 1: 3–8.

Clark, G.M., Tong, Y.C., Black, R.C., Forster, I.C., Patrick, J.F. and Dewhurst, D.J. (1977c) A multiple electrode cochlear implant. Journal of Laryngology and Otology 91: 935–45.

Clark, G.M., Tong, T.C., Martin, L.F.A., Busby, P.A., Dowell, R.C., Seligman, P.M. and Patrick, J.F. (1981d) A multiple-channel cochlear implant: an evaluation using nonsense syllables. Annals of Otology, Rhinology and Laryngology 90: 227–30.

Clark, G.M., Crosby, P.A., Dowell, R.C., Kuzma, J.A., Money, D.K., Patrick, J.F., Seligman, P.M. and Tong, Y.C. (1983) The preliminary clinical trial of a multi-channel cochlear implant hearing prosthesis. Journal of the Acoustical Society of America 74:1911–13.

Clark, G.M., Dowell, R.C., Pyman, B.C., Brown, A.M., Webb, R.L., Tong, Y.C., Bailey, Q. and Seligman, P.M. (1984) Clinical trial of a multi-channel cochlear prosthesis: results on 10 postlingually deaf patients. Australian and New Zealand Journal of Surgery 54: 519–26.

Clark, G.M., Blamey, P.J., Brown, A.M., Busby, P.A., Dowell, R.C., Franz, B.K-H., Pyman, B.C., Shepherd, R.K., Tong, Y.C. and Webb, R.L. (1987a) The University of Melbourne/Nucleus Multiple Electrode Cochlear Prosthesis. In Pfaltz, C.R. (Ed) Advances in Oto-Rhino-Laryngol. Vol. 38. Basel: Karger.

Clark, G.M., Busby, P.A., Roberts, S.A., Dowell, R.C., Tong, Y.C., Blamey, P.J., Nienhuys, T.G., Mecklenburg, D.J., Webb, R.L., Pyman, B.C. and Franz, B.K. (1987c) Preliminary results for the Cochlear Corporation multi electrode intra-cochlear implant in six prelingually deaf patients. American Journal of Otology 8: 234–9.

Clark, G.M., Blamey, P.J., Busby, P.A., Dowell, R.C., Franz, B.K-H., Musgrave, G.N., Nienhuys, T.G., Pyman, B.C., Roberts, S.A., Tong, Y.C., Webb, R.L., Kuzma, J.A., Money, D.K., Patrick, J.F. and Seligman, P.M. (1987b). A multiple electrode intracochlear implant for children. Archives of Otolaryngology 8: 825–8.

Clark, G.M., Tong, Y.C., Bailey, Q.R., Black, R.C., Martin, L.F., Millar, J.B., O'Loughlin, B.J., Patrick, J.F. and Pyman, B.C. (1978) A multiple electrode cochlear implant. Journal of the Otolaryngological Society of Australia 4: 208–12.

Clifford, A.R. and Gibson, W.P.R. (1987) Anatomy of the round window with respect to cochlear implant surgery. Annals of Otology, Rhinology and Laryngology Suppl. 128, 96: 17–19.

Cooper, F.S., Delattre, P.C., Liberman, A.M., Borst, J.M. and Gerstman, L.J. (1952) Some experiments on the perception of synthetic speech sounds. Journal of the Acoustical Society of America 24: 597–606.

Craig, W. (1964) Effect of preschool training on the development of reading and lipreading skills of deaf children. American Annals of the Deaf 109: 280.

Davis, H. and Silverman, S.R. (1970) Hearing and Deafness. New York: Holt, Rinehart and Winston.

Dawson, P.W., Blamey, P.J., Rowland, L.C., Dettman, S.J., Clark, G.M., Busby, P.A., Brown, A.M., Dowell, R.C. and Rickards, F.W. (1992) Cochlear implants in children, adolescents and prelinguistically deafened adults: speech perception. Journal of Speech and Hearing Research 35: 401–17.

De Filippo, C. L. and Scott, B. L. (1978) A method for training and evaluating the reception of ongoing speech. Journal of the Acoustical Society of America 63: 1186–92.

Delattre, P.C., Liberman, A.M., Cooper, F.S. and Gerstman, L.J. (1952) An experimental study of the acoustic developments of vowel colour observations on one and two formant vowels synthesized from spectrographic patterns. Word 8: 195–210.

Djourno, A., and Eyries, C. (1957). Prosthese auditive for excitation electrique a distance du nerf sensoniel a l'aide d'un bobinage inclus a demeure. Presse Med. 35:14–17.

Dooley, G.J., Blamey, P.J., Seligman, P.M., Alcantara, J.I., Clark, G.M., Shallop, J.K., Arndt, P., Heller, J.W. and Menapace, C.M. (1993) Combined electrical and acoustical stimulation using a bimodal prosthesis. Archives of Otolaryngology 119: 55–60.

Dormer, K.J., Richard, G., Hough, J.V.C. and Hewell, T. (1980) The Cochlear Implant (auditory prosthesis) utilizing rare earth magnets. American Journal of Otology 2: 22–7.

Dowell, R.C. (1991) Speech perception in noise for multichannel cochlear implant users. Doctor of Philosophy thesis, University of Melbourne.

Dowell, R.C., Mecklenburg, D.J. and Clark, G.M. (1986) Speech recognition for 40 patients receiving multi-channel cochlear implants. Archives of Otolaryngology 112:1054–9.

Dowell, R.C., Seligman, P.M., Blamey, P.J. and Clark G.M. (1987) Speech perception using a two-formant 22-electrode cochlear prosthesis in quiet and in noise. Acta Otolaryngologica (Stockholm) 104: 439–446.

Dowell, R.C., Whitford, L.A., Seligman, P.M., Franz, B.K-H. and Clark, G.M. (1990) Preliminary results with a Miniature Speech Processor for the 22-electrode Melbourne/Cochlear Hearing Prosthesis. 14th World Congress of Otology. Amsterdam: Kugler and Ghedini.

Doyle, J.D., Doyle, J.B. and Turnbull, F.M. (1964) Electrical stimulation of eighth cranial nerve. Archives of Otolaryngology 80: 388–91.

Eddington, D.K. (1983) Speech recognition in deaf subjects with multichannel intracochlear electrodes. Annals of the New York Academy of Sciences 405: 241–58.

Fant, G. (1956) On the predictability of formant levels and spectrum envelopes from formant frequencies. In Halle, H. Lurnt, M. and Maclean, H. (Eds) For Roman Jakobson. The Hague: Mounton.

Forster, I.C. (1978). The Biological Development of a Hearing Prosthesis for the Profoundly Deaf. Doctor of Philosophy Thesis, University of Melbourne.

Fourcin, A.J., Rosen, S.M., Moore, B.C.J., Douek, E.E., Clarke, G.P., Dodson, H. and Bannister, L.H. (1979) External electrical stimulation of the cochlea: clinical, psychophysical, speech-perceptional and histological findings. British Journal of Audiology 13: 85–107.

Franz, B.K-H.G. and Clark, G.M. (1987) Refined surgical technique for insertion of banded electrode array. Annals of Otology, Rhinology and Laryngology Suppl. 128, 96:15–17.

Gantz, B.J., McCabe, B.F., Tyler, R.S. and Preece, J.P. (1987) Evaluation of four cochlear implant designs. In International Cochlear Implant Symposium and Workshop – Melbourne; Eds Clark, G.M., and Busby, P.A. Ann. Otol. Rhino. Laryngol. Suppl. 128, 96:145–7.

Gersuni, G.V. and Volokhov, A.A. (1936) On the electrical excitability of the auditory organ: on the effect of alternating currents on the normal auditory apparatus. Journal of Experimental Psychology 19:370–82.

Gisselsson, L. (1950) Experimental investigation into the problem of humoral transmission in the cochlea. Acta Otolaryngologica (Stockh). Supp 82,16.

Hallworth, R.J. (1976) An Implantable Multi-Micro-Electrode Array Fabricated by Thin Film Methods. Master of Engineering Thesis, University of Melbourne.

Hochmair-Desoyer, I.J., Hochmair, E.S., Fischer, R.E. and Burian, L. (1980) Cochlear prostheses in use: recent speech comprehension results. Archives of Otolaryngology 229: 81–9.

House, W.F. and Urban, J. (1973) Long term results of electrode implantation and electronic stimulation of the cochlea in man. Annals of Otology, Rhinology and Laryngology 82: 504.

House, W.F., Berliner, K., Graham, M., Luckey, R., Norton, N., Selters, W., Tobin, H., Urban, J. and Wexler, M. (1976) Cochlear implants. Annals of Otology, Rhinology and Laryngology Suppl. 27, 85:3-6.

Jansen, C. (1968) The combined approach for tympanoplasty. Journal of Laryngology and Otology 82:779–93.

Johnsson, L.G., House, W.F. and Linthcum, T.H. (1982) Otopathological findings in a patient with bilateral cochlear implants. Annals of Otology, Rhinology and Laryngology 91:74–9.

Jones, R.C., Stevens, S.S., and Lurie, M.H. (1940). Three mechanisms of hearing by electrical stimulation. Journal of the Acoustical Society of America 12: 281–90.

Kerr, A. and Schuknecht, H.F. (1968) The spiral ganglion in profound deafness. Acta Otolaryngologica (Stockh) 65: 586–98.

Laird, R.K. (1979) The Bioengineering Development of a Sound Encoder for an Implantable Hearing Prosthesis for the Profoundly Deaf. Master of Engineering Thesis, University of Melbourne.

Lawrence, M. (1964) Direct stimulation of auditory nerve fibres. Archives of Otolaryngology 80: 367–8.

Liberman, A.M., Delattre, P.C., Cooper, F.S. and Gerstman, L.J. (1954) The role of consonant-vowel transitions in the perception of the stop and nasal consonants. Psychology Monographs 68:1–13.

Martin, L.F.A., Tong, Y.C. and Clark, G.M. (1981) A multiple-channel cochlear implant: evaluation using open-set CID sentences. Laryngoscope 91: 628–34.

McDermott, H.J. (1989) An advanced multiple channel cochlear implant. IEEE Transactions in Biomedical Engineering 36: 789–97.

McKay, C.M., McDermott, H.J., Vandali, A.E. and Clark, G.M. (1991) Preliminary results with a six spectral maxima sound processor for The University of Melbourne/Nucleus multiple-electrode cochlear implant. Journal of the Otolaryngological Society of Australia 6: 354–9.

McKay, C.M., McDermott, H.J., Vandali, A.E. and Clark, G.M. (1992) A comparison of speech perception of cochlear implantees using the spectral maxima sound processor (SMSP) and the MSP (Multipeak) processor. Acta Otolaryngologica (Stockh) 112: 752–61.

Merzenich, M.M. (1974) Studies on electrical stimulation of the auditory nerve in animals and man: cochlear implants. In Tower, The Nervous System, 3. New York: Raven Press. pp 337–548.

Michelson, R.P. (1971) Electrical stimulation of the human cochlea – a preliminary report. Archives of Otolaryngology 93: 317–23.

Moxon, E.C. (1967) Electric Stimulation of the Cats Cochlea: A Study of Discharge Rates in Single Auditory Nerve Fibres. Master of Science Thesis, Massachusetts Institute of Technology.

Moxon, E.C. (1968) Auditory nerve responses to electric stimuli. MIT QPR 90: 270–6.

Moxon, E.C. (1971) Neural and Mechanical Responses to Electrical Stimulation of the Cat's Inner Ear. Doctor of Philosophy Thesis, Massachusetts Institute of Technology.

Nienhuys, T.G., Musgrave, G.N., Busby, P.A., Blamey, P.J., Noll, P., Tong, Y.C., Dowell, R.C., Brown, L.F. and Clark, G.M. (1987) Educational assessment and management of children with multichannel cochlear implants. Annals of Oto-Rhino-Laryngology Suppl. 128, 96:80–3.

Ormorod, F.C. (1960). The pathology of congenital deafness. Journal of Laryngology and Otology 74: 919–50.

Owens, E. and Telleen C. (1981) Speech perception with hearing aids and cochlear implants. Archives of Otolaryngology 107:160–2.

Patrick, J.F. and MacFarlane, J.C. (1987) Characterization of mechanical properties of single electrodes and multielectrodes. Annals of Otology, Rhinology and Laryngology Suppl. 128, 96: 46–8.

Plomp, R. (1976) Aspects of Tone Sensation. In Carterette, E.C. and Friedman, M.P. (Eds) Series in Cognition and Perception. London: Academic Press. p 109.

Plomp R. and Steeneken, H.J.M. (1971) Pitch versus timbre. Proceedings 7th International Congress of Acoustics, Budapest 3,377–80.

Potter, R.K., Kopp, G.A. and Green, H.C. (1947) Visible Speech. New York: van Nostrand.

Powell, T.P.S. and Erulkar, S.D. (1962) Transneuronal cell degeneration in the auditory relay nuclei of the cat. Journal of Anatomy 96: 249–68.

Schuknecht, H.F. (1953) Lesions of organ of Corti. Transactions of the American Academy of Ophthalmology and Otolaryngology 57: 366–83.

Schuknecht, H.F. (1964) Further observations on the pathology of presbyacusis. Archives of Otolaryngology 80: 369–82.

Shepherd, R.K. (1977) Platinum Transportation from the Inner Ear of a Cat: A Spectrophotometric Technique. Bachelor of Science Thesis, Deakin University.

Shepherd, R.K., Clark, G.M. and Black, R.C. (1983a) Chronic electrical stimulation of the auditory nerve in cats: physiological and histopathological results. Acta Otolaryngologica (Stockh) Suppl. 399,19–31.

Shepherd, R.K., Clark, G.M., Black, R.C. and Patrick, J.F. (1983b) The histopathological effects of chronic electrical stimulation of the cat cochlea. Journal of Laryngology and Otology 97: 333–41.

Shepherd, R.K., Clark, G.M., Pyman, B.C. and Webb, R.L. (1985) Banded intracochlear electrode array: evaluation of insertion trauma in human temporal bones. Annals of Otology, Rhinology and Laryngology 94: 55–9.

Simmons, F.B., Mongeon, C.J., Lewis, W.R. and Huntington, D.A. (1964) Electrical stimulation of acoustical nerve and inferior colliculus. Results in man. Archives of Otolaryngology 79: 559–67.

Simmons, F.B., Epley, J.M., Lummis, R.C., Guttman, N., Frishkoff, L.S., Harmon, L.D. and Zwicker, E. (1965) Auditory nerve: electrical stimulation in man. Science 148: 104–6.

Simmons, F.B. (1966) Electrical stimulation of the auditory nerve in man. Archives of Otolaryngology 84: 2-4.

Simmons, F.B. (1967) Permanent intracochlear electrodes in cats, tissue tolerance and cochlear microphonics. Laryngoscope 77: 171–86.

Skinner, M.W., Holden, I.K., Holden, T.A., Dowell, R.C., Seligman, P.M., Brimacombe, J.A. and Beiter, A.I. (1991) Performance of postlingually deaf adults with the wearable speech processor (WSPIII) and mini speech processor (MSI) of the Nucleus multi-electrode cochlear implant. Ear and Hearing 12: 3–22.

Staller, S.J., Dowell, R.C., Beiter, A.L. and Brimacombe, J.A. (1991) Perceptual abilities of children with the Nucleus 22-channel cochlear implant. Ear and Hearing Suppl, 4 12: 34–47.

Stevens, S.S. and Jones, R.C. (1939) The mechanisms of hearing by electrical stimulation. Journal of the Acoustical Society of America 10: 261–9.

Stevens, S.S. and Volkmann, J. (1970) The relation of pitch to frequency: a revised scale. American Journal of Psychology 53: 329–53.

Tong, Y.C., Busby, P.A. and Clark, G.M. (1986) Psychophysical studies on prelingual patients using a multiple-electrode cochlear implant. Journal of the Acoustical Society of America 80: Suppl, 1, 530.

Tong, Y.C., Busby, P.A. and Clark, G.M. (1988) Perceptual studies on cochlear implant patients with early onset of profound hearing impairment prior to normal development of auditory, speech and language skills. Journal of the Acoustical Society of America 84: 951–62.

Tong, Y.C., Clark, G.M., Seligman, P.M. and Patrick, J.F. (1980a) Speech processing for a multiple-electrode cochlear implant hearing prostheses. Journal of the Acoustical Society of America 68: 1897–9.

Tong, Y.C., Dowell, R.C., Blamey, P.J. and Clark, G.M. (1984) Two-component hearing sensations produced by two electrode stimulation in the cochlea of a deaf patient. Science 219: 993–4.

Tong, Y.C., Clark, G.M., Blamey, P.J., Busby, P.A. and Dowell, R.C. (1982) Psychophysical studies for two multiple-channel cochlear implant patients. Journal of the Acoustical Society of America 71: 153–60.

Tong, Y.C., Clark, G.M., Dowell, R.C., Martin, L.F.A., Seligman, P.M. and Patrick, J.F. (1981). A multiple-channel cochlear implant and wearable speech-processor. Acta Otolaryngologica (Stockh) 92: 193–8.

Tong, Y.C., Millar, J.B., Clark, G.M., Martin, L.F., Busby, P.A. and Patrick, J.F. (1980b) Psychophysical and speech perception studies on two multiple channel cochlear implant patients. Journal of Laryngology and Otology 94: 1241–56.

Tyler, R.S., Tye-Murray, M., Preece, J.P., Gantz, B.J. and McCabe, B.F. (1987) Vowel and consonant confusions among cochlear implant patients: do different implants make a difference? Annals of Otology, Rhinology and Laryngology 96: suppl 128: 141–44.

Van Hoesel, R.J.M, Tong, Y.C., Hollow, R.D. and Clark, G.M. (1993) Psychophysical and speech perception studies: a case report on a cochlear implant subject. Journal of the Acoustical Society of America 94: 3178–89.

Van Hoesel, R.J.M., Tong, Y.C., Hollow, R.D., Huigen, J.M. and Clark, G.M. (1990) Preliminary studies on a bilateral cochlear implant user. Abstract of presentation at the 120th meeting of the Acoustical Society of America, San Diego, 26–28 November.

Williams, A.J., Clark, G.M. and Stanley, G.V. (1976) Pitch discrimination in the cat through electrical stimulation of the terminal auditory nerve fibres'. Physiology and Psychology 4: 23–7.

10

The Cochlear Implant: A Weapon to Destroy Deafness or a Support for Lipreading? A Personal View

ANITA WALLIN

Introduction

Cochlear implants are advanced electronic 'hearing aids' for deaf people. Unfortunately many culturally deaf (or more properly Deaf) people see the cochlear implant as an attempt by hearing professionals to destroy the rich language and culture of the Deaf community. As a result they are antagonistic towards cochlear implants in general. This antagonism seems to represent a failure to recognize differences between the needs of Deaf people and those with an acquired hearing loss who might best be described as deafened or even deaf. In short the Deaf need habilitation and the deafened need rehabilitation.

People who are born deaf or those who have a strong association with the Deaf community see the cochlear implant as a threat to their identity and to their culture. The origins of this view lie in the United States where cochlear implants were first introduced. Quite possibly, mistakes and misrepresentations were made in these early days of cochlear implantation, and these may have contributed to this antagonism. Whatever the causes, this highly negative view is now widespread among Deaf people throughout the world. But much of this negativity is based, I believe, on ignorance. Many Deaf and Hard-of-Hearing people have never met anyone who uses a cochlear implant, and have little knowledge of the benefits and potential of cochlear implants.

In Sweden we have had the same debate over cochlear implants. It is to be hoped that this has led to better knowledge about implants in general and specifically about their potential for many deafened people. Prior to this debate the needs of the deafened community were not well recognized. It is now accepted that the Deaf have rights to their specific identity and culture. The deafened also need to have their claims to the same rights and privileges recognized.

If we are to understand why cochlear implants are appropriate for many deafened people we need first to understand what it means for a hearing person to be deafened.

Deafness

Daniela Gabizon is an Israeli doctor who is also a deafened adult. At the Fourth International Congress of Hard of Hearing People in Israel she attempted to describe what it is like to be deafened.

> Physicians say that nobody seems to be dying through his ears, at least not by lack of hearing. Wrong! It is a killer! It kills silently. This killer does not leave any sign on the victim's body, he just takes the soul away from it. Hearing loss imposes the most overwhelming threat to a person's self. It severely affects a person's capability in every aspect of life, more than any other disability, to perform in the simplest situations. It undermines the status of the person in society and within the family, and it also severely affects the capacity to earn a decent living.

As a deafened adult I can only agree with this viewpoint. When one becomes deaf one loses one's foothold in existence. Much of what has been built up in life is razed. Every aspect is affected – job, status, self-confidence, finances, personal relations, etc. To be deaf is to suffer a great loss, and this gives rise to a complicated change in a person's life.

My initial experience of my own deafness was that it accelerated my ageing. My body and my soul were both ageing. My deafness resulted from ageing of my hair cells. Through some genetic deficiency they had lost their elasticity or their ability to repair. I started to wear glasses so that I could pick up lipreading cues more accurately. My soul was starving because I was lacking stimuli from my surroundings. My aged parents saw me as a child once again. Worse, I became a child to my own children. The glint in my eyes disappeared. My initiative decreased and my tiredness increased. All of me was sad. My resistance to infections was increased. I aged many years in just a few months. I was ageing much faster than my hearing friends of the same age. My life shifted from one phase to another. The first part of my life had been very effective and was dedicated to goal oriented tasks. With the onset of deafness I entered a time of life more concerned with getting to know myself. I agree with the deafened Swedish author Bo Andersson who said at a meeting in Uppsala that 'being profoundly hard of hearing or deafened has so many similarities to being retired'.

What remains for the person who has been deafened? What can be done? There appear to be some characteristics which make some people better able to cope with deafness. It helps to be strong-willed, creative, and, if possible, patient. If the person is outgoing with a keen sense of humour this will also help. Similarly, someone who possesses great skill in some area and is recognized for this by her/his family, and by society at large, will also be better able to cope with acquired deafness. Supportive family and friends are also a great asset for any deafened person to possess. It also seems to help if the person has had some experience with deafness in a family member or close friend prior to her/his own loss.

Society has certain different expectations for men and women. These expectations in the workplace and in social interactions create unique problems for deafened men. I believe that men face a more difficult situation when they are deafened, because of these societal expectations. There is, however, one group whom, I believe, face the biggest problems of all deafened people. These are children who are deafened before they have mastered reading and writing skills. At this time linguistic skills are also not fully developed. To be deafened at this time in one's life is to face the most terrible situation of all.

When I became deaf I started to examine how other deafened people reacted to their disability. I discovered that there are a number of different ways of confronting hearing loss: some positive and some negative. It seems that deafened people fall into a number of distinct categories. There are those who possess some outstanding ability in a specific field. They might be artists, authors, crafts people, specialists or academics. They retain their status in their specific field despite their deafness. Interpreters and assistants provide satisfactory assistance for such people.

There is another group which consists of those who build up a new status and regain their self-esteem by working within the deafened community. They find a new life working for deafened people's rights, and fighting for a better position for the deafened in society. Their deafness provides them with a new interest in life, and they seize it.

Other deafened people adjust their lifestyle to adapt to their new situation. In some cases this may involve coming into closer contact with the Deaf and embracing aspects of Deaf culture. Others may seek solace in closer contact with nature.

There is a final group who go into an extended and perhaps permanent state of mourning. They see their deafness as overwhelming and can see no way of improving their situation. Deafness for these people represents a form of living death.

Identity

In spite of my total deafness I can never be a full member of Deaf society. My signing skills will never be sufficiently developed to enable me to express all that I would wish. Signing will always be a 'second language' for me. At best I will be partially accepted by the Deaf community. I will always be an 'immigrant' in Deaf society. Deaf culture is a fascinating culture with many unique and exciting characteristics. But I have my roots in the culture of the hearing world and spoken Swedish is my mother tongue. Deafened people have very strong contacts with hearing people. Their families are mostly hearing and most of their friends and workmates are usually hearing. It is within this community that we feel safest and most secure. It is also the society where we have obligations – to our children, to our elderly parents, sick friends, and our jobs. We cannot turn our backs on all of these.

As a deafened person I can ask my family to learn sign language so that they can communicate easily with me. Close friends may also learn it. But the sign language that they learn will almost certainly never be used with other hearing people. It will be used with me and perhaps any other deafened people my family and friends happen to come across. In a perfect world everyone – Deaf, deafened and hearing – would be able to communicate using sign language. But we do not live in Utopia, so this will never be achieved.

Those of us who have become deafened after having acquired spoken language need to able to communicate effectively with all people. If we are to achieve this we need all types of support. We need cochlear implants. We need signs. We need anything and everything that can enhance our communication with the world around us. We need anything and everything that will help overcome isolation and any feeling of handicap.

What Supports are Available?

There is no doubt that signing, either by itself or as a support for speech, does enhance communication. But both parties have to be familiar with it. It is more natural for deafened adults to use signs in patterns that follow the rules of spoken language. In this way, signs are a support for spoken language rather than another language with its own rules and forms.

When one of our senses fails, the others have to assume a higher importance. The eyes and the nose have to compensate for the impressions that the ears previously gave. We have to listen with our eyes, our nose, with our whole body.

Bodily contact such as hugs can, in some situations, say more than words to a deaf person. In Sweden it is far more common for deaf and hard of hearing people to hug each other than it is for hearing people. Even when people are not close friends hugs act as an accepted communication method.

Vibrotactile aids and cochlear implants offer technical support to facilitate communication. Tactiling as used by Gustaf Söderlund (see Chapter 3) can provide a very useful supplement to lipreading. The cochlear implant also provides lipreading support, but in addition it offers access to environmental sounds. Gustaf is a close friend of mine and we have had many opportunities to compare the effectiveness of our two approaches. In noisy situations, such as a restaurant on a busy street, Gustaf's performance is superior. The signals he receives are not disturbed by traffic, other conversations, or by the clatter of china. In a silent room, with good acoustics, my implant provides me with so much information that I am at an advantage. The implant combined with a tactile aid does give me better understanding in a noisy environment, but the improvement is not so great that it outweighs the practical difficulties. Finally, the text telephone should be mentioned. It really improves communication.

But above all we need human support in the form of understanding!

What Support do I Receive from my Implant?

Before I received my implant I was told that if everything went well it would assist my lipreading. It does help my lipreading, but I have found that it offers me much more than that. Before I became deaf, listening provided me with speech information, music, environmental sounds, and the sound of silence. Once I became deaf I lost all of these. The cochlear implant has given me the opportunity to:

- Hear environmental sounds.
- Hear what one person says in a quiet environment.
- Listen to music again, at least to some extent.
- Feel silence, for the implant interrupts the sounds of tinnitus.
- Get feedback of my own voice.

My tinnitus did not vanish with my implant but it has been interrupted to some extent. Coupled to this is my enhanced quality of life, which makes it easier for me to repress the sounds of tinnitus and get on with my daily life. The quality of sound that I receive through my implant would appear to be very poor to any normally-hearing person. Why then do I feel that I have got back half of my life?

The Happiness of Hearing Again

It is as difficult or impossible for a hearing person to understand what it is like to be deaf (Gabizon, 1992) as it is for a deaf person to understand what it is like to 'hear' again with a cochlear implant (Wallin, 1992). It is an indescribable feeling when the barriers to information created by deafness are torn down. This is what happens when the cochlear implant is activated in a deafened person's ear. It will not give back complete hearing, but it provides the possibility to be once again part of a living world. The isolation is broken! One gains an added appreciation of the sounds of life. Our ears are a fantastic resource. We receive sounds in many more situations than any normally-hearing person can appreciate. It was only after I received my implant that I realized how much sounds meant to me and how much they contributed to the quality of my life.

The joy of cochlear implant users at hearing the sound of bird song and other sounds from nature seems strange to many Deaf people. Here we implantees are at an advantage because we have experienced this joy first-hand. We have discovered the happiness of hearing sounds again. The happiness of being able to see again or being able to walk again is accepted. It is time to accept that the same joy is experienced when we can hear again. Deafened people don't long to hear environmental sounds when they are deaf. They have a memory of these sounds. But once the implant is activated the implantee embarks on a voyage of discovery and recovers a source of great happiness. Instead of listening to the internal sounds of tinnitus, interesting external sounds are stimulating our brains.

What sounds are the best? The basic ability to communicate with one person is of course invaluable. When I was deaf what I really missed was casual conversation, social chats, gossip and jokes. Being able to sit on my children's beds and listen to them talk provides me great satisfaction. So does the opportunity to be able to discuss equally and easily with my husband, or to share joys or anxieties with close friends.

In spite of this primary need to be able to talk with one person, the ability to once again hear environmental sounds may just be the most important benefit provided by the cochlear implant. There are no signs or written words which can substitute for the environmental sounds which can still fill my eyes with tears. The ability to once again hear bird song is a wonderful experience, but there are many other sounds which also provide great joy. The sounds of water running, the wind, snow, laughter and crying all provide valuable and interesting information about the world around me. Even trivial things such as the sound of typewriting, the whisk in a bowl, the clatter of china, the rustle of a newspaper, and the sound of the motor of my car or other cars provide me with great satisfaction. These and other sounds can also provide important warning sounds. There are other even more sophisticated insights provided by the implant. Listening to my daughter playing jazz piano as she waits for me to prepare dinner provides me with some information about her state of mind at that moment.

After three years as an implantee I am still learning new sounds.

Recently, quite by chance, I placed my external microphone close to the nose of my sleeping husband. I was rewarded with a terrible noise. He was snoring! I didn't know that he did. Is this interesting information? Scarcely, but it is informative! The cochlear implant acts as an ice breaker. Once again you can take part in the social chit-chat that is so important for us human beings. This builds on itself and results in more spontaneous social contacts and with it an improved view of your own self-worth. Loneliness decreases and everything seems to change for the better. You feel that you have more power, and you regain your status within your group. The implant's influence pervades your whole life, offering new beginnings and the return of many old possibilities. The change from totally deaf to hard-of-hearing has been very well described using poems and photographs in Franz Wimmer's 'Wenn der Nebel Fallt' (When the Mist is Lifting).

My own personal experience and my observations of implants in others have shown me the great value of implants for many deafened people. Sometimes I feel that I overestimate the benefits of my implant and then I have a cable breakdown or I'm stuck without batteries. Once again I am totally deaf for a little while, and I am immediately struck by how much my implant gives me and how frustrated I am without it. Becoming hard of hearing after being totally deaf was a wonderful experience for me, and yet I remember how depressing it was when I was hard-of-hearing before I became totally deaf. The difference now is that I can compare being hard-of-hearing to being totally deaf. Since my implant I have been continually improving but before the implant my situation was steadily deteriorating. I have seen many similarities to my situation in those of a 3-year-old girl deafened by meningitis. The reaction to being deafened is common to all of us, irrespective of our age, but we express our feelings in different ways. There is, however, one important difference between the situation of a deafened adult and that of a deafened child. The child deafened at this age may lose the ability to speak. Adults will have at least expressive communication, and we can always rely on the printed word for reception of language.

Initial Feelings and Expectations

To hear with your implant for the first time is a very exciting experience. You can never really predict how it will sound and how much help it will provide. You can talk to other implantees before you receive your implant, but no one really knows how *you* will perform with it. There are so many factors which will influence how you perform with your implant that it is impossible to predict your own outcome.

Initially I was partly disappointed with my implant, but I never regretted having the operation. Six months later, however, after I'd had a chance to learn how to interpret those electrical signals, I could see

..nuch it had contributed to my quality of life. And I was not the only one who could see the benefits. My family and my friends could all see how much help it gave me.

Looking back, I see now that the implant has in fact exceeded my expectations. It provides support in areas that I did not anticipate. Many of these improvements involve the use of the implant in conjunction with other support systems such as lipreading, body language, and signs. The cochlear implant has given me a positive outlook, and has greatly improved my everyday life. The end result is that I am quite dependent on my implant and would not like to live without it.

Limitations of the Cochlear Implant

The cochlear implant is not a perfect substitute for real ears. No piece of technical equipment can achieve that. The support provided by the implant varies considerably from individual to individual. In common with many other implant users I receive great assistance when my implant supplements lipreading. In face-to-face communication with one person speaking Swedish, I understand most of what is being said to me. But put me in a group of three people or ask me to follow a conversation going on between two other people and I am in trouble. At best I have difficulties in understanding and in some cases I'm totally lost. Thus, I have to have special help if I'm to understand conversations taking place in coffee breaks or at a dinner party. I have extreme difficulty in having a conversation in a big hall. I find it almost impossible to understand what is being said in this situation. When it happens, I am still deaf and very dependent on others if I am to follow what is going on. I need to have another form of communication available to me such as writing or signs.

In most communication situations with normally-hearing people, I find that I am able to get around any problems some way or other. Someone will usually give me some signs or gestures to help me follow the conversation, or they might clarify what was said if I have misunderstood. One situation where I did experience great difficulty with my implant was in attempting to talk with a group of elderly confused patients. These people were apt to start a conversation in unexpected ways, or to deviate from their original topic in a most unpredictable fashion. In this situation I found that I could not rely on anyone for help, and I just felt confused. Today I am prepared to move in closer and make the effort to understand what is being said. When I am older perhaps I will be more inclined to just sit there and let the conversation wash over me. In some of these situations signs may be a real help. As a result I am learning signs as an insurance policy for my old age! I feel that it may be easier at that time to live with other hearing-impaired people regardless of whether or not they have a cochlear implant. Then a true Total Communication approach could be used, combining both sounds and signs.

There are occasions when the sound from my implant does not give me enough information to understand what is being said. There are other times when I have to listen for a long period of time, and I find that my concentration starts to waver. I find that even having a glass of wine at these times can lead to a failure to understand what is being said. Conversely, a cup of coffee may be enough to increase my concentration. The quality, rhythm and loudness of a person's voice or whether the speaker is male or female can also be critical to me. Small differences in a speaker's voice can lead to large differences in understanding.

Unfortunately, I can rarely predict how well I will be able to perform. This can be very confusing, not only to me but the people around me. There are some consonants, for example, [f] and [h], which I find I always miss. I need to be aware that this is going to happen.

When I am having trouble following what is being understood, I need some form of supplementary assistance. Which of the possible support systems do I prefer? At a meeting of the Swedish National Association for Hearing Impaired People I had the chance to select the method I preferred. The meeting was held in a large hall and I could select between a number of possible alternatives. There were interpreters using Swedish Sign Language, while others used signs as a support for speech, the Mouth Hand System (a Danish system which provides the lipreader with hand cues to the consonants) was also available, and a real time written display was also available. Spontaneously, I moved as close as I could to the speaker so I could pick up as much of the speech as possible. When I missed what the speaker said I caught up by following the written words. Why did I adopt this approach? Quite simply I wanted to get as much as possible directly from the speaker. If I was looking at an interpreter I wouldn't be able to pick up the speaker's body language and gestures. It is not just what a speaker says that is important, it is how she or he says it. But this is a personal choice. It is up to the individual person to select the system which is best for her/him. The system I adopted required a good signal from the implant, coupled with fast reading.

I use this approach when I watch television with subtitles, and I find it very satisfying. I almost feel that I am hearing every word. What I miss with my hearing is available via the written word. Other people, however, prefer other methods.

The implant does not give directional hearing. All sound comes from the same direction. I found this very confusing at first. The chatter of sea birds seemed to come from the forest, not the seashore. Over time I have learned to correct some of these problems. Now if I hear a 'car' which never arrives I know it was probably a plane or a helicopter!

Some implantees are very good at telephone conversations. Unfortunately, I am not one of them! I look forward to the availability of video phones so that I will be able to both see and hear the speaker.

In the future I hope that we'll see further improvements to the cochlear implant. Things that I'd like to see include: better microphones, better reproduction of music, a cordless link between the speech processor and the implanted coil, long-life batteries, better telecoils. More consideration should be given to providing implantees with the same options available to hearing aid users. I would like my implant to be able to pick up the signals from telecoils and phones designed for use by the hearing-impaired. In summary, implantees want to see any risks minimized, and the development of a technically better implant.

Shared Responsibility – Duties in Both Directions

Hearing people have an obligation to make society accessible for deaf people. Deaf people, however, also have an obligation to attempt, wherever possible, to communicate with other people. Many hearing-impaired people derive great benefit from conventional hearing aids. There are very often problems but they do give significant support. Deafened people may find it necessary to learn signs to facilitate communication. At the same time they should seek to find out about cochlear implants to see if this approach would be of potential benefit to them. As a deafened friend of mine said, 'My family has willingly learned signs and actively contributed in many ways to improving our communication. An implant may be an alternative for me to help facilitate communication with them.'

One of the best ways to help communication is to inform people that you are profoundly hard-of-hearing or deaf. It's annoying to have to do it, and at times it frightens people away, but it is necessary. As an implantee I have taken to introducing myself as being a 'hearing deaf'. It certainly gains the other person's attention and is an easy way to make her/him aware of my disability. In the future, as the use of the cochlear implant becomes more common, it may not be so necessary to make such an introduction.

It Is Easier to be Deaf When You Can Hear a Little

I once had a very interesting conversation with a profoundly hard-of-hearing woman. Many members of her family were deaf and she had been brought up within the Deaf culture. Perhaps not surprisingly, she was opposed to cochlear implants. However, she said that she thought that her situation was much easier than that of her brothers and sisters, as she received some help from a hearing aid. I feel much the same way about my cochlear implant when I am with other deafened people. It is easier to be deaf when you are able to hear at least a little!

Who Should get a Cochlear Implant? Who Makes the Decision?

There should be freedom of choice for anyone who wants to have an implant. Before someone can make such a choice, however, she or he needs to receive accurate information about the potential benefits and problems of implants. This information needs to come from a variety of expert sources. These should include experts from the fields of medicine, medical engineering, psychology, and rehabilitation. There should be opportunities to meet those deafened people who already have implants. On the other side of the coin, potential implantees should also meet those who are against implantation. Both sides of the argument have to be considered.

Children who have been deafened should have the same rights to the implant as adults. Their situation might be even more critical than adults with acquired deafness. They have the right to all available support. Once a decision has been made it should be supported by all sides. I recognize that sometimes doctors and the relatives of deafened people sometimes overestimate the potential benefit of cochlear implantation for a particular individual. On the other hand, however, many members of associations for the Deaf and the Hard-of-Hearing tend to underestimate or even trivialize the potential benefits of implantation. There are many factors which have to be considered before a decision is made to have or not to have a cochlear implant. For some people it is a very difficult decision to make. Personally, I never hesitated in my decision. I wanted sounds back in my ears, so I had the implant!

It is important that potential implantees and their families have realistic expectations about the potential benefits of the implant. People who expect too much are going to be disappointed. People who are interested in, and accepting of, technological solutions to the problems of hearing disability will probably be most satisfied by the implant. Those people who search for more humanistic solutions to their problems will probably be less satisfied. Those who have trouble accepting and using conventional hearing aids should think long and hard before they make a decision to have an implant.

Some people who work with the deafened feel that before a person has an implant she or he should accept deafness. In reality this will mean waiting for several years. I am not sure that this is a reasonable demand. We don't expect people who have a broken leg to adjust to life in a wheelchair before we deign to put their leg in plaster! A long wait before a decision can be made may create difficulties which will be difficult to repair.

Conclusions

In the end, a cochlear implant is just an advanced hearing aid, but it does offer a great deal to deafened people. The cochlear implant does not give back normal hearing, but it does help many people to live a more meaningful life and help them come to terms with their disability. If my fate was to be deafened, I feel that I am lucky that it happened in this decade when implants are available. I also feel lucky that my type of hearing loss made me a suitable candidate for implantation. Finally, I am glad that I live in a country where the cochlear implant is available to deafened people.

Cochlear implants can change the lives of many deafened people. I hope that in time members of the Deaf culture can appreciate and understand the many benefits we deafened people can derive from cochlear implants. It may not be a suitable solution for their situation, but that is no reason to stand in the way of those of us who have been hearing, and wish to regain at least some access to sound.

References

Gabizon, D. (1992) Becoming deaf. In Congress book from the International Congress of Hard-of-Hearing People, 9–14 August, Jerusalem, Israel.

Wallin, A. (1992) A user's experience of a cochlear implant. In Risberg, A., Felicetti, S., Plant, G. and Spens, K-E. (Eds) Proceedings of the Second International Conference on Tactile Aids and Cochlear Implants, 9–11 June, Stockholm.

Wimmer, K.F. (1991) Wenn der Nebel fällt.

11

Speech Perception and Production Skills in Children with Cochlear Implants

MARY JOE OSBERGER

Introduction

Roughly 10 years have passed since the first clinical trials began with cochlear implants in children (Berliner and Eisenberg, 1985). Since that time, numerous advances have been made in implant technology and in the application of this technology to clinical populations. Even though researchers strive to develop even more effective implant devices (Wilson *et al.*, 1991), the performance of children with the current technology has far surpassed the expectations of professionals involved in this field of study, as well as those of most parents whose children have been implanted. No other sensory aid has had the same impact on improving the viability of oral communication for children with profound hearing impairments as have cochlear implants, not even acoustic hearing aids. Yet, while the literature contains a number of studies on children's performance with implants, this field of study is still in its infancy. Research has shown that the performance of children improves beyond three years of multichannel implant use and, thus, the upper limit of performance with commercially available implants has not been established (Miyamoto *et al.*, 1993; Osberger *et al.*, 1993). As the performance of implanted children continues to improve, initial criteria used to determine implant candidacy have been challenged. Moreover, implants are now being recommended for very young, preverbal children which poses unique challenges in determining candidacy and evaluating device benefits.

The purpose of this chapter is to review some of the major findings that have been reported on children's performance with implants. The goal is not to provide an exhaustive review of studies in the literature because this is available in other publications (see Tyler, 1993a). Rather, the intent is to present current results to highlight research directions in the clinical application of implants with children.

Evaluation of Speech Perception Abilities

Outcome measures

Selection of outcome measures (dependent variables) has posed an enormous challenge because few appropriate measures existed at the time that implant research began with children. New measures were developed but test construction was affected by the limited language abilities of the children who were implant candidates. The restricted word knowledge of children with profound hearing impairments limits the number of lexical items on a test, especially if the items must be pictured to elicit a response from the child. A limited number of items requires relatively large changes in performance for statistical significance to be reached and reduces the number of equivalent lists or forms that can be developed. The latter problem increases the potential that there might be long-term test learning effects if children are evaluated with the same test items over time. Moreover, at the time that many tests were implemented with implanted children, relatively little was known about the performance of children with hearing aids on the same measure.

Since paediatric implant work began, a number of new procedures have been developed to evaluate children's pre- and post-implant performance (Boothroyd, 1991; Geers and Moog, 1990; Osberger et al., 1991a; Tyler, 1993b). A complete description of these measures appears in Tyler (1993a). The measures used most often to assess auditory speech perception abilities in implanted children can be divided into three major categories. One group of tests assesses recognition of words on the basis of non-phonetic or prosodic cues. Performance on these measures presumably reflects perception of temporal and amplitude changes in speech. Examples of these measures are the Discrimination After Training (DAT) Test (Thielemeir, 1984), the Monosyllable-Trochee-Spondee Test (MTS) (Erber and Alencewicz, 1976) and the Early Speech Perception (ESP) tests (Geers and Moog, 1990).

The Change/No Change Test (Carney et al., 1993; Osberger et al., 1991a) was designed to assess detection of changes in speech features without requiring a word recognition response. The stimuli consist of syllables spoken by an adult male, digitized and manipulated to equalize overall syllable duration and intensity within a trial, and then recorded on audiotape. Each trial consists of a sequence of 10 syllables. All 10 syllables are the same on a no-change trial, whereas the last five syllables differ from the first five on a change trial. The test contains seven subtests each of which contrasts a different speech feature (syllable length, intonation, fundamental frequency, talker gender, vowel height, vowel place and consonant manner). The children are instructed to respond 'same' on a no-change trial, and 'different' on a change trial. Chance performance is 50%.

A second group of measures assess word recognition abilities in a closed set. That is, the child has a set of alternatives from which to chose the answer. Examples of these tests are the Monosyllable-Trochee-Spondee Test (Erber and Alencewicz, 1976) (word recognition based on phonetic distinctions can be assessed on this measure as well as word recognition based on non-phonetic distinctions), the Word Intelligibility by Picture Identification (WIPI) (Ross and Lerman, 1971), Northwestern University Children's Perception of Speech (NU-CHIPS) (Elliott and Katz, 1980), and subtests of the ESP tests (Geers and Moog, 1990). A measure developed in our laboratory is the Minimal Pairs Test (Robbins *et al.*, 1988). It consists of pairs of pictured words, with members of a pair differing in terms of a single vowel or consonant. The test consists of 20 word pairs, 12 with consonant contrasts and 8 with vowel contrasts. Each word in a pair is presented as a test item but in random order, totalling 40 different items. Each item is presented two times, also in random order, totalling 80 items on the entire test. The test is administered via live voice. Performance on the test is analysed in terms of vowel and consonant features (vowel height, vowel place, consonant voice, manner and place). Chance performance is 50%.

The third category of tests are those that assess speech recognition in an open-set. A great deal of emphasis is placed on these measures because they require that the child have stored representations of spoken words to repeat the items back correctly. That is, the child must match a spoken word to an underlying representation of that word in his or her mental lexicon. This process requires that implant processing schemes encode enough detail for the child to establish phonetic categories, a formidable task given the impoverished speech signal that is transmitted by the implant relative to that provided by the normal ear.

An open-set measure commonly used is the Phonetically Balanced Kindergarten Test (PBK) (Haskins, 1949) which assesses recognition of monosyllabic words. The Common Phrases Test (Osberger *et al.*, 1991a) was developed in our laboratory to assess understanding of familiar phrases used in everyday situations. This test was motivated by the notion that children would be better able to recognize familiar phrases than monosyllabic words in an open-set, a notion based on the assumption that children would make use of linguistic redundancy to aid their speech understanding as do listeners with normal hearing. The test employs a pre-test familiarization of item topics to orient the child to the task. The child is shown a set of 10 pictured items and told that simple questions, commands, or statements will be said about the items. The card with the pictured items is then removed before testing begins. Performance is scored in terms of the percentage of phrases correctly understood. That is, the child must repeat correctly all words in a phrase to receive credit for that item (if a question is asked, the child is given full credit if answered appropriately). The child must demonstrate *comprehension* of each test item. If the examiner is uncertain about this, the child is queried to determine if the item was comprehended correctly. If not, the child receives no credit for the item. This strict scoring system is used because the high predictability and familiarity of the phrases and the pretest familiarization might yield spurious scores. This test is administered with auditory cues only, visual cues only, or combined auditory plus visual cues.

A problem with most of the measures developed for implant evaluation, however, is that relatively little is known about their psychometric properties, especially test–retest reliability. This information is essential to determine if within- and between-subjects differences reflect random variations in performance or real improvement on a measure. Collecting test–retest reliability data is difficult in this population because most children do not live in the same city as the implant centre and time constraints make repeated administrations of the tests within a short time interval difficult. One approach to this problem is to establish test–retest reliability with data collected from children with profound hearing impairments who use conventional hearing aids. Carney and her colleagues (Carney *et al.*, 1991) collected test–retest data on selected speech perception measures from 11 subjects with profound hearing impairments who used conventional hearing aids. The subjects were tested two times on the measures within a 2–3 week period. Table 1 shows the means and standard deviations of the differences between the initial tests and the retests for the 11 subjects. The data in Table 1 suggest greater variability on the MTS: Stress (word recognition based on non-phonetic cues) and the Common Phrases Test than for the other measures. Carney *et al.* (1991) also reported that test–retest reliability varied among tests more than it varied within individual subjects, and, similarly, scores within a single test varied more than scores within individual subjects. The investigation of Carney and colleagues is still underway with test–retest data being collected from more subjects. These additional data will provide important information on the reliability of many of the speech perception measures used to evaluate implant performance.

Table 1. Means and standard deviations for differences between initial test and retest scores in per cent correct (after Carney *et al.*, 1991).

Test	Mean	SD
Change/No Change	2.5	2.5
Minimal Pairs	5.0	2.7
MTS:Word	9.8	11.6
MTS:Stress	11.2	11.0
Common Phrases: Auditory + Visual	8.2	8.7
Common Phrases: Auditory	5.4	12.1

Because the validity of most of the speech perception measures is unknown, Robbins and colleagues (Robbins *et al.*, 1991) developed the Meaningful Auditory Integration Scale (MAIS) to assess use of sound in everyday situations. The MAIS is designed to assess children's: (1) bonding to their sensory aid; (2) alerting to sound in the environment, and (3) ability to derive meaning from auditory phenomena. 'Bonding' to the device is included because it is assumed the child must have a consistent routine for wearing the device to derive maximum benefit from it, and it is assumed that the greater the benefit derived from the device, the more willing the child will be to wear it. Alerting to sound is assessed in situations in which the child is not in a 'listening set', reflecting spontaneous responses to sound in everyday situations. Deriving meaning from sound examines the child's ability to associate sounds with their events in the environment.

The MAIS consists of a series of 10 items which are used as probes to query the parents about the frequency of occurrence of observed behaviour. An interview technique rather than direct questioning is used to avoid biasing the parents' responses and eliminate the possibility of yes–no responses. The responses to each probe are scored on a scale from 0 to 4, based on the frequency of the reported behaviour (0 = never, 1 = rarely, 2 = occasionally, 3 = frequently, 4 = always). Detailed scoring criteria were developed and inter- and intra-judge reliability data reported (Robbins *et al.*, 1991). The investigation by Robbins *et al.* (1991) revealed that there were differences in MAIS scores as a function of the type of sensory aid used by the children. Subjects who used conventional hearing aids (mean three-frequency pure tone average in the better ear was 91 dB HL) had the highest score (mean score = 28, range = 15 to 37), followed by Nucleus users (mean score = 19, range = 8 to 30), then single-channel implant users (mean = 13, range = 2 to 33), and users of a two-channel vibrotactile aid (Tactaid II) had the lowest score (mean score = 5, range = 0 to 8).

Figure 1 shows recent data collected with the MAIS, plotted as a function of duration of implant use. Data are reported for 51 prelingually deafened children who received the Nucleus implant before age 9. The data plotted in Figure 1 are cross-sectional in that scores were averaged across all subjects who had been evaluated at a particular interval. Scores on questions 1 and 2, 3 to 6, and 7 to 10 reflect device bonding, alerting to sound, and deriving meaning from sound, respectively. In the pre-implant condition, the mean score on device-bonding was the highest which reflects hearing aid or tactile aid use. The steady improvement in device bonding following implantation was due to: (1) the increased amount of time that the implant was used over the pre-implant sensory aid (i.e., hearing aids or tactile aid), and (2) an increase in detecting and identifying device problems. The pre-implant scores on the questions that probed alerting to and deriving meaning from sound were lower than those that assessed device-bonding, reflecting the very limited auditory abilities of these subjects before they were implanted. After 6 months, there was a sharp increase in alerting to sound in the environment which appeared to reach a plateau after 2 years of implant use. Deriving meaning from sound improved at a slower rate than did improvement in the other two areas. The data also suggest that the MAIS was most sensitive to these global changes in auditory performance during the first two years of implant use. Improvement on the MAIS after that time was more limited. This latter finding might reflect the fact that other types of auditory skills were developing beyond 2 years of implant use, such as word recognition, that were not assessed by the MAIS (Fryauf-Bertschy, 1992; Miyamoto *et al.*, 1992; Osberger *et al.*, 1991a).

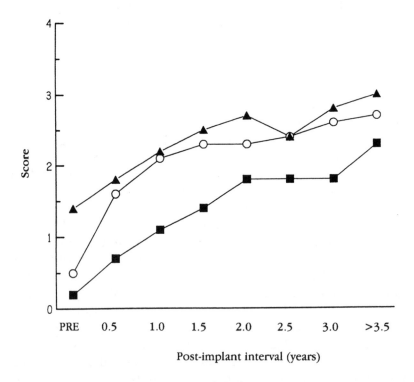

Figure 1. Mean scores of 51 prelingually deafened subjects with Nucleus cochlear implant on the Meaningful Auditory Integration Scale (MAIS) as a function of duration of implant use. The number of Nucleus subjects tested at each interval was: 39, 34, 27, 25, 21, 15 and 15 at the pre, 0.5, 1.0, 1.5, 2.0, 2.5 and 3.0 year post-implant interval, respectively. The mean score at the last interval is the average of the data collected at the 3.5, 4.0, 4.5 and 5.0 years post-implant intervals. At these intervals, 20 scores were averaged from 15 different children. ▲ Device bonding, O Alert to sound, ■ Derive meaning.

Variables Affecting Performance with Implants

Research has shown that there are large individual differences among implanted children on speech perception measures. Some children demonstrate relatively high levels of speech recognition, whereas others perceive primarily prosodic speech information from their devices (Osberger *et al.*, 1991a; Staller *et al.*, 1991a, 1991b; Waltzman *et al.*, 1990, 1992). The independent variables that have most often been examined to explain such performance differences are age at onset of deafness, duration of deafness before implantation, and educational setting. Studies by Staller and colleagues (Staller *et al.*, 1991a, 1991b) reported that two factors, age at onset of deafness and duration of deafness, were significantly related to speech perception performance in children who used the Nucleus multichannel cochlear implant. Specifically, they found that subjects with later onset and shorter duration of deafness tended to perform better on measures of speech perception than did subjects with early onset of deafness but relatively long duration of deafness at the time of implantation.

A recent study by Miyamoto and colleagues (Miyamoto *et al.*, 1993) revealed that age at onset of deafness was not a significant factor in implant performance if the deafness occurred before age 3 years and children were implanted before the age of 10 years. This study compared the speech perception skills of prelingually deafened children with congenital deafness or deafness acquired before age 3 years from meningitis. The results showed no statistically significant difference between the scores of the two groups of subjects on nearly every speech perception measure. Data reported by other investigators have provided additional information about the relationship between age at onset and duration of deafness and implant performance. These data suggested that if the onset of deafness was early and implantation did not occur until the teen years, improvements in speech perception were much more limited than if implantation occurred at an earlier age and after a shorter duration of deafness (Osberger *et al.*, 1993). Now that more children are being implanted between the ages of 2 and 4 years, it will be important to determine if their performance with an implant exceeds that of children who have been implanted at an older age (i.e., after age 5 or 6).

The post-implant performance of children with postlingual deafness (i.e., onset of deafness at age 5 years or later) differs from that of children with prelingual deafness in several important respects. Children with relatively late onset of deafness typically show rapid and marked improvement in speech perception abilities with an implant (Fryauf-Bertschy *et al.*, 1992; Osberger *et al.*, 1991a, 1993)). This finding suggests that these children developed underlying representations of spoken language before they became deaf, whereas prelingually deafened children must rely on the information from the implant to develop such representations. Because of this difference, the performance of prelingually deafened children improves at a much slower pace than that of postlingually deafened children. At this time, it is not known if the performance levels achieved by prelingually deafened children with an implant will eventually match those of postlingually deafened children.

The results of several investigations have shown a significant relationship between the communication method used by the child and performance on speech perception measures. In these studies, more children who used oral communication achieved higher levels of implant performance than did children who used Total Communication (Berliner *et al.*, 1989; Osberger *et al.*, 1991a; Somers, 1991). The relationship between communication mode and implant performance is less clear in other studies. For example, Miyamoto *et al.* (1993) found that children who used oral communication obtained significantly higher scores on only 2 of the 13 speech perception measures in their study. Clearly, additional research is needed to clarify this issue.

A variable that needs to be considered in implant performance in the pediatric population is the length of time that the child has used the device. As noted above, research has shown that perceptual skills develop over a relatively long time-course in prelingually deafened children (Fryauf-Bertschy *et al.*, 1992; Miyamoto *et al.*, 1992; Waltzman *et al.*, 1990, 1992). A recent study by Miyamoto *et al.* (in press) examined the relationship between this variable, as well as other demographic and device variables, and four measures of speech perception (two closed- and two open-set speech recognition measures) in 61 children who used the Nucleus multichannel cochlear implant. The results of a series of multiple regression analyses revealed that the variables of processor type (Wearable Speech Processor III or MiniSpeech Processor), duration of deafness, communication mode (oral or total communication), age at onset of deafness, duration of implant use, and age implanted accounted for roughly 35% of the variance on two tests of closed-set word recognition, and 40% of the variance on measures that assessed recognition of open-set speech recognition. A finding of significance was that duration of implant use accounted for the most variance on all of the speech perception measures. This finding supports a number of previous studies which showed that substantial improvements in closed-set word recognition usually did not occur until after the children had used the implant for more than one year, and improvements in open-set speech recognition occurred after an even longer period of device use (Fryauf-Bertschy *et al.*, 1992; Miyamoto *et al.*, 1992; Osberger *et al.*, 1991a; Waltzman *et al.*, 1990, 1992).

Speech Perception Results with Cochlear Implants

Single versus multichannel cochlear implants

Evaluation of different implant devices (i.e., single and multichannel implants) has been dictated by the chronology of implant technology. The first implant used with children was a single-channel one, the 3M/House device in 1980 (Berliner and Eisenberg, 1985). In 1986, worldwide clinical trials began with a multichannel device, the Nucleus 22-Channel Cochlear Implant System (Mecklenburg *et al.*, 1991). Most investigations with children have reported on the performance of either single- or multichannel implant users, whereas relatively few studies have compared performance as a function of implant type. A study conducted by Miyamoto and colleagues (Miyamoto *et al.*, 1992) is one of the few that compared the performance of matched groups of children who used either the 3M/House device or the Nucleus multichannel cochlear implant over time. The results revealed that the performance of the Nucleus users was higher on every speech perception measure, even on those measures that assessed aspects of speech purportedly transmitted the best by the single-channel device (i.e., selected suprasegmental information). Thus, the multichannel implant not only permitted better word recognition without lipreading, but it also conveyed better information about the time-intensity cues in speech. This finding suggests that the relative benefit of a multichannel over a single-channel device is realized in the perception of suprasegmental, as well as segmental speech information. Even though some reports have shown that a small percentage of children demonstrated open-set speech recognition with the 3M/House implant (Berliner *et al.*, 1989; Geers and Moog, 1989), the highest level of performance achieved by the *majority* of single-channel users was the perception of stress pattern and syllable number in speech. Moreover, even those subjects who demonstrated high levels of performance with a single-channel implant would probably have demonstrated even higher levels of performance with a multichannel device.

Even though there is abundant evidence that shows users of multichannel devices obtain more benefit from their devices than do single-channel users (Gantz *et al.*, 1988; Cohen *et al.*, 1993; Miyamoto *et al.*, 1992), the issue of single versus multichannel implants is still controversial outside the United States. This is an issue of particular importance in Europe since the introduction of the MED-EL broadband analogue single-channel cochlear implant systems (Hochmair-Desoyer and Steinwender, 1993). At this time, however, there are few data to support the use of single-channel implants over multichannel ones, especially in prelingually deafened children. The following case study further illustrates the advantages of single-channel devices over multi-channel ones. Jennifer became deaf at 1.3 years of age from meningitis and she was implanted with the 3M/House single-channel implant when she was 4½ years old. She used that device for roughly four years and then she received the Nucleus implant when she was about 8½ years of age. The functioning single-channel implant was removed and the Nucleus device was implanted in the same ear in which the single-channel device had been used. The removal of the functioning 3M/House device and implantation of the same ear with the multichannel implant was made by Jennifer's parents.

Table 2 shows her performance over time with the single- and multi-channel device on the Minimal Pairs and Common Phrases Tests, described above. With the single-channel device, she identified some words correctly on the basis of vowel distinctions but her scores even on these items were far from perfect. Her scores on the consonant items remained no better than chance for the 4 years of single-channel implant use. There was, however, improvement in her lipreading skills over time with the single-channel implant, evidenced by her score on the Common Phrases test when the stimuli were presented in the audi-tory-plus-visual condition. In contrast, her score remained at zero when the phrases were presented with only auditory cues. After 6 months of multichannel use, Jennifer demonstrated a large improvement in her recognition of words based on vowel distinctions and there was grad-ual improvement in her recognition of words that differed in terms of manner distinctions, as shown by her scores on the Minimal Pairs Test. Her recognition of words on the basis of consonant place and voicing features, however, remained poor even after 2 years of multichannel use. Jennifer demonstrated open-set speech recognition after 6 months of multichannel implant use, as shown by her performance on the Common Phrases Test when it was administered with only auditory cues. A noteworthy finding is that her performance on this measure increased from 20 to 90% between the 6 and 18 months post-implant intervals.

Speech perception results with multichannel cochlear implants

Within-subjects design

The approach that has been used most often to evaluate implant bene-fit in children is a within-subjects design wherein the subject serves as his or her own control in the pre-and post-implant conditions. The largest studies of this type have been conducted by Cochlear Corporation as part of the clinical trials of the Nucleus multichannel implant in children (Staller *et al.*, 1991a, 1991b). Staller *et al.* have used a single-subject repeated-measures approach and determined

Table 2. Scores (per cent correct) for one subject who initially was implanted with the 3M/House device and later upgraded to the Nucleus device in the same ear

Test	3M/House implant use (yrs)				Nucleus implant use (yrs)		
	1.0	2.0	3.0	4.0	0.5	1.5	2.0
[a]Minimal Pairs: Vowel Place	19	69	69	81	88	94	94
Minimal Pairs: Vowel Height	50	63	88	56	100	94	100
Minimal Pairs: Consonant Voice	56	56	63	50	56	56	56
Minimal Pairs: Consonant Manner	38	44	44	38	81	75	100
Minimal Pairs: Consonant Place	63	50	63	31	50	63	50
Common Phrases: Auditory + Visual	20	80	100	100	100	100	100
Common Phrases: Auditory	0	0	0	0	20	90	100

[a]Chance performance = 50%.

statistical significance of the changes between the pre- and post-implant scores using the binomial model (Thorton and Raffin, 1978).

A unique aspect of the Staller *et al.* (1991a) investigation was that subjects were tested before and after an 8-week training period with their pre-implant sensory aid (i.e., conventional hearing aids or tactile aid). The results showed that none of the mean differences between pre- and post-training were statistically significant for the Monosyllable-Trochee-Spondee test (MTS) (Erber and Alencewicz, 1976) or for the Auditory Numbers Test (ANT) (Erber, 1980), a test similar in concept to the MTS but designed for young children. Thus, these results suggested that improvement in performance following implantation was not likely to be due to the effects of training alone. Mean scores reported after 12 months of multichannel implant use were 39% (n = 84) on the MTS word recognition test, 23% (n = 42) on the GASP sentences (Erber, 1982), an open-set sentence recognition task, and 12% (n = 25) on the PBK test (Staller *et al.*, 1991b). Examination of performance changes of individual subjects after 12 months of implant use revealed that 13% of the subjects demonstrated significantly above chance closed-set word identification on the MTS test before implantation, whereas postoperatively, 62% could perform the task at significantly above chance levels. Preoperatively, the subjects showed no open-set speech recognition, but 12 months after implantation, 45% of the subjects recognized one or more words in the GASP sentences.

For research purposes, it is important to analyse pre-and post-implant performance with statistical analyses. Such analyses, however, may not always reveal changes that are of *clinical* significance. Geers and Moog (1989) have developed a classification system that describes performance along a hierarchy of speech perception abilities: (1) detection/inconsistent pattern perception, (2) consistent pattern perception, (3) inconsistent word identification, (4) consistent word identification, and (5) open-set word recognition. Staller *et al.* (1991b) reported that the percentage of children reaching category 3 and above increased from 12% preoperatively to 80% postoperatively, and roughly half of the subjects demonstrated open-set speech recognition and were assigned a category rating of 5. Osberger *et al.* (1991a) developed a similar classification scheme, modified to describe performance on the tests in their assessment battery, and also found that about one-half of the subjects demonstrated open-set speech recognition with their implants. Classifications schemes such as the one developed by Geers and Moog (1989) are extremely useful in counseling parents about potential implant benefits as well as monitoring post-implant progress.

Between-subjects design

A criticism of the within-subjects design is that it is difficult to interpret the results relative to the performance of other children with profound hearing impairments who have not received an implant. Even though there might be statistically significant differences between pre-and post-implant scores, it, nevertheless, can be difficult to determine the significance of these changes. Comparison of implanted children's performance with that of a control group can address this issue. In our laboratory, we have compared the performance of implanted children with that of children with profound hearing impairments who use conventional hearing aids (Miyamoto *et al.*, 1993; Osberger *et al.*, 1993). Previous research has shown that children with profound hearing impairments demonstrate a wide range of auditory capabilities (Boothroyd, 1984; Erber, 1972). Using the results of previous investigators as a guide, hearing aid users have been divided into three groups based on the unaided better-ear pure tone thresholds at 500, 1000, 2000 Hz. Subjects classified as *Gold* hearing aid users demonstrated pure tone thresholds of 90 to 100 dB HL at two of the three frequencies (with none of the thresholds greater than 105 dB HL). *Silver* hearing aid users demonstrated hearing levels of 101 to 110 dB HL at two of the three frequencies, whereas *Bronze* hearing aid users demonstrated two of three thresholds greater than 110 dBHL. Using this approach, the Gold hearing aid users were viewed as setting the 'gold standard of performance' for children with profound hearing impairments because previous research has shown that children with this amount of residual hearing develop the most intelligible speech (Smith, 1975; Ling and Milne, 1981; Monsen, 1978). At the other end of the continuum were Bronze hearing aid users who appeared to respond to auditory stimuli on the basis of vibrotactile sensation (Boothroyd and Cawkwell, 1970). To date, the majority of children who have received implants would be classified as Bronze hearing aid users. The unaided pure tone thresholds of the Silver hearing aid users are intermediate to those of the other two groups.

Figure 2 shows the cross-sectional data for 62 Nucleus users compared to the mean scores of the three groups of hearing aid users on two tests of closed-set word recognition. The subjects were prelingually deafened (i.e., before age 3 years) and they were implanted before age 9 years. Their mean age at onset of deafness was 0.8 years and the mean age that they were implanted was 5.8 years. Whenever possible, subjects were tested in the pre-implant condition and at 6-month intervals thereafter. Some subjects, however, entered the study after they had already received their implant or they were not available at every post-implant interval. Therefore the data were analysed on a cross-sectional basis. Data also are shown for 21 Gold hearing aid users (mean PTA of 94 dB HL; mean chronological age = 10.2 years) and 10 Silver hearing aid users (mean PTA of 104 dB HL; mean chronological age = 8.2 years), and 28 Bronze hearing aid users (mean PTA > 110 dB HL, mean chronological age = 7.0 years). Recall that all of the Bronze hearing aid users received a Nucleus multichannel implant, and were subsequently followed as implant subjects. In our research programme, the performance of the hearing aid users is being evaluated over time on these measures, but the data in Figure 2 and in all subsequent figures reflect the mean score at one interval for these subjects (i.e., the most recent evaluation interval).

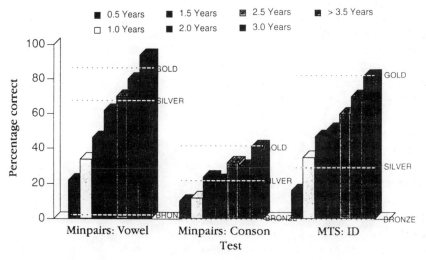

Figure 2. Mean scores of 62 prelingually deafened subjects with Nucleus cochlear implant on the vowel and consonant items on the Minimal Pairs test and the Monosyllable-Trochee-Spondee (MTS) test as a function of duration of implant use. The number of Nucleus subjects tested at each interval was: 31, 17, 24, 20, 15 and 14, at the 0.5, 1.0, 1.5, 2.0, 2.5 and 3.0 year post-implant intervals, respectively. The mean score at the last interval is the average of the data collected at the 3.5, 4.0, 4.5 and 5.0 years post-implant intervals. At these intervals, 25 scores were averaged from 15 different children. The dashed lines show the mean score for three groups of hearing aid subjects, Bronze (*n* = 28), Silver (*n* = 10) and Gold (*n* = 21) at one test interval.

Performance on the Minimal Pairs test (Figure 2) has been analysed in terms of word recognition based on vowel and consonant contrasts. The results show relatively large and rapid improvement in the implanted children's recognition of words based on vowel distinctions. After 2.5 years of implant use, the mean score of the Nucleus subjects was the same as that of the Silver hearing aid users, and after 3 years of implant use, the performance of the implant subjects was better than that of the Silver hearing aid users. At the last interval, the mean score of the Nucleus group was actually slightly higher than that of the Gold group. A similar pattern of performance was present on the MTS word identification test except that the performance of the Nucleus users surpassed that of the Silver hearing aid users after only one year of device use. Scores for all groups were lower on the consonant items of the Minimal Pairs test than for the vowel items and the word recognition score on the MTS. However, the pattern of performance among the groups of subjects was the same as that observed for the vowels items on the Minimal Pairs test and the MTS word recognition.

Figure 3 compares the performance of the four groups of subjects on the consonant items of the Minimal Pairs test plotted as a function of feature. These data show that the manner feature was perceived the

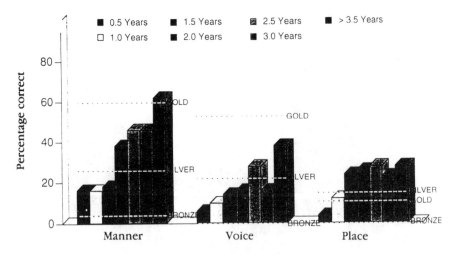

Figure 3. Mean scores of 62 prelingually deafened subjects with Nucleus cochlear implant on the consonant features of the Minimal Pairs test as a function of duration of implant use. The number of subjects tested at each interval was: 31, 17, 24, 20, 15 and 14, at the 0.5, 1.0, 1.5, 2.0, 2.5 and 3.0 year post-implant intervals, respectively. The mean score at the last interval is the average of the data collected at the 3.5, 4.0, 4.5 and 5.0 years post-implant intervals. At these intervals, 25 scores were averaged from 15 different children. The dashed lines show the mean score for three groups of hearing aid subjects, Bronze ($n = 28$), Silver ($n = 10$) and Gold ($n = 21$) at one test interval.

best by all groups. An interesting finding is that there was very little difference between the hearing aid groups in their perception of place information. Moreover, after 1.5 years of implant use, the mean score of the Nucleus users was higher on this feature than that of both the Silver and Gold hearing aid users. The mean score of the Nucleus users was higher than that of the Silver hearing users on consonant voice but was about 15% lower than that of the Gold hearing aid users on this feature.

Figure 4 summarizes the performance of the groups on the Common Phrases test. When the test was administered with auditory cues only, the mean score of the Nucleus users was relatively low, although there was improvement in this condition over time. At the one-year post-implant interval, the mean score of the Nucleus users was higher than that of the Silver hearing aid users. In contrast, the mean score of the Nucleus users remained lower than that of the Gold hearing aid users, even after 3.5 years or more of multichannel implant use. When the test was administered with auditory-plus-visual cues, there were large and rapid improvements in the scores of the Nucleus users which surpassed the mean score of the Silver hearing aid users

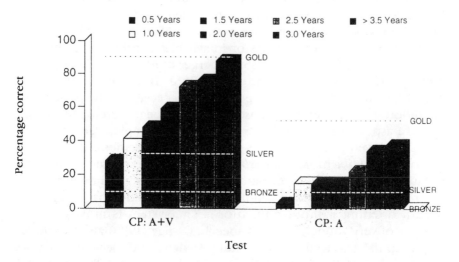

Figure 4. Mean scores of 62 prelingually deafened subjects with Nucleus cochlear implant on the Common Phrases (CP) test as a function of duration of implant use. The test was administered with combined auditory and visual (A + V) cues or auditory (A) cues only. The number of Nucleus subjects tested at each interval was: 31, 17, 24, 20, 15 and 14, at the 0.5, 1.0, 1.5, 2.0, 2.5 and 3.0 year post-implant intervals, respectively. The mean score at the last interval is the average of the data collected at the 3.5, 4.0, 4.5 and 5.0 years post-implant intervals. At these intervals, 25 scores were averaged from 15 different children. The dashed lines show the mean score for three groups of hearing aid subjects, Bronze (n = 28), Silver (n = 10) and Gold (n = 21) at one test interval.

after one year of device use and matched that of the Gold hearing aid users at the last evaluation interval.

The results of this study revealed that improvement in speech perception skills occurred beyond 3 years of implant use in children with prelingual deafness. After one-to-two years of device use, the performance of the implanted subjects surpassed that of the Silver hearing aid users on the measures. Moreover, the scores of the implanted subjects gradually improved to approximate those of the Gold hearing aid users on almost every measure. These data not only illustrate the long time-course over which learning occurs but further suggest that children classified as Silver hearing aid users might benefit more from a multi-channel cochlear implant than from use of only hearing aids. These findings are in general agreement with those of other investigators who have compared the performance of implanted subjects to hearing aid users (Somers, 1991; Geers and Moog, 1992).

Evaluation of Speech Production Abilities

Outcome measures

The speech production abilities of children with cochlear implants have been studied less extensively than their speech perception abilities. The majority of studies have examined *phonetic* production skills in spontaneous speech samples or in syllables elicited on an imitative basis (Kirk and Hill-Brown, 1985; Osberger *et al.*, 1991b; Tobey *et al.*, 1991a, 1991b; Tye-Murray and Kirk, 1993). Because of the limited speech production skills of these children, especially in the pre-implant condition, new methods of transcription have been developed to characterize aspects of the children's speech. For example, Osberger *et al.* (1991b) developed an analysis scheme that classifies utterances as *speech*, *speechlike* or *non-English/non speech*. The system also includes notation of undesirable articulatory gestures that should be eliminated from a child's speech (for example, lip smacking and pops, exaggerated mouth opening without phonation). The system is most useful in analysis of very young children's speech. Carney (1990) also developed a system, the Reduced Aspect Feature Analysis (RAFT), which involves transcription of the features heard in each utterance. This approach eliminates the problem of having to assign a phonetic label to sounds that do not fit clearly into existing categories. Also, examination of features might be more sensitive to changes that occur in the speech of implanted children than are traditional methods of phonetic transcription.

Another approach that is used commonly to assess the speech of implanted children is elicitation of CV syllables with an imitative task. Examples of this type of measure are the Phonetic Level Speech

Evaluation (Ling, 1976) and The Central Institute for the Deaf (CID) Phonetic Inventory (Moog, 1989). The utterances are broadly transcribed and performance is expressed in terms of: (1) per cent correct production of consonants and vowels (Geers and Moog, 1992), (2) a coding scheme wherein different numeric values are assigned to the production skills (Kirk and Hill-Brown, 1985; Tobey *et al.*, 1991a), or (3) the results are classified according to descriptive categories (Tobey, *et al.*, 1991a). Select non-segmental or suprasegmental skills also are assessed on these measures. These items, which sample vocal control of loudness and pitch, however, do not necessarily predict use of intonation and stress changes during spontaneous speech. This type of task (i.e., imitation of syllables) and the procedures used to analyse the samples are unique to work with hearing-impaired children. More traditional approaches, such as picture articulation tests, are problematic to use with profoundly hearing-impaired children because of the children's limited speech and language skills. An imitative syllable task can provide useful information about emerging speech skills following implantation but recent data suggest that performance on a measure such as this does not reliably predict phonemic use of the sounds in spontaneous speech (Tye-Murray and Kirk, 1993).

One limitation of phonetic procedures is that this type of analysis provides no information about the use of sounds to signal differences in meaning. To determine if the sounds are used according to the rules of spoken language, a phonological analysis is needed. A measure used frequently with hearing-impaired children is the Phonologic Level Speech Evaluation (Ling, 1976). Using this technique, spontaneous speech samples are analysed to determine if speech sounds are used consistently, inconsistently, or not at all. Again, a measure such as this might yield useful information about changes in the speech of children following implantation, but this analysis scheme is very different from that typically used by linguists and phonologists to develop phonemic inventories and examine a child's phonology (Stoel-Gammon and Dunn, 1985).

The measure that is most important in evaluating the viability of oral communication for implanted children is overall speech intelligibility. The most rigorous method of intelligibility assessment is an open-set response format in which a panel of judges writes down what they think the child has said, and their responses are scored in terms of the percentage of key words correctly understood (McGarr, 1983; Smith, 1975), or a weighting system is used to assign words different values depending on their contribution to the linguistic message conveyed (Monsen, 1983). The advantage of using an open-set item identification, or 'write down' task, is that it has high face validity (Samar and Metz, 1988), but data collection and analyses are time-consuming and not practical in most clinical situations, factors that might account for the dearth of intelligibility studies with implanted children.

A scale similar to the MAIS has been developed by Robbins and Osberger (1990) to assess use of speech in everyday situations. Similar to the MAIS, the Meaningful Use of Speech Scale (MUSS) contains 10 probes, and responses to each probe are scored on a continuum of zero to 4. Three areas of behaviour are assessed, reflecting: (1) vocal control, (2) use of speech alone without sign or gesture, and (3) use of repair and clarification strategies to aid listeners' comprehension of their speech. Figure 5 shows changes on the MUSS over time. Data are reported for the same sample of 51 children whose performance was analysed on the MAIS, as described above. The scores improved gradually during the first 2 years of implant use in all three areas and then appear to reach a plateau after 2.5 years of device use. Long-term use data are needed from a larger group of subjects to determine if this trend continues. Additional data also are needed to examine vocal control after 2.5 years of implant use to determine if there is a true decrement in this area or if the decrease in scores reflects a sampling problem. The data show that even though there is an increase in the use of speech alone, the children still do not frequently communicate without signs and gestures. Also, they fail to use frequently oral repair and clarification strategies, a problem area for many hearing-impaired children.

Speech Production Results with Cochlear Implants

Single versus multichannel cochlear implants

Kirk and Hill-Brown (1985) reported that children who used the 3M/House device showed improvement in their imitative and spontaneous productions of non-segmental and segmental aspects of speech, with the greatest improvements observed in the production of vowels and diphthongs and simple consonants. Relatively few studies have compared the speech production abilities of single- and multichannel implant users. Osberger et al. (1991b) reported that the phonetic repertoires of both single- and multichannel implant users increased relative to the size of the subjects' repertoires in the pre-implant condition. However, the multichannel users demonstrated the more dramatic changes in the diversity of their phonetic repertoires than did the single-channel users. Specifically, the multichannel users showed a greater increase in their acquisition of front vowels, fricatives, liquids, glides and voiceless consonants than did the single-channel users.

Osberger et al. (1993) examined the speech intelligibility of single- and multichannel implant users and found no obvious differences as a

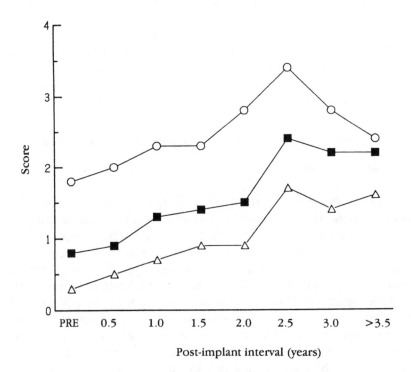

Figure 5. Mean scores of 51 prelingually deafened subjects with the Nucleus cochlear implant on the Meaningful Use of Speech Scale (MUSS) as a function of duration of implant use. The number of subjects tested at each interval was: 39, 34, 27, 25, 21, 15, and 15 at the pre, 0.5, 1.0, 1.5, 2.0, 2.5 and 3.0 year post-implant interval, respectively. The mean score at the last interval is the average of the data collected at the 3.5, 4.0, 4.5 and 5.0 years post-implant intervals. At these intervals, 20 scores were averaged from 15 different children. ○ Vocal control, ■ Speech alone, △ Modify to aid comprehension.

function of implant type. On the average, the post-implant speech intelligibility of the subjects with prelingual deafness was similar to that of hearing aid users with unaided hearing levels between 100 and 110 dB HL (i.e., a mean intelligibility score of roughly 20%). Given that research has shown that perception skills are superior with a multichannel than a single-channel device, it is surprising that Osberger *et al.* (1993) did not find differences in the speech intelligibility of these two groups of children. There are several explanations for this finding. First, there was a number of subjects in the study with prelingual deafness who did not receive an implant until they were in their teens. It is not unexpected that these children would show limited improvements in their speech intelligibility even with a multichannel implant. Secondly, prelingually deafened subjects who were implanted at an earlier age had only about two years of experience with the Nucleus implant at the time the study was completed. Longer experience with the multi-channel implant might have revealed differences between single- and multichannel users. A finding of interest reported by Osberger and colleagues (1993) was the trend of higher speech intelligibility in those subjects who demonstrated good speech perception skills with their device, and who used oral communication.

Speech production results with multichannel cochlear implants

Within-subjects design

Most studies have employed this type of design to examine changes in phonetic speech skills in imitative and spontaneous speech samples following implantation with a multichannel device. The results of these studies have shown improvement in the production of vowels, diphthongs, consonants, and select non-segmental speech skills (Tobey *et al*, 1991a, 1991b; Tobey and Hasenstab, 1991; Tye-Murray and Kirk, 1993). Tobey *et al.* (1991a) also examined improvement in the intelligibility of key words produced in sentences by multichannel implant users. Her results showed that after one year of Nucleus device use, the mean intelligibility score of the subjects was 34% compared to a pre-implant score of 18%. The results also showed that 63% of the subjects showed an improvement in intelligibility during the first year of multichannel implant use.

Between-subjects design

In our laboratory, the speech production skills of multichannel implant users and hearing aid users have been compared in a manner similar to that described above for the studies of speech perception. The subjects' production of consonant and vowel features has been examined in an imitative syllable task, and speech intelligibility measured with the write-down procedure.

Figures 6 and 7 summarize the performance of multichannel implant and hearing aid users on the syllable imitation task. The speech corpus consisted contained a total of eight vowels and diphthongs, sampled in a /bV/ context and 20 consonants in the initial position of a consonant–vowel (CV) syllable, where V = /i a u/. Each syllable was elicited imitatively from the examiner's model and repeated three times. The samples were recorded on audiotape and later transcribed by a group of speech–language pathologists who used broad transcription. The transcriptions were then analysed in terms of the percentage of vowel and consonant features produced by the child that matched the features of the examiner's target. For example, if the target was /ta/ and the child produced /ba/, the consonant feature of manner was counted as correct, but no credit was given for place of articulation or voicing. Production of the correct syllable shape (i.e., CV) also was examined. To receive credit for this feature, the child only had to produce a CV syllable, irrespective of the intended consonant and vowel targets. The percentage of features produced correctly was then averaged across repetitions and subjects within each group. For the consonant features, data were averaged across vowel environment.

Figure 6 summarizes the children's production of syllable shape, vowels and diphthong features. Data were collected from 45 prelingually deafened children who were implanted with the Nucleus device before age 9. The hearing aid subjects consisted of 10 Gold and 12 Silver hearing aid users, and 38 Bronze hearing aid users who were subsequently implanted with the Nucleus device. The data in Figure 6 show large and rapid improvements in the production of the correct syllable shape and vowel targets following implantation with a multi-channel implant. The production of these features by the implant users was better than that of the Silver hearing aid users after only 6 months of implant use, and eventually the implanted subjects' scores matched those of the Gold hearing aid users. The acquisition of diphthongs

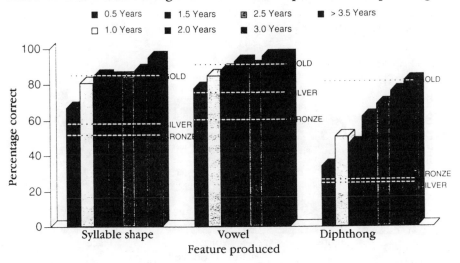

Figure 6. Mean scores of 45 prelingually deafened children with the Nucleus cochlear implant on the production of syllable shape, vowel and diphthong features in an imitative syllable task as a function of duration of implant use. The number of Nucleus subjects tested at each interval was: 31, 25, 19, 14, 9 and 11 at the 0.5, 1.0, 1.5, 2.0, 2.5 and 3.0 year post-implant intervals, respectively. The mean score at the last interval is the average of the data collected at the 3.5, 4.0, 4.5 and 5.0 years post implant intervals. At these intervals, 15 scores were averaged for 7 different subjects. The dashed lines show the mean score for three groups of hearing aid subjects, Bronze (n = 38), Silver (n = 12) and Gold (n = 10) at one test interval.

occurred at a slower rate than the other features but the trends were the same with respect to group comparisons. It is noteworthy that the production scores for syllable shape and diphthongs were similar for the Bronze and Silver hearing aid users. Thus, even though the Silver hearing aid users had more hearing than the Bronze hearing aid users, the auditory input and feedback was not sufficient for the Silver hearing aid users to acquire diphthongs or learn to produce syllable shape with a high degree of accuracy.

Figure 7 shows the data for production of consonant features over time in the same groups of children. The same group trends observed for the production of vowels was apparent in their production of consonant features. That is, there were relatively rapid improvements in the Nucleus users' production of consonant features. The production scores of the implant subjects exceeded those of the Silver hearing aid users after only 6 months of the multichannel implant use and matched those of the Gold hearing aid users within several years of device use. In fact, the scores of the Nucleus users were actually higher than those of the Gold hearing aid users at the later test intervals. Again, there was little difference between the scores of the Silver and Bronze hearing aid users. These data, and those plotted in Figure 6, suggest that children

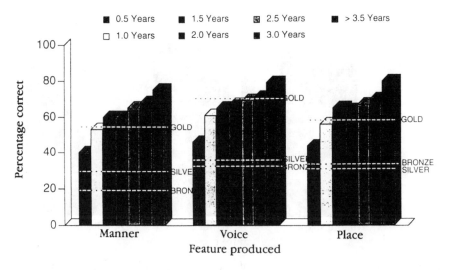

Figure 7. Mean scores of 45 prelingually deafened children with the Nucleus cochlear implant on the production of consonant features in an imitative syllable task as a function of duration of implant use. The number of Nucleus subjects tested at each interval was: 31, 25, 19, 14, 9 and 11 at the 0.5, 1.0, 1.5, 2.0, 2.5 and 3.0 year post-implant intervals, respectively. The mean score at the last interval is the average of the data collected at the 3.5, 4.0, 4.5 and 5.0 years post implant intervals. At these intervals, 15 scores were averaged for 7 different subjects. The dashed lines show the mean score for three groups of hearing aid subjects, Bronze (n = 38), Silver (n = 12) and Gold (n = 10) at one test interval.

with unaided thresholds between 100 to 110 dB HL are most readily able to acquire vowels and have considerable difficulty in the acquisition of diphthongs and consonants. The data also suggest that Silver hearing aid users might develop better speech skills if they had received a multichannel cochlear implant.

The next study is an extension of the Osberger et al. (1993) investigation of speech intelligibility in implanted children. Given that research has shown large improvements in speech perception skills, and selected production skills over time, the speech intelligibility was examined in Nucleus users who had used their device for as long as 5 years. Speech intelligibility was measured in 29 prelingually deafened subjects (mean age onset of deafness = 5.7 years; mean age when implanted = 5.7 years). Roughly half of the subjects used total communication, whereas the other half used oral communication. Intelligibility also was measured in 14 Gold (mean PTA = 93 dB HL; mean chronological age = 10.4 years) 8 Silver (mean PTA = 103 dB HL; mean chronological age = 8.7 years), and 28 Bronze (mean PTA > 110 dB HL; mean chronological age = 7 years) hearing aid users. The Bronze hearing aid users all received the Nucleus multichannel cochlear implant.

Each subject produced 10 sentences that were repeated after an examiner's spoken model. The sentences were tape recorded and subsequently digitized, randomized, and played to panels of listeners who had no prior experience in listening to the speech of hearing-impaired talkers. Each set of 10 sentences produced by a single subject was evaluated by a panel of three listeners. The listeners were instructed to write down what they thought the subject had said. Intelligibility was measured as the mean percentage of words correctly, understood, averaged across the three listeners.

The speech intelligibility results are summarized in Table 3. The mean speech intelligibility score of the Bronze hearing aid users was low, only 4%, whereas the score of the Gold hearing aid users was relatively high. The speech intelligibility score of the Silver hearing aid users was only about 15% higher than that of the Bronze group. Postimplant, there was a gradual improvement in the speech intelligibility of the Nucleus users. In fact, the average speech intelligibility scores of the Nucleus users remained low through the first 2 years of multichannel implant use. After 2.5 years of implant use, the average speech intelligibility of the implanted subjects began to exceed that of the Silver hearing aid users. After 3.5 to 4 years of device use, the average intelligibility of the implant users speech was about 40% which was roughly 20% higher than that of the Silver hearing aid users. In contrast, the mean intelligibility score of the implant users remained below that of the Gold hearing aid users. In fact, the average intelligibility of the Gold hearing aid users' speech was about 30% higher than that of the implant users, and about 50% higher than that of the Silver hearing aid users.

The results of this study revealed clear improvements in speech intelligibility in prelingually deafened children after they received a multichannel cochlear implant. The largest changes in intelligibility did not occur until after the subjects had used their implant for 2 or more years. The mean speech intelligibility of the implanted subjects was higher than that of subjects who had no residual hearing (i.e., Bronze hearing aid users), as well as that of subjects with hearing levels between 100 to 110 dB HL (i.e., Silver hearing aid users). This finding differs from that of our previous research (Osberger *et al.*, 1993) which showed that the speech intelligibility of multichannel implant users was similar to that of Silver hearing aid users. However, the subjects had used the multichannel implant for a shorter period of time in the previous than in the current study. The results are similar to that of our previous study in that the speech intelligibility of the Gold hearing aid users was higher than that of the Nucleus users. The speech intelligibility of the implanted subjects, however, might have matched that of the Gold hearing aid users if they had received their implant at an earlier age. The majority of children in this study were not implanted until they were 5 to 8 years old, whereas the Gold hearing aid users received their sensory aids when they were around 2 years of age. Studies are

Table 3. Mean speech intelligibility scores (percentage correct) for 29 prelingually deafened children who used the Nucleus cochlear implant compared to three groups of hearing aid users

Hearing aid subjects

	n	Mean	Range
Gold	14	80	63–97
Silver	8	18	0–67
Bronze	28	4	0–22

Nucleus users

Length of use (yrs)	n	Mean	Range
0.5	16	8	0–21
1.0	6	10	0–29
1.5	6	14	0–36
2.0	10	18	0–46
2.5	12	26	3–53
3.0	11	30	0–49
3.5	4	41	0–79
≥ 4.0	6	37	12–66

now underway to examine changes in speech intelligibility in children who are implanted between ages 2 and 4 years.

Summary of Research Findings

The research conducted to date reveals that great strides have been made in determining the benefits that children with profound hearing impairments derive from cochlear implants. Available data suggest the following conclusions about children's performance with cochlear implants.

1. Higher levels of speech perception and production performance are demonstrated by pediatric users of multichannel than single-channel implants. Even though a small percentage of single-channel implant users demonstrate open-set speech recognition, the majority do not.

2. Children with postlingual deafness (i.e., onset at or after age 5 years) show the most rapid and dramatic improvements in their speech perception and production skills following implantation. Most of these children demonstrate high levels of open-set speech recognition with multichannel cochlear implants.

3 Children who derive the least amount of benefit from an implant are those with early onset of deafness who were not implanted until they were teenagers. The greatest perceptual benefits derived by these children are improved sound detection, awareness and alerting to sounds in the environment, and enhanced speechreading performance. Selected speech production skills might also improve following implantation, including improved timing and phrasing, loudness control, and production of word-final consonants. These children are still implant candidates but they and their parents must receive extensive counselling regarding the relatively limited improvements that are to be expected following implantation.

4 The speech perception and production skills of children with prelingual deafness (i.e., onset before age 3 years) who are implanted between the ages of 4 and 8 years improve over an extended period of time following implantation with a multichannel device. Duration of implant use is the most important factor in explaining performance differences among these children.

5 On the average, the implant performance of children with congenital deafness is similar to that of children who acquired deafness before age 3 years from meningitis.

6 Following implantation of prelingually deafened children with multichannel devices, the first improvements are observed in global auditory skills (i.e., detecting and alerting to sounds in the environment). Even though word recognition skills may begin to emerge in these

children during the first year of implant use, substantial improvements in speech understanding without speechreading are not evident until after 2 or more years of multichannel implant use. Improvement in recognition of words based on vowel distinctions emerges before word recognition based on consonant distinctions. Recognition of simple phrases in an open-set emerges before recognition of monosyllabic words. Roughly half of these subjects demonstrate open-set speech recognition, some of whom achieve performance levels comparable to those of postlingually deafened children.

7   A similar pattern of performance is found in speech production changes in prelingually deafened children. Improvement is first noted in the use and control of vocalizations. Large improvements in the children's phonetic speech skills also occur, with the first changes noted in acquisition of simple vowels. Phonemic speech skills are acquired at a slower rate than phonetic skills. Improvements in speech intelligibility do not occur until after 2 or more years of multichannel implant use.

8   There is a trend for higher performance levels among implanted children who use oral rather than Total Communication. Interpretation of this finding should be made with caution when selecting an educational programme for an implanted child, given that a number of factors influence this decision.

9   The number of children who are implant candidates appears to be higher than originally projected when pediatric implant work began over 10 years ago. Initially, only children who demonstrated essentially no response to sound (i.e., Bronze hearing aid users) were considered to be candidates for an implant. Recent data suggest, however, that children who demonstrate unaided thresholds between 100 to 105 dB HL (i.e., Silver hearing aid users) would benefit more from a multichannel cochlear implant than from continued use of only conventional hearing aid amplification. These children demonstrate low frequency hearing and are able to perceive prosodic aspects of speech and, in some cases, demonstrate limited closed-set word recognition with their hearing aids. Because their hearing aided responses to high frequency sounds (i.e., 1500 Hz and higher) are at levels of 55 dB HL or higher, they have limited access to consonant information, especially in everyday listening situations. With the implant, they gain better information to consonant information which should improve their speech understanding without lipreading and overall speech intelligibility.

Research Needs in Pediatric Cochlear Implants

As noted earlier, implant work is still in its infancy, especially with respect to pediatric issues. Many questions remain unanswered and need to be addressed to better document and understand the benefits that children with profound hearing impairments derive from cochlear implants. The following are suggested areas of research.

1. The upper limits of speech perception and production performance with the commercially available implant technology have not been determined in prelingually deafened children. Existing data suggest the need to continue to monitor the progress of children who have used the Nucleus multichannel cochlear implant with the MPeak strategy beyond 3 years of use. Unless longitudinal study of these children is continued beyond this time, the impact of this implant processing scheme on improving those skills most important for oral communication (i.e., open-set speech recognition and speech intelligibility) will not be established.

2 There is a need for careful and systematic comparison of different processing schemes in children. Work with adults suggests that continuous interleaved sampling processors result in higher levels of speech perception performance than compressed analogue or feature extraction schemes. It is not known if similar performance differences as a function of processing strategy also will be observed in prelingually deafened children.

3 As more younger children are implanted between the ages of 2 and 3, it will be important to compare their performance over time to that of children who were implanted at later ages (i.e., between 4 and 8). In Europe, a number of children under the age of 2 have been implanted with the Nucleus device. Anecdotal evidence suggests that these children will achieve performance levels even higher than those of children implanted between ages 2 and 3.

4 Children who have some residual hearing (i.e., Silver hearing aid users) are now being implanted with multichannel devices. Within-subjects comparisons are important to determine the benefit that they derive from the implant relative to their performance with hearing aids. Between-subjects studies also are important to determine if children who were Silver hearing aid users demonstrate higher levels of implant performance than children who were implanted as Bronze hearing aid users. Silver hearing aid users might demonstrate higher levels of performance with an implant than Bronze hearing aid users because the former have better nerve survival, thereby permitting better use of information transmitted by the implant.

5 Longitudinal studies of children with conventional hearing aids need to be continued. It is important to document *rate* of skill acquisition in children with hearing aids and compare learning rates to those demonstrated by children with multichannel implants. These data are essential to document implant benefit and refine candidacy criteria.

6 Studies need to be initiated that provide more insight into the *processes* underlying the development of perception and production skills of children with implants. Most of the data collected to date has provided *descriptive* information on children's performance with implants. This, of course, is important and necessary information but it provides limited insight into processes underlying the observed changes in performance.

7 Finally, only limited data are available on the effect of implants on the acquisition of spoken language and academic performance. Longitudinal studies are needed to document changes in language acquisition and those skills underlying reading and academic success.

Acknowledgements

Preparation of this manuscript was supported, in part, by grant DC00423 from the National Institutes of Health, National Institute on Deafness and Other Communication Disorders.

References

Berliner, K.I. and Eisenberg, L.S. (1985) Methods and issues in the cochlear implantation of children: An overview, Ear and Hearing 6 (Suppl.), 6S-13S.

Berliner, K.I., Tonokawa, L.L., Dye L.L. and House, W.F. (1989) Open-set speech recognition in children with a single-channel cochlear implant. Ear and Hearing 10: 237–42.

Boothroyd, A. (1991) Assessment of speech perception capacity in profoundly deaf children. American Journal of Otology 12: Suppl., 67–72.

Boothroyd, A. (1984) Auditory perception of speech contrasts by subjects with sensorineural hearing loss. Journal of Speech and Hearing Research 27: 134–44.

Boothroyd, A. and Cawkwell, S. (1970) Vibrotactile thresholds in pure-tone audiometry. Acta Otolaryngologica 69: 384–7.

Carney, A.E. (1990) Reduced aspect feature transcription (RAFT). Journal of the Acoustical Society of America 87 (Suppl.): S89 (A).

Carney, A.E., Osberger, M.J., Carney, E; Robbins, A.M., Renshaw, J.J. and Miyamoto, R.T. (1993) A comparison of speech discrimination with cochlear implants and tactile aids. Journal of the Acoustical Society of America 94: 2036–49.

Carney, A.E., Osberger, M.J., Miyamoto, R.T., Karasek, A., Dettmann, D. and Johnson, D.L. (1991) Speech perception along the sensory aid continuum: From hearing aids to cochlear implants. In Pediatric Amplification: Proceedings of the 1991 National Conference, edited by J. Feigin and P. Stelmachowicz (Boys Town National Research Hospital, Omaha, NE).

Cohen, N.L., Waltzman, S.B. and Fisher, S.G. (1993) A prospective, randomized study of cochlear implants. New England Journal of Medicine 328: 233–7.

Elliott, L.L. and Katz, D.R. (1980) Northwestern University Children's Perception of Speech (NU-CHIPS). (Auditec, St. Louis).

Erber, N.P. (1972) Auditory, visual and auditory-visual recognition of consonants by children with normal and impaired hearing. Journal of Speech and Hearing Research 15: 413–22.

Erber, N.P. (1980) Use of auditory numbers to evaluate speech perception abilities of hearing-impaired children. Journal of Speech and Hearing Disorders 45: 527–32.

Erber, N.P. (1982) Auditory Training. Washington, DC: Alexandra Graham Bell Association for the Deaf.

Erber, N.P. and Alencewicz, C.M. (1976) Audiologic evaluation of deaf children, Journal of Speech and Hearing Disorders 41: 256–67.

Fryauf-Bertschy, H., Tyler, R.S., Kelsay, D.M. and Gantz, B.J. (1992) Performance over time of congenitally deaf and postlingually deafened children using a multichannel cochlear implant. Journal of Speech and Hearing Research 35: 913–20.

Gantz, B.J., Tyler, R., Knutson, J., Woodworth, G., Abbas, P., McCabe, B., Hinrichs, J., Tye-Murray, N., Lansing, C., Kuk, F. and Brown, C.J. (1988) Evaluation of five different cochlear implant designs: Audiologic assessment and predictors of performance. Laryngoscope 98: 1100–6.

Geers, A.E. and Moog, J.S. (1989) Evaluating speech perception skills: Tools for measuring benefits of cochlear implants, tactile aids and hearing aids. In Owens, E. and Kessler, D. (Eds) Cochlear Implants in Young Deaf Children. San Diego: College-Hill Press.

Geers, A.E. and Moog, J.S. (1990) Early Speech Perception Battery. St. Louis: Central Institute for the Deaf.

Geers, A.E. and Moog, J.S. (1992) The Central Institute for the Deaf cochlear implant study: A progress report. Journal of Speech Language Pathology and Audiology 16: 129–40.

Haskins, H. (1949) A Phonetically Balanced Test of Speech Discrimination for Children. Unpublished master's thesis, Northwestern University, Evanston, IL.

Hochmair-Desoyer, I. and Steinwender, G. (1993) Results from better postlingual adult users of the MED-EL device. Paper presented at the 3rd International Cochlear Implant Conference (Austria, April 4–7, 1993).

Kirk, K.I. and Hill-Brown, C.J. (1985) Speech and language results in children with a cochlear implant. Ear and Hearing 6 (Suppl.): 36S–47S.

Ling, D.D. (1976) Speech and the Hearing-Impaired Child: Theory and Practice. Washington, DC: Alexander Graham Bell Association for the Deaf.

Ling, D.L. and Milne, M. (1981) The development of speech in hearing-impaired children. In Bess, F., Freeman, B. and Sinclair, J. (Eds) Amplification in Education. Washington, DC Alexander Graham Bell Association for the Deaf.

McGarr, N. (1983) The intelligibility of deaf speech to experienced and inexperienced listeners. Journal of Speech and Hearing Research 26: 451–8.

Mecklenburg, D., Demorest, M.E. and Staller, S. J. (1991) Scope and design of the clinical trial of the Nucleus multichannel cochlear implant in children. Ear and Hearing 12 (Suppl.): 3S–9S.

Miyamoto, R.T., Osberger, M.J., Robbins, A.M., Myres, W.A. and Kessler, K. (1993) Prelingually deafened children's performance with the Nucleus multichannel cochlear implant. American Journal of Otology 14: 437–45.

Miyamoto, R.T., Osberger, M.J., Robbins, A.M., Myres, W.A., Kessler, K. and Pope, M.L. (1992) Longitudinal evaluation of communication skills of children with single- or multichannel cochlear implants. American Journal of Otology 13: 215–22.

Miyamoto R.T., Osberger, M.J., Todd, S.L., Robbins, A.M., Stroer, B.S., Zimmerman-

Phillips, S. and Carney, A.E. (in press) Variables affecting implant performance in children. Laryngoscope.

Monsen, R.B. (1978) Toward measuring how well hearing-impaired children speak. Journal of Speech and Hearing Research 21: 197–219.

Monsen, R.B. (1983) The oral speech intelligibility of hearing-impaired talkers. Journal of Speech and Hearing Disorders 48: 286–96.

Moog, J.S. (1989) The CID Phonetic Inventory. St Louis: Central Institute for the Deaf.

Osberger, M.J., Maso, M. and Sam, L.K. (1993) Speech intelligibility of children with cochlear implants, tactile aids or hearing aids. Journal of Speech and Hearing Research 36: 186–203.

Osberger, M.J., Miyamoto, R.T., Zimmerman-Phillips, S., Kemink, J., Stroer, B.S., Firszt, J.B. and Novak, M.A. (1991a) Independent evaluation of the speech perception abilities of children with the Nucleus 22-Channel cochlear implant system. Ear and Hearing 12 (Suppl.): 66S–80S.

Osberger, M.J., Robbins, A.M., Berry, S.W., Todd, S.L., Hesketh, L.J. and Sedey, A. (1991b) Analysis of spontaneous speech samples of children with cochlear implants or tactile aids. American Journal of Otology 12 (Suppl.): 151–64.

Robbins, A.M. and Osberger, M.J. (1990) The Meaningful Use of Speech Scale (MUSS). Indiana University School of Medicine, Indianapolis, IN.

Robbins, A.M., Renshaw, J.J. and Berry, S.W. (1991) Evaluating meaningful auditory integration in profoundly hearing-impaired children. American Journal of Otology 12 (Suppl.): 144–51.

Robbins, A. M., Renshaw J.J., Miyamoto R.T., Osberger, M.J. and Pope, M.L. (1988) Minimal Pairs Test. Indiana University School of Medicine, Indianapolis.

Ross, M. and Lerman, J. (1971) Word Intelligibility by Picture Identification. Pittsburgh: Stanwix House, Inc.

Samar, V. and Metz, D. (1988) Construct validity of speech intelligibility – rating scale procedures for the hearing-impaired population. Journal of Speech and Hearing Research 31: 307–16.

Smith, C.R. (1975) Residual hearing and speech production in deaf children, Journal of Speech and Hearing Research 18: 795–811.

Somers, M.N. (1991) Speech perception abilities in children with cochlear implants or hearing aids. American Journal of Otology 12 (Suppl.): 174–8.

Staller, S.J., Beiter, A.L., Brimacombe, J.A., Mecklenburg, D.J. and Arndt, P. (1991a) Pediatric performance with the Nucleus 22-Channel Cochlear Implant System. American Journal of Otology 12 (Suppl.): 126–36.

Staller, S.J., Dowell, R.C., Beiter, A.L. and Brimacombe, J.A. (1991b) Perceptual abilities of children with the Nucleus 22-channel cochlear implant. American Journal of Otology 12 (Suppl.): 34S–47S.

Stoel-Gammon, C. and Dunn, C. (1985) Normal and Disordered Phonology in Children. Austin, TX: Pro-ed.

Thielemeir, M.A. (1984) The Discrimination After Training (DAT) Test. Los Angeles: House Ear Institute.

Thorton A.R. and Raffin, M.J.M. (1978) Speech-discrimination scores modeled as a binomial variable. Journal of Speech and Hearing Research 21: 507–18.

Tobey, E.A., Angelette, S., Murchinson, C., Nicosia, J., Sprague, S., Staller, S., Brimacombe, J. and Beiter, A.L. (1991a) Speech production performance in children with multichannel cochlear implants. American Journal of Otology 12 (Suppl.): 165–73.

Tobey, E.A., Pancamo, S., Staller, S.J., Brimacombe, J. and Beiter, A.L. (1991b)

Consonant production in children receiving a multichannel cochlear implant. Ear and Hearing 12 (Suppl.): 23–31.

Tobey, E.A. and Hasenstab, S. (1991) Effects of a Nucleus multichannel cochlear implant upon speech production in children. Ear and Hearing 12 (Suppl.): 55S–65S.

Tye-Murray, N. and Kirk, K.I. (1993) Vowel and diphthong production by young users of cochlear implants and the relationship between the phonetic level evaluation and spontaneous speech. Journal of Speech and Hearing Research 36: 488–502.

Tyler, R.S. (Ed) (1993a) Cochlear Implants. San Diego: Singular Publishing Group.

Tyler, R.S. (1993b) Speech perception by children. In Tyler, R.S. (Eds) Cochlear Implants. San Diego: Singular Publishing Group.

Waltzman, S.B., Cohen, N.L. and Shapiro, W.H. (1992) Use of multichannel cochlear implants in the congenitally and prelingually deaf population, Laryngoscope 102: 395–9.

Waltzman, S.B., Cohen, N.L., Spivak, L., Ying, E., Brackett, D., Shapiro, W. and Hoffman, R. (1990) Improvement in speech perception and production abilities in children using a multichannel cochlear implant. Laryngoscope 100: 240–3.

Wilson, B.S., Finley, C.C., Lawson, D.T., Wolford, R.D., Eddington, D.K. and Rabinowitz, W.M. (1991) Better speech recognition with cochlear implants. Nature 352: 236–8.

12
Speech Perception for Adults Using Cochlear Implants

RICHARD C. DOWELL

Introduction

A mere 16 years ago, the title of this chapter would have created considerable consternation in audiological circles. A high proportion of otologists and audiologists would have wondered, with good reason, about the potential content of such a chapter. In 1977, there were certainly cochlear implants in use with reported benefits, but reliable documentation of any useful speech perception under controlled conditions was difficult to find. The rapid development of cochlear prostheses since that time has led to thousands of profoundly hearing-impaired adults obtaining benefits for speech perception, and there is now no doubt regarding the efficacy of such devices. This chapter will provide a brief overview of this rapid improvement in the speech perception of adult cochlear implant users, consider some of the reasons for this improvement, and discuss some of the factors that may influence speech perception performance for the individual user.

Speech Perception

Speech perception is part of the communication process. Speech and language provides the vehicle for the transmission of ideas from one person to another and speech perception plays a key role in this process. On the other hand, speech perception can occur in some forms without communication. For instance, it is possible to repeat, with varying difficulty, words and sentences in a foreign language without any knowledge of their meaning. Indeed, some tests of speech perception involve nonsense syllables or artificially constructed sentences without true meaning. Thus, there are aspects of speech perception which do not involve communication. Similarly, there are many aspects of communication which do not involve speech perception, including sign languages, gesture and facial expressions.

For a profoundly hearing-impaired adult using a cochlear implant, we are most interested in providing improvements in speech perception which improve communication. This may seem a trivial statement, but there are some speech discrimination abilities that do not necessarily lead to improvements in communication. For example, various tests have been designed to assess the ability to discriminate between male and female speakers, for example, male/female speaker identification test from the Minimal Auditory Capabilities (MAC) battery (Owens *et al.*, 1981). It is difficult to see how this ability has any direct relevance to understanding speech and therefore communication. Such a test is intended to provide information about discrimination of prosodic or suprasegmental aspects of speech and this ability may lead, in turn, to improved speech understanding, but the link is tenuous, or at least indirect.

A similar argument can be applied to vowel and consonant confusion tests using nonsense syllables. They do provide useful information about speech perception but the link to improved communication is again indirect. To illustrate this point, we can ima-gine two profoundly deaf subjects, one using a multichannel tactile aid such as the 'Tickle-Talker' (see Chapter 5) and the other using a multichannel cochlear prosthesis. On a particular series of nonsense syllable tests, the tactile subject may score 80% for vowels and 60% for consonants, whereas the cochlear implant subject may score 60% for vowels and 40% for consonants under the same conditions. In a limited sense, the tactile aid user is demonstrating better speech perception than the implant user. If, however, we then test the same subjects using an open-set sentence test, we may find that the tactile subject scores poorly (0%) while the implant user is able to recognize around 50% of the sentence material. We would have no hesitation, based on this result in claiming that the implant user has far better speech perception. To any student of speech and language processing there is no conflict here. The apparent inconsistency in the test results is probably due to the rate at which phonemic information must be processed to understand connected speech. The tactile aid user in this case may be able to identify phonemes presented one at a time but have problems processing the string of phonemes in sentence or discourse material at the rate required for understanding. I have not included this example of inconsistency in speech perception testing in order to discuss the complexities of speech and language processing, but merely to highlight the difficulties that arise in the assessment of all types of aids for hearing-impaired people when we ask 'which one is better?' The next section of this chapter will discuss the various approaches that have been taken in assessing speech perception in cochlear implant subjects and some of the strengths and weaknesses in these methods.

Measurement of Speech Perception

Assessment of lipreading (speechreading) ability

The need for assessment of lipreading ability in cochlear implant users arose from the relatively poor speech perception obtained by the early implant users using auditory input alone. The standard speech testing techniques used in audiology usually involved recognition of monosyllabic words in an open-set context (e.g. the various phonetically balanced word lists such as the Northwestern University Auditory test number 6 (Tillman and Carhart, 1966), the Consonant-Nucleus-Consonant word lists (Peterson and Lehiste, 1962), and the AB word lists (Boothroyd, 1968) which used a fixed set of phonemes for each list). In the 1970s, the main clinical application of cochlear implants involved the single-channel device developed by William House in Los Angeles. Anecdotal reports suggested that many of these patients obtained communication benefit from this device despite limitations on the amount of speech information transmitted by the device. Even an independent study of a group of patients using the House device in 1977 (Bilger *et al.*, 1977) concluded that users did obtain benefit in their everyday communication despite very poor results on standard speech perception tests.

At this time there was also an increasing interest in attempting to help profoundly hearing-impaired subjects with improving hearing aid technology. Here too was a group who did not perform well on standard auditory tests but could benefit greatly from enhanced lipreading. Researchers and clinicians became more interested in lipreading ability and how it could be aided.

One development at this time which has now been used very widely in cochlear implant research and rehabilitation is continuous discourse tracking (CDT, also known as speech tracking). This was developed as a rehabilitative technique by De Filippo and Scott at the Central Institute for the Deaf in St Louis, and aimed to provide a measure of communication speed in hearing-impaired subjects (De Filippo and Scott, 1978). Continuous discourse tracking involved a clinician reading from an appropriate text (a novel, newspaper article, etc.) and the subject attempting to repeat verbatim the delivered message. A hierarchy of specific strategies was used to clarify words or phrases when errors were made. This continued for a fixed time interval and the total number of words completed was recorded. From this, a score in words per minute could be calculated which provided a measure of communication speed under these rather unnatural conditions. These scores could then be compared for visual alone, auditory–visual and auditory alone conditions (when possible) and with scores from previous test sessions.

In the context of cochlear implant rehabilitation, CDT provides a useful tool for the clinician as the scores can provide a guide to a particular patient's progress both in using the auditory input from the cochlear implant to enhance their lipreading and their overall improvement over time. The task involved in CDT for subjects, although it is a little unnatural, has direct relevance to communication, so that clinicians and implant users can be confident that improved scores represent genuine changes in communication ability. CDT has been well accepted in this context and has become an important tool in the rehabilitation of hearing-impaired subjects. It is, however, difficult to use the measures obtained with CDT for research purposes as the absolute scores reflect many variables that are unrelated to the speech perception of the subject. For instance, the material used can vary in difficulty, clinicians vary in their use of clarification strategies, and tracking rates improve with familiarity both with the task itself and the particular speaker. This unfortunately means that a tracking rate of 40 words per minute at two different centres may not mean that the subjects involved are equivalent in speech perception ability. An example of the effect of different speakers on CDT rates is shown in Figure 1. In this case, the same subjects were tested with the same material using the same procedure but the two speakers involved were very different in the amount of experience they had in communicating with profoundly hearing-impaired subjects. Note that the absolute scores obtained for speaker 1 are on average double those for speaker 2 although the proportional differences obtained between lipreading alone and lipreading with cochlear implant conditions remained similar for particular subjects.

CDT does provide useful information for the rehabilitationist working with individual cochlear implant users. In this situation, the material, technique and speaker remain fixed and scores can provide a record of the subject's progress over time and the improvement obtained when using the cochlear implant. This record can often help with motivation of subjects who are learning to use the implant and are frustrated with their progress. Figure 2 shows CDT results for a series of rehabilitation sessions following cochlear implant surgery. Note the improvement in scores over time and the increased difference between conditions over time.

Even in this rehabilitative context, CDT may only be useful when scores are between approximately 20 and 70 words per minute. In general, a score below 20 words per minute means that the interaction proceeds rather tediously and the task may be more of a frustration than a useful learning exercise. On the other hand, once subjects reach approximately 70 words per minute, although higher rates are certainly possible, the actual rate obtained tends to depend on whether one or two difficult words are encountered which hold up progress for ten or

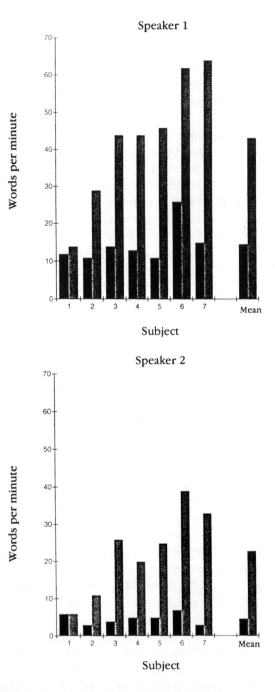

Figure 1. Results for continuous discourse tracking for seven subjects using a multichannel cochlear implant with lipreading (shaded columns) and for lipreading alone (solid columns) with two different speakers. Note that results for speaker 1, who was more familiar with the task, are much better than for speaker 2. ■ Lipreading alone, ▓ Lipreading with implant

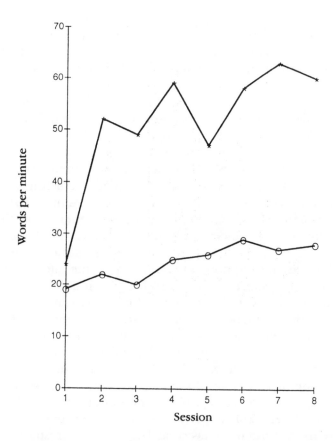

Figure 2. Results for continuous discourse tracking for a multichannel cochlear implant user over a series of postoperative rehabilitation sessions. Open circles (-⊖-): lipreading alone; asterisks ⊀ : lipreading with implant.

twenty seconds. Thus rates between 70 and 110 words per minute tend to give an inverse measure of how many particularly difficult words are encountered within the particular passage of text, rather than the overall speed of communication during most of the session.

There have been attempts to devise methods of scoring for CDT that deal with some of the problems (Levitt *et al.*, 1986; Rosen *et al.*, 1980). For instance, the improvement obtained for one condition over another can be expressed as a proportion of the lower score, the higher score or a measured ceiling tracking rate. These have some value, but it remains difficult to compare CDT results across different research groups. A more detailed discussion of the CDT procedure and its inherent problems can be found in an excellent review article by Nancy Tye-Murray and Richard Tyler (Tye-Murray and Tyler, 1988).

A more formal way to assess the enhancement of lipreading skills provided by cochlear implants is by using standard speech perception tests presented in the auditory–visual mode. Sentence materials are most often used as these are more relevant to everyday conversational speech understanding. There are also problems that arise with this approach. Most of the sentence materials that have been used in cochlear implant work for such testing have been standardized as auditory tests and not for the auditory–visual modality. When used as a lipreading assessment, different sentence lists may differ in difficulty. In addition, the particular speaker presenting the test, either live voice or videotaped, may influence the absolute scores obtained and even which lists are more difficult due to individual lip movement characteristics. If tests are not presented using videotaped recordings, test results can be influenced (even unknowingly) by the presenter, particularly if it is desirable that one condition produces a better result than another. Even when these problems are controlled, there remains a statistical problem in comparing scores on lipreading assessments. In the auditory–visual mode, the addition of variances from the auditory and visual inputs and their interaction will lead to larger variability between one test and another than would be expected for auditory input alone.

In addition, a typical sentence test may consist of 10 sentences from which 50 key words are chosen as scoring words. However, in statistical terms, these 50 items are not strictly independent. For instance, in an everyday sentence such as 'I walked to the store after breakfast and bought the morning paper', most of the words are linked by syntactic and/or semantic context. The correct recognition of one word helps in the recognition of others. This is particularly true when the sentence material is more natural and using everyday language. The result is that a 50 item sentence test may have the test/retest variability of a 20 or 30 item test with strictly independent items (e.g. monosyllabic words). This is not something that applies only to lipreading assessment but to sentence testing in general.

In assessing cochlear implant users we are often interested in the improvement obtained when the device is switched on in the auditory visual mode. As with any test score that is a proportion, variance is not equal across the range of scores. This is most obvious in the so-called 'ceiling effect' where a high score is usually much more difficult to improve upon than a mid-range score. Mathematical transformations can be used to deal with this problem within certain limits (Thornton and Raffin, 1978), but in practice, it is desirable to choose a test or test conditions which give a mid-range score so that a retest will be sensitive to improvement.

Closed-set speech perception tests

As mentioned in the previous section, speech perception for cochlear implant users in the early years of their clinical use was poor relative to normal listeners and the standard tests of speech perception were not appropriate for evaluating these subjects. A way of making a speech perception test easier is by restricting the number of alternatives from which the subject has to choose. This can be done in a variety of ways, either by providing a fixed list of alternatives to the subject or providing contextual clues. This type of approach has provided the field of speech perception assessment with a large array of tests of varying difficulty, applicability and utility. The strength of well-designed closed-set tests has been their ability to target specific aspects of speech perception in cochlear implant users. This type of testing can provide important information about speech processing for cochlear implants. For instance, if a particular speech processing scheme purports to provide information about a particular acoustic phonetic feature, it is possible to determine how well this information is perceived and the proportion of subjects able to the use it effectively. This type of approach has been used in many batteries of tests that have been designed for profoundly hearing-impaired subjects.

The Minimal Auditory Capabilities battery (MAC) has been used consistently for implant users (Owens *et al.*, 1981) and incorporates a number of closed-set tests that target specific features in this way. Particular tests assess discrimination of speaker sex, syllable pattern, vowels and consonants and provide a hierarchy of difficulty in acoustic feature discrimination.

Another way of looking at the discrimination of particular acoustic features is to use a set of nonsense syllables which differ in only one particular phoneme. A set of syllables can then be constructed which differ in the initial, final or medial consonant or vowel. A typical test will require the subject to listen to a test item and identify from a list which particular syllable they perceived. The strength of this approach is that the discriminations required by the subject are very well defined and the type of errors can be analysed in addition to obtaining an overall score for correct responses. A confusion matrix of responses can be constructed which can be analysed using a number of mathematical procedures including information transmission analysis (Miller and Nicely, 1955), multidimensional scaling (Tyler *et al.*, 1987) and hierarchical clustering (Busby *et al.*, 1984). Although these techniques differ in their approach and do not always provide identical information from the same data, they all aim to describe how subjects use information to recognize phonemes. There are two aspects to this process: the information contained in the stimuli and the strategies employed by subjects to use this information.

It is generally assumed that subjects group phonemes according to acoustic phonetic features such as voicing, nasality, formant structure, etc. In multidimensional scaling and hierarchical clustering, the grouping of phonemes according to acoustic features is not imposed on the data but derived from the analysis. In information transmission analysis, the phonetic features are decided prior to the analysis. Caution must be exercised in drawing conclusions from these types of analyses as problems can arise with assessing the statistical significance of particular results. The analysis of these types of phoneme confusion tasks, however, has provided important information about speech processing for cochlear implants (Blamey *et al.*, 1987, Dowell *et al.*, 1990a), and about the way profoundly deaf subjects use information to discriminate between phonemes (Van Tasell *et al.*, 1987).

It should be remembered that closed-set tests in general and phoneme confusion tasks in particular do not assess overall speech perception ability. They are useful for assessing the perception of certain acoustic features and are usually correlated with the ability to understand connected speech but as already mentioned, the ability to recognize phonemes in isolation may be a necessary, but not sufficient, condition for the perception of connected speech.

Open-set speech perception tests

It can be argued that there is no such thing as an open-set speech test. There are a finite number of words in the English (or any other) language and by combining words together and applying the rules of syntax, there is a finite (but rather large) set of possible sentences. Thus whatever test we create, we are dealing with a large but finite closed-set of possible responses. In a practical sense, however, most researchers would agree that once the number of possible responses exceeds 100 or so, the test can be considered an open-set assessment. Open-set testing is of great interest in cochlear implant work as the ultimate efficacy of a device designed for speech perception must be strongly related to the amount of speech that subjects can understand. Until ten or so years ago, many workers were sceptical that any cochlear implants produced open-set results with auditory input alone. The few reports of such performance (Clark *et al.*, 1980; Eddington *et al.*, 1978; Hochmair-Desoyer *et al.*, 1980) tended to be explained away by suggesting that subjects were looking into mirrors or had good residual hearing. The weight of evidence soon became overwhelming, however, and it was clear that many profoundly or totally deaf subjects using cochlear implants were able to understand substantial amounts of unknown connected speech and use this ability effectively in their daily lives.

This still did not help the situation regarding the reporting of speech perception results for cochlear implant users as now that open-set performance was a reality, it became very important to be able to claim that subjects could obtain such performance. Despite open-set testing being perhaps the best measure of overall performance it is also subject to many biases and interpretation and it has been difficult for cochlear implant researchers to resist the temptation to enhance the quality of their open-set results. For this reason, it is important when interpreting open-set results in particular, to know exactly how the test was performed, and to refrain from comparing results for different devices or different researchers if the test conditions are unknown.

I would suggest that open-set testing should be performed using unknown, untrained, non-contextual, recorded material without repeats using an unfamiliar speaker and free-field presentation (i.e. not direct interface with the cochlear implant). This provides a conservative measure of open-set performance which is comparable with results obtained with hearing-impaired subjects and with other implants.

Cochlear Implants and Speech Perception

The first serious attempts to look at speech perception in cochlear implant users occurred in the late 1970s. Bilger and colleagues undertook a comprehensive study to investigate the performance of subjects using the House single-channel cochlear implant (Bilger *et al.*, 1977). They concluded that although many subjects reported benefit for speech perception particularly with speechreading, performance on standard speech perception tests with auditory input alone showed no useful results.

Fourcin and others assessed a small number of subjects using a single-channel promontory stimulator which provided F0 (fundamental frequency) information directly as electrical stimulation rate (Fourcin *et al.*, 1979). The speech perception results obtained showed clear improvement when this device was used in conjunction with speechreading, particularly in a closed-set consonant test. This system did not show any useful speech perception with auditory input alone, and was not designed for this purpose. However, this study did show how a feature extraction approach could provide useful information. Hochmair-Desoyer and colleagues showed that some subjects using a single-channel implant with a full speech waveform analogue coding scheme obtained significant scores on speech perception tests with auditory input alone (Hochmair-Desoyer *et al.*, 1981) although it was not clear what proportion of adult subjects could achieve this performance. Eddington and colleagues (Eddington *et al.*, 1983) showed impressive open-set speech perception for one subject with a four electrode intracochlear implant using four bandpass filters and compressed analogue stimulation. Clark and colleagues (Clark, Tong and Dowell, 1983) showed modest open-set speech perception scores for two subjects implanted with a 10-channel intracochlear device. This used a feature extraction speech processor which provided F0 (fundamental frequency) information as stimulation rate, F2 (second formant or more accurately, the main mid-frequency spectral peak) information as site of electrical stimulation within the cochlea, and amplitude as stimulation current scaled between the subject's threshold and maximum comfortable level. Results for other devices were reported as promising but were often difficult to interpret.

These early speech perception results raised more questions than they answered and debate continued as to whether intracochlear electrodes were better than extracochlear, multichannel systems were better than single-channel, analogue stimulation was better than pulsatile, transcutaneous transmission was better than using a percutaneous connector, and so on. The speech perception results at this stage could not answer any of these questions as the numbers of subjects were too small and were often selected to reflect the best performance (i.e. 'star' patients). There was also a lack of consistency in the tests themselves and their administration. The development of the Australian (Nucleus) multichannel cochlear prosthesis as a potential commercial product during 1981 and 1982 provided one of the first controlled, unselected clinical trials of a cochlear implant system using some of the newly-developed speech perception assessment techniques (MAC battery, speech tracking, etc.). The results of the initial clinical trial (Dowell *et al.*, 1985) and later studies with a larger group of subjects (Dowell *et al.*, 1986) provided other researchers and clinicians with objective data on what could be expected from this prosthesis when applied to a general population of adults with acquired profound hearing loss. With the 22 electrode implantable device and original F0F2 speech processor (known as the WSP 2, for Wearable Speech Processor, version 2) the clinical results can be summarized as follows: over 90% of subjects obtained significant benefit when the prosthesis was used with lipreading. Approximately 70% of subjects were able to understand some speech without lipreading and around 30% were able to understand enough speech without speechreading to conduct simple conversations without visual clues (Dowell *et al.*, 1985, Dowell *et al.*, 1986, Brown *et al.*, 1985). Figures 3 and 4 show results obtained for the first 15 subjects implanted in Melbourne with the Nucleus 22-electrode prosthesis for open-set sentence perception with audition alone (Figure 3), lipreading alone and lipreading with audition (Figure 4). These results were obtained after approximately 3 months of experience with the speech processor which used an F0F2 coding scheme.

Independent studies, notably at the University of Iowa, confirmed the potential of the Australian multichannel cochlear prostheses to provide some deaf subjects with useful open-set speech perception (Tyler *et al.*, 1984). The group at the University of Iowa were also able to help answer one of the long standing questions in cochlear implant research regarding the use of multiple or single electrode systems. After reviewing the speech perception results for groups of subjects using the 3M-

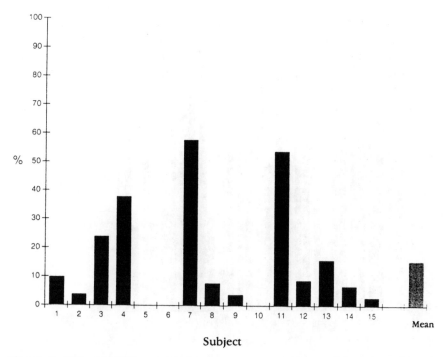

Figure 3. Open-set (CID everyday) sentence scores using audition alone for subjects using the F0F2 speech processor (WSP 2) with the Nucleus 22 electrode cochlear prosthesis. These were obtained after approximately 3 months of experience with the device.

House and 3M-Vienna single-channel cochlear implants, and the Nucleus and Ineraid multichannel systems, they concluded that only the multichannel systems offered the potential for open-set auditory alone performance for adults with acquired deafness (Gantz *et al.*, 1987). Although there is some continuing debate about whether the Austrian single-channel system (known originally as the Vienna system, but now manufactured by MED-EL medical electronics in Innsbruck) is able to provide open-set speech perception for typical patients (as opposed to isolated 'stars'), there have not been reliable independent studies supporting the results reported by the developers of the device (Hochmair-Desoyer *et al.*, 1980) in unselected subjects.

With clear evidence that multichannel intracochlear systems could provide useful auditory alone speech perception, the Nucleus prosthesis came into widespread clinical use from around 1985. This was not simply because this system provided better speech perception, as other multichannel systems had been shown to provide a similar range of performance (the Ineraid system developed originally in Salt Lake City, and the device developed at the University of California, San Francisco). These other systems either ran into reliability problems or

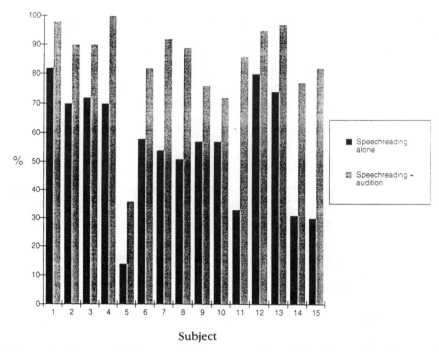

Figure 4. Open-set (CID everyday) sentence scores using lipreading alone and lipreading with audition for subjects using the F0F2 speech processor (WSP 3) with the Nucleus 22 electrode cochlear prosthesis. These were obtained after approximately 3 months of experience with the device.

involved the use of percutaneous connectors which, in the opinion of the regulatory bodies (USA Food and Drug Administration), carried increased medical risks. Another advantage of the Nucleus system was the ability of the audiologist to programme each prosthesis for the individual user using a PC-based software and hardware package. This type of flexibility proved to be vital for the general clinical application of cochlear implant systems.

In 1985, a new signal coding scheme was introduced for the Nucleus prosthesis which used an additional electrode position to code the frequency and amplitude of the main spectral peak between 250 and 1000 Hz (the first formant in voiced speech). The investigation of the effect on speech perception of this new coding scheme (known as F0F1F2) was hampered by a number of problems. The performance of implanted subjects varies over a wide range (Figure 3) and improves with experience for at least two years after implantation and probably over longer periods for some subjects (Brown *et al.*, 1987; Tye-Murray *et al.*, 1992). These factors make it difficult to show a statistically significant improvement in performance as they introduce additional variance into most studies. An initial study of seven subjects in 1985 showed very promising results after changing to the new speech processor (Dowell *et al.*, 1987a). The mean scores for open-set sentences with auditory input alone improved from 30.4% to 62.9%, but this result was confounded by experience effects, as the subjects were tested up to four weeks later with the new scheme and were all within 18 months of implant surgery. Unequivocal evidence of the effectiveness of the new scheme was only obtained after 2 years of clinical use of the new system when results could be compared for larger groups of subjects tested after the same amount of implant experience (Dowell *et al.*, 1987b). Clinical results eventually showed an improvement from a mean open-set sentence score of 15.9% for the F0F2 speech processor to 35.4% for the F0F1F2 processor for adult patients assessed after 3 months of experience with the prosthesis. Additional studies showed that the F0F1F2 coding provided increased information at an acoustic phonetic level (Dowell *et al.*,1990a) and improved the performance in moderate levels of background noise. Figure 5 shows individual results for subjects implanted in Melbourne who used the F0F1F2 coding scheme. These were obtained using the CID everyday sentence test after 3 months experience with the prosthesis and are directly comparable with the results in Figure 3.

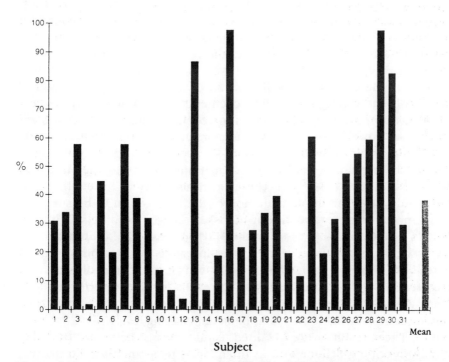

Figure 5. Open-set (CID everyday) sentence scores using audition alone for subjects using the F0F1F2 speech processor (WSP 3) with the Nucleus 22 electrode cochlear prosthesis. These were obtained after approximately 3 months of experience with the device.

By 1987, speech perception results with multichannel cochlear implants had exceeded expectations. With more adults implanted and those implanted gaining continual experience, scores approaching 100% for open-set sentence testing in quiet were now commonplace. The new challenge became the improvement of performance in background noise. The original Nucleus system using feature extraction to provide F0 and F2 information had not performed well in moderate levels of noise and the analogue processing used in the Ineraid device and the San Francisco implant appeared to be more robust in noisy conditions (Gantz *et al.*, 1987). The F0F1F2 coding scheme improved this situation for the Nucleus system by providing better performance, particularly in noise (Dowell *et al.*, 1987b).

Despite the encouraging scores, even the better subjects reported difficulty in understanding speech in everyday environments (for example, while driving, at restaurants, etc.). It was felt that improved speech perception in noise would require more redundancy in the processed signal and a departure from the feature extraction approach that had been used in the Nucleus system. The next development to take place in speech processing for the Nucleus device was a new coding scheme which added high frequency information to the existing F0F1F2 scheme. This became known as the Multipeak coding scheme and was implemented in a new clinical speech processor (known as the MSP for Miniature Speech Processor) in 1989. As this change involved both the hardware (from WSP-3 to MSP) and the coding scheme, the analysis of speech perception results again proved to be difficult. Initial research studies in Melbourne (Dowell *et al.*, 1990b) and St Louis (Skinner *et al.*, 1991) showed significant improvements in open-set speech perception in quiet and in noise, but showed little change in results for closed-set vowel and consonant assessments. Additional studies indicated that the improvement in open-set speech perception was largely due to the extra high frequency information provided by the Multipeak scheme (Dowell, 1991), but it was again necessary to review the clinical results after the implementation of the new system to be sure that this improvement was evident across a range of subjects. Figure 6 shows results for subjects using the MSP processor and Multipeak coding scheme for open-set sentence testing after 3 to 4 months experience with their implant. These results can be compared directly with Figures 3 and 5. Figure 7 shows the results for five experienced subjects tested with the F0F1F2 and Multipeak processing schemes using open-set monosyllabic words in quiet and varying levels of background noise. These results were obtained using the same hardware (the MSP for both coding schemes) and unchanged programming parameters (the thresholds, maximum levels and frequency allocation for each electrode) with a balanced design to control for experience effects. In both the clinical results (Figure 6) and the research studies (Figure 7), a significant improvement in open-set speech perception was evident for subjects using the Multipeak coding.

In a little more than ten years, the speech perception performance for adults with acquired deafness using cochlear implants has progressed from little or no open-set word or sentence recognition to a situation where interactive conversation is possible for 70% of subjects using audition alone (based on sentence scores exceeding 40%). Additional improvements are also on the way for adult implant users. Wilson and colleagues have shown (Wilson *et al.*, 1992) substantial improvements in speech perception for a series of experienced subjects using a CIS (for Continuous Interleaved Sampling) speech processor with the Ineraid implant compared with the four channel compressed analogue scheme that is currently used with this system. The CIS processor separates the electrical stimulation pulses in time such that electrode current interaction is avoided and runs at a high overall rate, thus increasing the potential information transmitted. Results for 11 subjects for open-set monosyllabic words show a mean word score of 47%. Two subjects score over 80% correct for monosyllables, performance that is comparable to that of hearing-impaired subjects with a moderate high frequency hearing loss.

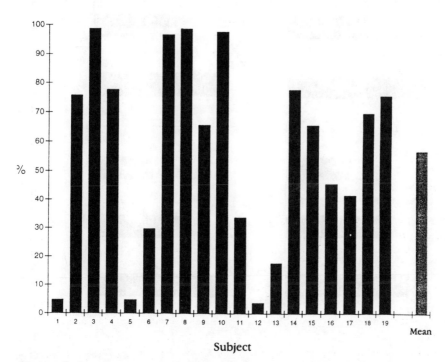

Figure 6. Open-set sentence scores using audition alone for subjects using the Multipeak speech processor (MSP) with the Nucleus 22 electrode cochlear prosthesis. These were obtained after approximately 3 months of experience with the device.

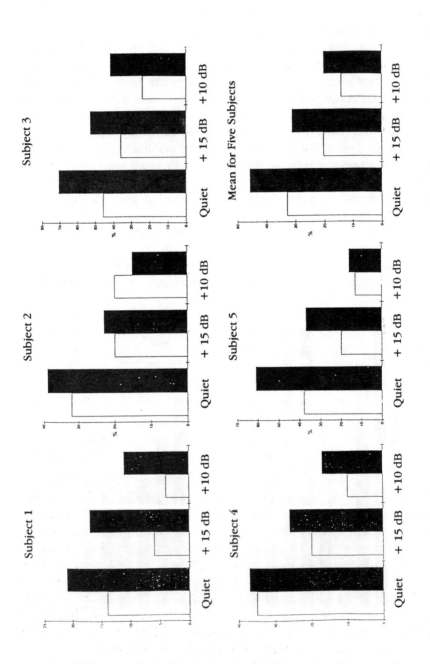

Figure 7. Open-set monosyllabic word scores using audition alone in quiet and at various signal-to-noise ratios for five experienced subjects using the Multipeak (solid columns) and F0F1F2 (open columns) speech coding schemes.

McDermott and colleagues have shown similar speech perception results for subjects using a Spectral Maxima Speech Processor (SMSP) with the Nucleus 22 electrode implant system (McKay *et al.*, 1991). This coding scheme selects the six maximum outputs from an array of 16 bandpass filters and uses the output from the filters to stimulate at six different places in the cochlea based on the frequency of the selected filters. This potentially provides additional spectral information about the incoming signal compared with the MSP/Multipeak processor. Results for 10 subjects show a mean word score for open-set monosyllables of 54% with several subjects also scoring over 80% correct on individual tests.

A new implant system developed by the MINIMED corporation based on work at the University of California San Francisco, shows promise in providing a flexible implanted device allowing substantial changes in signal coding without a connector through the skin (e.g. the Ineraid implant). Clinical trial results have shown open-set speech perception similar to the other multichannel implant systems (Kessler, 1993).

Despite these encouraging results, clinicians working with implanted adults still face a number of difficulties. The extraordinary performance for some subjects is balanced by disappointment for others who are not able to understand speech as easily as they would like. All results from clinical implant programmes show a wide range of performance and the ability of clinicians to predict postoperative performance is crucial to preoperative counselling of these subjects, particularly now that many patients with useful residual hearing are being considered for cochlear implantation. The factors influencing this wide range of performance will be discussed in the next section.

Factors Affecting Speech Perception Performance

It has become increasingly important to be able to provide a reasonable prediction of postoperative performance for adult cochlear implant candidates. It is important, not only in deciding whether a particular candidate is likely to be better off with an implant, but also to provide realistic expectations for the postoperative rehabilitation programme. As discussed in the previous section, both the average results and the performance of the best subjects have improved consistently over the last 10 years, but results for open-set sentence testing still range from 0% to 100%. A number of studies have provided some insight into the reasons for this large range of performance, although much of the variation in performance remains unexplained.

If we consider the chain of information transmission in a multichannel cochlear implant system, it is possible to identify crucial stages where specific factors may influence overall performance. At the beginning of this chain is the speech processing hardware. Obviously, any fault at this level will affect speech perception. For instance, simple problems such as broken cables, faulty microphones and broken battery contacts will have a profound effect on the input to the implant system. Another factor at the hardware level is the speech processing scheme which, as shown in the previous section, has a significant influence on the speech perception results. Coupled with these engineering and maintenance factors are the application of the system for the particular user. For instance, the Nucleus 22 electrode implant system is individually programmed for each subject by measuring thresholds, maximum comfort levels and other parameters which alter the actual signal delivered to the electrodes in the cochlea. If this programming is done poorly, or not attended to regularly, the signal may not be optimal for speech perception.

Next in the chain of information transmission is the interface between the electrodes within the cochlea (in most cases) and the auditory neurons. As cochlear implants are applied in cases of profound hearing loss, we are invariably dealing with damaged cochleas. The degree of damage and the type of pathology influence the number of surviving auditory neurons that are available for stimulation and the surgical placement of the electrode array within the cochlea. For instance, bacterial meningitis can often lead to new bone growth within the cochlea and in the worst cases the cochlea may be totally obliterated by new bone formation. Cochlear otosclerosis can also lead to gross changes in the structure of the cochlea providing problems for electrode placement. Other pathologies may not show obvious changes to the bony cochlea structures, but may lead to degeneration of the neural elements with a consequent effect on the efficacy of intra-cochlear electrical stimulation. It is difficult to know the exact state of the cochlea from current preoperative assessment techniques, however, CT scans and magnetic resonance imaging can provide some idea of the structural state of the cochlea, and electrical stimulation of the promontory may provide some information about the surviving neural elements. Blamey and colleagues have shown that the results of preoperative promontory stimulation tests (when looked at from a psychophysical point of view) were significantly correlated with postoperative speech perception results (Blamey *et al.*, 1992). They also showed that the number of electrodes used in the speech processor (related to the number of electrodes placed successfully into the cochlea at surgery) and the postoperative dynamic range of electrical stimulation were also correlated with speech perception performance. These three factors are probably all related in some way to the amount of damage to cochlea structures and/or neural elements and as such represent indirect measurements of the efficacy of the electrode–neuron interface.

The final requirement for implant users to obtain useful speech perception is for them to be able to use the information provided by the prosthesis effectively. That this is important in overall performance is clearly demonstrated by the improvement over time evident for cochlear implant users (Dowell *et al.*, 1986; Brown *et al.*, 1987, Tye-Murray *et al.*, 1992). Many users continue to improve their scores on speech perception tests for years after implantation showing that considerable learning is required to make the best possible use of the information. Results have also suggested that the duration of profound hearing impairment prior to implantation has a significant effect on postoperative speech perception (Blamey *et al.*, 1992). This implies that certain skills needed for processing auditory information deteriorate with lack of use over long periods of time. It is likely that individual cognitive ability and other special skills may also have a significant effect on performance, but these particular skills have not been identified as yet. For instance, lipreading ability also varies over a wide range, and as this involves integrating incomplete information, it was expected by some researchers that people who were good speechreaders would perform well with a cochlear implant. However, virtually no correlation has been found between these abilities. Similarly, no studies have shown that intelligence (as measured by psychological tests) is correlated with speech perception performance.

There remains much to learn before speech perception results with cochlear implants can be predicted with any accuracy. On the other hand, we now have some useful trends that can give an approximate prediction based on the preoperative history, audiological and medical assessments. We can expect results to continue to improve, not only due to improvements in the speech processing and electrical stimulation hardware, but also due to the changing population being treated. There will be fewer candidates with long-term profound deafness and more with residual hearing in the non-implanted ear so that sensory deprivation, and the subsequent loss of auditory processing skills, will not be as much of a factor in postoperative performance.

References

Bilger, R.C., Black, R.O., Hopkinson, N.T., Meyers, E.N., Payne, J.L., Vega, A. and Wolf, R.V. (1977).. Evaluation of subjects presently fitted with implanted auditory prosthesis. Annals of Otology, Suppl 38.

Blamey, P.J., Dowell, R.C., Brown, A.M., Clark, G.M. and Seligman, P.M. (1987) Vowel and consonant recognition of cochlear implant patients using formant-estimating speech processors. Journal of the Acoustical Society of America 82(1): 48–57.

Blamey, P.J., Pyman, B.C., Gordon, M.B., Clark, G.M., Brown, A.M., Dowell, R.C. and Hollow, R.D. (1992) Factors predicting postoperative sentence scores in postlinguistically deaf adult cochlear implant patients. Annals of Otology, Rhinology and Laryngology 101: 342–8.

Boothroyd, A.(1968) Developments in speech audiometry. Sound 2: 3–10.

Brown, A.M., Dowell, R.C. and Clark, G.M. (1987) Clinical results for postlingually deaf patients implanted with multichannel cochlear prostheses. Annals of Otology, Rhinology and Laryngology 96, Suppl 128: 127–8.

Brown, A.M., Clark, G.M., Dowell, R.C., Martin, L.F.A. and Seligman, P.M.(1985) Telephone use by a multi-channel cochlear implant patient: an evaluation using open-set CID sentences. Journal of Laryngology and Otology 99: 231–8.

Busby, P.A., Tong, Y.C. and Clark, G.M. (1984) Underlying dimensions and individual differences in auditory, visual and auditory visual vowel perception by hearing impaired children. Journal of the Acoustical Society of America 75: 1858–65.

Clark, G.M., Tong, Y.C. and Dowell, R.C. (1983) Clinical results with a multichannel pseudobipolar system. Annals of the New York Academy of Sciences 405: 370–6.

De Filippo, C.L. and Scott, B.L. (1978) A method for training and evaluating the reception of ongoing speech. Journal of the Acoustical Society of America 63: 1186–92.

Dowell, R.C. (1991) Speech perception i.ι noise for multichannel cochlear implant users. Doctoral thesis, University of Melbourne.

Dowell, R.C., Brown, A.M. and Mecklenburg, D.J. (1990a) Clinical assessment of implanted deaf adults. In Clark, G.M., Tong, Y.C. and Patrick, J.F. (Eds) Cochlear Prostheses. Edinburgh: Churchill Livingstone.

Dowell, R.C., Mecklenburg, D.J. and Clark, G.M. (1986) Speech recognition in 40 multichannel cochlear implant patients in the USA and Australia. Archives of Otolaryngology 112: 1054–9.

Dowell, R.C., Martin, L.F.A., Clark, G.M. and Brown, A.M. (1985) Results of a preliminary clinical trial on a multiple channel cochlear prosthesis. Annals of Otology, Rhinology and Laryngology 94(3): 244–50.

Dowell, R.C., Seligman, P.M., Blamey, P.J. and Clark, G.M. (1987a) Evaluation of a two-formant speech processing strategy for a multichannel cochlear prosthesis. Annals of Otology, Rhinology and Laryngology 96 (Suppl. 128): 132–4.

Dowell, R.C., Seligman, P.M., Blamey, P.J. and Clark, G.M. (1987b) Speech perception using a two-formant 22-electrode cochlear prosthesis in quiet and in noise. Acta Otolaryngologica 104: 439–46.

Dowell, R.C., Whitford, L.A., Seligman, P.M., Franz, B.K.-H. and Clark, G.M. (1990b) Preliminary results with a miniature speech processor for the 22 electrode Melbourne/Cochlear hearing prosthesis. In Sacristan T,, et al. (Eds) Proceedings of the XIV World Congress of Otorhinolaryngology – Head and Neck Surgery. Amsterdam: Kugler and Ghedini.

Eddington, D.K. (1983) Speech recognition in deaf subjects with multichannel intracochlear electrodes. Annals of the New York Academy of Sciences 405: 241–58.

Eddington, D.K., Dobelle, W.H., Brackman, D.E., Mladejovsky, M.G. and Parkin, J.L. (1978) Auditory prosthesis research with multiple channel intracochlear stimulation in man. Annals of Otology, Rhinology and Laryngology 87 (Suppl. 53): 5–39.

Fourcin, A.J., Rosen, S.M., Moore, B.C.J., Douek, E.E., Clarke, G.P., Dodson, H. and Bannister, L.H. (1979) External electrical stimulation of the cochlea: clinical, psychophysical, speech perceptual and histological findings. British Journal of Audiology 13: 85–107.

Gantz, B.J., McCabe, B.F., Tyler, R.S. and Preece, J.P. (1987) Evaluation of four cochlear implant designs. Annals of Otology, Rhinology and Laryngology 96 (Suppl. 128): 145–7.

Hochmair-Desoyer, I.J., Hochmair, E.S., Fischer, R.E. and Burian, K. (1980) Cochlear prostheses in use: recent speech comprehension results. Archives of Otorhinolaryngology 229: 81–98.

Kessler, D.K. (1993) Clinical results for the Clarion cochlear implant. Paper presented at the 3rd International Cochlear Implant Conference, Innsbruck, April.

Levitt, H., Waltzman, S., Shapiro, W.H. and Cohen, N.L. (1986) Evaluation of a chochler prosthesis using connected discourse tracking. Journal of Rehabilitation Research and Development 23: 147–153.

McKay, C., McDermott, H., Vandali, A. and Clark, G. (1991) Preliminary results with a six spectral maxima sound processor for the University of Melbourne/Nucleus multiple-electrode cochlear implant. Journal of the Otolaryngological Society of Australia 6(5): 354–9.

Miller, G.A. and Nicely, P.E. (1955) An analysis of perceptual confusions among some English consonants. Journal of the Acoustical Society of America 27: 338–52.

Owens, E., Kessler, D.K. and Schubert, E.D. (1981) The Minimal Auditory Capabilities (MAC) battery. Hearing Aid Journal 34: 9–34.

Peterson, G.E. and Lehiste, I. (1962) Revised CNC lists for auditory tests. Journal of Speech and Hearing Disorders 27: 62–70.

Rosen, S., Fourcin, A.J. and Moore, B.C.J. (1980) Lipreading connected discourse with fundamental frequency information. British Society of Audiology Newsletter 42–43.

Skinner, M.W., Holden, L.K., Holden, T.A., Dowell, R.C., Seligman, P.M., Brimacombe, J.A. and Beiter, A.L. (1991) Performance of postlingually deaf adults with the wearable speech processor (WSP III) and mini speech processor (MSP) of the Nucleus multielectrode cochlear implant. Ear and Hearing 12(1): 3–22.

Thornton, A.R. and Raffin, M.J.M. (1978) Speech discrimination scores modeled as a binomial variable. Journal of Speech and Hearing Research 21: 507–18.

Tillman, T.W. and Carhart, R. (1966) An expanded test for speech discrimination utilizing CNC words: Northwestern University auditory test no. 6. Technical report No. SAM-TR-66-55. USAF School of Aerospace Medicine, Brooks Air Force Base, Texas.

Tye-Murray, N. and Lowder, M.W. (1990) Comparison of the F0F2 and F0F1F2 processing strategies for the Cochlear Corporation cochlear implant. Ear and Hearing 11: 195–200.

Tye-Murray, N. and Tyler, R.S. (1988) A critique of continuous discourse tracking as a test procedure. Journal of Speech and Hearing Disorders 53: 226–31.

Tye-Murray, N., Tyler, R.S., Woodworth, G.G. and Gantz, B.J. (1992) Performance over time with a Nucleus or Ineraid cochlear implant. Ear and Hearing 13: 200–9.

Tyler, R.S., Lowder, M.W., Otto, S.R., Preece, J.P., Gantz, B.J. and McCabe, B.F. (1984) Initial Iowa results with the multichannel cochlear implant from Melbourne. Journal of Speech and Hearing Research 27(4): 596–604.

Tyler, R.S., Tye-Murray, N., Preece, J.P., Gantz, B.J., McCabe, B.F. (1987) Vowel and consonant confusions among cochlear implant patients: do different implants make a difference. Annals of Otology, Rhinology and Laryngology 96, Suppl 128: 141–4.

Van Tasell, D.J., Soli, S.K., Kirby, V.M. and Widin, G.P. (1987) Speech waveform envelope cues for consonant recognition. Journal of the Acoustical Society of America 82: 1152–61.

Wilson, B.S., Lawson, D.T., Finley, C.C. and Zerbi ,M. (1992) Speech processors for auditory prostheses. Final report. NIH project NO1-DC-9-2401.

13
Speech Production by Adults Using Cochlear Implants

DAVID HOUSE

Introduction

When an adult with normal speech and language skills is confronted ‚with a sudden profound or total loss of hearing, the primary concern is to regain the ability to perceive speech. Speech production is not as immediately and dramatically affected. Cochlear implants are generally designed with this fact in mind and are meant to optimize the perception of the speech of others. A large part of current research involving cochlear implants has been devoted to evaluating the perceptual performance of cochlear implant users.

Over a period of time, however, speech production can also be affected by deafness, sometimes quite severely. There are a considerable number of studies which document the deterioration of speech production after the onset of hearing loss in postlingually deafened speakers (for example, Cowie and Douglas-Cowie, 1983; Plant, 1983; Plant and Hammarberg, 1983; Waldstein, 1990; Lane and Webster, 1991; and Cowie and Douglas-Cowie, Chapter 23). Speech production problems can be quite diverse affecting individuals very differently. Harsh or breathy voice quality, inappropriate intonation, loss of laryngeal and timing control leading to devoicing or intrusive voicing, hypernasality, vowel reduction and lengthening, and omission or substitution of consonants are some of the features reported in the speech production of postlingually deafened speakers. A growing body of research is now being carried out to explore effects of the auditory feedback provided by a cochlear implant on such deviant features in speech production.

There are a number of good reasons for focusing on the speech production of cochlear implant users. First of all, speech production is an integral part of speech communication. Improved production should necessarily lead to a better communication situation in general for the implant user and thus indirectly facilitate speech perception. An increased understanding of how speech features are influenced in production may also give us insights into how these features are perceived by the implant users. This could tell us something about those particular features which are less successfully conveyed by the implant leading to improvements in implant design. Speech training programmes can be fashioned to concentrate on particular areas of production which in turn may also lead to enhanced awareness and improved perception. Another aspect of production studies more related to basic research can be found in addressing the question of the role of auditory feedback as crucial to speech production control (cf. Lane and Tranel, 1971; Sherrard, 1982). Finally, studies of the speech production of adult implant users should help us in defining what to look for when assessing the performance of the increasing number of children being fitted with cochlear implants.

The goal of this chapter is to present a general overview of some of the current research investigating the speech of adult implant users. A brief description of some of the commonest features of postlingually deafened adult speech is followed by an account of several methods used to investigate these features before and after implant activation. The results of a number of investigations are discussed, and the chapter concludes with a look at some of the questions that future research may address.

Changes in speech following acquired deafness

One of the most prominent features of speech following loss of hearing seems to be the loss of laryngeal control (Lane and Webster, 1991). This results in individual voice quality aberrations which can be perceived by listeners as ranging from breathiness to harsh, grating or pressed voice quality (Penn, 1955; Cowie and Douglas-Cowie, 1983; Plant, 1983; Plant and Hammarberg, 1983; House and Willstedt, 1993). Another consequence of loss of laryngeal control is less control of voice fundamental frequency (F0). Speakers are reported to have uncontrolled or monotonous pitch (Penn, 1955), inappropriate intonation (Cowie and Douglas-Cowie, 1983), reduced F0 range (Plant, 1983; Plant and Hammarberg, 1983), and higher average F0 levels and greater F0 variability than normal hearing subjects (Leder, Spitzer and Kirchner, 1987a; Lane and Webster, 1991). Thus considerable individual variation is demonstrated in the literature in terms of the resulting F0 level, range and variation. However, maintaining laryngeal control often seems to be dependent upon some type of auditory feedback.

Other features of speech which can be related to loss of laryngeal control involve excess stress, excessive pause time and devoicing of voiced obstruents and voicing of voiceless obstruents (Cowie and Douglas-Cowie, 1983; Plant, 1983; Waldstein, 1990). Voice intensity is also a feature related to loss of laryngeal control and can either be too loud (to enable kinaesthetic feedback) or too soft (for fear of being too loud) (Kirk and Edgerton, 1983).

Hypernasality is another feature commonly reported in the speech of adults with acquired deafness (Penn, 1955; Cowie and Douglas-Cowie, 1983; Plant, 1983; Plant and Hammarberg, 1983; House and Willstedt, 1993). It would appear that control of the velum, in much the same way as control of the larynx, is also dependent upon auditory feedback.

The features reported on above mostly affect the prosody of speech (e.g. intonation, rhythm, stress patterns, voice quality). Segmental abnormalities have also been documented for both consonants and vowels. Where consonants are concerned, fricatives and especially the frequency of sibilant noise seem to be most affected by loss of hearing. Some segmental substitution has been reported particularly for /s/ which is sometimes produced more like [t] (Read, 1989). Consonant cluster reduction is common (Plant, 1983) as is consonant omission (Cowie and Douglas-Cowie, 1983) and reduced differentiation of obstruent contrasts (Lane and Webster, 1991). As mentioned above, voicing and devoicing of obstruents may also occur. Vowel substitutions are rarer, with vowel reduction (i.e. a more constricted vowel space) and longer vowel durations being the primary features of vowel change associated with loss of hearing (Cowie and Douglas-Cowie, 1983; Waldstein, 1990; and Economou et al., 1992). Speaking rate can also be affected and tends to be longer than normal after loss of hearing (Leder et al., 1987c) which may reflect both segmental and prosodic difficulties.

In summary, the speech of postlingually deafened adults can deteriorate substantially in a great number of ways. The severity of this deterioration is, however, very individual in nature. Some speakers show very little change after several years, while the speech of others deteri-orates comparatively rapidly (Cowie et al., 1982; Read, 1991). One general finding seems to be that the segmental aspects of speech are more resistant to change than are the suprasegmental and prosodic aspects, although this was not substantiated by Waldstein (1990). Lane and Webster (1991, page 861) speculate that the control of fundamental frequency 'may represent a slow tracking movement with relatively large degrees of freedom and relatively poor access to alternate afferent feedback,' while plosives and fricatives may entail a larger degree of afferent feedback. Zimmerman and Rettaliata (1981, page 177), in a cinefluorographic study of tongue and jaw movements of one deafened speaker, suggest that 'overlearned motor patterns' may take a long time to degenerate but that 'auditory information plays a critical role in the long-term monitoring and maintenance of coordinative structures'. The crucial question is then, if some form of auditory information is restored by means of a cochlear implant, will this lead to improvements in speech production?

Methods of Investigation

How can the question of changes in speech production following cochlear implantation be approached? The methodologically appealing aspect of working with the speech production of implant users is that recordings and measurements can be made prior to the implant operation, after the operation but immediately before activation of the implant (there is often a time lag of about one month between the operation and activation of the implant to allow for recovery after the surgical procedure), and immediately following processor activation. Recordings and measurements can then be repeated at certain time intervals following processor activation. The processor can also be turned off for various intervals with recordings being made after a period of auditory deprivation. Aspects of recordings and measurements can then be compared to ascertain the effect of auditory feedback. This type of before and after methodology is common to most studies of speech production and implant users. However, apart from this common denominator in methodology, there appears in the literature a wealth of different approaches to investigating the speech of implant users.

One approach involves an auditory analysis of audio recordings, often of read text passages or word lists. This method is most suited to studies of features of speech production which are difficult to analyse acoustically such as perceived aspects of voice quality or overall ratings of speech acceptability. A panel of listeners is often used in such studies, either trained listeners (see Öster 1988) to evaluate features such as aspects of voice quality, or untrained listeners (see Economou *et al.*, 1992) to evaluate general acceptability and perceived deviation. Questionnaires are also used where members of the user's family are asked to comment upon changes in speech production (East and Cooper, 1986; Öster, 1988).

The other major approach involves an acoustic analysis of audio recordings. A substantial number of studies have concentrated on the analysis of fundamental frequency. This is in line with the data on speech changes following deafness where loss of laryngeal control results in aberrations of fundamental frequency. Calculating the average F0 in a read text passage before and after processor activation can give an indication of changes in voice control and provide information on a possible change to a more normal and appropriate F0. To assess more carefully how fundamental frequency is used by the speaker, measurements of average F0 can be complemented with measurements of the range of F0 and actual intonation contours. Such measurements include maximum and minimum values thus giving a better picture of the speaker's control of F0 (see House and Willstedt, 1993).

Another way of analysing fundamental frequency is to record a laryngeal signal either with contact microphones (Plant and Öster, 1986; Öster 1988) or using a laryngograph (Ball and Faulkner, 1989; Ball *et al.*, 1990; Read, 1991). The signal, containing information on the rate of vibration of the vocal folds, is then analysed producing data on the frequency distribution. The data is often displayed in the form of a histogram producing a visual display of mean fundamental frequency, range and variation. This display can also reveal aspects of voice quality such as creak or other irregularities in the periodicity of the voice source (see Abberton *et al.*, 1989 and Ball *et al.*, 1990) and can thus comprise a quantitative measurement of changes of voice quality following an implant. Voice quality differences can also be assessed by analysing speech waveform perturbations. Large perturbations (i.e. large changes in period to period frequency or amplitude) are often evidence of aberrant voice quality (Hammarberg, 1986; Öster, 1988; Ball *et al.*, 1990).

. The analysis of vowel production usually involves a spectrographic analysis where the frequencies of the first and second formants are plotted in terms of an F1-F2 vowel space (Plant and Öster, 1986; Tartter *et al.*, 1989; Perkell *et al.*, 1992; Economou *et al.*, 1992). A change in the quality of different vowels will be indicated by changes in the F1-F2 plots and can reveal a possible shift in the speaker's overall vowel articulation. Vowel durations are often measured, and differences in amplitude between the first two harmonics in the acoustic spectrum of vowels have also been measured as an indication of the 'breathiness' of the voice (see Perkell *et al.*, 1992).

Consonant production has generally been analysed in terms of voicing, place of articulation and manner of articulation (see Tartter *et al.*, 1989 and Economou *et al.*, 1992). Spectrograms can be used to measure voice onset time as an indication of voicing, burst or frication spectrum as an indication of place of articulation, and transition duration for glides and stops and nasal resonances as acoustic indicators of manner of articulation.

Measurements involving more general aspects of the speech of implant users include speech duration, rate of articulation in syllables per second (Öster, 1988), sound pressure level (SPL) to compare overall speech intensity before and after implantation (Perkell *et al.*, 1992) and average air flow and volume of air expended per syllable as a measurement of speech breathing (Lane *et al.*, 1991). An additional factor in many studies is the use of speech and voice training and therapy in connection with implant activation (see Waters, 1986). Furthermore, different types of implants process and present the speech signal in different ways, possibly leading to differences in the relative strengths of speech cues available to the implant user (Economou *et al.*, 1992).

In summary, the diversity of methods used to assess the speech of implant users combined with the great individual variation found in this group of speakers does not facilitate a very unified picture of changes in speech following a cochlear implant. It is difficult to compare studies where quite different methods have been used. Finally, with the exception of a few studies involving speakers of Swedish, the bulk of published research has been carried out on speakers of English. This fact can give rise to questions of language specificity, that is, how well do results for English speakers generalize to other languages?

Results

Although difficulties are involved in comparing results from different studies, certain general trends can be observed. Most studies do report some changes in speech parameters after implant activation, and these changes are usually in the direction of more normal values. Changes are, however, for the most part difficult to predict, and vary considerably from individual to individual. This section presents some of the findings organized in terms of the various speech parameters that have been investigated.

Changes in fundamental frequency

Changes in the mean fundamental frequency used by a speaker is a fairly straightforward measurement used in many investigations. The general trend is toward a lowering of an abnormally high F0 (Leder, Spitzer and Kirchner, 1987a; Öster, 1988; Ball and Faulkner, 1989; Perkell et al., 1992; House and Willstedt, 1993). It appears that lack of laryngeal control, often resulting in a high F0, can be somewhat alleviated by the feedback provided by the implant. It is also common for an abnormally low F0 to be raised to a more appropriate level after an implant (Kirk and Edgerton, 1983; Öster, 1988). Some speakers, however, demonstrate no change in F0, even if they show abnormal values both before and after implant activation (Ball and Faulkner, 1989; Perkell et al., 1992).

Changes in the range of fundamental frequency have also been documented in a number of studies. Here the general trend is from a wide F0 range to a more controlled, narrow range (Ball and Faulkner, 1989; Öster, 1987) although the opposite has also been reported (Plant and Öster, 1986). A more appropriate range of F0 after implantation also bears witness to the role of auditory feedback in helping speakers improve laryngeal control.

Changes in the use of F0 have also been studied. Leder et al. (1986) report on the reacquisition of contrastive stress in one implant user.

Plant and Öster (1986) show more appropriate accentuation patterns in one implant user after activation. House and Willstedt (1993) documented changes in both F0 mean and range in the use of these parameters to signal speaker mood. Three speakers changed F0 mean and range to more appropriate values after implant activation to differentiate between anger (low F0 mean, narrow F0 range) and happiness (high F0 mean, wide F0 range). These results were also corroborated by the results of a listening test where happiness was only identified by the listener panel in utterances produced after implant activation. Speaker mood has also been shown to pose difficulties for perception for both hearing-impaired subjects (Öster and Risberg, 1986) and implant users (House, 1992).

Changes in voice quality

Improvements in voice quality after implant activation have been documented using ratings provided by panels of listeners. A lesser degree of creaky voice is one of the improvements often reported as are improvements concerning grating, hyperfunctional voice and hypernasality (Waters, 1986; Öster, 1988; Read, 1989; House and Willstedt, 1993). Improvements concerning primarily creak have been documented by means of histograms produced from laryngograph recordings (Ball and Faulkner, 1989) and by means of waveform perturbation analysis (Öster, 1988). These general improvements in voice quality, however, are individual and do not occur in all implant users (Plant and Öster, 1986; Waters, 1986; Ball and Faulkner, 1989). These changes often involve not only implant activation but also voice training. Perkell *et al.* (1992) showed evidence of a reduction of breathiness in one subject (toward normal values) and a reduction in press in two subjects (toward normal values). These positive changes applied to three of four subjects.

Changes in the production of vowels and consonants

The production of vowels and consonants among implant subjects are topics which are not represented by a great number of studies. Plant and Öster (1986) report a generalized backwards shift of the vowel space for one subject which has both positive and negative effects on vowel production. Perkell *et al.* (1992) found changes in the normative direction in vowel space (particularly the F2 dimension) in two of their subjects. Tartter *et al.* (1989), however, report an adverse effect after one year of implant use on one subject's vowel production. The vowel space steadily constricted toward lower first and second formant frequency values.

The same subject did improve in production of some segmental consonant distinctions. She shortened voiceless stop onsets, reduced word-final aspiration, lengthened voice offset times for final voiced stops, and was able to produce better burst and frication spectra. Few studies have specifically dealt with consonant production changes in adults, although changes in production in children have also been documented (Economou *et al.*, 1992).

Other aspects of speech production

Some other, more general aspects of speech production that have been investigated involve speech duration, rate of articulation, intensity and speech breathing. In some implant users these aspects have changed toward the more normal, for example, slow articulation speeding up and fast articulation slowing down (Öster, 1988), more normal intensity (Perkell *et al.*,1992), and more normal speech breathing (Lane *et al.*, 1991). Here again, however, these trends were not found in all subjects. Perkell *et al.*, (1992) established certain relationships between measured parameters suggesting that it is not adequate to analyse each parameter separately. Results of questionnaires testify to the general improvement of speech production as perceived by the implant users themselves and their families with improved self-confidence being listed as one of the most valued aspects of implant use (East and Cooper, 1986; Öster, 1988).

Discussion and Conclusions

It is clear from the results presented in the literature that the restoration of auditory information by means of a cochlear implant can lead to improvements in speech production. Improvements can be in specific areas such as control of fundamental frequency or in more general terms such as changes in intensity or rate of speech. Evidence suggests, however, that auditory feedback has perhaps the greatest effect in restoring laryngeal control leading to better control of fundamental frequency and improvements in voice quality. This is in line with the suggestion by Lane and Webster (1991) concerning the relatively poor access to afferent feedback available for control of fundamental frequency. It may also be the case that implants are more successful at transmitting information about fundamental frequency than, for example, information concerning vowel space, at least in terms of self-hearing. The possible relationship between perceptual gains and changes in production among implant users is an exciting area for future research (cf. Perkell *et al.*, 1992).

The large individual variation in changes in speech production is another question that arises when looking at the data. Some users demonstrate large improvements in production while others show little change. It is also very difficult to predict what changes will occur after implant activation. A relationship may exist between prior linguistic experience and production, whereby greater changes in production could be expected the older the implant user was at age of onset of deafness (Perkell *et al.*, 1992). More data needs to be gathered to substantiate this speculation. This idea is also related to the question of prelingually deaf implant users. Busby *et al.* (1991) report some improvements for consonant production in prelingually deaf implant users. Here, however, the relevant questions concerning perception and production seem to be quite different than for postlingually deaf implant users since prelingually deaf users lack developed auditory speech and language skills.

A third question involves the use of speech and language training and therapy. Such training is often seen as an integral part of the fitting of an implant and as such it is difficult to separate effects of the implant from effects of training (Waters, 1986; House and Willstedt, 1993). While laryngograph displays have been used to train intonation in deaf adults (see Abberton and Fourcin, 1972; Abberton *et al.*, 1977) the use of an implant makes speech and voice training possible in a much different way via the use of auditory feedback. Here, again, future research may approach interesting questions in this area.

Other questions involve changes in production over time, changes in the speech production of children, and possible language specific speech changes. Some subjects do improve or change their production over time, especially during the first 6 months (Perkell *et al.*, 1992; House and Willstedt, 1993), but this is also highly dependent on the individual. Öster (1988) and Svirsky *et al.* (1992) showed that rapid speech changes can occur as a result of switching off the implant. To what degree speech changes are learned over time is indeed an interesting area for future work. In working with children, can we find the same changes that occur for adults? Furthermore, if fundamental frequency control is one of the most apparent changes after implant activation, more studies on the use of intonation by implant subjects would serve to enhance our knowledge of how this control is integrated into a linguistic system.

These results and questions, taken as a whole, are very encouraging for the users of cochlear implants, even though many new questions need to be answered. This is indeed a field where much research is needed. To conclude, a short personal comment on the three speakers studied by House and Willstedt (1993). The speakers could not only convey happiness when asked to do so, they are genuinely happy with their implants.

Acknowledgements

Many thanks are due to Arne Risberg for personal inspiration in this field of research. Preparation of this chapter was supported in part by the Bank of Sweden Tercentenary Foundation.

References

Abberton, E., Howard, D.M. and Fourcin, A.J. (1989) Laryngographic assessment of normal voice: a tutorial. Clinical Linguistics and Phonetics 3: 281–96.

Abberton, E. and Fourcin, A.J. (1972) Laryngographic analysis and intonation. British Journal of Disorders of Communication 7: 24–9.

Abberton, E., Parker, A. and Fourcin, A.J. (1977) Speech improvement in deaf adults using laryngograph displays. In Pickett, J. (Ed) Papers from the research conference on speech-processing aids for the deaf. Gallaudet College, Washington D.C. pp 172–88.

Ball, G. and Faulkner, A. (1989) Speech production of postlingually deafened adults using electrical and acoustic speech pattern prosthesis. Speech, Hearing and Language: Work. Prog. (U.C.L.) 3: 13–32.

Ball, V., Faulkner, A. and Fourcin, A. (1990) The effects of two different speech-coding strategies on voice fundamental frequency control in deafened adults. British Journal of Audiology 24: 393–409.

Busby, P.A., Roberts, S.A., Tong, Y.C. and Clark, G.M. (1991) Results of speech perception and speech production training for three prelingually deaf patients using a multiple-electrode cochlear implant. British Journal of Audiology 25: 291–302.

Cowie, R.I. and Douglas-Cowie, E. (1983) Speech production in profound post-lingual deafness. In Lutman, M.E and Haggard, M.P. (Eds) Hearing Science and Hearing Disorders. New York: Academic. pp 183–231.

Cowie, R., Douglas-Cowie, E. and Kerr, A.G. (1982) A study of speech deterioration in post-lingually deafened adults. Journal of Laryngology and Otology 96: 101–12.

East, C.A. and Cooper, H.R. (1986) Extra-cochlear implants: the patient's viewpoint. British Journal of Audiology 20: 55–9.

Economou, A., Tartter V.C., Chute, P.M. and Hellman, S.A. (1992) Speech changes following reimplantation from a single-channel to a multichannel cochlear implant. Journal of the Acoustical Society of America 92: 1310–23.

Engelman, L.R., Waterfall, M.K. and Hough, J.V.D. (1981) Results following cochlear implantation and rehabilitation. Laryngoscope 91: 1821–33.

Hammarberg, B. (1986) Perceptual and acoustic analysis of dysphonia. Doctoral dissertation, Huddinge University Hospital, Dept. of Logopedics and Phoniatrics, Stockholm.

House, D. (1992) Cochlear implants and the perception of mood in speech. British Journal of Audiology 26: 198.

House, D. and Willstedt, U. (1993) Changes in control of fundamental frequency and voice quality following cochlear implant activation and speech training. In Proceedings of the second international conference on tactile aids, hearing aids and cochlear implants, edited by A. Risberg, S. Felicetti, G. Plant and K. Spens, Dept. of Speech Communication and Music Acoustics, KTH (Stockholm), pp 201–10.

Kirk, K.I. and Edgerton, B.J. (1983) Effects of cochlear implant use on voice parameters. Otolaryngological Clinics of North America 16: 281–92.

Lane, H., Perkell, J., Svirsky, M. and Webster, J. (1991) Changes in speech breathing following cochlear implant in postlingually deafened adults. Journal of Speech and Hearing Research 34: 526–33.

Lane, H. and Tranel, B. (1971) The Lombard sign and the role of hearing in speech. Journal of Speech and Hearing Research 14: 677–709.

Lane, H. and Webster, J.W. (1991) Speech deterioration in postlingually deafened adults. Journal of the Acoustical Society of America 89: 859–66.

Leder, S.B. and Spitzer, J.B. (1990) Longitudinal effects of single-channel cochlear implantation on voice quality. Laryngoscope 100: 395–8.

Leder, S.B., Spitzer, J.B. and Kirchner, J.C. (1987a) Speaking fundamental frequency of postlingually profoundly deaf adult men. Annals of Otology, Rhinology and Laryngology 96: 322–4.

Leder, S.B., Spitzer, J.B., Milner, P., Flevaris-Phillips, C., Richardson, F. and Kirchner, J.C. (1986) Reacquisition of contrastive stress in an adventitiously deaf speaker using a single-channel cochlear implant. Journal of the Acoustical Society of America 79: 1967–74.

Leder, S.B., Spitzer, J.B., Milner, P., Flevaris-Phillips, C., Kirchner, J.C. and Richardson, F. (1987b) Voice intensity of prospective cochlear-implant candidates and normal-hearing adult males. Laryngoscope 97: 224–7.

Leder, S.B., Spitzer, J.B., Kirchner, J.C., Flevaris-Phillips, C., Milner, P. and Richardson, F. (1987c) Speaking rate of adventitiously deaf male cochlear implant candidates. Journal of the Acoustical Society of America 82: 843–6.

Öster, A. (1987) Some effects of cochlear implantation on speech production. Speech Trans. Lab. QPSR (Stockholm) 1: 81–9.

Öster, A. (1988) Changes in speech with use of an implant. Speech Trans. Lab. QPSR (Stockholm) 4: 13–22.

Öster, A. and Risberg, A. (1986) The identification of the mood of a speaker by hearing impaired listeners. Speech Trans. Lab. QPSR (Stockholm) 4: 79–90.

Penn, J.P. (1955) Voice and speech patterns of the hard of hearing. Acta Oto-Laryngologica, Suppl. 124.

Perkell, J., Lane, H., Svirsky, M. and Webster, J. (1992) Speech of cochlear implant patients: A longitudinal study of vowel production. Journal of the Acoustical Society of America 91: 2961–78.

Plant, G. (1983) The effects of a long-term hearing loss on speech production. Speech Trans. Lab. QPSR (Stockholm) 1: 18–35.

Plant, G. and Hammarberg, B. (1983) Acoustic and perceptual analysis of the speech of the deafened. Speech Trans. Lab. QPSR (Stockholm) 2–3: 85–107.

Plant, G. and Öster, A. (1986) The effects of cochlear implantation on speech production. A case study. Speech Trans. Lab. QPSR (Stockholm) 1: 65–86.

Read, T. (1989) Improvement in speech production following use of the UCH/RND Cochlear Implant. Journal of Laryngology and Otology, Suppl. 18: 45–9.

Read, T. (1991) Speech production in postlinguistically deafened adult cochlear implant users. In Cooper, H. (Ed) Cochlear Implants: A Practical Guide. London: Whurr Publishers.

Sherrard, C.A. (1982) 'Auditory feedback' or 'sidetone'? The effects on speech production and intelligibility of auditory stimulation from the larynx. Language and Speech 25: 283–92.

Svirsky, M.A., Lane, H., Perkell, J.S. and Wozniak, J. (1992) Effects of short-term auditory deprivation on speech production in adult cochlear implant users. Journal of the Acoustical Society of America 92: 1284–300.

Tartter, V., Chute, P. and Hellman, S. (1989) The speech of a postlingually deafened teenager during the first year of use of a multichannel cochlear implant. Journal of the Acoustical Society of America 86: 2113–21.

Waters, T. (1986) Speech therapy with cochlear implant wearers. British Journal of Audiology 20: 35–43.

Waldstein, R. (1990) Effects of postlingual deafness on speech production:

Implications for the role of auditory feedback. Journal of the Acoustical Society of America 88: 2099–114.

Zimmerman, G. and Rettaliata, P. (1981) Articulatory patterns of an adventitiously deaf speaker: Implications of the role of auditory information in speech production. Journal of Speech and Hearing Research 24: 169–78.

Part III
Speech Perception and Testing

14
Speech Related to Pure Tone Audiograms

GUNNAR FANT

Introduction

A prerequisite for speech perception is that a sufficient part of the speech signal is above the threshold of hearing. The extent to which this is the case, assuming reference speech power and spectral distribution at a certain distance to a human receiver, may be visualized by superimposing the spectral distribution of speech on a pure tone audiogram. An example is given in Figure 1, which is taken from Lidén and Fant (1954). The shaded frequency-intensity area is the reference distribution of speech power and is often referred to as the 'speech banana'. Although this representation of speech has been widely accepted and used in audiological circles, its origins are not well known and were not discussed in the Lidén and Fant (1954) work. The graph was the result of speech analysis work I carried out at the Ericsson Telephone Company in the period 1946–1949. Prior to this material being published (Fant, 1959) I made the results available to Erik Wedenberg who used them in his studies of auditory training programmes for severely hard-of-hearing children (Wedenberg, 1951, 1953). It is the purpose of this chapter to review the derivation and applications of the 'speech banana'.

The Speech Analysis Data

One of the aims of my work at Ericsson was to provide a background for understanding the consequences of reserving parts of the available bandwidth in telephone lines for signalling purposes. The problem is analogous to the evaluation of the degradation caused by a specific hearing loss. In addition to direct perceptual tests it was considered important to study the actual frequency locations and intensities of the major formants of Swedish speech sounds.

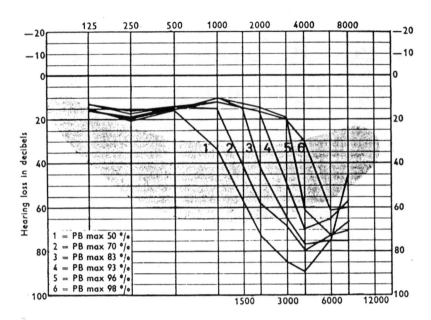

Figure 1. Maximum scores for PB (phonetically balanced word lists) in some cases of high frequency hearing loss. From Lidén and Fant (1954).

The speech analysis was carried out with considerable care to preserve absolute calibration of the intensity data. A composite graph of speech formants from all Swedish vowels and consonants was constructed and this is shown in Figure 2 (from Fant, 1959). The frame is an intensity (sound pressure level) versus frequency diagram in which the standardized free field threshold of hearing and a 40 dB equal loudness contour are shown. All sound pressure levels pertain to a speaking distance of one metre. The French and Steinberg (1947) average speech spectrum, modified to represent intensity in successive 250 Hz bands, was also included. It fits well into the formant data which shows a distribution of approximately +10 dB to –20 dB around the long term average data. The maximum sound pressure levels were of the order of 65 dB corresponding to the first formant (F1) of vowels with F1 values around 500 Hz.

In Figure 3 (Fant, 1959) these data have been transformed to sensation levels above the standardized free field threshold at a distance of 1 metre and summarized to show regions occupied by voice fundamental frequency (F0), and the first, second, third and fourth formants. Also shown are the main consonant area and the high frequency consonants region. In audiological applications of this work the divisions are usually left out and only the outline contour of the 'speech banana' is retained.

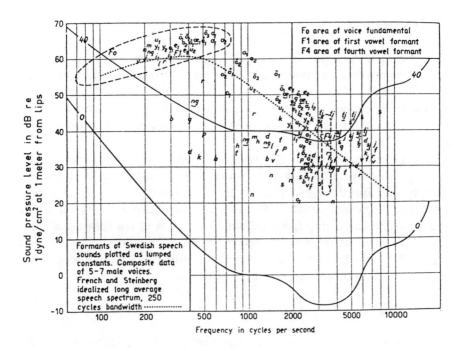

Figure 2. Sound pressure level versus frequency plot of Swedish vowel and consonant formant data. From Fant (1959).

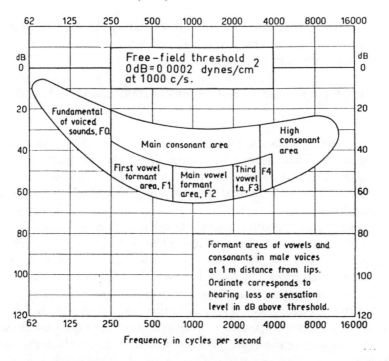

Figure 3. Speech spectrum data schematized in terms of formant areas. The ordinate is sensation level versus free field threshold at 1 metre distance. From Fant (1959).

Applications

We can return to Figure 1. This includes data on articulation scores for various high frequency hearing losses derived from speech audiometry with phonetically balanced monosyllabic (PBM) word lists. It may be seen that only when a substantial part of the formant region is below the subject's threshold of hearing is there an appreciable reduction of the articulation score.

The potential value of the spectral information transmitted in a speech communication link is quantified by the Articulation Index (A_i, French and Steinberg, 1947) which includes the receivers hearing threshold. A_i, which equals 1 for an ideal communication system, and which can be calculated from the weighted sum of contributions from each part band of the speech spectrum in proportion to its relative importance and the extent to which the intensity in a band exceeds the subjects masked or unmasked threshold. Thus,

$$A_i = \Sigma\, a_n\, W_n$$

where a_n is the relative importance of the band number n and W_n is an intensity factor which varies between 0 and 1, the latter when the sound pressure level in a band is 30 dB or more above the threshold.

The following tabulation derived from data published by Beranek (1947) shows the Articulation Index a_n per octave band centred at each of seven audiometric frequencies.

Frequency (Hz)	125	250	500	1000	2000	4000	8000
a_n (%)	2	7	14	23	32	19	3

Corresponding data for Swedish are not available but should not differ too much from these. Given a total Articulation Index the corresponding articulation score depends upon the specified test used, its vocabulary, and its level of difficulty (Beranek, 1947; French and Steinberg, 1947).

The simplified procedure above has been applied to typical hearing losses of four categories: (1) conductive loss, (2) sensorineural loss, (3) combined loss and (4) noise induced loss. The examples shown in Figure 4 are taken from a statistical survey I carried out in 1944 in connection with my electrical engineering thesis work. They were extracted from a sample of 377 audiograms taken in a Stockholm audiological clinic. Thirteen per cent were classified as conductive hearing loss, 39% as sensorineural, 37% as mixed whilst 11% were noise induced.

A calculation of the Articulation Index for the examples presented in Figure 4 yielded the following values. Conductive loss $A_i = 0.9$, sensorineural loss $A_i = 0.5$, mixed loss $A_i = 0.4$ and noise induced loss $A_i = 0.7$.

This is merely a formal exercise stressing the basic fact that a certain signal-to-noise or signal-to-threshold distance is required for speech reception and that the relative importance of different frequency regions varies. In addition we have to consider the qualitative impairments in several auditory functions and in more central stages of speech information processing and, cognitive functions. But this is another domain in which Arne Risberg and his associates contributed a lifetime of productive studies.

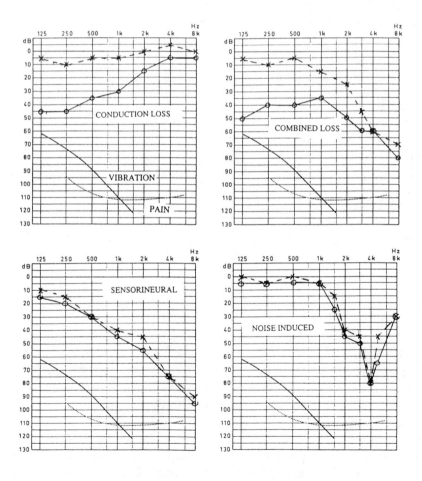

Figure 4. Pure tone audiograms illustrating four typical types of hearing loss. Crosses and broken lines pertain to supplementary bone conduction measures.

References

Beranek, L. (1947) The design of speech communication systems. Proceedings I.R.E. 35: 880.

Fant, G. (1959) Acoustic analysis and synthesis of speech with applications to Swedish. Ericsson Technics No.1, 1–108.

French, N.R. and Steinberg, J.C. (1947) Factors governing the intelligibility of speech sounds. Journal of the Acoustical Society of America 19: 90–119.

Lidén, G. and Fant, G.(1954) Swedish word material for speech audiometry and articulation tests. Acta Otolaryngologica, Suppl. 116, 189–204.

Wedenberg, E. (1951) Auditory training of deaf and hard of hearing children. Acta Otolaryngologica, Suppl. XCIV.

Wedenberg, E. (1953) Auditory training of severely hard of hearing pre-school children. Acta Otolaryngologica.

15

What Makes a Good Speech Test?

HARVEY DILLON AND TERESA CHING

Introduction

The characteristics of speech tests vary enormously in a large number of dimensions. When one wishes to select a speech test for some new purpose, there is a bewildering array of tests from which to choose. How does one know if the test one chooses is a good one? In this chapter we will review the attributes of speech tests and then link those attributes to the requirements of particular applications of speech tests. There are no speech tests which are intrinsically good; there are, however, applications that are better suited by some speech tests than by others. The first step in finding a good speech test is to have a well thought out application. This will involve answering questions like:

- Why do I want to use a speech test?
- Do I want to predict real life speech understanding?
- Do I want to compare two or more scores?
- Do I need to know which phonemes the person cannot hear?
- Do I need to find a maximum score or a speech threshold?

From questions like these, one can then make up a list of attributes that the desired speech test should have. From a complete list of attributes, one can then choose a speech test which possesses as many as possible of those attributes. If no existing test comes close enough, then one can modify an existing test, or make up an entirely new one.

For convenience, we will refer to the person to whom the test is to be administered as 'the subject'. In all cases the reader can substitute 'the client' or 'the patient', depending on one's perspective, without any change of meaning.

In the next sections we will review the attributes of speech tests which must be considered when selecting a speech test. The first section contains attributes which are implicit in the items chosen to comprise the speech test. Once a test is selected, the experimenter or clinician has no control over these attributes. The second section contains attributes related to the recording and presentation of test materials, over which the experimenter or clinician has considerable control. The third section contains attributes which are the consequence of the attributes outlined in the first two sections. Following that we will review some common applications for speech tests and will suggest which choices are appropriate for some of those attributes. The concluding section consists of a table which lists a range of speech tests and their implicit attributes.

Attributes of Speech Test Materials

Redundancy and context

Due to its redundant nature, speech is a highly efficient means of communication, despite interferences and noise. This arises from the superfluity of rules in the system: phonological rules which constrain the occurrence of phonemes to form words, syntactic rules which govern the structure of sentences, and semantic rules which restrict the co-occurrence of words in a sentence. The rules facilitate speech reception by enabling us to make intelligent guesses when part of the acoustic signal is masked or missing. We supplement bits of information in a manner consistent with our knowledge – knowledge of the world in which we communicate, and knowledge of the language in which we communicate.

The redundancy in speech can be exploited to construct speech test materials which range from those with negligible contextual information to those which contain all the redundancy inherent to real speech. At one extreme are tests comprised of nonsense syllables, such as CV (consonant–vowel), V, VC, CVC, or VCVs. There is minimal contextual information, and if an inventory of 24 consonants and 20 vowels were used in the construction of the stimuli, there is only 1 chance in 24 of guessing what a consonant was, or 1 chance in 20 of getting the vowel correct, in the absence of any acoustic information about the item. Nonsense syllable tests may be made easier by an increase in phonetic context, such as when the vowel context is known in a VCV test; or by limiting the number of phonemes tested, such as the Ling 7 sound test (Ling, 1976).

If the test material comprises words, such as the CNC word lists (Peterson and Lehiste, 1962), phonological and lexical information contribute to reception. If the material is made up of words of more than one syllable, then possible responses can be narrowed down by drawing on rules which govern admissible sound combinations across syllables and syllable combinations to form words; and in the case of the Monosyllabic-trochee-spondee test (Erber and Alencewicz, 1976), alternatives are further limited to words with the appropriate stress patterns. When phrases or sentences are used, the effect of syntactic and semantic contexts can vary depending on whether the words are strung in a random order (e.g. the zero predicability sentences in Boothroyd and Nittrouer, 1988), or arranged in a syntactically correct sequence (such as the BKB lists). Furthermore, sentences can range from meaningful to semantically anomalous, such as the high and low predictability sentences in the SPIN test (Kalikow *et al.*, 1977). Finally, tests which use paragraph material are similar to everyday speech in their redundancy and contextual information.

We need to remember that predictability from context rests in the listener's mind, not in the acoustic signal. Speech tests comprising material that is rich in contextual cues taps the subject's knowledge of the world, knowledge of the language, and the ability to use contextual information to perceive speech, in addition to the auditory ability to hear and process acoustic cues. Material with low redundancy and low context tests the listener's ability to perceive acoustic cues. This is an important consideration especially when subjects may or may not have the requisite knowledge and linguistic and cognitive abilities.

Acoustic context

To discuss the role of acoustic features in the design of speech tests, we need to distinguish between the acoustic level and the phonetic level of description of speech sounds. In acoustic analyses, we refer to the measurable properties of the speech waveform, such as fundamental frequency or presence of random excitation, formant frequencies and amplitude. In phonetic description, we classify sounds into categories such as vowels, consonants, stops, fricatives, glides and nasals.

All phonetic contrasts are cued by a multiplicity of interacting acoustic cues. For example, vowels are known to vary in terms of formant frequencies, amplitudes and durations. A subject who successfully discriminated between 'key' and 'car' in a speech test may do so on the basis of intensity cues alone, rather than differences in formant structure, or vowel quality, in phonetic terms. It is thus not surprising if the same subject could not distinguish other vowel quality differences, such as that between 'bee' and 'boo'. In a similar way, voicing distinction for stops, for instance, can be marked by the timing of low frequency periodicity, burst intensity, presence or absence of aspiration, the first formant onset frequency (initial position) and the duration of the preceding vowel (in certain final positions). A subject who hears the voicing distinction in a stimulus may rely on the detection of periodicity only, without the benefit of the entire range of features.

The richness of acoustic context of the test item, or the number of cues present in an item, is related firstly to the phonetic context in which it is presented and secondly to the way in which it is recorded.

For example, an intonation test may be based on voice pitch changes in isolated nonsense monosyllables only, such as in the THRIFT test (Boothroyd, 1986). By comparison, in the SPAC test (Boothroyd, 1984) intonation patterns in connected discourse are cued by semantic information, variations in relative intensity and duration, in addition to differences in voice pitch.

The way in which the stimuli were recorded affects the amount of acoustic information contained in the test material. The enunciation of the speaker is known to affect the relative difficulty of a test, especially when monosyllables were used (e.g. the Hughes recording of the PB-50 word lists, see Davis and Silverman, 1978). When a test item occurs in an accented syllable, it has greater clarity than that in an unaccented syllable due to the inherent changes in frequency, amplitude and duration associated with the accent. Test items spoken in a freely flowing sentence and then edited out to form the isolated stimuli also contain prosodic information characteristic of connected speech. When larger units, such as phrases or sentences are used as stimuli, acoustic cues for signalling individual phonemic contrasts may be reduced as the speed of articulation increases, but prosodic information will contribute to overall speech processing.

The acoustic context of the stimuli can also be varied for assessing the perception of particular acoustic features. Natural speech could be modified with computer manipulation to neutralize some cues to a phonetic contrast while retaining others (Revoile et al., 1982). Alternatively, carefully designed and controlled synthetic speech closely modelled on natural speech may be used to test perception of major acoustic cues (Hazan and Fourcin, 1985).

When test material is presented in the same carrier phrase in which it was recorded, the co-articulation effects in phonemes adjacent to the test item can help identify the target (Lynn and Brotman, 1981). The carrier phrase also carries acoustic information about the speaker source that would contribute to the labelling of phonetic categories, as it facilitates normalization processes.

Phonemic balance

Test material having a reasonable proportional representation of the sounds that occur in everyday speech is said to be phonetically balanced or PB (Egan, 1948). PB is normally measured separately for initial and final consonants, and is based only on the distribution of phonemes in monosyllables in spoken language. As such it is constrained by the phonological rules operating in the sound system, and is more aptly described as phonemic balance. A PB list is one in which all phonemes are represented in the list with the frequency of occurrence representative of everyday speech (e.g. Denes, 1963; Mines et al.,

1978). Because there are only a limited number of words that satisfy the balance requirement, equivalent lists are difficult to compile. An alternative way to obtain PB scores is to use word lists which contain the same proportion of phonemes (iso-phonemic) in each list (e.g. Boothroyd, 1968). The score obtained for each phoneme can then be weighted by its frequency of occurrence in everyday speech.

The rationale for using phonemically balanced test material is that if the listener were unable to perceive a particular phoneme which occurs infrequently in normal everyday speech, the handicap experienced is not as severe as it would have been had the phoneme been a more common one. This assumes that the spectral composition of a sound (physical realization of a phoneme) is invariant. However, a given phoneme can have different phonetic realizations in the neighbourhood of different sounds. Transitions from one sound to another are often important cues for identification, especially in sound sequences in which there may or may not be a steady state pattern, such as those in connected speech. The relevance of precise fulfilment of phonemic balance in speech test material to predicting communicative difficulties in everyday life due to hearing loss is questionable.

Visual context

There is a growing appreciation of the crucial importance of visual information to speech perception, not only in hearing aid users, but also in normal listeners, especially under less than ideal listening conditions (Summerfield, 1983). Some subjects who perform with open-set recognition in the laboratory would be unable to function in the real world of interfering noise and multiple speakers without the help of visual clues. Hearing-impaired persons, even successful hearing aid users with moderate losses, rely heavily on visual information (Walden et al., 1990). Information arises from articulatory movements in particular, but other paralinguistic information such as facial expressions, sex, age, identity, and attitude of the speaker is also conveyed.

Many of the consonantal ambiguities in auditory perception can be resolved when visual clues are available. The use of audio and audiovisual presentations makes it possible to compare speech processing using auditory cues only, and also in combination with visual information. Ability to integrate auditory with visual cues can also be assessed.

Word familiarity

Words which are encountered more frequently in real life tend to be recognized better in speech tests than words which are not. The familiarity of a word obviously needs to be viewed in the context of the people to whom the test is to be administered. While words which are infrequently used in general language will not be familiar to most people, even words used frequently may not be familiar to young children. Furthermore, children who have had a profound hearing loss since birth will usually have a much narrower vocabulary than normal-hearing children of their own age. Myklebust (1964) compared reading vocabulary of school age children, and reported higher scores for 9-year-old hearing children than for 15-year-old hearing-impaired children.

The familiarity of words, to the target subjects, will have several effects on the difficulty of speech tests. First, if a test contains a high proportion of relatively unfamiliar words, then the total score will be lower than if more familiar words had been used. Second, if word familiarity is, on the average, higher in one list than in another, then the equivalence of lists for difficulty will be adversely affected. Third, within a list, the range of familiarity of words will affect the range of difficulty of the items within that list. As we shall discuss below, each of these effects on difficulty has important implications for the application of speech tests.

Response set

Speech tests are often categorized as open response or closed response. In an open response format, the listeners repeat verbally or write down the sound or word(s) that they thought they heard. Restrictions on the allowable responses may be non-existent, or they may be minimal. For example, the subject may be advised only that the words are real words, or perhaps that they are monosyllabic, but not necessarily real words.

In a closed response format, listeners are presented with a list of responses from which to choose. Usually, but not necessarily, the response alternatives are revealed to the listeners before the stimulus is presented. Closed response formats can differ greatly in the degree to which the allowable responses are restricted. For example, a minimal pairs test may allow only two response alternatives. These are usually chosen so that the two alternatives differ in a way that makes the test appropriately difficult. A test designed for adults with a mild hearing loss, for example, might use responses of 'fin' and 'thin' when the stimulus is 'fin'. Test difficulty is greatest when the response foils differ from the stimulus by only one articulatory feature, especially when that feature is place of articulation, as in the preceding example. A much easier test is created if the responses differ by several features. A test for children with profound hearing loss, for example, might use 'elephant' and 'shoe' as the alternatives when the stimulus is 'shoe'. Tests with four to six response alternatives are most common (for example, House et al., 1965). The greater the number of alternatives in the response set, the more likely it is that any actual misperception will be available to the subject as a possible response. As the size of the response set increases, however, responding becomes more difficult for the subject and scores decrease (Miller *et al.*, 1951). The subject has to 'remember' his or her perception while scanning a list of response alternatives. It is possible that the resulting test scores are influenced by the subject's short-term acoustic memory and reading skills.

One advantage of the open response set format is that the tester is able to find out exactly what the subject heard, not the closest alternative from amongst a predefined set of items. One disadvantage is that scores will increase if the same material is repeated to the subject at a later time, especially if the material includes meaningful words. This will also happen to some extent for closed response set tests (for example, Walker *et al.*, 1982), but the extent to which the subject becomes familiar with the test material is much greater for open-set material. Learning of open-set material can probably be minimized by ensuring that only material which resulted in very low scores on the first presentation is re-used, but the scope for arranging multiple tests in this way is limited.

The distinction between open and closed response tests becomes blurred when the 'closed' response set actually includes all the items that would be possible in an open response set. One example would be a CV nonsense syllable in which the vowel was known to the subject, and the response set included all the consonants. Another example would be a test where the test items, and the response set, comprised all the single digits. For this reason, and because of the limitations on answers imposed by any context in the material, or by the size of a closed response set, the 'openness' of a response set should really be considered to be a continuum, rather than just comprise the categories of open and closed.

Number of items per list

The number of items per list is the primary determinant of test reliability and is thus one of the most important characteristics of a speech test. Test reliability will be discussed further below. For some tests, the number of items can be interpreted as the number of phonemes, or words, or sentences, and this is also discussed further below.

Number of lists

In clinical applications, one rarely needs a large number of lists, because clinical time constraints preclude a large amount of speech testing. In experimental settings, however, one frequently wishes to compare a large number of experimental conditions. For tests with meaningful material, subjects learn the material, and scores increase with repeated application of particular items. The alternative is to use 'equivalent' lists so that any item is presented only once. The greater the number of equivalent lists available, the more flexibly can the test be applied in experiments with many conditions.

Ability tested: detection, discrimination, recognition or understanding

Speech tests have traditionally been called 'speech discrimination tests'. More recently, this use has been criticized on the grounds that discrimination involves differentiating between two or more things, whereas in most speech tests, only one stimulus is presented, and the subject is asked to identify the sound. Accordingly, speech tests are increasingly being referred to as speech identification, or speech recognition, or speech intelligibility tests. The distinction is useful in that some speech tests really do fit the definition of discrimination tests. In one form, two stimuli are presented and the subject is required to say whether the stimuli are the same or different. In another form (odd-one-out paradigm), three stimuli are presented and the subject is asked which one is different from the other two. In a simpler version of this (A-B-X paradigm), the first two stimuli are different, and the subject is asked whether the third stimulus is the same as the first or the second stimuli. For none of these tests does the subject have to recognize or label the test stimulus. Discrimination tests (as opposed to recognition tests) may be useful as indicators of potential recognition ability. This would be the case where the subject has had limited exposure to the types of sounds being tested, or possibly to any sounds. The basis of this is that while discrimination does not guarantee eventual recognition, an absence of discrimination ability makes the development of recognition ability unlikely. The ability to discriminate speech sounds has been measured in infants as young as 4 days (Bertoncini *et al.*, 1987).

In addition to discrimination and recognition there are two other abilities which speech tests can be used to assess. If the subject is required only to indicate when speech is present or absent, speech detection ability is being assessed. If the subject is asked to carry out some task, or to answer a question appropriately, after hearing the speech item, speech understanding or message comprehension is being tested. This is further discussed below under Response Method.

Monaural/binaural stimulus presentation

Any test comprising a single audio channel can be presented under headphones either monaurally or binaurally. Some tests, however, such as the Staggered Spondaic Word Test (SSW; Katz, 1977), are specifically designed for binaural presentation and present different information to each ear. Such tests have application in testing central processing disorders.

Attributes of Test Recording and Presentation Methods

Response method

Subjects can indicate their perceptions in several ways. Most commonly, the subject verbally repeats what they thought they heard. For open response set tests, the only alternative to this is for the subject to write down the answer. Either approach can create additional errors. Verbal answers can be misheard by the tester (especially if the tester has an expectation of what the subject is going to say). Written answers, unless the subject can write phonetically, can contain spelling errors which can be misinterpreted by the tester as errors of perception. Similarly, for nonsense syllable items, the lack of a one-to-one correspondence between phonemes and spelling conventions, such as /s/ and /z/, can result in uncertainty for the tester. For subjects with no speech production disorders, the best solution is to have the subject respond verbally and by writing, and for the tester to watch the subject's lips as well as listen. (Most errors made by normal hearers are place errors, which can mostly be resolved by lipreading.) Ideally, the tester should be unaware of the correct answer. In critical applications, the subject's response can be videotaped, and a second tester can transcribe the response. Data on the extent of errors made by the tester is scarce, but the combination of listening, watching, and where necessary, having the subject write down their perception seems a satisfactory solution for most purposes.

Responding is simpler for closed response set tests. The subject can indicate the number of the chosen response, or can point to it. In some cases, the test items can be presented as pictures, to which the subject points, so that the test subject needs no expressive language at all (for example, Wilson and Antablin, 1980). For tests administered on computer, the pointing can be via a touch sensitive screen, or done with a mouse or keyboard. It is possible for response biases to be introduced by the spatial arrangement of the response foils, but this can be controlled for by rearrangement of the foils when multiple testing with the same foils is used.

An alternative response method is to ask the subject to make a response appropriate to the stimulus, rather than simply repeat the stimulus. For example, in the COT test (Common Objects Test, Plant and Moore, 1992), the subject may be instructed to 'pick up the red plane'. The stimulus is considered to be heard correctly if the subject performs the task as directed. Choosing response methods of this type may be motivated by the desire to avoid the use of expressive language by the subjects, or to help maintain the interest of the subjects. Alternatively, the motivation may be to measure whether the message has been correctly *understood*, rather than to measure whether sounds can be correctly recognized and repeated. In the Helen test (Ewertson, 1973) for example, the stimuli are questions, and a response is counted as correct if the answer given by the subject is appropriate to the question asked.

Quantity scored

For speech identification tests, one can measure and express the score in a variety of ways. For a monosyllabic word test, for example, the items can be scored as proportion of words correct or as proportion of phonemes correct. Phoneme scoring will always lead to a higher score than word scoring, because a word cannot be correct unless all its phonemes are correct. A difference in average score is not, however, the most significant difference between these two methods. Because each word contains more than one phoneme, the score will be based on a higher number of items for phoneme scoring than for word scoring. As discussed below, increasing the number of scored items increases test reliability. The only disadvantage of phoneme scoring is that it places additional demands on the concentration of the tester. When the material is isolated monosyllabic words, the additional difficulty for the tester is not significant. When the material consists of sentences with several key words per sentence, scoring becomes difficult for the tester unless the subject is perceiving nearly everything correctly.

Phoneme and word scoring are the two methods most commonly used. Another scoring method is to count complete sentences as items. This occurs when the response task requires the subject to follow an instruction or answer a question, and when the subject's actions are then judged as either right or wrong. Alternatively, one can increase the number of items into units even smaller than phonemes by counting the number of distinctive features by which the stimulus and the response differ (McPherson and Pang-Ching, 1979). Feeney (1990) has shown that this increased number of items improves test reliability and provides additional information about the errors made.

A variation to counting items occurs in connected discourse tracking (De Filippo and Scott, 1978). In this method, the talker presents and re-presents words or phrases until the listener is able to repeat them correctly. In this case, the number of words per minute, rather than the proportion of words correct, is scored.

Quantity expressed: per cent correct versus threshold

Frequently, the quantity counted (distinctive features, phonemes, words, sentences, words per minute) is also the quantity used to express the result of the test. The percentage of speech units correct is the most appropriate way to express the results whenever the purpose of the speech test is to find the maximum achievable score, or the score obtained under some specified conditions, such as a particular presentation level and/or signal to noise ratio (SNR). For many applications, however, it is more useful to find a speech threshold. That is, the speech level or SNR at which some specified level of performance (such as 50 % correct) is achieved.

Method of level and SNR adjustment

The level of an item in a speech test is normally controlled in some way. The crudest method is for the talker to be instructed to speak with 'normal vocal effort' for all items. A slightly more sophisticated method is to provide the talker with an SPL monitor while the recording takes place. For greater control of levels, the level of each item can be measured after recording, and an attenuator used to correct each item to the same level. Of course, there is really no such thing as 'the level' of an item, because whether the item is a nonsense syllable or a sentence, its level varies continuously during the duration of the item. Speech levels are most frequently measured as the maximum level attained by a VU meter during the course of the item. More recently, Leq measurement has become easy to do and is more reproducible than watching a moving VU needle. Leq refers to equivalent continuous level, and is equal to the level of a constant intensity sound which has the same intensity as the average speech item intensity. Averaging of the speech intensity is normally performed over the entire duration of the speech word or sentence. (The averaging could, however, be restricted to just the vowel portion of a word.) For both the VU and Leq methods, the resulting level is much more influenced by the level of vowels than by the level of consonants in the item.

Range of intensity levels presented, and adaptive testing

The range of intensity levels in speech test items has traditionally been minimized at the time of recording. For some applications, a wider range of intensity levels is required. This can be achieved in the recording by using a wide range of stresses in sentence material, or by recording dialogue between two talkers who are talking with different overall levels or at different distances from the microphone.

For material recorded with a relatively constant intensity level, the levels of presentation can be selected in one of several ways. For non-adaptive testing with a single list, some rule can be used to select a single level. This may be a level which is typical of everyday speech, or it may be a level which is believed will result in maximum percentage correct for that person. Most comfortable level is frequently used but this will not result in maximum speech identification (Ullrich and Grimm, 1976; Beattie and Warren, 1982).

For adaptive testing, the level of each item can be increased or decreased depending on whether the previous item was perceived incorrectly or correctly, respectively (Levitt, 1971; Dirks et al., 1982). Alternatively, items can be grouped into threes or fours, and the level of each group determined on the basis of the number of items correct in the preceding group. If several lists are to be presented, then each list can be presented at a different level or SNR, and an entire psychometric function (or performance intensity curve) generated. The levels (or SNRs) can be chosen adaptively so that the lists result in performance ranging from a low score up to the maximum score achievable by the subject.

Adaptive tests have the advantage that measurement time is used most efficiently. That is, the number of items presented at levels which do not provide useful information (because of ceiling or floor effects) is minimized. Adaptive procedures are most efficient if all presentations are close to the level and/or SNR required to achieve the criterion level of performance. This requires variation of the level/SNR after each item, and is most effective if the speech test items are homogeneous in difficulty.

Spectral characteristics of signal and noise

Information about speech is potentially available to a subject whenever the power of the speech in a frequency region exceeds both the subject's thresholds in that frequency region and the power of any masking noise or competing signal in that frequency region. Consequently, the spectral shape of the signal and any masking noise are key attributes of a speech test (e.g. Danhauer et al., 1985). Naturally, the spectral shape of a speech signal varies from instant to instant, but we can gain much understanding about performance if we know only the long-term rms spectrum of the speech and the noise. If the speech has been recorded and played back by amplification systems with a flat frequency response, then the long-term average spectrum will be determined mainly by the particular person chosen as the talker. Unless the material is highly constrained, such as nonsense syllables with only a few vowels, or words with an abnormally high proportion of /s/, /z/, /ʃ/ or /ʒ/, then the choice of material will not affect the spectrum of the speech.

Considerably more choice is available for the spectrum of the noise. Some noises will have a spectrum similar to that of the speech. These include a babble of talkers, and random (Gaussian) noise which has intentionally been spectrally shaped to match the long-term average speech spectrum. Traffic noise is likely to be more weighted towards low frequencies, and noise with a lot of impulsive content is likely to be more weighted towards the high frequencies. White noise is strongly weighted more towards high frequencies than is speech.

For a given noise spectrum, speech spectrum, and hearing threshold contour, and a given signal and noise overall SPL, one can calculate the proportion of the time that the signal will be audible in each frequency region. The results obtained with a speech test may depend a great deal on whether the particular combination of signal and noise results in a preponderance of low frequency or high frequency energy being available.

Temporal characteristics of competing noise

The statement in the preceding paragraph, that one can calculate the proportion of time the signal is audible at each frequency, is strictly only true if the amplitude of the noise does not fluctuate with time. If the noise level fluctuates, then subjects will be able to extract a greater amount of information when the noise level momentarily reduces. Subjects with normal hearing are able to take advantage of brief reductions of masker intensity. As hearing loss becomes greater, subjects become less able to take advantage of such fluctuations (Festen and Plomp, 1990).

Spatial location of signal and noise

Most speech testing is performed with the speech and noise coming from the same loudspeaker. In real life, speech and noise rarely come from the same direction, and in some test situations it is desirable to physically separate the speech and noise sources to reflect this. Normal-hearing listeners, and to a lesser extent, hearing-impaired listeners, will in general find the test easier for separated sources than for coincident sources. The decreased difficulty will occur partly because of head diffraction effects, especially if the orientation of speech and noise relative to one ear of the listener results in a head baffle effect for the speech (increased speech SPL) and a head shadow effect for the noise (decreased noise SPL).

As well as the orientation of the speech and noise, the distance of the source(s) from the listener will also be important in any environment other than an anechoic chamber. As the distance from the speech source to the listener decreases, the ratio of direct sound intensity to reverberant sound intensity increases. Unless this ratio is either much greater than 0 dB or much less than 0 dB, the easiness of the test also increases with the direct to reverberant intensity ratio. The relative intensities of the direct and reverberant fields will also affect the types of confusions made by a subject (Danhauer and Johnson, 1991).

Live voice versus recordings

Clinicians sometimes speak the test materials themselves, presumably either because they consider it is more interesting for the client or because they consider the client will need visual cues to be able to attain a satisfactory score. Unfortunately, the results obtained will depend on who is doing the talking (House *et al*, 1965; Penrod, 1979; Hood and Poole, 1980). Even for a particular talker, the manner in which speech sounds are produced can affect the score obtained (Brandy, 1966). Random variations in the intensity or clarity of enunciation will thus decrease test reliability. If the clinician has a bias about which of several measurement conditions should produce the highest score, then the clinician could consciously or unconsciously vary his clarity of presentation, either auditorily or visually, across conditions to help achieve a desired result. Using recorded versions of speech tests prevent such biases from affecting results. In addition, recorded tests can be edited to ensure uniformity of presentation level, can be standardized with normal hearers to ensure that all items have been correctly produced by the talker, and their acoustic characteristics can be analysed. Recorded tests (including audiovisually recorded tests) should thus be used whenever reliable results are needed. The use of interactive video laser discs coupled with adaptive presentations can make recorded stimuli suitable even for small children.

Dependent Attributes of Speech Tests

The above list of attributes all represent more or less independent choices which the tester can make when choosing, designing, or using a test. (Choices for some of the attributes obviously place restrictions on choices that can be made for some of the other attributes.) The following attributes all represent consequences of the attributes already discussed. For example, one cannot *choose* a certain reliability; it is the unavoidable result of other attributes, the most important of which is the number of items per list.

Reliability

Because the difficulty of words within a list varies, and because repeated presentation of the same word will not always produce the same response, test scores have to be viewed as a statistical estimate of speech intelligibility rather than as an exact measurement. Reliability refers to the degree to which repeated application of the speech test under identical conditions results in identical scores. Actually this is a rather theoretical definition. In practice, if reliability is assessed by repeating a particular list, then test conditions are not identical, as the subject is more familiar with the test items for the second administration. Alternatively, if a different list is used for the second administration, then any true differences in difficulty between the two lists will affect the measurement of reliability.

Unless the items of a speech test differ widely in difficulty, the test score (for repeated applications of the test) is distributed as a binomial variable (Hagerman, 1976; Thornton and Raffin, 1978; Dillon, 1982). Consequently the standard deviation of a test score can be calculated to be: $SD = \sqrt{(P(1 - P)/N)}$, where P is the probability of getting an item correct, and N is the number of items in the test. Clearly, increasing the number of items in a list always increases the reliability of a list. When using an established test with lists of a certain length, reliability can obviously be increased by combining several lists for each measurement condition. There are two disadvantages. First, testing time is increased, and subject fatigue may be more likely. Secondly, the use of several lists for one measurement condition may leave an inadequate number of lists for the other measurement conditions to be tested.

List equivalence

The lists of a speech test are equivalent if any list would result in the same score as any other list when tested under the same test conditions. To achieve list equivalence, test items need to be distributed among the lists such that the items in each list have similar redundancy, phonemic balance and word familiarity. (Naturally, all the other attributes of the speech test mentioned above would also need to be held constant across lists, but it would be unusual for these other attributes to vary across lists.)

One approach to achieving list equivalence is to use the same words in every list with only the order changed. For meaningful stimuli, this approach only seems suitable when the speech test is to be used to determine the speech recognition threshold, rather than the maximum attainable intelligibility, because learning of the stimuli by the subject is inevitable. Hagerman (1982, 1984) used 10 sentences of five words each, with the same 50 words re-edited to form different sentences for each list. In a more extreme example, Plant (1991) restricted the stimulus set to only five words and presented them repeatedly in random order with the test level varied adaptively. When the stimuli are meaningful, the measured speech reception threshold reduces as the size of the stimulus set is reduced (Punch and Howard, 1985). Repetition of the same stimuli from list to list is also suitable when the stimuli are nonsense syllables, and in this case, the potential for learning of the stimuli is less (Edgerton *et al.*, 1981), although some learning still does occur (Walker *et al.*, 1982).

Difficulty range within lists

Although the score obtained with a particular list is usually summarized with a single number representing the overall percentage of items correct, the items giving rise to this score may vary widely in difficulty (e.g. Campbell, 1965). In one list, for example, all the items may have a probability of correct identification of 50%. In another list, half the items may be difficult items with a probability of identification of 10%, and the other half may be easy items with a probability of 90%. Both lists will result in a score of 50%, but there the similarity between the lists ends. The list with items of widely varying difficulty will provide the more reliable score, because the test–retest standard deviation should be calculated from the binomial distribution using a value for p of 0.9 or 0.1. Conversely, the list with items of more uniform difficulty will provide scores which change more readily as the measurement conditions. This is discussed further below under 'Sensitivity' (below).

For lists to be equivalent for all applications, the difficulty range within lists also needs to be held constant across lists. All of the attributes of speech tests mentioned in the previous section can affect the difficulty of items.

Slope of the performance intensity function

The percentage of items correctly identified is affected by the presentation level of the items and by the signal to noise ratio (SNR) if a background noise is present. When percentage correct is plotted against either presentation level (for speech in quiet) or SNR (for speech in noise), the result is called the performance intensity (PI) function. The slope of the PI function (in percentage per dB) thus describes how much the test score is affected by level or noise. It is an important parameter for determining and understanding the reliability of adaptive speech tests, and for determining the sensitivity of speech tests to changes in signal level and SNR. Several factors affect the slope of the PI function, which can range from 2% per dB to 20% per dB.

First, tests with items of homogeneous difficulty have steeper slopes. A PI function for a test can be viewed as the average of the PI functions for each item in the test. When items of widely varying difficulty are mixed together, the slope for the entire test will be much less than the slope of any item because at any one level or SNR, some items will be at their ceiling performance level (with zero slope), some will be at their floor performance level (also with zero slope), and some will be at their mid performance level (with maximum slope). Examples of PI functions for individual consonants can be found in Kent *et al.* (1979).

Second, tests where the long-term average spectrum of the speech matches that of the noise (for speech in noise), or that of the subject's threshold (for speech in quiet), will have steeper slopes (e.g. Beattie and Warren, 1983). Consider a speech test in quiet administered to a subject with a steeply sloping high frequency loss. At low test levels the subject will be able to hear only low frequency information and will achieve some less than perfect score. As test level is increased, the sensation level of the low frequency information will increase, and the score will increase slightly. Because the high frequency information is still well below threshold, test level must be increased by many decibels before the high frequency information becomes audible, and hence before test scores can reach close to 100%. Consequently, the slope of the PI function is small.

Third, tests which contain highly redundant information, high word familiarity, and for which limited response sets are available, have steeper slopes. For such a speech test, the listener requires very little acoustic information to correctly perceive an item. That is, scores of close to 100% correct will be obtained at relatively low sensation levels or poor SNRs. As the level or SNR is decreased to the point at which the speech is just inaudible, the score will decrease to 0% correct. Consequently, the score changes rapidly with level or SNR. The rapid change of performance with level or SNR for highly redundant items can also be viewed as a process of positive feedback. When the speech is inaudible, the redundancy of the speech is of no use to the listener, because the listener cannot extract any information, and is thus not aware of the redundancies present. As soon as a little of the speech signal is audible, the listener will first perceive the easiest phonemes or words, and these will provide clues about the identity of the remaining phonemes or words, thus making the remaining items easier to perceive. They will therefore be perceived at a lower level or poorer SNR than if they had been presented in a lower redundancy context.

The last two points are well summarized by the articulation index (AI) method of predicting speech intelligibility (French and Steinberg, 1947). The AI value increases most rapidly with signal level when the signal spectrum matches the noise spectrum (point 2). Percentage correct increases most rapidly with AI value for highly redundant (easy) material (point 3). The AI method has successfully been used to predict speech intelligibility scores for people with mild and moderate hearing losses (Dubno *et al.*, 1989)

Shape of the importance function

Because the AI method provides many useful insights into the results of speech tests, the shape of the importance function of the speech material is an important attribute of the speech test. The importance function describes the relative contribution to intelligibility of audible signal in each frequency region. For nonsense syllable tests, the importance function has a maximum at 2500 Hz, and decreases to zero at 200 and 8000 Hz. For tests comprising 'easy' continuous discourse, the importance function has a maximum at 500 Hz and decreases to zero at 125 Hz and 10 kHz (Pavlovic, 1987). Despite these apparently large differences in the location of the importance function maximum, the degree and type of redundancy which is required to produce an importance function different from that of nonsense syllables is not yet fully understood, and Bell *et al.* (1992) have queried the effects of procedural details on the various functions derived. They showed that the importance function for high context sentences is only slightly different from that for low context sentences. The overall shape of the importance function can be summarized by the crossover frequency – the frequency above and below which equal amounts of information is carried. When the data reviewed in Studebaker *et al.* (1987) are averaged and compared to that in Bell *et al.* (1992), it appears that the crossover frequency averages 1747 Hz for nonsense syllables, 1577 Hz for words, 1520 Hz for low context sentences, 1340 Hz for high context sentences, 1189 Hz for continuous discourse, and 725 Hz for synthetic sentences (the SSI test). With the exception of the SSI result, these values progress monotonically downwards as context is added. The very low value for the SSI test may be because its closed response sentence format allows the correct answer to be determined by correct perception of the vowels alone.

Although a particular speech test is usually considered to have a single composite importance function, it is possible to calculate the importance function for individual subtests. For the Diagnostic Rhyme Test, for example, Duggirala *et al.* (1988) have shown that the importance function for the nasality subtest is weighted towards low frequencies, while that for the sibilance subtest is weighted towards the high frequencies. This process could presumably be extended to derive an importance function for individual sounds.

Validity

A speech test can be considered to be valid if the score obtained reflects the proportion of information which would be correctly perceived in some real life situation. Most of the speech material and presentation attributes discussed above need to be selected to match a particular real life situation if the score obtained is to reflect the difficulty experienced in the actual situation.

Sensitivity

For a test to be sensitive, we need the test score to change as the measurement conditions change, and we need the direction and extent of such changes to be reliable. As mentioned earlier, reliability can be maximized either by increasing the number of items or by choosing items that are very easy or very hard (for which P is close to 1 or 0 respectively). Unfortunately, these extreme values of P also result in the score being relatively unaffected by changes in measurement conditions. As shown in Dillon (1982), test sensitivity can be maximized by choosing the test score to be about 90%, or lower if the items vary much in difficulty. As well as these statistical aspects to sensitivity, many of the other test attributes discussed above will affect sensitivity in particular applications.

Applications of Speech Tests

The uses to which a speech test can be put fall into two broad classes. In the first class are all applications in which a subject is tested under two or more conditions. The tester is primarily interested in whether the score obtained under each condition is higher or lower than the score obtained under each other condition. How that subject scores relative to other people to whom the test may be administered is of secondary or no importance. Conversely, in the second class are all applications in which the tester is primarily interested in how a subject scores relative to the 'usual' score for members of the population from which the subject comes. Of course, it is possible for a tester to be interested in both aspects of test scores obtained on a subject, but in such cases the tester is invariably asking two separate questions of the data, and is therefore using the test for two different applications.

Applications in which the tester wishes to compare two listening conditions are reviewed first.

Evaluating the relative effectiveness of hearing aid electroacoustics

Speech tests can be used to determine the relative effectiveness of different hearing aid electroacoustic characteristics. These characteristics include variations in gain-frequency response, compression parameters, adaptive filtering for noise reduction or loudness compensation, and a wide variety of more complex signal processing schemes.

Because there are usually several conditions to be compared, a prime requisite for such testing is the ability to repeat tests on each subject. This either requires the availability of a sufficient number of equivalent lists, or the use of nonsense syllables. The following points will be applicable to many measurements of hearing aid effectiveness.

- If the best amplification scheme is to be found for each individual subject, a high degree of reliability is usually required. Scoring at the lowest possible unit (phonemes, or even speech features) is thus desirable to maximize the number of items scored. Similarly, a low level of redundancy or context constraints between items is desirable so that the number of *independent* items scored is as high as possible.
- If the amplification schemes differ in the amount of gain given to low versus high frequency regions, then speech material with an importance function similar to that of everyday speech should probably be used (Kamm *et al.*, 1982). (More research is required to identify how speech tests have to be constructed to meet this criterion, but the issue is discussed in Bell *et al.*, 1992).
- If the signal processing being tested is time dependent (for example, compression, adaptive filtering) then the results may only be valid if the speech material has prosody similar to that of real speech.
- The above constraints combine to call for a speech test with realistic prosody, a high number of scored items per unit of presentation time, and a low level of context between scored items. The most suitable type of tests thus appears to be nonsense sentences, with multiple key words per sentence. Some tests meeting these constraints have been mentioned in Lippmann *et al.* (1981), Gatehouse (1990) and Neuman *et al.* (in preparation). The use of multiple words per presentation phrase has been reviewed by Harris (1980), but the tests reviewed are mostly lists of monosyllables, which lack normal sentence prosody.
- If the experimenter wishes to find the lowest signal level or poorest SNR at which some criterion level of performance is achieved, then the signal level or SNR should be varied adaptively from item to item during the testing for greatest efficiency. For such adaptive testing, the performance intensity function should have a high slope. That is, the items should have a homogeneous difficulty (e.g. Plomp and Mimpen, 1979).
- If the testing is to reveal the types of confusions made with each amplification characteristic (as well as the overall score), then the response set for each item should either be open or else include all likely confusions.
- If any of the amplification conditions cause speech to sound highly unfamiliar to the subject, then it may be more appropriate to test speech discrimination rather than speech identification, unless the

subject can receive sufficient listening experience with the novel amplification scheme prior to testing taking place.

- The particular signal processing being investigated may imply that particular noise types and levels, or ranges of signal intensities (rather than a constant intensity), should be used if the advantages of the processing scheme are to be measured. If the testing must be performed in poor SNRs, then an easy test may be necessary so that scores are not at floor level. Conversely, if the testing must be performed at good SNRs, then a hard test may be necessary so that scores are not at ceiling level.
- Addition of noise will reduce differences in speech scores between devices with different gain-frequency responses (e.g. Edgerton *et al.*, 1986).

Evaluating monaural/binaural and side of fitting differences

Hearing aid fittings can be performed monaurally in either the better or worse ear, or binaurally. Speech tests may be employed to examine which arrangement is preferable.

The most important variable for such tests is the location of the speech and noise sources. Indeed, almost any outcome about the relative effectiveness can be assured by a judicious choice of where the speech loudspeaker and where the noise loudspeaker are placed relative to the aided and unaided ears. No single arrangement of speech and noise adequately simulates the range of speech and noise source locations and reverberation conditions found in real life. The issue is too complex to further consider in this chapter (see Siegenthaler and Craig, 1981; Nabalek and Mason, 1981; Nabalek and Robinson, 1982; Feuerstein, 1992).

Evaluating aided/unaided differences

If a hearing loss is mild, the advantages of a hearing aid may be uncertain, and one may wish to measure the increase in speech perception offered by the hearing aid.

- If testing is to be performed in quiet, then the most important determinants of the increased intelligibility is the presentation level chosen for the test and the range of intensity levels in the test material at a particular presentation level. As all hearing aids increase the sensation level of speech, at least in some frequency regions, and as a low sensation level of speech guarantees a sub-optimal speech identification score, a very low presentation level will maximize the aided/unaided difference and a very high presentation level will minimize, eliminate, or even reverse it.

- If testing is to be performed in noise, then the level and spectral shape of the noise and signal relative to the subject's threshold will be the most important determinant of aided/unaided benefit. For noise with any particular spectral shape, if the level chosen for the noise is significantly greater than threshold in every critical band, then the aided/unaided benefit will be very small or zero for any type of speech test. (This occurs because at each frequency, the hearing aid will amplify the speech and noise by the same amount and the amount of signal audible at that frequency will be unchanged by amplification.) Any small aided advantage which occurs at high noise and signal levels probably arises because the frequency dependent amplification minimizes the extent of upward spread of masking by the low frequency components of the noise and signal.
- If the hearing aid fitting is monaural, then the degree of aided versus unaided benefit will depend on the location of the speech relative to the aided ear, especially if noise from another source is also used in the testing.

Relative to these effects of speech and noise levels, location, and spectral shape, the other attributes of speech tests are of secondary importance in this application.

Relative intelligibility and the rating method

Although in this chapter we have restricted our discussion to traditional types of speech tests, in which the tester (or a computer) decides whether the response of the subject is correct or incorrect, there is an alternative way to use speech material for each of the above three applications. During the past decade, much use has been made of speech rating tasks. In such tests, the subject is presented with a sentence or a passage, in quiet or in noise, and is asked to rate the proportion of words which are understandable (see Walker and Byrne (1985) for a review). In an adaptive version of the test, the subject is asked to adjust the speech or noise level until some criterion proportion of the words are believed by the subject to be understandable (Speaks *et al.*, 1972; Walker and Byrne, 1985). Although the experimenter does not know whether the subject is making over- or under-optimistic assessments of intelligibility, it seems reasonable to assume that the subject adopts a consistent criterion for repeated measurements, so the method is particularly well suited for comparisons of intelligibility across different counterbalanced experimental conditions. Other variations on rating of intelligibility by the subject are paired comparisons (for example, Studebaker *et al.*, 1982) and magnitude estimations of intelligibility (e.g. Studebaker and Sherbecoe, 1988). The sensitivity of these methods relative to each other and relative to traditional speech tests has been investigated in several studies (e.g. Tecca and Goldstein, 1984; Cox *et al.*, 1991b), but the position is not as yet clear, especially if test time is held constant in the comparison. One disadvantage of subjective rating methods is that misperceptions made by the subjects cannot be deduced by the experimenter. One advantage is that the ease of understanding can be directly assessed by the subject, even when speech identification performance is at too high a level for different experimental conditions to result in significantly different scores. (It has been suggested by Ross (1975) that the use of speech identification tests for comparing amplification conditions should be supplemented by ratings of ease of understanding, because the concentration required for listening can be fatiguing for hearing-impaired people, even when they can achieve near-perfect identification performance.)

We will now review applications in which the tester wishes to compare performance of an individual against the performance achieved by some population or populations.

Confirming the audiogram

Speech tests can be used to confirm the pure tone audiogram assessment of hearing loss. This is particularly valuable when non-organic hearing loss (malingering) is suspected. The speech test can be used in an informal way by checking for gross discrepancies between the average pure tone loss and the level at which speech is audible and/or identifiable. More quantitatively, the level at which the subject scores 50% of the maximum score achievable at any level can be determined and the probable average pure tone loss estimated. For this procedure the prime requirement is a speech test for which the expected relationship between speech test results and the audiogram is known! Suitable data for children has been published by Markides (1980). In terms of speech test attributes, a steep PI function and a high number of (independent) items are desirable. The high number of items leads to a small test–retest standard deviation for percentage correct, and the steeply sloping PI function enables this small standard deviation to be translated into a small test–retest standard deviation for speech level.

Establishing hearing aid candidacy

Performance on a speech test is sometimes used clinically to help predict the likely success of a hearing aid fitting. The rationale apparently is that people who achieve low speech identification scores are less likely to benefit from a hearing aid. We are not aware of any data to support this application of speech tests, and we are aware of several reasons why speech tests should not be used in this way. First, it is likely that an optimally shaped hearing aid response will result in a higher score than is obtainable with a flat frequency response system, at least for subjects with sloping losses. Secondly, considerable testing may be necessary to ensure that the level which results in the highest possible score has been used. Thirdly, and more fundamentally, how does one choose an appropriate cut-off score and a speech test of appropriate difficulty? Even a person who obtains very little speech information through a hearing aid may find the signal beneficial as an aid to lipreading, or as a means of monitoring environmental sounds.

Diagnosing retrocochlear versus peripheral disorders

Speech tests have long been used to distinguish retrocochlear from peripheral disorders. Of key importance is the shape of the PI function, and in particular, the presence of roll-over at high intensities. Because individual points on the PI function can only be measured with the precision appropriate to the length of the lists used, the degree of curvature of the PI function for hearing-impaired subjects can most accurately be assessed if the PI function slopes steeply (for normal hearers). As neither of the authors is particularly knowledgeable about diagnostic uses of speech tests, we will not say any more about it. The reader is referred to more specialized texts, such as Jerger and Jerger (1971), Dirks (1977), Hurley (1980) and Hannley and Jerger (1981).

Determining auditory training required

Auditory training aims to enable hearing-impaired persons to make maximal use of sound cues audible to them, so as to enhance their speech understanding abilities and their speech-monitoring abilities. One may wish to know how well the subjects understand speech in an everyday situation, and why they do what they do.

- If testing aims to obtain a global measure of speech communicative ability of subjects in a natural situation, material with high redundancy, such as sentences and connected discourse, should be used. One may wish to compare audio and audiovisual performance, and also listening in quiet and listening with competing stimuli.
- If testing is for determining the starting point of training, test material should include prosodic as well as segmental contrasts with well defined acoustic patterns and minimal redundancy. This enables the tester to determine what acoustic cues were and were not used, so that auditory training could start at a level at which some success was achieved, and yet some systematic errors were made. If the aim is to identify target phoneme errors, nonsense syllable tests are useful for obtaining and analysing confusion patterns. These tests

require task familiarization, but numerous equivalent lists can be generated easily for further testing.

- If the subject has speech production or related difficulties, response methods have to be adjusted so that results are not confounded. Selected subtests from the Minimal Auditory Capabilities (MAC) battery (Owens, Kessler, Raggio and Schubert, 1985) can be useful in this application. In children, highly restricted response sets are necessary, such as the Early Speech Perception tests (Moog and Geers, 1990) or the PLOTT tests (Plant, 1984).

- If testing for auditory training is associated with the use of a new sensation, such as that provided by a new signal-processing auditory assistive device, detection and discrimination abilities, rather than identification should be tested until the subject is familiarized with the task. Audiovisual procedures need to be used to ensure that assessment and training tasks are understood, and that maximum benefit can be obtained from the device through integration of auditory and visual information.

Predicting real world communication effectiveness

While tests appropriate for determining auditory training are often analytic in nature, phoneme and word scores in speech tests are limited in their predictive power for performance in connected speech (Giolas and Epstein, 1963). Material that is high in redundancy and rich in acoustic and visual contexts is appropriate for assessing communication effectiveness in everyday situations. This is because the material contains contextual information which is likely to be found in real life. Audio only and audiovisual presentations of stimuli can be used to obtain a measure of the relative effectiveness of the subjects' use of auditory cues and the ability to integrate auditory with visual cues. Electronic addition of noise and reverberation can be used to simulate the noise and reverberation that would be found in any particular real world environment (Cox *et al.*, 1991a).

Tables 1 and 2 list several of the attributes applicable to many available speech tests. The attributes included in the tables are those which are implicit to the test material, rather than those which result from particular methods of recording or presentation. A detailed discussion of the significance of each attribute can be found earlier in the chapter.

Table 1. Tests on sentence perception

Test name	Context		Target hearing-impaired group	Response		Ability tested	No. of items per list	No. of lists
	Linguistic	Acoustic		set	method			
Auditory test no. 12 (PAL) (Hudgins et al., 1947)	simple open questions requiring one-word answers	natural intonation	adults	open	answer question	understanding and answering	S = 20 W = 20	8
Bamford-Kowal-Bench Lists (BKB-A) (Bench et al., 1979; Bench and Doyle, 1979)	everyday sentences, varying from 4 to 7 words in length	natural intonation	> 8 yrs, mild–severe	open	repeat	identification	S = 16 W = 77 Kw = 50	21
CID Everyday Sentences (Silverman and Hirsh, 1955)	everyday sentences, 4 sentence types, 2–12 words in length	natural intonation	adults, suitable for subjects with severe recognition problems	open	repeat	identification	S = 10 W = 67 Kw = 50	10
CUNY Sentence Lists (Boothroyd, 1991)	sentences related to 12 known topics, varying from 3 to 14 words in length	natural intonation	adults	open	repeat	identification	S = 12 W = 102	72
HELEN Lipreading test (Ewertsen, 1973)	questions based on sentences using alternative-question forms	natural intonation	adults	open	answer question	understanding and answering questions	S = 25 W = 25	8

Test	Stimuli	Speech quality	Population	Mode	Response	Measure	Scoring
Australian adaptation (Plant, Phillips and Tsembis, 1982)	open questions related to self, relatives, home, favourite things, and those with easy answers	natural intonation	adults	open	answer question	understanding and answering questions	S = 20 4 W = 20
Iowa Sentence Tests (Tyler, Preece and Tye-Murray, 1986)	sentences, varying from 4 to 7 words in length	natural intonation	adults	open	repeat	identification	S = 30 6 rand. W = 153 Kw = 88
Paediatric Speech Intelligibility Test (Jerger, et al., 1980)	familiar sentences	natural speech	3–9 years	closed	picture pointing	discrimination	S = 10 2
Speech Perception in Noise (SPIN) (Kalikow, Stevens and Elliot, 1977)	sentences, half containing high predictability and half low predictability words, varying from 5 – 8 words in length	Natural speech in babble noise	adults	open	repeat last word in each sentence	identification	S = 50 8 Kw = 50
Synthetic Sentence Identification Test (SSI) (Speaks and Jerger, 1965)	4 level approximations of syntactically correct sentences	Synthetic sentences with discourse as competing noise	adults	closed, 10-choice	repeat	identification	S = 10 24

Key:S: sentence; P: phoneme; W: word; Kw: keyword.

Table 2. Tests on phoneme and word perception

Test name	Context Linguistic	Context Phonemic Balance	Context Acoustic	Target hearing-impaired group	Response set	Response method	Ability tested	No. of items per list	No. of lists
AB Isophonemic word test (Boothroyd, 1968)	monosyllabic words	no	CVC words in isolation, built from the same 10 vowels and 20 consonants	adults, mild–severe	open	repeat	identification	P = 30, W = 10	15
Auditory numbers test (Erber, 1980)	numbers	no	single number or sequence of numbers 1–5	> = 3 yrs	closed, 5-choice	picture pointing	identification	W = 5	1
CID Auditory tests W-1, W-2 (Hirsh et al., 1952)	familiar spondee words	no	2-syllable words in carrier phrase	adults	open	repeat	identification	W = 36	1
CID W-22 (Hirsh et al., 1952)	monosyllabic words	yes	CVC words in isolation	adults	open closed	repeat multiple choice	identification discrimination	P = 150, W = 50	4
CNC (Peterson and Lehiste, 1962)	monosyllabic words	yes	CVC in isolation	adults	open	repeat	identification	P = 150, W = 50	10

Test	Stimulus		Description	Population	Response	Method	Task	Score	
CUNY Nonsense Syllable Test (NST) (Levitt and Resnick, 1978)	nonsense syllables	no	CV, VC in carrier phrase. V = /i a u/ C = different place and manner, voicing constant can be randomized	adults	closed, 7 to 9-choice	mark on response sheet	identification	P = 55	
CUNY Modified NST (Gelfand et al.., 1992)	nonsense syllables	no	CV, VC in isolation V = /i a u/ 22 initial C 16 final C can be randomized	adults	closed, 22 or 16-choice	mark on response sheet	identification	P = 38	
Early Speech Perception (ESP) (Moog and Geers, 1990)	speech patterns- 1- to 3-syllable-words	no	3 each of monosyllables, trochees, spondees and 3-syllable words	> = 6 yrs	closed, 12-choice	picture pointing	discrimination	S = 24	1
	spondee words	no	spondees with differing vowels and consonants in isolation				identification	W = 24	1
	monosyllabic words	no	monosyllabic words beginning with /b/ and ending in a plosive				identification	W = 24	1

Test	Stimuli		Description	Population	Response set	Task	Measure	N	
FAAF: Four Alternative Auditory Feature Test (Foster and Haggard, 1987)	Monosyllabic words	no	CVC words in a carrier phrase	adults	closed, 4-choice	mark on response sheet	identification	W = 80	5 rand.
Glendonald Auditory Screening Procedure Erber, 1982)	mono, spondee, trochee, tri-syllabic words	no	words in isolation	>= 4 years, mild to profound loss	closed, 4-choice	picture pointing	detection, discrimination	W = 24	1
	sentences		questions		open	answer question	understanding and answering questions	S = 10	1
Iowa medial consonant recognition test (Tyler, et al., 1983)	nonsense syllables	no	/aCa/ where C = /b d g p t k f v s z m n/	adults	closed, 14-choice	repeat	identification	P = 70	6 rand.
Iowa vowel recognition test (Tyler et al., 1983)	monosyllabic words	no	/h V d/ where V = /i e ae 3 u o/	adults	closed, 9-choice	repeat	identification	P = 45	6 rand.
Kendall Toy test (Kendall, 1953)	monosyllabic words formed from the most common vowels and consonants	no	monosyllabic words in carrier phrase	3-5 years, mild-severe	closed, 10-choice	object pointing	identification	W = 10	3

Test									
Modified Rhyme Test (House, et al., 1965)	monosyllabic words	no	CVC, CV in isolation	adults	closed, 6-choice	mark response	identification	P = 50	6
Monosyllabic Trochee Spondee test (MTS) (Erber and Alencewicz, 1976)	1–2 syllable words	no	mono and disyllabic words in carrier phrase	> = 4 yrs	closed, 12-choice	picture pointing	identification	W = 12	1
Northwestern University Children's Perception of Speech – NUCHIPS (Elliott and Katz, 1980)	monosyllabic words formed from the most frequently occurring phonemes	no	Monosyllabic words in carrier phrase	> = 3 yrs, (measured by the Peabody Picture Vocabulary Test)	closed, 4-choice	picture pointing	identification	W = 50	4
NU-4 (Tillman, Carhart and Wilbur, 1963)	monosyllabic words	yes	CVC in isolation	adults	open	repeat	identification	P = 150, W = 50	2
NU-6 (Tillman and Carhart, 1966)	monosyllabic words	yes	CVC in isolation	adults	open	repeat	identification	P = 150, W = 50	4
Paediatric Speech Intelligibility Test (Jerger, et al., 1980)	familiar monosyllables	no	words in carrier	3–9 years	closed, 5-choice	picture pointing	discrimination	W = 20	1

Test	Stimuli	Feedback	Description	Age	Open/Closed	Response	Task	Score
Phonetically balanced Kindergarten Test (PBK) (Haskins, 1964)	monosyllabic words	yes	words in isolation	> = 6 yrs	open	repeat	identification	P = 150 W = 50 4
PLOTT test (Plant, 1984)	sounds in isolation	no	11 vowels and 11 consonants in isolation	> = 5 years	closed, 2-choice	Yes/no response by pointing	detection	score = 22 1
	numbers		Numbers 1–5		closed, 5-choice	picture pointing	discrimination	score = 5
	1 – 3 syllable words		3 of each monosyllables, trochees, spondees, 3-syllable words in carrier phrase		closed, 12-choice		discrimination identification	stress pattern score = 12 Word score = 12
	Monosyllabic words		12 monosyllabic words in carrier phrase		closed, 12-choice		identification	Word score = 12
			2 vowel subtests and 3 consonant subtests: 5 pairs of CVC words in each subtest		closed, 2-choice		discrimination	50 in each subtest
Psychoacoustic Laboratory Lists PB-50 (Egan, 1948)	reasonably common monosyllabic words	yes	Monosyllabic words in carrier phrase	adults	open	repeat	identification	W = 50 20

Test										
Rhyme test (Fairbanks, 1958)	words drawn from 250 common word list	no	words in isolation	adults	closed	insert missing sound in word frame	identification	P = 50	1	
SPAC (Boothroyd, 1984)	speech patterns carried by meaningful phrases: suprasegmental contrasts	no	3-word phrase with different word stress	> 9 years post lingually-deaf	closed, 3-choice	mark on response sheet	discrimination	P = 12	4 forms	
			short phrases with a rising or falling intonation		closed, 2-choice			Intonation score = 12		
			phrases spoken by talkers of different sex					correct sex = 12		
			sentences with monotone vs natural intonation					pitch score = 12		
	CVC words in carrier phrase: segmental contrasts		Segmental contrasts: 2 vowel subtests and 6 consonant subtests					speech pattern score for each subtest = 12		
THRIFT (Boothroyd, 1986)	speech patterns carried by pure tone	no	Synthetic tones for long short distinctions	> = 6 years	closed, 3-choice	mark on response sheet	discrimination	Duration score = 24	4 forms	

speech patterns carried by synthetic vowels	Synthetic constant or changing fundamental frequency patterns on 'ah' and 'oh'							Intonation score = 24
Nonsense syllables	CV and VC in isolation: 2 vowel subtests in different consonant contexts, 6 consonant subtests in different vowel contexts							P = 24 for each subtest
Word Intelligibility by picture identification (WIPI)(Ross and Lerman, 1970)	monosyllabic words	no	monosyllabic words in carrier phrase	> 5 years moderate loss, > 7 years severe loss	closed, 6-choice	picture pointing	discrimination	W = 25 4

Key: S: sentence; P, phoneme; W, word; Kw, keyword.

References

ANSI (1969) ANSI S3.5-1969. American national standard method for the calculation of the articulation index. American National Standards Institute, New York.

Beattie, R.C. and Warren, V.G. (1982) Relationships among speech threshold, loudness discomfort, comfortable loudness, and PB max in the elderly hearing impaired. American Journal of Otology 3: 353–8.

Beattie, R.C. and Warren, V. (1983) Slope characteristics of CID W-22 word functions in elderly hearing-impaired listeners. Journal of Speech and Hearing Disorders 48: 119–27.

Bell, T.S., Dirks, D.D. and Trine, T.D. (1992) Frequency-importance functions for words in high- and low-context sentences. Journal of Speech and Hearing Research 35: 950–9.

Bench, J. and Doyle, J. (1979) The BKB/A (Bamford Kowal Bench) Sentence Lists for Speech Audiometry – Australian version, Lincoln Institute, Victoria, Australia.

Bench, J., Kowal, A. and Bamford, J. (1979) The BKB (Bamford-Kowal-Bench) sentence lists for partially hearing children. British Journal of Audiology 13: 108–12.

Bertoncini, J., Bijeljac, Babic R., Blumstein, S.E. and Mehler, J. (1987) Discrimination in neonates of very short CVs. Journal of the Acoustical Society of America 82: 31–7.

Boothroyd, A. (1968) Developments in speech audiometry. Sound 2: 3–10.

Boothroyd, A. (1984) Auditory perception of speech contrasts by persons with sensorineural hearing loss. Journal of Speech and Hearing Research 27: 134–44.

Boothroyd, A. (1986) A three-interval, forced-choice test of speech pattern contrast perception. City University of New York and Lexington Center, New York.

Boothroyd, A. (1991) CASPER: a user-friendly system for Computer Assisted Speech Perception Testing and Training. City University of New York, New York.

Boothroyd, A. and Nittrouer, S. (1988) Mathematical treatment of context effects in phoneme and word recognition, Journal of the Acoustical Society of America 84: 101–14.

Brandy, W. T. (1966) Reliability of voice tests of speech discrimination. Journal of Speech and Hearing Research 9: 461–5.

Campbell, R. A. (1965) Discrimination test word difficulty. Journal of Speech and Hearing Research 8, 13–22.

Cox, R.M., Alexander, G.C. and Rivera, I.M. (1991a) Accuracy of audiometric test room simulations of three real-world listening environments. Journal of the Acoustical Society of America 90: 764–72.

Cox, R.M., Alexander, G.C. and Rivera, I.M. (1991b) Comparison of objective and subjective measures of speech intelligibility in elderly hearing-impaired listeners. Journal of Speech and Hearing Research 34: 904–15.

Danhauer, J.L., Doyle, P.C. and Lucks, L. (1985) Effects of noise on NST and NU 6 stimuli. Ear and Hearing 6: 266-9.

Danhauer, J.L. and Johnson, C.E. (1991) Perceptual features for normal listeners' phoneme recognition in a reverberant lecture hall. Journal of the American Academy of Audiology 2: 91–8.

Davis, H. and Silverman, H.R. (1978) Hearing and Deafness. New York: Holt, Rinehart and Winston.

De Filippo, C.L. and Scott, B.L. (1978) A method for training and evaluating the reception of on-going speech. Journal of the Acoustical Society of America 63: 1186–92.

Denes, P.B. (1963) On the statistics of spoken English. Journal of the Acoustical Society of America 35: 892–904.

Dillon, H. (1982) A quantitative examination of the sources of speech discrimination test score variability. Ear and Hearing 3: 51–8.

Dillon, H. (1983) The effect of test difficulty on the sensitivity of speech discrimination tests. Journal of the Acoustical Society of America 73: 336–44.

Dirks, D.D. (1977) Use of performance-intensity functions for diagnosis. Journal of Speech and Hearing Research 42: 408–15.

Dirks, D.D., Morgan, D.E., and Dubno, Y.R. (1982) A procedure for quantifying the effects of noise on speech recognition. Journal of Speech and Hearing Disorders 47: 114–23.

Dubno, J.R., Dirks, D.D. and Schaefer, A.B. (1989) Stop-consonant recognition for normal-hearing listeners and listeners with high-frequency hearing loss. II: Articulation index predictions. Journal of the Acoustical Society of America 85: 355–64.

Duggirala, V., Studebaker, G.A., Pavlovic, C.V. and Sherbecoe, R.L. (1988) Frequency importance functions for a feature recognition test material. Journal of the Acoustical Society of America 83: 2372–82.

Edgerton B.J., Danhauer, J.L. and Rizzo, S. (1981) Practice effects for normal listeners' performance on a nonsense syllable test. Journal of Audiology Research 21: 125–31.

Edgerton, B.J., Danhauer, J.L. and Simmons, F.J. (1986) Use of the California Consonant Test in evaluating hearing aids. American Journal of Otology 7: 104–9.

Egan, J. (1948) Articulation testing methods. Laryngoscope 558: 955–91.

Elliott, L. and Katz, D. (1980) Development of a New Children's Test of Speech Discrimination. St Louis: Auditec.

Erber, N. (1980) Use of auditory numbers test to evaluate speech perception abilities of hearing impaired children. Journal of Speech and Hearing Disorders 41: 256–67.

Erber, N. (1982) Auditory Training. Washington D.C.: Alexander Graham Bell Association.

Erber, N. and Alencewicz, C. (1976) Audiologic evaluation of deaf children. Journal of Speech and Hearing Disorders 41: 256–67.

Ewertsen, H.W. (1973) Auditive, visual and audio-visual perception of speech. The Helen Group, State Hearing Centre, Copenhagen.

Fairbanks, G. (1958) Test of phonemic differentiation: The Rhyme Test. Journal of the Acoustical Society of America 30: 596–600.2

Feeney, M.P. (1990) Distinctive feature scoring of the California Consonant Test. Journal of Speech and Hearing Disorders 55: 282–9.

Festen, J.M. and Plomp, R. (1990) Effects of fluctuating noise and interfering speech on the speech-reception threshold for impaired and normal hearing. Journal of the Acoustical Society of America 88: 1725–36.

Feuerstein, J.F. (1992) Monaural versus binaural hearing: ease of listening, word recognition, and attentional effort. Ear and Hearing 13: 80–6.

Foster, J.R. and Haggard, M.P. (1987) 'The four alternative auditory feature test (FAAF)–linguistic and psychometric properties of the material with normative data in noise. British Journal of Audiology 21: 165–74.

French, N.R. and Steinberg, J.C. (1947) Factors governing the intelligibility of speech sounds. Journal of the Acoustical Society of America 19: 90–119.

Gatehouse, S. (1990) The contribution of central auditory factors to auditory disability. Acta. Otolaryngologica Suppl. Stockh. 476: 182–8.

Gelfand, S.A., Schwander, T., Levitt, H., Weiss, M. and Silman, S. (1992) Speech recognition performance on a modified nonsense syllable test. Journal of Rehabilitation Research and Development 29: 53–60.

Giolas, T.G. and Epstein, A. (1963) Comparative intelligibility of word lists and continuous discourse. Journal of Speech and Hearing Research 6, 349–358.

Hagerman, B. (1976) Reliability in the determination of speech discrimination. Scandinavian Audiology 5, 219–228.

Hagerman, B. (1982) Sentences for testing speech intelligibility in noise. Scandinavian Audiology 11, 79–87.

Hagerman, B. (1984) Clinical measurements of speech reception threshold in noise. Scandinavian Audiology 13: 57–63.

Hannley, M. and Jerger, J. (1981) PB rollover and the acoustic reflex. Audiology 20: 251–8.

Harris, J. D. (1980) On the use of a three-words-per-item format in tests for the hearing of speech. Journal of the Acoustical Society of America 67: 345–7.

Haskins, H.A. (1964) Kindergarten PB word lists. In Newby, H.A. (Eds) Audiology. New York: Appleton-Century-Crofts.

Hazan, V. and Fourcin, A.J. (1985) Microprocessor-controlled speech pattern audiometry. Audiology 24: 325–35.

Hirsh, I.J., Davis, H., Silverman, S.R., Reynolds, E.G., Eldert, E. and Bensen, R.W. (1952) Development of materials for speech audiometry. Journal of Speech and Hearing Disorders 17: 321–37.

Hood, J. D. and Poole, J. P. (1980) Influence of speaker and other factors affecting speech intelligibility. Audiology 19: 434–55.

House, A.S., Williams, C.E., Hecker, M.H.L. and Kryter, K.D. (1965) Articulation testing methods: consonantal differentiation in a closed-response set. Journal of the Acoustical Society of America 37: 158–66.

Hudgins, C.V., Hawkins, J.E., Karlin, J.E. and Stevens, S.S. (1947) The development of recorded auditory tests for measuring hearing loss for speech. Laryngoscope 47: 57–89.

Hurley, R.M. (1980) Speech protocols in the central auditory nervous system evaluation. In Rupp, R.R. and Stockdell, K. G. (Eds) Speech Protocols in Audiology. New York: Grune & Stratton.

Jerger, J. and Jerger, S. (1971) Diagnostic significance of PB word functions. Archives of Otolaryngology 93: 573–80.

Jerger, S., Lewis, S., Hawkins, J. and Jerger, J. (1980) Paediatric speech intelligibility test, I. Generation of speech materials. International Journal of Paediatric Otolaryngology 2: 217–30.

Kalikow, D.H., Stevens, J.N., and Elliott, L.L. (1977) Development of a test of speech intelligibility in noise using sentence materials with controlled word predicability. Journal of the Acoustical Society of America 61, 1337–51.

Kamm, C.A., Dirks, D.D., and Carterette, E.C. (1982) Some effects of spectral shaping on recognition of speech by hearing-impaired listeners. Journal of the Acoustical Society of America 71, 1211–24.

Katz, J. (1977) The staggered spondaic word test. In Keith, R. (Ed) Central Auditory Dysfunction. New York: Grune and Stratton. pp 103–21.

Kendall, D. C. (1953) Audiometry for young children: part 1. Teacher of the Deaf 51: 171–8.

Kent, R.D., Wiley, T.L. and Strennen, M.L. (1979) Consonant discrimination as a function of presentation level. Audiology 18: 212–24.

Levitt, H. (1971) Transformed methods in psycho-acoustics. Journal of the Acoustical Society of America 49: 467–77.

Levitt, H. and Resnick, S.B. (1978) Speech reception by the hearing impaired: Methods of testing and the development of new tests. Scandinavian Audiology 6 (Suppl.):107–30.

Ling, D. (1976). Speech for the hearing impaired child. A.G. Bell Association, Washington, D.C.

Lippmann, R.P., Braida, L.D. and Durlach, N.I. (1981) Study of multichannel amplitude compression and linear amplification for persons with sensorineural hearing loss. Journal of the Acoustical Society of America 69: 524–34.

Lynn, J.M. and Brotman, S.R. (1981) Perceptual significance of the CID W-22 carrier phrase. Ear and Hearing 2: 95–9.

Markides, A. (1980) The relation between hearing loss for pure tones and hearing loss for speech among hearing-impaired children. British Journal of Audiology 14: 115–21.

McPherson, D.F. and Pang-Ching, G.K. (1979) Development of a distinctive feature discrimination test. Journal of Auditory Research 19: 235–46.

Miller, G.A., Heise, G.A., and Lichten, W. (1951) The intelligibility of speech as a function of the context of the test materials. Journal of Experimental Psychology 41: 329–35.

Mines M.A., Hanson, B. F. and Shoup J.E. (1978) Frequency of occurrence of phonemes in conversational English. Language and Speech 21: 221–41.

Moog, J.S. and Geers, A.E. (1990) Early speech perception for profoundly hearing-impaired children. Central Institute of the Deaf, Missouri.

Myklebust, H. (1964) The Psychology of Deafness. New York: Grune and Stratton.

Nabalek, A.K. and Mason, D. (1981) Effect of noise and reverberation on binaural and monaural word identification by subjects with various audiograms. Journal of Speech and Hearing Research 24: 375–83.

Nabelek, A.K. and Robinson, P.K. (1982) Monaural and binaural speech perception in reverberation for listeners of various ages. Journal of the Acoustical Society of America 71: 1242–8.

Neuman, A.C., Levitt, H., Dillon, H. and Rubin-Spitz, J. (In preparation) Evaluation of speech materials for hearing impaired assessment.

Owens, E., Kessler, D.K., Raggio, M.W. and Schubert, E.D. (1985) Analysis and revision of the Minimal Auditory Capabilities (MAC) battery. Ear and Hearing 6(6): 280–90.

Pavlovic, C.V. (1987) Derivation of primary parameters and procedures for use in speech intelligibility predictions. Journal of the Acoustical Society of America 82: 413–22.

Penrod, J. P. (1979) Talker effects on word-discrimination scores of adults with sensorineural hearing impairment. Journal of Speech and Hearing Disorders 44: 340–9.

Peterson, G.E. and Lehiste, I. (1962) Revised CNC lists for auditory tests. Journal of Speech and Hearing Disorders 27: 62–70.

Plant, G. (1984) A diagnostic speech perception test for severely and profoundly hearing impaired children. Australian Journal of Audiology 6: 1–9.

Plant, G. (1991) The development of speech tests in Aboriginal languages. Australian Journal of Audiology 13: 30–40.

Plant, G. and Moore, A. (1992) The Common Objects Token (COT) test: a sentence test for profoundly hearing-impaired children. Australian Journal of Audiology 14: 76–83.

Plant, G., Phillips, D. and Tsembis, J. (1982) An auditory-visual speech test for the elderly hearing-impaired. Australian Journal of Audiology 4: 62–8.

Plomp, R. and Mimpen, A.M. (1979) Improving the reliability of testing the speech reception threshold for sentences. Audiology 18: 43–52.

Punch, J.L. and Howard, M.T. (1985) Spondee recognition threshold as a function of set size. Journal of Speech and Hearing Disorders 50: 120–.

Revoile, S., Pickett, J.M., Holden, L.D. and Talkin, D. (1982) Acoustic cues to final stop voicing for impaired- and normal-hearing listeners. Journal of the Acoustical Society of America 72: 1145–54.

Ross, M. (1975) An evaluation of hearing aid evaluations. American Speech and Hearing Association, Washington, D.C.

Ross, M. and Lerman, J. (1970) A picture identification test for hearing impaired children. Journal of Speech and Hearing Research 13: 44–53.

Siegenthaler, B.M. and Craig, C.H. (1981) Monaural vs binaural speech reception threshold and word discrimination scores in the hearing impaired. Journal of Audiology Research 21: 133–5.

Silverman, S.R. and Hirsh, I. (1955) Problems related to the use of speech in clinical audiometry. Annals of Otology, Rhinology and Laryngology 64: 1234–44.

Speaks, C. and Jerger, J. (1965) Method for measurement of speech identification. Journal of Speech and Hearing Research 8: 185–94.

Speaks, C., Parker, B., Harris, B. and Kuhl, P. (1972) Intelligibility of connected discourse. Journal of Speech and Hearing Research 15: 590–602.

Studebaker, G.A., Bisset, J.D., Van, Ort D.M. and Hoffnung, S.U. (1982) Paired comparison judgments of relative intelligibility in noise. Journal of the Acoustical Society of America 72: 80–92.

Studebaker, G.A., Pavlovic, C.V. and Sherbecoe, R.L. (1987) A frequency importance function for continuous discourse. Journal of the Acoustical Society of America 81: 1130–1138.

Studebaker, G.A. and Sherbecoe, R.L. (1988) Magnitude estimations of the intelligibility and quality of speech in noise. Ear and Hearing 9: 259–67.

Summerfield, Q. (1983) Audio-visual speech perception, lipreading and artificial stimulation. In Haggard, M.P. and Lutman, M.E. (Eds) Hearing Science and Hearing Disorders. London: Academic Press. pp 131–82.

Tecca, J.E. and Goldstein, D.P. (1984) Effect of low-frequency hearing aid response on four measures of speech perception. Ear and Hearing 5: 22–9.

Thornton, A.R. and Raffin, M.J.M. (1978) Speech discrimination scores modeled as a binomial variable. Journal of Speech and Hearing Research 21: 507–18.

Tillman, T.W. and Carhart, R. (1966) An expanded test for speech discrimination utilising CNC monosyllabic words, N.U. Auditory Test No. 6, USAF School of Aerospace Medicine, Texas.

Tillman, T.W., Carhart, R. and Wilber, L. (1963). A test for speech discrimination composed of CNC monosyllabic words, Northwestern University Auditory Test No. 4, USAF School of Aerospace Medicine, Texas.

Tyler, R., Preece, J. and Lowder, M. (1983) Iowa cochlear implant tests. University of Iowa, Iowa.

Tyler, R., Preece, J.P. and Tye-Murray, N. (1986) The Iowa phoneme and sentence tests, University of Iowa, Iowa.

Ullrich, K. and Grimm, D. (1976) Most comfortable listening level presentation versus maximum discrimination for word discrimination material. Audiology 15: 338–47.

Walden, B.E., Montgomery, A.A., Prosek, R.A. and Hawkins, D.B. (1990) Visual biasing of normal and impaired auditory speech perception. Journal of Speech and Hearing Research 33: 163–73.

Walker, G. and Byrne, D. (1985) Reliability of speech intelligibility estimation for measuring speech reception thresholds in quiet and in noise. Australian Journal of Audiology 7: 23–31.

Walker, G., Byrne, D. and Dillon, H. (1982) Learning effects with a closed response set nonsense syllable test. Australian Journal of Audiology 4: 27–31.

Wilson, R. H. and Antablin, J. K. (1980) A picture identification task as an estimate of the word recognition performance of nonverbal adults. Journal of Speech and Hearing Disorders 45: 223–37.

16

Speech Perception Tests and Hearing-impaired Children

ARTHUR BOOTHROYD

Introduction

For the purposes of this chapter, speech perception will be defined as the making of inferences about language patterns (phonemes, words, phrases, and sentences) represented by the speech of a talker. This is a narrow definition that does not include the extraction of meaning or intent from the language patterns. Note that the inferences made by the perceiver are based not only on sensory evidence derived from the speech movements and sounds of the talker, but also on contextual evidence. Successful inference also depends on the knowledge and skills that the perceiver brings to the task (Boothroyd, 1993b).

Much of the impact of sensorineural hearing loss depends on the extent to which it affects speech perception. A primary goal of management is, therefore, to improve speech perception. Approaches include the use of hearing aids and other sensory aids to increase access to the sound and movement patterns of speech; educational intervention designed to develop the necessary world and language knowledge; and rehabilitation designed to develop or improve speech perception skills (Boothroyd, 1988a). For effective selection, planning, implementation, and evaluation of these approaches, information is required about individual speech perception capacity and performance, hence the need for speech perception tests.

The issues that need to be addressed in the design of speech perception tests are the same as for any test, namely validity, reliability and efficiency (Crocker and Algina, 1986). In other words, the tests must measure what they are intended to measure, the results should be repeatable, and administration should be easy and fast. These issues are not easily addressed in tests of speech perception and the difficulties become acute when dealing with severely and profoundly deaf children. My purpose in this chapter is to explore these difficulties. By way of illustration, I shall present evaluative data on a specific test of speech perception designed for use with prelingually deafened children.

The Nature of Speech Perception

Speech perception, even when defined as narrowly as it is in this chapter, is a complex process involving the integration of many components. These components can be divided into three major groups: the evidence available to the perceiver, the perceiver's knowledge, and the perceiver's skills. Each of these groups can be further subdivided, as follows (see also Figure 1).

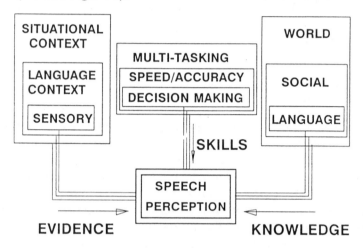

Figure 1. Schematic model of the principal factors contributing to speech perception.

Evidence

Sensory evidence

Sensory evidence is generated by the perceiver's sense organs in response to the talker's speech movements and the resulting sounds. For hearing persons, the ear is the principal source of sensory evidence, but the eyes can play a valuable secondary role, especially in noisy surroundings. For hearing-impaired persons, the eyes often play the major role via speechreading. Hearing aids, cochlear implants, other sensory aids, and direct tactile contact may also be used to enhance sensory evidence.

Linguistic contextual evidence

Surrounding language patterns provide valuable contextual evidence by virtue of phonotactic, lexical, syntactic, semantic and topical constraints. Speech sounds, for example, are more easily recognized when in the context of meaningful words (Boothroyd and Nittrouer, 1988).

Similarly, words are more easily recognized in meaningful sentences (Miller, Heise and Lichten, 1951), and sentences are more easily recognized in conversational or paragraph context (Hnath-Chisolm, Hanin and Boothroyd, 1985). The effect of context is to change the a priori probabilities associated with various possible interpretations of the sensory evidence. Exactly how the perceiver takes advantage of this information is not clear, but its impact is considerable. For normally-hearing subjects listening in difficult conditions, the combined effect of phonological, lexical, sentential, and topical context appears to be equivalent to a 5- to 10-fold increase in the sources of sensory evidence (Boothroyd, 1991b).

Situational contextual evidence

Spoken language input always occurs in a context. The context includes objects, people and events, and extends in both space and time. Like linguistic context, the situational context alters the relative probabilities for possible interpretations of a given speech input and aids the perceiver in the task of formulating and choosing among these possibilities. Unlike linguistic context, access to which is compromised by hearing impairment, the situational context is fully accessible to the hearing-impaired person.

Knowledge

Language knowledge

Everything the perceiver knows about spoken language can contribute to perception. This includes knowledge of such things as the relationships among speech movements and speech sounds (phonetics), the sound patterns of the language and the ways in which these patterns are used to determine and modify meaning (phonology), the words of the language (vocabulary), the ways in which words are combined to make sentences (syntax), the ways in which sentences are used to express meaning (semantics), and the ways in which people use language to satisfy intent (pragmatics). It is this knowledge which enables the perceiver to take advantage of both sensory and contextual evidence.

World knowledge (or general cognition)

Everything the perceiver knows about the objects, substances, events, attributes and rules of the physical world plays a role in speech perception. It is easy to forget that spoken language is a code, that language stands for something else. Without knowledge of that 'something else', language has no value. Even though the extraction of meaning has been excluded from our current definition of speech perception, the fact that meaning contributes to the utility of contextual evidence, and, therefore, to the perception of spoken language patterns, cannot be ignored.

People knowledge (or social cognition)

Everything the perceiver knows about the special attributes, events and rules of the world of people can aid in perception. People knowledge includes knowledge of the ways in which people use language to satisfy communicative intent and, therefore, overlaps with the pragmatic level of language knowledge.

Skills

Decision making

Even with adequate knowledge and sensory data, speech perception cannot occur unless the perceiver can use this knowledge to formulate, and make choices among, possible interpretations of the sensory input. We know very little about this skill, how it is accomplished, how it is acquired and refined, and what subskills are involved. Most clinical speech perception tests, however, are based on the assumption that the skill has been mastered. This assumption is seldom justified in the case of young deaf children.

Speed

Successful speech perception calls for high speed. The speed of speech transmission is controlled, not by the perceiver, but by the talker, and the perceiver must complete decision making at a rate that equals or exceeds that of the incoming information. To do so may involve some loss of accuracy. Finding a compromise between speed and accuracy is, probably, one of the most important aspects of speech perception skill development. Perceptual speed, however, is largely ignored in clinical speech perception tests.

Multi-tasking

Closely related to the issue of speed is the need to complete the speech perception process while simultaneously extracting meaning, deducing significance, and, perhaps, formulating a response. This, again, is an aspect of the process that has largely been ignored in the development of clinical tests.

Validity of Speech Perception Tests

Because speech perception has so many components, we cannot address issues of validity without deciding which components are to be evaluated. Do we wish to know, for example, how much sensory evidence is available from a damaged ear, or provided by some sensory aid? Do we wish to know how well the subject is able to take advantage of linguistic context? Do we need information about speech skills and their susceptibility to fatigue? Or are we concerned only with overall performance?

The answers to the foregoing questions depend, in turn, on the purpose of the testing. If the purpose is to establish the need for various forms of sensory assistance, or to determine their effectiveness, then our interest is in sensory evidence. If the goal is to plan a programme of habilitative or rehabilitative intervention, then we may also be concerned with knowledge and skills. If the purpose is to decide whether a subject can function effectively in a particular educational or work environment, we may need also to evaluate overall performance in a real or representative setting.

Unfortunately, even if we can be clear about the purpose of testing, this information does not automatically translate into task or stimulus selection. Consider, for example, the goal of assessing the adequacy of the sensory evidence available to a hearing-impaired child. To meet this goal we need to remove contextual cues from the test stimuli and to devise a task in which the child's speech perception skill does not affect performance. By using isolated words as the language patterns to be perceived, the confounding effects of sentence-level and situational context can, indeed, be removed. Other effects remain, however, including those of lexical context, phonological and lexical knowledge, and decision-making skills. If these residual effects could be rendered constant across subjects, their contributions to differences among test scores would be eliminated. Such is the goal of using simple vocabularies and forced-choice response tasks in tests for children. Hearing-impaired children, however, form a heterogeneous population and inter-subject differences of knowledge and skill are large, especially in those with prelingual onset of deafness. We may seek to minimize the influences of these differences, but it is difficult to eliminate them.

Consider, also, the design of global tests that are intended to measure overall performance. Here, the problem is to create an appropriate balance among the components of speech perception so as to preserve ecological validity, while, at the same time creating the control needed for reliable, quantitative evaluation. Tests using everyday sentences may go part way towards meeting this goal, but they do not adequately tap the skills of speed and multi-tasking. Moreover, the effects of fatigue after prolonged listening are seldom addressed. Connected discourse tracking has become popular for adult testing, and it appears to meet many of the criteria for a truly global test (De Filippo and Scott, 1978). Here, however, talker skill, text difficulty, and talker–subject interaction are confounding factors (Hochberg, Rosen and Ball, 1987; Tye-Murray and Tyler, 1988). Moreover, the test measures the speed of a talker/listener pair for a fixed accuracy level of 100%. It does not measure accuracy. Nor does it assess an individual perceiver's ability to find a compromise between speed and accuracy.

In short, the complex nature of speech perception, the number of components that are involved, the interactions among them, and our general lack of understanding of the process make it difficult to design speech perception tests that either probe single components, or balance their contributions in an ecologically valid way.

The foregoing discussion has been about construct validity, that is, the demonstration that a test should measure what it is intended to measure under the assumptions of a plausible theoretical construct. The empirical approach is to measure the correlation between the test measure and some independent measure that is known to assess what it is intended to assess. In speech perception testing, we seldom have such independent measures. It is possible, however, to devise a global test with high construct validity, such as word recognition in sentences of known topic, and then determine the predictive value of simpler, speedier tests such as nonsense syllable recognition. Such determinations are, unfortunately, specific to the population tested, which returns us to our principal concern, the testing of hearing-impaired children.

Population Factors Affecting Validity

Four factors contribute to the special difficulties of devising valid speech perception tests in hearing-impaired children: age at onset of hearing loss, current age, degree of loss, and learning opportunity.

Age at onset

Among subjects whose hearing loss was acquired in adult life, it is usual to assume uniformity of knowledge and skill, at least as they apply to auditory speech perception. With such uniformity, any test of speech perception accuracy should serve to rank subjects in terms of both access to sensory evidence and overall speech perception performance. The only problems to be expected would be ceiling and floor effects from tests that are too easy or too difficult. Under the homogeneity assumption, the long-established use of word repetition tests, as an index of both sensory evidence and overall speech perception performance, seems appropriate.

One could argue, however, that, even in a postlingually deafened population, the assumption of homogeneity is not justified. Inter-subject differences are to be expected in any area of human performance, and elderly subjects are known to have more difficulty with speech perception than can be explained solely on the basis of access to sensory evidence. Moreover, if we move from the auditory to the visual domain, there are obvious and dramatic differences of speechreading skill among subjects who may be assumed to have similar access to sensory evidence and similar prior knowledge (Hanin, 1988). There is, apparently, much to be learned about the interactions of evidence, knowledge, skill and perceptual modality, even in an adult population.

When a hearing loss is acquired postlingually but during childhood, the assumption of uniformity is, clearly, unjustified. Childhood is a time for expanding and refining world knowledge, social knowledge, language knowledge, and the skills of speech production and perception. We should, therefore, expect the results of word recognition tests to reflect not only access to sensory evidence but also knowledge and skill. Knowledge and skill will, in turn, reflect exact age at onset, degree of hearing loss, appropriateness of sensory assistance and educational management, and individual aptitudes. As indicated earlier, attempts to eliminate these effects by the use of simplified word lists and/or multiple choice testing are unlikely to be effective.

When a hearing loss is present at birth, or acquired prelingually, all aspects of knowledge and skill are at considerable risk, and marked population heterogeneity should be assumed. It becomes very important, in this population, to be clear about what aspect of speech perception is to be tested and to design tests accordingly. It also becomes very difficult to accomplish these goals because few assumptions can be made about the existence of the knowledge and skills needed to perform various speech perception tasks.

Current age

So far, issues of validity have been discussed only in relation to the speech perception task. There are, however, other aspects of testing that need to be taken into account when working with children. In particular, test tasks should be within the cognitive capabilities of young subjects, they should be interesting enough to guarantee full participation, and the attentional demands should not be too great. The younger the child, the more difficult it becomes to meet these criteria. If they are not met, there is no way of knowing whether poor performance is due to poor speech perception capacity or to task-related difficulties.

Degree of hearing loss

Age at onset interacts with magnitude of hearing loss in terms of their effects on speech perception. A prelingually acquired severe or profound hearing loss, for example, is likely to have more serious long-term effects on knowledge and skill than is a moderate hearing loss. Moreover, the role of prosthetic and educational management in the years between onset and testing becomes critical for a severe or profound loss. Note, also, that 'floor' effects are potentially more serious with profoundly deaf subjects. A score of zero on a word recognition test, for example, is often incorrectly assumed to reflect the absence of auditory sensory evidence. It has been shown, however, that some profoundly deaf subjects, without open-set word recognition ability, demonstrate significant access to phonologically significant information when presented with phonetic contrast tests (Boothroyd, 1984).

Learning opportunity

Finally, in those children for whom considerable time has elapsed since the onset of deafness, the intervening learning opportunity is crucial to the development of the knowledge and skills involved in speech perception. The importance of learning opportunity increases with earlier age at onset and increasing hearing loss. Learning opportunity, however, is almost impossible to quantify. One possible approach is to classify children according to the educational/communication philosophy of the intervention programme in which they have been enrolled. The underlying assumption is that the opportunities for acquiring speech perception skills, and other aspects of spoken language knowledge and competence, will increase to the extent that the programme espouses such acquisition as a goal. In oral programmes it is a primary goal. In total communication programmes, it is a secondary goal. And, in the emerging sign language programmes, it is not a goal. Associations between programme type and speech perception performance would be expected and have, in fact, been reported (Geers and Moog, 1992). The translation of educational philosophy into educational practice, however, is an uncertain pursuit and the label used to categorize an educational environment is often a poor guide to the nature, quality, and appropriateness of an individual child's learning opportunity. We cannot, therefore, use programme labels as an infallible guide to opportunity.

In summary, earlier age at onset of deafness increases population heterogeneity in terms of the knowledge and skills required for speech perception; lower current age may be assumed to involve a reduction of knowledge and skills, even in the absence of a hearing loss; lower current age also places increasing demands on the cognitive and motivational suitability of test tasks; increasing hearing loss is likely to exaggerate the effects of age at onset and to render standard tests too difficult and, therefore, non-discriminatory; and knowledge and skill will depend, in part, on learning opportunity. For all of these reasons, it becomes increasingly difficult to satisfy validity requirements in populations with earlier age at onset, lower current age, greater hearing loss, and inadequate learning opportunity.

Reliability

In a general sense, a test's reliability is a measure of the extent to which repeated administrations yield identical results. Reliability can be assessed in two different but related ways. The first is as the standard deviation of repeated scores for an individual subject, from which one can derive confidence limits for a single score. Such an approach is useful if the test is to be used for within-subject assessment of the effects of different forms of sensory assistance or training.

The second approach to reliability assessment is to measure the correlation between scores obtained on two presentations of the test to a representative sample of subjects. The resulting correlation coefficient is, essentially, a measure of the test's ability to make distinctions among subjects.

The two measures of reliability are related but not identical. It is possible, for example, for test scores to have narrow confidence limits but a low test–retest correlation if the test population has little variability. In such a case, the test is unnecessary for inter-subject performance evaluation but may be useful for measuring intra-subject changes.

Test–retest variability and confidence limits of test scores can, to a certain extent, be predicted from binomial theory (Boothroyd, 1968; Thornton and Raffin, 1978). One underlying assumption is that the probability of a correct response (i.e., the probability of the perceiver's inferred language patterns corresponding with those of the talker) is constant from trial to trial. This assumption is seldom met in practice. Fortunately, however, the resulting errors are often small enough to be ignored (Dillon, 1982, 1983). A second assumption is that the probability of error on each trial does not depend on success or failure on other trials. This assumption is valid for lists of unrelated words, and for phonemes in nonsense syllables, but not for words in sentences, or phonemes in real words. There are, however, quantitative methods for dealing with violations of the independence assumption (Boothroyd and Nittrouer, 1988). The estimation approach, when used with care, can be an effective substitute for empirical measures of variability.

Even in adult populations, the reliability of speech perception test scores tends to be low. Word recognition scores in the region of 50%, for example, have 95% confidence limits in the region of ±14% when measured with a list of 50 words, and over 20% when based on only 25 words. The dangers of using such tests for clinical hearing aid comparisons were demonstrated many years ago when it was shown that hearing aid differences tend to be of the same order of magnitude as the uncertainty in individual test scores (Shore, Bilger and Hirsh, 1960).

It is more difficult to ensure adequately low test–retest variability when evaluating children than when evaluating adults. One reason is that subject performance is more likely to change over time because of differences of motivation, compliance, attention, alertness, and so on. Another is that the amount of time available for testing a young child is often incompatible with the number of trials needed for adequate precision.

Efficiency

An efficient test is one that provides all the necessary information, with adequate reliability, in a clinically feasible amount of time. The inverse relationship between information and reliability on the one hand and speed on the other creates serious difficulties of test design, and these difficulties increase with decreasing age of the test population.

Solutions

Researchers and clinicians have produced many solutions to the problems of speech perception testing in hearing-impaired children. A thorough review will be found in a recent chapter by Tyler (1993). Most of the resulting tests have been intended to measure the amount of sensory evidence available via amplification, speechreading, cochlear implants, tactile aids, or some combination of these. The approaches have been of three basic types: single figure of merit, descriptive/analytic, and classificatory.

Figure of merit

Figure-of-merit approaches generate a single score to represent speech perception performance. Such approaches are, usually, adaptations of the word recognition testing that has become standard with adult populations. The simplest adaptation is to use age-appropriate word lists such as the PBK lists, so as to minimize the effects of word knowledge on test scores (Haskins, 1949). A further adaptation is to use a pointing response to pictured alternatives, as in the WIPI (Ross and Lerman, 1970) and the NUCHIPS (Elliott and Katz, 1980), so as to avoid the confounding effects of the speech output problems of prelingually deafened children. It is unreasonable to expect, however, that absolute scores obtained with these tests will be in any sense equivalent, or that they will correspond with adult scores on word recognition tests. It is also unreasonable to expect that the scores will be insensitive to differences of language knowledge and speech perception skill. Nevertheless, each test can serve, within limits, to differentiate among subjects and to register intra-subject changes.

Descriptive/analytic

The descriptive/analytic test provides more detailed information than is a available from a single figure of merit. Such tests, typically, seek to determine the kinds of sensory evidence to which the subject has access. The question is usually asked in terms of phonologically significant features such as voicing and place of articulation. Examples are Risberg's diagnostic rhyme test (Risberg, 1976), Boothroyd's SPAC test (Boothroyd, 1984, 1988b), Erber's vowel and consonant identification tests (Erber, 1972; Hack and Erber, 1982), and sections of Plant's PLOTT test (Plant, 1984). The first three tests require the subject to choose among a closed set of printed words or pictures in order to assess the perception of several phonetic features. Erber's tests call for the closed-set identification of vowels and consonants and use confusion matrices to determine access to specific contrasts. More recent variants, designed to further reduce the confounding effects of linguistic knowledge, include Osberger's 'change/no change' test of feature perception (Osberger *et al.*, 1991), the Audiovisual Feature test of Tyler *et al.*, (Tyler, Fryauf-Bertschy and Kelsay, 1991), and Boothroyd's THRIFT and IMSPAC tests (Boothroyd, 1991a, 1991b). The THRIFT will be discussed in more detail later. In all cases, the aim is to derive a profile showing the relative access to different phonetic contrasts in such a way as to determine the need for, and success of, various forms of sensory assistance. These tests can also be used to provide an overall single figure of merit.

Classificatory

A major drawback to the first two kinds of test is the time taken to administer them. Both adequate reliability and analytic detail call for many trials. A pragmatic approach to this problem, in the case of the profoundly deaf, has been to seek only a simple classification. Erber's MTS test (Erber and Alencewicz, 1976), for example, seeks to distinguish subjects who can differentiate among words on the basis of spectral and fine temporal detail from those who can only make distinctions on the basis of gross syllabic pattern. It does, however, provide figures of merit for these two abilities. The ANT test is intended to distinguish children who can differentiate the numbers one through five from those who can only count the number of syllables (Erber, 1980). Geers and Moog have also advocated classifying children into four categories on the basis of the details they are able to perceive in the acoustic patterns of speech (Geers and Moog, 1987), and their

Early Speech Perception test (ESP) is designed to make this possible (Moog and Geers, 1990).

Researchers have shown considerable ingenuity in addressing the problems of speech perception testing in children, and each of the resulting tests has merit. In general, however, there has been little standardization or evaluation of these tests, most having been developed to address urgent research or clinical needs. Moreover, the problem of separating sensory factors from cognitive and linguistic factors has seldom been adequately addressed. The remainder of this chapter is devoted to the presentation of evaluative data obtained with THRIFT. In addition to describing an approach to evaluation, this material also serves to illustrate the magnitude of the difficulties encountered in developing and standardizing paediatric speech perception tests.

A three-interval forced-choice test of speech pattern contrast perception (THRIFT)

Purpose

THRIFT has two purposes. One is to generate a profile of an individual's access to several phonologically significant speech pattern contrasts. The other is to provide a single figure of merit. This figure of merit should quantify sensory capacity in a manner that is predictive of the potential for development of sentence-level speech perception performance while remaining insensitive to current knowledge and skill. In other words, the test is intended to measure the amount of sensory evidence that the subject obtains from speech, regardless of such things as current age, age at onset of deafness, listening experience, motor speech skill, and language development. This test evolved from work with the Speech Pattern Contrast test (SPAC) (Boothroyd, 1988b), the design of which was based on Risberg's rhyme test (Risberg, 1976). The SPAC test has been used successfully in studies of orally-trained hearing-impaired teenagers and adult cochlear implantees (Boothroyd, 1984, 1993a; Waltzman and Hochberg, 1990). Performance, however, is heavily dependent on lexical knowledge and reading ability and the test is, therefore, unsuitable for young children. THRIFT was designed to avoid the need for vocabulary knowledge and reading skills.

Description (see also Boothroyd (1991a, 1991b) and Boothroyd et al. (1988))

THRIFT uses an oddity task. Each stimulus consists of three utterances. Two are repetitions of the same syllable (consonant(C)–vowel(V), VC, or CVC). One differs from the other two along a single phonologically significant dimension of one of its components. In 'taw taw daw', for example, the difference is in the voicing of the initial consonant. The subject's task is to decide whether the odd-man-out was first, second, or third in the sequence of three utterances. Response can be verbal, by pointing, or by key press.

THRIFT is divided into subtests. Within a subtest, the contrasting dimension remains constant but its phonetic context changes from trial to trial. Following 'taw taw daw', for example, a subject might hear 'voo foo voo'. The contrast is still of initial consonant voicing but the consonant context has changed from alveolar stop to labial fricative and the following vowel has changed. Note, also, that the consonant in the odd-man-out has changed from voiced to voiceless. This variation of phonetic context was introduced to increase face validity of the test as a predictor of the potential for development of sentence-level speech perception skills.

There are nine subtests, as follows:

1. Intonation (e.g. 'peh?' versus 'peh!')
2. Vowel height (e.g. 'saw' versus 'sue')
3. Vowel place (e.g. 'doo' versus 'dee')
4. Initial consonant voicing (e.g. 'taw' versus 'daw')
5. Final consonant voicing (e.g. 'eez' versus 'eece')
6 Initial consonant continuance (e.g. 'seh' versus 'teh')
7. Final consonant continuance (e.g. 'awz' versus 'awd')
8. Initial consonant place (e.g. 'foo' versus 'soo')
9. Final consonant place (e.g. 'eeg' versus 'eed')

Scores for the nine contrasts are also averaged to generate a composite score which serves as a single figure of merit. In computing this composite score, no attempt is made to weight the contrasts in relation to their relative importance in the perception of running speech. The balance of six consonant contrasts to two vowel contrasts is probably appropriate, but the balance of eight segmental contrasts to one suprasegmental contrast probably underestimates the importance of the latter.

The test was designed with 12 trials per contrast for a total of 108 trials. The test can be administered with only 6 trials per contrast for a total of 54 trials, but at a cost to reliability. The number cannot be reduced below 6 because of the need to counterbalance the position of the odd-man-out and the direction of the contrast change (e.g. whether the odd-man-out is voiced or voiceless) within a subtest. Higher multiples of 6 can be used, however, if there is a need to increase test–retest reliability.

Administration

In its current form, the test uses a single female talker and is recorded on video laser disc. Stimulus presentation and scoring are under computer control (Figure 2). The purpose of the video recording is to permit assessment via speechreading, either alone or in combination with sound. For situations in which the visual component is not required, we have developed a version of THRIFT that requires only a personal computer fitted with an inexpensive sound board.

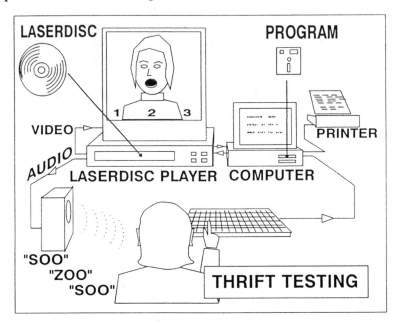

Figure 2. THRIFT is currently administered from a video laserdisc recording under computer control.

Construct validity

By using natural speech, phonologically significant contrasts, and a varying phonetic context, we have reduced the likelihood that a subject can obtain high scores on the basis of visual or acoustic cues that are irrelevant to the perception of running speech. At the same time, the influence of lexical and sentential context is removed by the use of nonsense syllables. Note also that the oddity task requires no phonemic recognition or classification, and it removes the need for reading ability.

On the negative side, the oddity task is cognitively, attentionally, and motivationally demanding and does not lend itself to application with very young children. Moreover, the use of phonologically-defined contrasts, together with a varying phonetic context, may put the prephonological child at a disadvantage. In theory, the oddity decision can be made on either an acoustic or a phonetic basis. The task is probably easier, however, for the individual who can first classify the stimuli phonetically before deciding which is the odd-man-out. Empirical validation is required to determine the exact importance of these theoretical threats to validity.

Empirical validity

Ideally, validity would be determined by comparing THRIFT with a criterion test whose validity was already established. In the absence of an adequate criterion, empirical evidence in support of validity must be accumulated piecemeal, in a variety of ways. The data summarized here were obtained with normally-hearing children, adults with simulated hearing losses, aided hearing-impaired children, and implanted hearing-impaired children.

Normally developing children

If THRIFT is valid as a test of sensory evidence, then normally-hearing children should score close to 100%, for auditory input, regardless of age. This prediction has been tested by administering the test to 44 children aged 5 to 11 (Laipply, 1990), and is supported, but only for children aged 8 years and older. Below age 8, mean scores fall rapidly with decreasing age, approaching chance levels (by extrapolation) at around age 4 (Figure 3). The age effect is more marked for some contrasts than for others, a finding that implicates both cognitive and phonological factors in the poorer performance of younger children. Between 8 and 11 years, the effect of age is still present but small. These results support the conclusion that THRIFT is reasonably valid as a measure of access to sensory evidence, independent of knowledge and skill, for normally developing children (and, by implication, recently deafened children) aged 8 years and older. They also suggest that a modified version, using only easier contrasts, might be valid for younger children. These findings cannot, of course, be extrapolated to prelingually deafened children in whom delays in the acquisition of phonological knowledge are to be expected.

Normally-hearing adults with simulated losses

To test the predictive validity of THRIFT, we have administered it, and a sentence test of speech perception, to a group of normally-hearing subjects with simulated hearing losses, created by low-pass filtering. The results show an orderly relationship between THRIFT scores and the recognition of words in sentences of known topic (Boothroyd, 1991b). Moreover, the form of the relationship is predicted from a theoretical model based on probability theory (Figure 4). This model assumes an

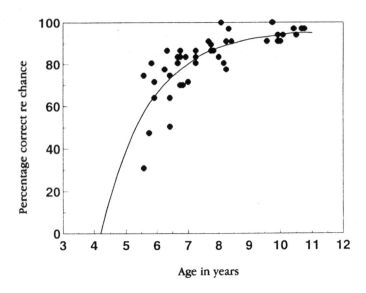

Figure 3. Composite THRIFT scores, obtained by hearing alone, as a function of age in normally-hearing children. Each datum is the mean of 54 trials. The curve is the least squares fit to an exponential growth function. The data are taken from Laipply (1990).

inherent ability to make phonemic distinctions, based on sensory evidence, and then accounts for the effects of word and sentence context with a series of empirically determined exponents. In addition to supporting the conclusion that THRIFT measures sensory capacity in a manner that is relevant to sentence-level speech perception, the findings of this study also point to a composite THRIFT score of 60% (after correction for guessing) as a minimal requirement for functional performance at the sentence level.

Aided hearing-impaired children

THRIFT was administered auditorily, under headphones, to the better ears of 71 hearing-impaired children who wear hearing aids. Three-frequency average pure tone thresholds ranged from 75 to 122 dBHL, with a mean of 99 dBHL. Ages ranged from 7 to 15 years with a mean of 10 years. Age at onset of deafness ranged from birth to 4 years with a mean of 0.6 years (the sample consisted almost entirely of prelingually deafened subjects). Forty-one of the children were from Oral programmes and 30 were from Total Communication programmes.

Composite THRIFT scores (based on 12 trials per subtest for a total of 108 trials) were expressed as a percentage and then corrected for guessing, using the following formula:

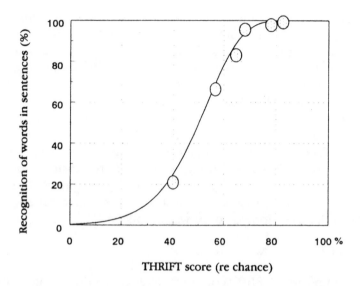

THRIFT score (re chance)

Figure 4. Per cent recognition of words in sentences of known topic, as a function of composite THRIFT scores, for normally-hearing adults listening with various amounts of low-pass filtering. Each datum is the mean of six subjects.

$$c = (r{-}33.33) / (100{-}33.33){*}100 \ldots \tag{1}$$

where c is the corrected score in %, and r is the raw score in %.

Composite THRIFT scores, after correction for guessing, ranged from −14 to 69% with a mean of 28% (note that, in a subject who is guessing on each trial, performance below the expected score of 33.3% can result in a negative value after correction). The standard deviation was 21%. In a linear correlational analysis, the best single predictor of THRIFT score was the 3-frequency average pure tone threshold of the test ear (r(69) = −0.65, p<0.001). THRIFT scores are shown as a function of hearing loss in Figure 5. Also shown is the regression function for score on loss. From this function we may conclude that the expected composite THRIFT score, in % after correction for guessing, is 1.25 times the amount by which the loss in dB is less than 121 dB. The standard error of prediction is ±16%.

The sensation level at which stimuli were presented (highest comfortable level minus detection level) was also a predictor of composite THRIFT score (r(62) = 0.65, p<0.001; note that sensation level data were not available for seven of the subjects). Sensation level was also correlated with pure tone threshold (r(62) = 0.70, p<0.001), as shown in the upper panel of Figure 5. Thus, one reason for the correlation between THRIFT scores and hearing loss could have been that the deafer subjects were listening at too low a sensation level. Sensation level was not, however, the only factor. In a multiple stepwise regression analysis, hearing loss alone accounted for 42% of the variance in THRIFT scores. The addition of sensation level accounted for another 7% (p = 0.005). These findings are in keeping with the conclusion that the deafer subject is doubly disadvantaged. First, greater cochlear damage reduces temporal and spectral resolution. Second, a reduced dynamic range deprives the subject of full audibility of the stimulus.

Composite THRIFT score was significantly correlated with age (r(69) = 0.33, p<0.005), as illustrated in Figure 6. In the regression analysis, age accounted for a further 6% of the variance in composite THRIFT score (p = 0.005) after loss and sensation level were taken into account. The full regression equation was as follows.

$$c = 43 - 0.67*t + 1.05*s + 2.78*a \dots \qquad (2)$$

where: c = composite THRIFT score in %, after correction for guessing,

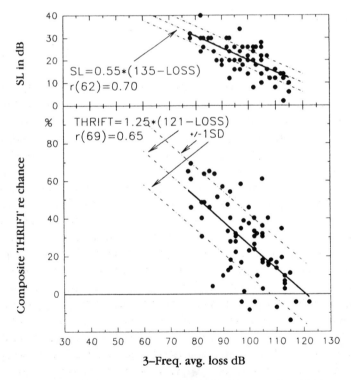

Figure 5. The top panel shows sensation level (highest comfortable listening level minus awareness threshold), as a function of hearing loss, for 71 hearing-impaired children listening to linearly amplified speech. The bottom panel shows composite auditory THRIFT score as a function of hearing loss. In a multiple regression analysis, loss and sensation level, together, accounted for 49% of the variance in THRIFT scores.

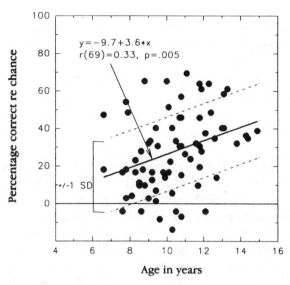

Figure 6. Composite auditory THRIFT score, as a function of age, for 71 hearing-impaired children.

t = 3-frequency average pure tone threshold in dBHL, s = sensation level in dB, and a = age in years.

The multiple correlation was 0.74, indicating that loss, sensation level and age could account for 55% of the variance in composite score. The standard error of prediction was 14%. It will be shown later that about 6% of this can be attributed to test–retest variability, leaving another 8% attributable to inter-subject differences beyond those accounted for by loss, sensation level and age.

In the multiple regression analysis neither educational environment (treated as a binary variable), nor age at onset of deafness, added significantly to the prediction of composite THRIFT score. Note, however, that almost all subjects were congenitally deaf and these data, therefore, provide little information about the possible effect of age at onset.

The fact that pure tone threshold and sensation level account for a major proportion of the variance in composite score support the conclusion that THRIFT is maximally sensitive to the sensory evidence available to the subject. The relatively small contribution of age and the absent contribution of educational environment support the conclusion that THRIFT is minimally sensitive to knowledge and skill. The presence of an age effect in the range of 7 to 15 years is in keeping with Laipply's data which showed a small age effect in normal children over age 8. In the hearing aid users, this effect amounted to almost 3% per year of age. Though small, the age effect is not insignificant. Its existence emphasizes the need for further work if we are to devise a test of sensory capacity that is completely insensitive to the effects of knowledge and skill.

Implanted hearing-impaired children

The test was also administered to 39 cochlear implant users. Thirty used the Nucleus 22-electrode device and 9 used the House-3M single-channel device. Ages ranged from 7 to 15 years with a mean of 10 years. Ages at onset of deafness ranged from birth to 6 years with a mean of 1.5 years. Duration from onset of profound deafness to implantation ranged from 0.6 to 10 years with a mean of 5 years. Duration of implant use ranged from 1 to 9 years with a mean of 4 years.

Composite THRIFT scores, after correction for guessing, ranged from -14 to 69% with a mean of 24%. (In passing, it is interesting to note that the ranges for aided and implanted children were identical.) In a correlational analysis, significant predictors of score were age at onset of deafness ($r(37) = 0.49$, $p < 0.001$) and type of device ($r(37) = 0.34$, $p < 0.033$), the latter being treated as a binary variable. In a multiple regression analysis for the 30 Nucleus subjects, only age at onset of deafness accounted for a significant proportion of the variance in the composite THRIFT scores, as shown in Figure 7 ($r = 0.53$, $p = 0.002$). The regression function from Figure 7 indicates that the expected composite score for a Nucleus implantee is 17% plus 6% for each year of hearing before the onset of deafness. The standard error of prediction is 16%, which is similar to that found for the hearing aid subjects, after accounting for the effects of loss, sensation level, and current age. The test–retest data, to be reported, suggest that only 6% of this residual variability is attributable to random effects, supporting the notion that the composite THRIFT score is sensitive to inter-subject differences, after the effects of device and age at onset are accounted for. Note that, in contrast to the aided subjects, test age was not a significant predictor of performance. Moreover, there was no significant effect of duration of device use, or of type of educational environment.

The data for the single-channel implant users are too few to draw conclusions about the effects of age at onset. The average composite score for the nine House-3M subjects, however, was 13%, compared with 27% for the Nucleus subjects. In a simple t test for uncorrelated means, the difference of 14% was significantly different from zero ($t(37) = 2.2$, $p = 0.033$).

The significant effect of device provides support for the conclusion that THRIFT is sensitive to the amount of sensory data available to the subject. The fact that there was also a significant effect of age at onset of deafness indicates that the test is not free of the effects of phonological knowledge and skill. In the present data, the effect of age at onset is more pronounced than that of device. It will be noted from Figure 7, however, that the distribution of age at onset is skewed. A few good performers with late onset may be artificially enhancing the coefficient of correlation. More data are required from children with later onset

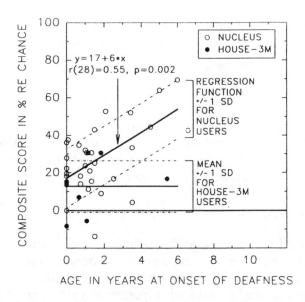

Figure 7. Composite auditory THRIFT score, as a function of device and age at onset of profound deafness, for 39 implanted children. The regression function is for 30 Nucleus implant users only. Data for nine House-3M implant users are shown for comparison.

before strong conclusions can be made about its relative importance. Nevertheless, this effect is in keeping with the age effect found in aided children and points to the potential limitations of the THRIFT procedure as a means of eliminating the effects of knowledge and skill. Concerns about this shortcoming are, however, somewhat reduced by the absence of measurable effects from current age and years of implant use among the implantees, and educational environment in both aid and implant users.

Reliability

THRIFT was administered twice to 110 child hearing aid and implant users. Each presentation used only 6 trials per contrast, so each composite score was based on only 54 trials. Figure 8 shows the relationship between the two scores which were significantly correlated $(p(108) = 0.81, p<0.001)$. From the error term in a repeated measures analysis of variance, it was found that the standard deviation of repeated scores was 9%. Note that this value relates to composite scores based on 54 trials. By increasing the number of trials to 108 (i.e., 12 per contrast), the standard deviation should be reduced by the square root of 2, to 6%. This value is less than the 14 and 16% residual standard error of prediction, respectively, reported above in the studies of aided and implanted children. Note, also, that the measured standard error of repeated scores is close to that estimated from binomial theory for a probability of 0.5 (before correction for guessing) and 108 trials, namely:

$$s = [\text{sqrt}](0.5*0.5/108)*100 \ldots. \tag{3}$$

which equals 4.8%, or 7.2% after correction for guessing. The fact that the measured test–retest variability is close to that predicted from binomial theory suggests that further improvements of reliability are unlikely without an increase in the number of test items.

Attribution of variance

It will be recalled that the composite THRIFT score is intended to provide a single figure of merit that is maximally dependent on the sensory evidence available to the subject and minimally dependent on the subject's language knowledge and speech perception skills. From the data obtained from child hearing aid and implant users, it is possible to attribute the group variance in THRIFT scores to various sources, as shown in Figure 9. In both cases, the percentage of variance that can be attributed either to random effects, or to factors known to be predictive of knowledge and skill, is small. This leaves a large percentage of the variance attributable to individual differences. Some of these differences are clearly related to factors known to be predictive of access to sensory evidence, namely hearing loss and sensation level in the case of

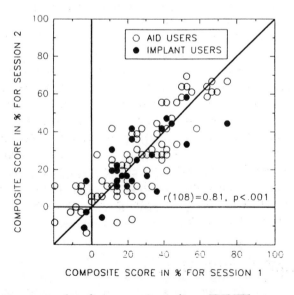

Figure 8. Test–retest data for composite auditory THRIFT scores of 110 implanted and aided children. Each score was based on 6 trials per subtest for a total of 54 trials.

the aided subjects, and implant device in the case of the implanted sub-jects. It seems reasonable to assume that a substantial proportion of the unexplained inter-subject variance is also a function of access to sensory data, in which case, the test meets its design goal, though not perfectly.

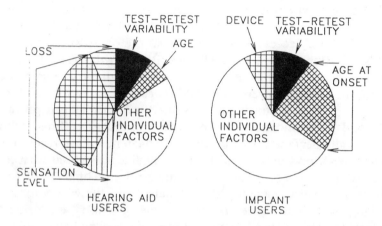

Figure 9. Pie charts showing the attribution of variance in the composite THRIFT scores of child hearing aid users (left) and child implant users (right).

Efficiency

The complete THRIFT, at 12 trials per subtest, takes approximately 20 minutes to administer. Testing time can be reduced by using only six trials per subtest but only at the expense of reliability. It is interesting to note that the standard deviation of repeated THRIFT scores, based on 108 trials and corrected for guessing, is almost identical to that for open-set word recognition scores, using 50 words per score, which can be obtained in 5 minutes. THRIFT, therefore, has only one-quarter the efficiency of the more standard word recognition test. To offset this weakness, however, it should be noted that THRIFT also provides a profile of the subject's access to several phonetic contrasts and that it can be used with subjects for whom word recognition testing is not appropriate. It also circumvents the floor effects, mentioned earlier, that are encountered when open-set word recognition tests are admin-istered to profoundly deaf subjects.

Summary and Conclusion

The empirical evidence supports the conclusion that THRIFT, or some similar test, should provide a reasonably valid measure of access to speech-related sensory evidence, without undue influence from cognitive or linguistic factors, in children aged 8 years or more. The test does not, however, eliminate cognitive and linguistic factors entirely, and it does not provide a solution to the problem of measuring sensory capacity in younger hearing-impaired children.

Experience in the use of THRIFT had already revealed its inadequacy for use with younger children, before the foregoing empirical data were obtained. As a result, we developed a parallel test, IMSPAC, in which sensory access is estimated from the objective evaluation of a child's imitations of nonsense syllables (Boothroyd, 1991a, 1991b). The results obtained using IMSPAC correlate well with those obtained using THRIFT in older children, and IMSPAC can be used with children as young as 3 years. Unfortunately, IMSPAC requires speech production skills and its application is, therefore, limited to children who are postlingually deafened or, if prelingually deafened, have received training in speech production and have intelligible speech, at least for the contrasts presented. In our continuing pursuit of tests of sensory speech perception capacity that remain valid for very young, non-speaking deaf children we are, at the time of writing, exploring three avenues. One is the development of interactive video games that probe contrast perception (Boothroyd et al., 1992). The second is the development of simpler oddity tasks based on successful work with normally-hearing infants (Kuhl, 1991; Kuhl, et al., 1992). The third is the use of electrophysiological responses to phonetic changes (Boothroyd, 1991b; Kraus et al., 1992, 1993).

In summary, speech perception is not a simple entity that can be evaluated with a single metric. Rather it is an inferential process involving interactions among several factors. Some of these factors are found in the speech stimulus, some in its context, and some in the knowledge and skills of the perceiver. The designer of a speech perception test must first have a clear concept of purpose, and that purpose must be translated into an understanding of what needs to be measured. Stimuli and tasks must then be selected which are theoretically sensitive to what is to be measured, insensitive to what is not to be measured, and appropriate for the population of interest. The resulting performance measures should be capable of detecting clinically significant inter- and intra-subject differences. Design should be followed by empirical investigations of validity, reliability and efficiency. Ideally, a new test will be validated by comparison with an existing test of known validity. In the absence of a criterion measure, validity can be investigated by indirect methods, as illustrated in the present chapter.

In spite of many years of productive research, the opportunity remains for the development of a battery of tests that can assess, separately and in combination, the many factors that contribute to speech perception and its development in young hearing-impaired children.

Acknowledgements

I am grateful to the many colleagues who provided assistance in either the preparation of this chapter or the collection of data. The list includes: Orna Eran, Jill Firszt, Joseph Fischgrund, Anne Geers, Laurie Hanin, Vardit Lichtenstein, Mary Rose McKinerny, Laura McKurdy, Jean Moog, David Shea, Lisa Tonakawa, Robin Waldstein, Susan Waltzman, and Eddy Yeung. Preparation supported, in part, by grant no. 2PO1DC00178 from the National Institutes of Health.

References

Boothroyd, A. (1968) Developments in speech audiometry. British Journal of Audiology (formerly Sound) 2: 3–10.

Boothroyd, A. (1984) Auditory perception of speech contrasts by subjects with sensorineural hearing loss. Journal of Speech and Hearing Research 27: 134–44.

Boothroyd, A. (1988a) Hearing Impairments in Young Children. Washington, D.C.: A. G. Bell Association for the Deaf. (Previously published in 1982 by Prentice Hall, Englewood Cliffs, NJ.)

Boothroyd, A. (1988b) Perception of speech pattern contrasts from auditory presentation of voice fundamental frequency. Ear and Hearing 9: 313–21.

Boothroyd, A. (1991a) Assessment of speech perception capacity in profoundly deaf children. American Journal of Otology 12(suppl): 67–72.

Boothroyd, A. (1991b) Speech perception measures and their role in the evaluation of hearing aid performance in a pediatric population. In Feigin J.A. and Stelmachowicz P.G. (Eds), Pediatric Amplification. Omaha, Nebraska: Boys Town National research Hospital. pp 77–91.

Boothroyd, A. (1993a) Profound deafness and cochlear implants. In Tyler, R. (Ed) Cochlear Implants: Audiological Foundations. San Diego, CA: Singular Publishing. pp 1–33.

Boothroyd, A. (1993b) Speech perception, sensorineural hearing loss, and hearing aids. In Studebaker, G. and Hochberg, I. (Ed.) Acoustical Factors Affecting Hearing Aid Performance. Boston, MA: Allyn and Bacon.

Boothroyd, A. and Nittrouer, S. (1988) Mathematical treatment of context effects in phoneme and word recognition. Journal of the Acoustical Society of America 84: 101–14.

Boothroyd, A., Hanin, L., Yeung, E. and Chen, Q. (1992) Video-game for speech perception testing and training of young hearing-impaired children. Proceedings of the Johns Hopkins National Search for Computing Applications to Assist Persons with Disabilities. Los Alamitos, CA: IEEE Computer Society Press.

Boothroyd, A., Springer, N., Smith, L. and Schulman, J. (1988) Amplitude compression and profound hearing loss. Journal of Speech and Hearing Research 33: 362–76.

Crocker, L.M. and Algina, J. (1986) Introduction to Classical and Modern Test Theory. Orlando, FL: Harcourt Brace.

De Filippo, C.L. and Scott, B.L. (1978) A method for training and evaluating the reception of ongoing speech. Journal of the Acoustical Society of America 63: 1186–92.

Dillon, H.A. (1982) A quantitative examination of the sources of speech discrimination test score variability. Ear and Hearing 3: 51–8.

Dillon, H.A. (1983) The effect of test difficulty on the sensitivity of speech discrimination tests. Journal of the Acoustical Society of America 73: 336–44.

Elliott, L. and Katz, D. (1980) Development of a New Children's Test of Speech Discrimination. St Louis, MO: Auditec.

Erber, N.P. (1972) Auditory, visual, and auditory-visual perception of consonants by children with normal and impaired hearing. Journal of Speech and Hearing Research 15: 413–22.

Erber, N.P. (1980) Use of the Auditory Numbers Test to evaluate speech perception abilities of hearing-impaired children. Journal of Speech and Hearing Disorders 45: 527–32.

Erber, N.P. and Alencewicz, C.M. (1976) Audiologic evaluation of deaf children. Journal of Speech and Hearing Disorders 41: 256–67.

Geers, A.E. and Moog, J.S. (1987) Predicting spoken language acquisition in profoundly deaf children. Journal of Speech and Hearing Disorders 52: 84–94.

Geers, A.E. and Moog, J.S. (1992) Speech perception and production skills of students with impaired hearing from oral and total communication education setting. Journal of Speech and Hearing Research, 35: 1384–1393.

Hack, Z. C., and Erber, N. P. (1982). Auditory, visual, and auditory-visual perception of vowels by hearing-impaired children. Journal of Speech and Hearing Research, 25: 100-107.

Hanin, L. (1988). The effects of experience and linguistic context on speechreading. Unpublished PhD dissertation, City University of New York.

Haskins, H. A. (1949). A Phonetically balanced test of speech discrimination for children. Unpublished MS Thesis, Northwestern University, Evanston, IL.

Hnath-Chisolm, T., Hanin, L. and Boothroyd, A. (1985) Speechreading with and without knowledge of sentence topic. Unpublished report, City University of New York.

Hochberg, I., Rosen, S. and Ball, V. (1987). Effect of text complexity upon connected discourse tracking. Annals of Otology, Rhinology, and Laryngology 96: 82–3.

Kraus, N., McGee, T., Sharma, A., Carrell, T. and Nicol, T. (1992) Mismatch negativity event-related potential elicited by speech stimuli. Ear and Hearing 13: 158–64.

Kraus, N., Micco, A.G., Koch, D.B., McGee, T., Carrell, T., Sharma, A., Wiet, R.J., and Weingaten, C.Z. (1993) The mismatch negativity cortical evoked potential elicited by speech in cochlear-implant users. Hearing Research 65: 118–24.

Kuhl, P.K. (1991) Human adults and human infants show a 'perceptual magnet effect' for prototypes of speech categories, monkeys do not. Perception and Psychophysics 50: 93–107.

Kuhl, P.K., Williams, K.A., Lacerda, F., Stevens, K.N. and Lindblom, B. (1992) Linguistic experience alters phonetic perception in infants by 6 months of age. Science 255: 606–8.

Laipply, E.M. (1990) Chronological age effects on the audiovisual perception of phonologically significant speech feature contrasts. Unpublished MS Thesis, University of South Florida: Tampa, FL.

Miller, G.A., Heise, G.A. and Lichten, W. (1951) The intelligibility of speech as a function of the context of the test material. Journal of Experimental Psychology 41: 329–35.

Moog, J.S. and Geers, A.E. (1990) Early Speech Perception Battery. St. Louis, MO: CID.

Osberger, M.J., Robbins, A.M., Miyamoto, R.T., Berry, S.W., Myres, W.A., Kesseler, K. and Pope, M.L. (1991) Speech perception abilities of children with cochlear implants, tactile aids, or hearing aids. American Journal of Otology 12: 105–15.

Plant, G. (1984) A diagnostic speech test for severely and profoundly hearing impaired children. Australian Journal of Audiology 6: 1–9.

Risberg, A. (1976) Diagnostic rhyme test for speech audiometry with severely hard of hearing and profoundly deaf children. Speech Transmission Laboratory Quarterly Progress and Status Report, 2-3. Stockholm: Karolinska Technical Institute. pp 40–55.

Ross, M. and Lerman, J. (1970) A picture identification test for hearing-impaired children. Journal of Speech and Hearing Disorders 13: 44–53.

Shore, I., Bilger, R.C. and Hirsh, I.J. (1960) Hearing aid evaluation: reliability of repeated measures. Journal of Speech and Hearing Disorders 25: 152-170.

Thornton, A.R. and Raffin, M.J.M. (1978) Speech discrimination scores modeled as a binomial variable. Journal of Speech and Hearing Research 21: 507–18.

Tye-Murray, N. and Tyler, R. S. (1988) A critique of continuous discourse tracking as a test procedure. Journal of Speech and Hearing Disorders 53: 226–31.

Tyler, R.S. (1993) Speech perception by children. In Tyler, R.S. (Ed) Cochlear Implants: Audiological Foundations San Diego, CA: Singular Publishing. pp 191–256.

Tyler, R.S., Fryauf-Bertschy, H. and Kelsay, D. (1991) Audiovisual Feature Test for Young Children. Iowa City, Iowa: University of Iowa.

Waltzman, S. and Hochberg, I. (1990) Perception of speech pattern contrasts using a multichannel cochlear implant. Ear and Hearing 11: 50–5.

17

Speech Perception Tests for Use with Australian Children

GEOFF PLANT

Introduction

This chapter concerns the development of speech tests for Australian children with varying degrees of hearing loss. The first section describes a test battery aimed at evaluating the auditory speech reception skills of children with profound hearing losses. This test battery was developed over a period of 10 years and the materials range in complexity from the detection of vowels and consonants in isolation to comprehension of simple sentences. The second section provides an overview of work carried out from 1988 to 1992. The project described was aimed at developing simple speech tests for hearing screening in Australian Aboriginal languages. In this case, the children tested had mild to moderate hearing losses resulting from otitis media. Both projects arose from a need to develop materials which were appropriate for Australian conditions and the specific needs of the target group. Although the tests were developed for Australian children many of the materials could be adapted for other dialects of English and other languages. The rationale behind the development of the tests could also prove useful for researchers developing similar materials.

Speech Tests for Profoundly Hearing-impaired Children

The first part of this chapter presents an overview of a battery of tests developed over the past decade to assess the auditory speech reception abilities of profoundly hearing-impaired Australian children. For the purposes of this paper profound deafness is defined as an average hearing loss (at 500, 1000 and 2000 Hz) in the better ear greater than 90 dB ISO. When the project commenced in the early 1980s there were very few materials available for this purpose. In many cases the only measure made of a child's auditory capacity at that time was the pure tone audiogram. Many audiologists, parents and teachers felt that this provided a very limited view of a child's auditory capabilities and potential. Tests were needed to assess a child's speech reception skills. Hearing aids were fitted to enhance the child's ability to perceive and produce speech, so measures were needed to assess their effectiveness.

In the early 1980s the Children's Auditory Test (Erber and Alcancewicz, 1976) and the Auditory Numbers Test (Erber, 1980) were the only materials being consistently used for assessment purposes in Australia. Both tests were useful in helping to determine whether a child was perceiving at least some of the spectral cues of speech, or whether the information available to her/him via her/his hearing aids was restricted to time and intensity cues. This judgement is critical in determining the intervention strategies adopted with a particular child. For example, the auditory training programme adopted with a child limited to time and intensity information from her/his hearing aids should be very different from that provided to a child who is able to understand, at least partially, speech presented via listening alone. It was obvious, however, that a more detailed assessment of a child's speech hearing was necessary.

The need to provide teachers with speech test information which would guide them in preparing appropriate auditory training strategies for individual children was one of the prime motivating factors in this project. Discussions with a number of congenitally, profoundly deaf young adults had highlighted the need to provide individualized auditory training approaches. One common theme in these discussions was the frustration auditory training had induced for many of these adults. They spoke of programmes containing materials that were either excessively easy or impossibly difficult. The end result of such approaches was that they rejected hearing aids as being of little, if any, benefit. In a few cases, circumstance had led to them trying hearing aids when they were adults, and finding that the aids did in fact provide some benefit. I remember being told by one young deaf man that his hearing aids provided him with access to environmental sound and suprasegmental cues which assisted his lipreading. When I asked why he had not worn hearing aids during his teenage years, if such information was available, his reply was simple and, in part, damning. 'Because all the teachers at school did in auditory training was to show me what I couldn't do. They never showed me what I *could* do with hearing aids!'

Another motivating force in the project throughout the 1980s was the development of tactile aids and cochlear implants, and their subsequent fitting to children. Before a decision is made to fit either a tactile aid or a cochlear implant, an extensive evaluation of a child's auditory status is critical. Wherever possible, this testing needs to go beyond the child's ability to detect pure tones. One of the themes of this chapter is that the pure tone audiogram is a poor predictor of a profoundly hearing-impaired child's ability to understand speech via listening alone. Tactile aids and cochlear implants are designed to provide the wearer with better access to the acoustic speech signal. A measure of the individual's speech test performance with conventional hearing aids can be compared to the performance range of children fitted with cochlear implants or tactile aids. If the child's speech test scores with hearing aids are equal to, or better than, the scores typically found among users of tactile aids or cochlear implants it would be difficult to justify either cochlear implantation or the fitting of a tactile aid. If, however, the child's performance is lower than those typically attained by implanted children or children fitted with tactile aids, consideration can then be given to adopting an alternative approach.

The PLOTT Test

This test was developed over two years in conjunction with Sharan Westcott who was, at that time, the National Acoustic Laboratories (NAL) paediatric audiologist at the North Rocks School for Deaf Children. Sharan was concerned that she had few tools available to assess adequately the speech hearing of the profoundly deaf children at the school. She felt that this lack of test materials severely limited her ability to make realistic suggestions to teachers regarding the auditory training activities that should be undertaken with individual children.

In 1981 we developed the first version of the PLOTT Test and Sharan administered it to many of the children at the North Rocks school. The results obtained (Plant and Westcott, 1982) were very encouraging, and indicated that many of the children had auditory capabilities far better than had previously been thought. We felt that the test had real potential, but also felt that there were a number of modifications which would greatly improve its effectiveness. Revised test items were selected which could be represented pictorially. In this way the child being tested could respond by pointing at the picture of the stimulus word. It was felt to be unrealistic to expect children to respond verbally, especially when the test items differed by only one phonetic feature. A signed response was also unsuitable, as the signing skills of many of the audiologists who would be presenting the test were not sufficiently well developed. Once the modifications to the original test format had been made, a professional artist drew the required pictures, and this second version of the PLOTT Test (Plant and Westcott, 1983; Plant, 1984) was given to a number of NAL paediatric audiologists throughout Australia for field trailing.

The modified test consisted of nine subtests of increasing difficulty. Subtest 1 looked at the ability of children to detect a number of vowels and consonants produced in isolation. Subtest 2 was based on Erber's

Auditory Numbers Test (Erber, 1980) and required the children to differentiate between the number strings 1, 12, 123, 1234, and 12345. Each pattern was presented twice for identification. Subtest 3 was also based on another of Erber's tests – the Children's Auditory Test. This test consisted of 12 words – 3 monosyllables, 3 spondees, 3 trochees, and 3 polysyllables. The test was scored for the number of words correctly identified and the number of syllables correctly categorized. Subtest 4 consisted of 12 consonant–vowel (CV) or consonant–vowel–consonant (CVC) words which include each of the 11 vowels of Australian English which can be produced in a stressed syllable. Each of the words in Subtests 3 and 4 were presented once for identification. The child's responses were recorded, enabling the audiologist to analyse any error patterns later.

Subtests 5–9 presented items which evaluated a child's ability to discriminate the segmental contrasts – vowel duration (Subtest 5), and formant frequency (Subtest 6), and consonant voicing (Subtest 7), manner of articulation (Subtest 8), and place of articulation (Subtest 9). Each subtest presented five pairs of words which differed along the phonetic dimension being contrasted. For example, the items contrasted in Subtest 5 (vowel identification) were: 'key/car', 'bin/bun', 'bee/boo', 'cat/cut', and 'black/block'. The test procedure adopted for Subtests 5–9 contrasted each word pair in turn. The child was initially familiarized with the test items, and then each word was presented five times in a random order. The child was encouraged to respond after each presentation, but no feedback was provided as to the correctness of the response. After each word in a pair had been presented five times, the total number of correct responses was counted, with a score of 8 or more correct significantly above chance at the 5% level.

Testing was performed in sound treated rooms with the phonemes and words presented via audition alone. The child being tested was encouraged to set her/his hearing aids at the recommended settings. To ensure that no lipreading cues were available, the tester placed a piece of thin card in front of his/her mouth before presenting each word.

The paediatric audiologists field trailing the test were asked to send in the results obtained using the test with severely (pure tone averages in the range 60–90 dB ISO) and profoundly hearing-impaired children. Eventually the results obtained with 100 children with a mean age of 11.5 years were analysed (Plant and Macrae, 1985). A number of striking features emerged in this analysis.

Very few of the children tested failed to detect all of the vowels presented in Subtest 1. Around 90% of the children were also able to detect the voiced consonants [ð], [v], [z], and [ʒ]. The only items which created difficulties were the voiceless consonants [θ], [f], [s], and [ʃ]. Similarly, only one child failed to discriminate between the number strings in Subtest 2.

The word identification and categorization scores obtained in Subtest 3 by the severely hard-of-hearing children were almost perfect. The results obtained by the profoundly deaf (average hearing losses at 0.5, 1, and 2 kHz greater than 90 dB ISO) were far more variable. Many of these children were able to utilize spectral cues in word identification while others appeared to be limited to time and intensity information. Children with very similar audiometric configurations differed widely in their ability to perform this task. The audiogram was a very poor predictor of speech reception ability. One feature of particular interest was that almost all of the children tested, even those with average hearing losses greater than 110 dB ISO, were able to categorize words correctly according to their syllable number and type. This was very encouraging given that this syllabic information can be an extremely useful adjunct to lipreading, and can assist in the development of speech production skills.

The identification scores obtained in Subtest 3 were relatively good predictors of a child's ability to perform Subtest 4. Those profoundly deaf children whose identification scores in Subtest 3 indicated an ability to utilize at least some spectral information performed relatively well on this subtest. Those who appeared to receive only time and intensity cues had much greater difficulty. It should be noted, however, that some of this latter group were able to use temporal information to differentiate reliably between those words which contained long vowels, and those with short vowels. Similarly, some children appeared to be able to use the intensity differences between open and closed vowels in their word identification. Although overall performance did decline as a function of increasing average hearing loss, the audiogram again proved to be a poor predictor of speech reception skills. The mean score of children with average losses in the range 100–109 dB ISO was poorer than that obtained by children with 90–99 dB losses, but within each group there was wide performance variability.

This trend was also evident in the remaining five subtests. Overall performance declined with increasing hearing loss, but subject-to-subject variability increased. Most children, regardless of their average hearing loss, were able to differentiate reliably between CVC words which differed only in vowel duration (Subtest 6). The only items which created difficulty at this level were the [i] vs [I] word pairs 'sleep/slip' and 'sheep/ship'.

Subtest 6 presented vowel contrasts for identification. Almost all of the children were able to discriminate between the high and low vowels in the word pairs 'key/car' and 'bin/bun'. Although the children may have been using first formant frequency differences to perform this task, there are also intensity differences between these vowels which may have enabled correct identification. The items at this level which created most difficulty were those which contrasted vowels with similar first formants but dissimilar second formants. In these cases the child does not have access to intensity cues and is forced to rely upon spectral cues for correct identification. Thus, items such as 'bee' vs 'boo', and 'cat' vs 'cut' created difficulties for many (around 40%) of the profoundly deaf children.

Subtest 7 examined the ability of the children to discriminate between initial voiced and voiceless stop consonants in word pairs such as 'path' vs 'bath', and 'coat' vs 'goat'. Almost all of the severely hearing-impaired children were able to perform this task very well. The performance of the profoundly deaf children, however, was extremely variable. Many children in this group scored at below chance level for this subtest, while others attained perfect or near perfect scores. For example, the scores of children with average hearing losses ranging from 100 to 109 dB ISO were from 26% to 100% correct.

The manner of articulation contrasts presented in Subtest 8 included items which differed in both voicing and manner of articulation ('one' vs 'sun' and 'tea' vs 'knee') and others which only differed in their manners of articulation ('tail' vs 'sail', 'mat' vs 'bat', and 'red' vs 'bed'). Not surprisingly the items which differed along two dimensions were easier to discriminate than those which differed only in their manner of articulation. The item creating the greatest difficulty was the 'tail/sail' contrast, whilst the 'one/sun' contrast proved to be the easiest.

The final subtest examined the ability of the children to discriminate place of articulation. This task proved to be difficult for almost all of the children tested. More than half of those with average hearing losses greater than 100 dB scored at or below chance level for this subtest. Again, however, in common with almost all of the subtests in the test, there was considerable variability in performance from subject-to-subject.

Overall, the results of the testing were very encouraging. The test could be used successfully with children as young as 6 years and it seemed to give a reliable picture of an individual child's speech reception skills. Unfortunately, the test did have some obvious deficiencies. The most obvious was the time taken to administer all nine subtests. The test required at least 30 minutes to test a child, but more often took around one hour. In many cases, and this was especially true with younger children, the test could take up to 2 hours to administer. A second problem was related to the type of material used for testing – isolated words. Many audiologists and teachers had concerns over the validity of isolated word perception scores, and felt that the use of sentence materials would be a more realistic way to measure a child's speech reception ability. Finally, it was found that some children were unable to complete any of the later subtests successfully (Subtests 5–9). This was not only unnecessarily time consuming, but it could also frustrate the child and present an unrealistically negative view of the child's auditory capacities to the child, her/his parents and teachers. It was these concerns which led to the development of the PLOTT Screening Test, the PLOTT Sentence Test, and the Common Objects Token (COT) Test.

The PLOTT Screening Test

The PLOTT Screening Test (Plant and Moore, 1992a, 1993) is again presented in auditory form alone (after auditory-visual familiarization) and consists of fourteen word level subtests. It was based, to an extent, on Thielemeir *et al.*'s (1985) Discrimination After Training (DAT) Test. There are, however, two important differences between the two tests. The PLOTT Screening Test has a number of higher level tests (consonant voicing, and manner, and place of articulation contrasts, for example) and it uses items which are appropriate for child speakers of Australian English.

Subtest 1 evaluated the ability of the child to discriminate between voiced and non-voiced speech. The syllable [ba] is produced with and without voice and the child has to indicate when she or he hears the syllable. A pass criterion of 8/10 correct (significantly above chance at the 5% level) was set for this task. If the child scored less than this some informal training was introduced before the subtest was readministered. If the child again failed to reach criterion the test was discontinued at that point. Subtest 2 required the child to differentiate between the number strings 1, 12, 123, 1234, and 12345. Subtests 3–7 required the child to differentiate between the following syllable contrasts: a monosyllable vs a trisyllable (Subtest 3), monosyllable vs a spondee (Subtest 4), a monosyllable vs a trochee (Subtest 5), a trochee vs a spondee (Subtest 6), and a trisyllable vs a spondee (Subtest 7). Each item in the syllable contrast was presented five times in a random order. The criterion for passing each of these subtests was a score of 8/10 correct (significantly above chance at near the 5% level).

Subtests 8 and 9 contrasted three items each. In Subtest 8 the contrasts were a monosyllable, a spondee and a trochee (dog vs football vs table) while those in Subtest 9 involved the contrast of three spondees (football vs toothbrush vs ice-cream). Thus, although the items in Subtest 8 can be discriminated using syllabic cues, those in Subtest 9 probably require at least some spectral information. Each item in the subtests was presented five times in a random order with the pass criterion being 9/15 correct (significantly above chance at the 5% level).

The final subtests (10–14) presented the easiest contrasts from Subtests 5–9 of the PLOTT Test. This was based on Plant and Macrae's (1985) analysis of the scores obtained by 100 children. These items were chosen because it was felt that if the children were unable to differentiate between them, the other items in a particular subtest would prove to be excessively difficult. Each of the two items in a subtest was presented five times in a random order, with the pass criterion again being 8/10 correct.

The test was presented live voice by a female speaker to 88 children (mean age = 9.5 years, range = 4–13 years) of whom 62 had an average hearing loss (at 0.5, 1 and 2 kHz in the better ear) greater than 90 dB ISO. The test was presented twice to each of the children, with one week between the two presentations. The results obtained showed that the test materials created few, if any, difficulties for children with mild and moderate hearing losses. The scores of children with severe hearing losses and average losses in the range 90–99 dB also indicated that they had few problems with the materials involving syllabic contrasts. The only subtests which consistently created difficulties were those involving consonant contrasts. The performance of the children with average hearing losses greater than 100 dB revealed that a number of them had difficulty with even the syllabic contrasts. This was especially true for children with losses greater than 110 dB. Around one-third of the children in this group were unable to differentiate between the syllabic contrasts. Almost all of the children (22 out of a total of 24) with average losses in the range 100–109 dB were able to differentiate between the high/low vowel contrast presented in the words 'key' and 'car'. Conversely, only two-thirds of the children with average losses of 110 dB+ were able to perform this task. The performance for the three consonant discrimination tasks was very poor for almost all of the children with average hearing losses greater than 100 dB. The item creating the most difficulty was, not surprisingly, the place of articulation contrast 'bun' vs 'gun'.

The test was presented twice to the children to determine if there was any test/retest variability in performance. The correlation coefficient between the scores obtained at the first and second presentations of the test was found to be 0.90. A t-test found no significant difference between the two presentations.

The results of this study again highlighted the need to administer speech tests to determine an individual child's auditory speech discrimination skills. The results for the PLOTT Screening Test obtained by children with similar audiometric configurations varied widely. These performance differences could not be predicted from either the child's aided or unaided audiograms.

The PLOTT Screening Test allows the tester to assess quickly the child's ability to detect speech, contrast syllable number and type in words, and to discriminate between a range of vowel and consonant contrasts. The test takes only about 15 minutes to present, and few of the children tested in the field trial had any difficulty understanding the task required. If the child is able to successfully complete all, or nearly all, of the subtests of the PLOTT Screening Test, the PLOTT Test can then be administered, to obtain a more complete picture of the child's ability to identify syllabic and segmental contrasts. The information obtained in this more detailed testing can then be used in planning appropriate individualized training activities and strategies to be adopted with the child. If a child scores poorly on the PLOTT Screening Test, however, the use of the full PLOTT Test is probably unwarranted.

The PLOTT Sentence Test

The aim of the PLOTT Sentence Test (Plant and Moore, 1992a) was to develop closed-set sentence length materials for use with profoundly deaf children. Although the use of open-set materials would obviously be more closely related to real-world performance, it was felt that such a task would prove to be impossible, and therefore threatening, for many profoundly deaf children. The use of closed-set materials provided an opportunity to measure a child's ability to perceive contrasts in sentences in a relatively unthreatening way.

In order to heighten the naturalness and interest level of the materials it was decided to use sentences which formed two short stories or test lists. One concerned a child's visit to the beach, while the other described a visit to the zoo. Each of the stories consisted of 11 separate contrasts – 11 stimulus sentences, each with three response foils. Each contrast was represented with both a pictorial and written version of the stimulus sentence and the three response foils, the child's task being to identify which of the four sentences was the test stimulus. Within each list there were a number of test contrasts which differed in their syllabic structure. An example of this type of contrast is: 'Bob has a football' vs 'Bob has a bike' vs 'Bob has one sister and two brothers' vs 'Bob has a baby brother' (Figure 1). It is possible to differentiate between these sentences using only time and intensity variations. There are, however, other contrasts in each list which have the same number of syllables. An example of this type of contrast is: 'Bob saw some red fish' vs 'Bob saw some blue fish' vs 'Bob saw some red birds' vs 'Bob saw some blue birds' (Figure 2). Such contrasts probably require at least some spectral information for correct identification.

The two lists of the PLOTT Sentence Test were presented to the same group of 88 children tested with the PLOTT Screening Test. The testing was conducted live voice by the same female speaker who had presented the PLOTT Screening Test. Analysis of the scores obtained found no statistically significant difference between the two lists. The correlation coefficient between the two lists was 0.87.

This test proved to be relatively easy for children with hearing losses in the range mild–severe, and it is probably unsuitable for use with this group. There was, however, great variability in the performance of the

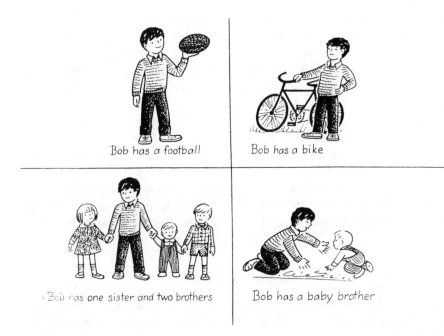

Figure 1. A sample page from the PLOTT Sentence Test showing contrasts which vary in sentence length, and syllabic patterns.

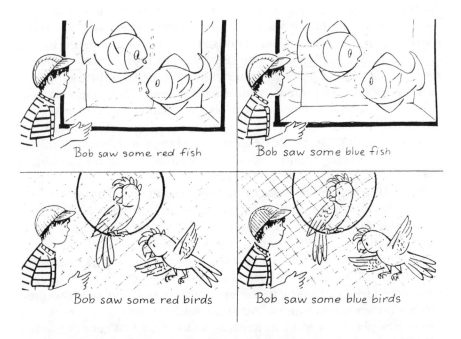

Figure 2. A sample page from the PLOTT Sentence Test showing contrasts which have the same sentence length and syllabic patterns.

children with profound hearing losses. Half of this group (32 out of 64 children) scored at or below chance level (less than 5/11) for the test. Neither the children's aided nor unaided hearing loss proved to be a good predictor of performance for this test. Of the 32 profoundly deaf children who scored significantly above chance for the PLOTT Sentence Test, 16 had scores of 8/11 correct or better. It is theoretically possible, with these test materials, to score above chance (6/11) on the basis of time and intensity cues alone, but to score eight or more correct strongly suggests the use of spectral information. This is not to say that the 50% of profoundly deaf children who scored less than 8/11 for the task were limited to time and intensity information. It is probable that many of the remaining profoundly deaf children did have access to some spectral information, but were still unable to score more than eight correct.

The Common Objects Token (COT) Test

The last test for profoundly deaf children to be described in this chapter is the Common Objects Token (COT) Test (Plant and More, 1992b). The aim in developing this test was to arrive at an instrument with a level of difficulty somewhere between the closed-set PLOTT Sentence Test and open-set sentence materials such as Bench, Doyle and Greenwood's (1987) Australian adaptation of Bench and Bamford's (1979) BKB Sentence Lists. It was felt that the move from a closed-set task to an open-set task would prove to be too large a step for many profoundly deaf children. Some children might be intimidated by the perceived complexity of the open-set task, and their scores could be unrealistically low as a result. Other children whose auditory input is restricted to time and intensity information would find open-set testing extremely difficult, if not impossible, to complete. As a result, their confidence in their ability to use auditory information might be reduced. The COT Test was designed to pinpoint children with the potential to correctly identify open-set materials, but to do so using a closed-set task of increasing complexity.

The COT Test comprises eight subtests, each consisting of ten sentences. A set of toys is used as the stimulus set for the test. This consists of four cars, four trains, four helicopters, four aeroplanes and a boat. In each set of four objects, one is coloured red, one blue, one green, and one yellow. Initially (Subtest 1) the child is presented with five objects and is asked: 'Where is the boat?' 'Where is the car?' etc. The child's task is to point to the appropriate toy. The task required becomes progressively more difficult. In Subtest 2 the child has the set of four cars placed in front of her/him and is asked 'Where is the red car?' 'Where is the yellow car?' etc. In Subtest 3 the set of helicopters is used but the child is now asked to 'Point to the yellow helicopter',

'Point to the blue helicopter' etc. Subtest 4 uses a set of eight items – the four cars and the four helicopters. The child is asked to either 'pick up' or 'point to' one of the objects. Subtest 5 uses the same instructions and the same set of objects as Subtest 4, but the child is now asked to either 'pick up' or 'point to' two objects. For example, the child may be asked to 'Pick up the red helicopter and the blue car'. In Subtest 6 the response set is increased to 16 objects – 4 cars, 4 planes, 4 trains, and 4 helicopters. The child is asked to 'pick up' or 'point to' one object. In Subtest 7 the same set of 16 objects forms the response set, but the child is now asked to either 'pick up' or 'point to' two objects. Finally, in Subtest 8 the child is asked to pick up one of the 16 items and to place it in a red, green, blue or yellow box.

The COT Test was presented live-voice without lipreading cues by a female native speaker of Australian English to a group of hearing-impaired children. Prior to presentation of the COT Test, the children were screened using the PLOTT Sentence Test. Only those children who scored above chance level for the PLOTT Sentence Test were included in the COT Test study. A total of 77 children were eventually tested using the COT Test. Of these 77 children, 25 had average losses in the range 61–90 dB while another 25 were profoundly deaf. That is, they had average hearing losses in the better ear greater than 90 dB.

The results of the testing revealed two distinct trends. First, overall performance declined as a function of increasing hearing loss, but there was a wide spread of scores for children with similar average hearing losses. For example, the scores obtained by children with average losses from 101 to 110 dB ranged from 37.5% to 84% correct. Neither aided nor unaided threshold averages provided an accurate estimate of a child's performance on the test. The mean score for the overall test for the 25 children with unaided average hearing losses greater than 90 dB was 55.75% correct, with individual scores ranging from 18.75% to 88.75%. This result again highlights the need to administer speech tests to determine the speech reception skills of individual profoundly deaf children.

The second observed trend was that the subtests which created the most difficulty were those which required the child to pick up or point to two objects (Subtests 5 and 7). There is a great deal of anecdotal evidence which indicates that many hearing-impaired people have difficulty understanding longer sentences. The task required of the child in Subtests 5 and 7 is to perceive five critical elements in each sentence. The child has to determine the motor response required, and the color and identity of the objects to be manipulated. If a child is able to perform relatively well for all but these two subtests, suggestions as to appropriate training can be made to the child's teacher. Goldberg Stout and Van Ert Windle's (1986) Developmental Approach to Successful Listening (DASL), for example, provides teachers and therapists with training exercises which gradually increase the number of critical elements in a single sentence.

The test was presented twice to 36 of the children to determine its test/retest reliability. The scores obtained in the two presentations were not significantly different. The correlation coefficient between the two presentations was found to be 0.94.

As part of a test battery for profoundly deaf children, the PLOTT Sentence Test can be used to gain a rough estimate of a child's ability to perceive sentence materials. If her/his score is 6/11 or better for the PLOTT Sentence test, the COT Test can be administered to assess the child's ability to perceive sentences of increasing complexity. If a child is able to score at a relatively high level (50% or more) the tester should consider presenting open-set sentence materials. For Australian conditions Bench, Doyle and Greenwood's (1987) adaptation of the BKB Sentences would seem to be the most suitable. They are relatively short, have an appropriate vocabulary, and use simple grammatical forms. For older children Tonisson's (1976) adaptation of the CID Everyday Sentence Lists could also be considered. Again, the information provided by this in-depth testing should prove invaluable in planning individualized training programmes.

Conclusion

The four tests presented in this overview represent a comprehensive test battery suitable for use with profoundly hearing-impaired Australian children. With relatively minor modifications they could also be adapted for use with other dialects of English. The materials used range from the detection of phonemes produced in isolation, to following complex instructions. When the project commenced, it was thought that only one test – the PLOTT Test – would be needed to provide an accurate picture of a child's speech reception skills. Within a few years, however, it became apparent that this test was too difficult for some children and quite often led to feelings of frustration for the child, parents, teachers and audiologists. A simpler test was developed to detect these children, and ensure that the testing was kept to the minimum necessary to obtain reliable results. Conversely there was a group of profoundly hearing-impaired children who were able to easily complete almost all of the subtests of the PLOTT Test. More difficult materials needed to be developed which. more accurately assessed the auditory potential of these children. Although the current test battery appears to meet the demands of these disparate groups, I have no doubt that the need to develop more and better tests will become apparent over the next few years.

Speech Tests in Aboriginal Languages

Introduction

The second part of this chapter is concerned with the development of speech tests to assess the hearing status of children with mild to moderate hearing losses.

It describes a project which was undertaken over the period 1988–1992 at Yuendumu and Nguiu in Australia's Northern Territory. The aim of the project was to develop reliable but simple-to-administer speech test materials in the languages of the communities – Warlpiri at Yuendumu and Tiwi at Nguiu. It was hoped that these tests could then be used as a screening procedure to be administered by teachers and health workers in the communities.

Mild to moderate hearing loss resulting from chronic otitis media represents a significant problem for many Aboriginal children throughout Australia. Quinn (1983), for example, reported that almost 50% of the ears of Aboriginal children in selected communities in Central Australia had an average hearing loss (at 0.5, 1 and 2 kHz) of 30 dB ISO or more. The long-term effects of such losses are not well understood, but there does seem to be 'an abundance of literature which supports the assumption that otitis-prone children are more susceptible to delays in speech-language, cognition and education' (Bess, 1985; page 43).

There are a number of reasons why speech testing should be conducted in community languages. The most obvious is that very many Aboriginal children, and this is especially true in remote communities such as Yuendumu and Nguiu, do not speak English as their first language. English is a *foreign language* and children at these, and many other communities, do not start to learn it until they enter school. Even when a child has started to learn English, the use of English speech tests may still be inappropriate. English speech tests may contain unfamiliar test items or difficult phonological contrasts. For example, neither Warlpiri nor Tiwi has consonant voicing distinctions. Thus, the Warlpiri word for man 'wati' can be realized as either [wat^{h}i] or [wadi]. Either production is acceptable and non-distinctive to a Warlpiri speaker. A 'simple' English contrast such as 'bin' vs 'pin' may prove to be extremely difficult for a Warlpiri speaker. Similarly, high frequency fricative sounds such as /s/ and /ʃ/ which are so important in English are not found in Aboriginal languages (see Dixon, Ramson and Thomas 1990 and Yallop, 1982 for excellent overviews of Aboriginal languages). Further, monosyllabic words and word final consonants do not occur in either Warlpiri or Tiwi and are rare in all Aboriginal languages, whereas monosyllabic word lists consisting of CVC words are a common speech test material in English. As a result, the score a child obtains for an English speech test may have a lot more to do with her/his English knowledge than her/his hearing status. The use of English speech tests may also prove to be very intimidating to many Aboriginal children especially if the tester is a non-Aboriginal. Finally, there is a need to recognize the *primacy* of the community language and its great social importance. The use of English speech tests in such circumstances may represent a non-too-subtle instance of *'linguistic imperialism'*.

Material collection

The first step in the development of an Aboriginal language speech test was to obtain a recorded version of a number of words in the language of the particular community. A set of 50 drawings depicting objects commonly found in or around Aboriginal communities was prepared for this purpose. These were shown one-by-one to an adult informant who spoke the community language as her/his mother tongue. The speaker was asked to name each object several times in her/his language, and these responses were recorded on high-quality audio cassette tape. Wherever possible, two speakers, one female and one male, were recorded saying each of the words. Once a recording session was completed the community's teacher/linguist or a literacy worker was asked to listen to the tape and comment on the adequacy and appropriateness of each word. They were also asked to write down each word using the accepted spelling conventions, and to note the number of syllables in the word. Although I am only presenting results for Warlpiri and Tiwi in this chapter, materials have been collected in a number of other languages. These include Eastern Aranda, North Queensland Creole and the Western Desert language.

Preparation of test materials and lists

The next step in the procedure was to select five words from each language to serve as the test items. The five words selected in a particular language had to have the same syllabic structure, but no attempt was made consciously to select items which contrasted minimal phonetic features. The words used for the Warlpiri test were the bisyllables: wati (man), parla (leaf), pingi (ant), warlu (fire) and jarlji (frog). The Tiwi test words consisted of the trisyllables miputi (fish), yikwani (fire), pijara (eye), japarra (moon) and yikara (hand).

The selected words were then computer edited using a system developed by Dermody, Katsch and Mackie (1983). The test words were equated for intensity using an Leq algorithm and test tapes were then prepared. Each test list contained 50 items, consisting of 10 quasi-random presentations of the five test words. That is, the five words were presented in blocks of five with the order within each block being randomized.

Testing using an adaptive speech test procedure

In the first part of this project (Plant, 1990) the materials were presented using a simple up–down adaptive speech threshold procedure based on that described by Mackie and Dermody (1986). The equipment used for testing consisted of:

1. An audio tape recorder with a pause control, VU meter, and provision for headphone monitoring.
2. An audiometer or a purpose built attenuator allowing the tester to raise or lower the test stimuli in 2 dB or 5 dB steps.
3. An amplifier which allowed free-field presentation of the test materials at 100 dB SPL at a distance of one metre.
4. A high quality loudspeaker.
5. A Sound Level Meter (SLM).

The child being tested was seated at a table one metre from the loudspeaker, and familiarized with the test materials. A sheet presenting clear and unambiguous pictures of the test items was placed on the table in front of the child. The advantage of only using five test words becomes obvious at this point. I was able to learn the five words in each of the languages and then present them live-voice to ensure that each child was familiar with the test items. I also found that my attempts to produce the test words tended to lessen the anxiety many children felt at being tested by a stranger. The child was asked to point at the appropriate picture after each word was said.

Once I was confident that the child was familiar with the test items and the task to be performed, the recorded test items were presented for identification. The SLM was used to measure the maximum rms level in dB SPL at the child's ear, prior to starting the test, and the first item was presented at 70 dB SPL. After the word was presented the tape was paused and the child asked to point at the appropriate picture. If the response was correct, the presentation level was decreased by 5 dB and the next word was presented. This procedure was repeated until the child made a mistake. At this point the level was increased by 5 dB and the step size reduced to 2 dB. If the child failed to respond correctly for the item presented at 70 dB SPL, the presentation level was increased in 5 dB steps until a correct response was given. Once this was achieved, the presentation level was lowered in 5 dB steps until the child again gave an incorrect response. The level was then increased by 5 dB and the step size of 2 dB was introduced.

Once the 2 dB steps were introduced, the presentation level was decreased after each item, until the child made an incorrect response.

At this point the presentation level was increased by 2 dB (the first reversal) until the child again gave a correct response. The presentation level was then decreased by 2 dB (the second reversal). A minimum of 12 reversals was obtained with each child, with the actual number being determined by the stability of the child's response pattern. Once I was satisfied that the child's response pattern was stable over at least 10 reversals, the child's Adaptive Speech Test (AST) Threshold (in dB SPL) was obtained by averaging the midpoints of the last 10 reversals. This can be taken as the 50% recognition point. To ensure test reliability the standard error of the midpoints was also calculated. This should be less than half the step size used in the testing – that is, less than 1 dB in this study.

On the same day I conducted the speech testing, pure tone audiometry was carried out with each child by an NAL audiologist. To minimize any possibility of tester bias, neither the audiologist nor I compared our respective test results until both of us had conducted our testing. Each child's Pure Tone Average (at 0.5, 1 and 2 kHz) was calculated and compared with the child's AST Threshold. For the Warlpiri testing a correlation coefficient of 0.76 was found between the two measures. When the testing was conducted in Tiwi a correlation coefficient of 0.73 was obtained.

Further testing using the AST procedure was carried out at Nguiu to compare the aided and unaided performance of children who had been fitted with radio frequency hearing aids (adapted Sony Walkmans and the Phonic Ear Easy Listener). This indicated that under normal classroom conditions the aids offered an advantage of approximately 10 dB at one metre. Additionally, it should be noted, the signal received via the radio frequency hearing aid will be relatively free of the effects of reverberation and classroom noise.

A modified screening procedure

Although the results obtained using the AST procedure were very encouraging, the method did not appear to be particularly suitable for screening purposes. It required considerable experience before the tester felt comfortable with the procedure. In the testing conducted with children at Yuendumu and Nguiu, I had noticed that the point at which children first made an error when the step size was 5 dB was very often close to their final AST Threshold. I decided to modify the procedure in the hope of arriving at a reliable measure which was relatively easy to administer. What I really wanted was a procedure that could be used by a teacher who was worried about the hearing status of a child in her/his class. The reality of life in isolated communities is that visits from audiologists are infrequent at best. Teachers may have children with a suspected loss in their classes for many months before it is finally confirmed.

The equipment and the test materials used in the modified procedure were the same as those described for the first study. The child was seated one metre from the speaker, with the paper showing the five response alternatives placed in front of her/him. Once the child was familiar with the test items and the picture pointing response task, testing was commenced. The first five items of the test tape were presented for identification at 70 dB SPL. If the child scored all items correct, the presentation level was lowered by 10 dB and the procedure repeated. If the child scored four out of five items correct (significantly above chance at the 1% level) the presentation level was reduced by only 5 dB for the next five test items. This procedure was continued (10 dB reduction for 5/5 correct and 5 dB reduction for 4/5 correct) until the materials were presented at a level which resulted in a score of 3/5 or less. The level was then raised by 5 dB and the next five items presented. If the child was able to score at least 4/5 the presentation level was decreased by 5 dB. This procedure continued until I was satisfied that I had located the lowest point at which a particular child could score at least 4/5 items correct.

Very few of the children tested failed to score at least 4/5 correct at 70 dB SPL. When this occurred, I raised the presentation level in 10 dB steps until the child was able to reach criterion (4/5 correct). Once this was attained I adopted the procedure outlined above.

As in the first study, a NAL audiologist performed pure tone audiometry with each of the children tested, using the speech test procedure. The results of the two forms of testing were not compared until both had been completed. A total of 28 children were tested using the Tiwi speech materials. This testing was carried out in approximately 4.5 hours, indicating that the procedure took only about 10 minutes per child to administer. When the lowest level at which an individual child scored at least 4/5 correct for the speech test was compared with the child's pure tone average (at 0.5, 1 and 2 kHz) a correlation coefficient of 0.91 was obtained. Similarly, testing of 50 Warlpiri children using the modified procedure yielded a correlation of 0.92 between the lowest 4/5 presentation level and pure tone average.

A final study using the modified procedure was carried out at Yuendumu. A total of 41 children were tested with the Warlpiri speech test presented via audiometric headphones. The results of this testing revealed a correlation of 0.84 between the children's lowest 4/5 level and their pure tone averages.

The future of the test procedures

The modified procedure seems to offer a simple, quick and reliable means of assessing a child's hearing, using test materials from her/his first language. The procedure is quite simple, and does not require long training for the potential tester. My experience in teaching the procedure to a number of teachers and audiologists indicated that it was possible to learn to use the procedure in about half an hour. The testing conducted using audiometric headphones indicated that the testing could be conducted using relatively simple equipment. I can envisage the development of a purpose-built screening audiometer for use in schools and health clinics. Such a device would enable teachers and health workers to screen the hearing of any children whose behaviour indicated that she or he may have a hearing problem. Once a hearing loss was confirmed by the testing some remedial steps could be immediately taken. The child could be given preferential seating in the classroom, and arrangements made for her/him to see an audiologist as quickly as possible to determine whether some form of amplification should be fitted.

Although there have been no studies investigating a possible link between fluctuating hearing losses and high rates of absenteeism in some Aboriginal community schools, there is at least some anecdotal evidence indicating that the two may be related. If they are, it is not at all surprising. Attempting to cope in noisy and reverberant classrooms must be difficult for any child with an undetected 30 dB hearing loss. Consider how much more difficult the situation must be if the language of instruction is a foreign language. It would not be surprising if a child's response to this situation was withdrawal. A reliable method of quickly detecting a child's hearing loss may help the teacher to provide the support needed to ensure that the loss does not result in classroom failure.

One important feature of the speech test procedures described is their high face validity for teachers and parents. It is quite often difficult for people to see the relationship between the detection of pure tones and speech reception. The use of speech materials allows the parent or teacher to immediately see how the hearing loss affects a child's speech reception. The use of materials in the child's home language increases the face validity of the test even further.

Much further work remains to be done in this area. The development of a simple, low cost speech audiometer would appear to be a critical need. The uses of such an audiometer would not be restricted to Aboriginal Australia. Otitis media represents a significant problem for many groups of indigenous people throughout the world. Stewart (1992) for example, reports that otitis media 'has ranked at or near the top in numbers of (medical) clinical visits' (Stewart, 1992; page 41) in Native American communities.

Materials also need to be gathered in as many Aboriginal languages as possible. It should be possible, for example, to have speech test materials in all Aboriginal languages with more than 500 speakers. The requirement of only five words from each language means that many different language tests could be stored on either audiocassette or compact disc. Compact disc would seem to have a number of advantages in this context. It is a durable medium which allows high fidelity reproduction with low noise and rapid access. Its only drawback would appear to be the cost of disc production.

Conclusion

The aim of the project was to develop a reliable and simple-to-administer hearing screening test with high face validity for use by health workers and teachers. These criteria appear to have been met using the speech test procedure outlined in this paper. If the procedure could be introduced into a number of communities, it would be possible to provide ongoing monitoring of school-age children. This would assist in the detection of children at risk for classroom failure, and allow teachers to implement appropriate remedial strategies. Such testing might also provide useful insights into any patterns of otitis media related hearing loss which will allow the development of better treatment and prevention strategies. The aim of any study in this area should be to reduce the incidence of otitis media to a minimum. Until this is achieved, however, procedures which allow the early detection of hearing loss should be introduced on a wide scale.

Acknowledgements

Many people contributed greatly to the development of the tests described in this chapter. At NAL these included Alessandra Moore, Sharan Westcott, Harvey Dillon, Greg Birtles, John Macrae, Philip Dermody, Kerry Lee, Richard Katsch, and Margaret Keogh. My sincere thanks to all of them for invaluable assistance. The speech tests in Aboriginal languages were inspired by two people greatly committed to overcoming the hearing problems confronting Aboriginal children. To Sue Quinn and Terry Nienhuys my thanks for urging me to become involved in this work and for ongoing support. Thanks are also due to Wendy Chan, Louise Skelt, Sue Brindall, Angela Hatfield, and Lew Leidwinger of NAL NT. Thanks also to the teachers, linguists, parents, and pupils of the community schools at Yuendumu and Nguiu. The chance to visit and work in these communities was inspiring and will always remain one of the highlights of my working life. Finally, thanks to Arthur Boothroyd for his valuable comments on an earlier draft of this chapter.

References

Bench, J. and Bamford, J. (1979) Speech Hearing Tests and the Spoken Language of Hearing-Impaired Children. London: Academic Press.

Bench, J., Doyle, J. and Greenwood, K.M. (1987) A standardisation of the BKB/A sentence test for children in comparison with the NAL-CID sentence test and the CAL-PBM word list. Australian Journal of Audiology 9: 39–48.

Bess, F. (1985) The minimally hearing-impaired child. Ear and Hearing 6: 43–7.

Dermody, P., Katsch, R. and Mackie, K. (1983) Amplitude equalisation techniques for use in word identification speech perception studies. In Cohen, A. and Broecke, M.P.R.v.d.(Eds) Abstracts of the 10th International Congress of Phonetic Sciences. Dordrecht Foris.

Dixon, R.M.W., Ramson, W.S. and Thomas, M. (1990) Australian Aboriginal Words in English. Melbourne: Oxford University Press.

Erber, N.P. (1980) Use of the Auditory Numbers Test to evaluate speech perception abilities of hearing-impaired children. Journal of Speech and Hearing Disorders 45: 527–32.

Erber, N.P. and Alencewicz, C.M. (1976) Audiological evaluation of deaf children. Journal of Speech and Hearing Disorders 41: 256–67.

Goldberg Stout, G. and Van Ert Windle, J. (1986) The Developmental Approach to Successful Listening (DASL). Developmental Approach to Successful Listening, Houston.

Mackie, K. and Dermody, P. (1986) Use of the monosyllabic adaptive speech test (MAST) with young children. Journal of Speech and Hearing Research. 29: 275–81.

Plant, G. (1990) The development of speech tests in Aboriginal languages. Australian Journal of Audiology (1984) A diagnostic speech test for severely and profoundly hearing-impaired children. Australian Journal of Audiology 6: 1–9.

Plant, G. and Macrae, J.H. (1985) An analysis of Plott Test results obtained with 100 hearing-impaired children. Paper presented at the NAL Hearing Aid Conference, Lindfield.

Plant, G. and Moore, A. (1992a) Two speech discrimination tests for profoundly hearing-impaired children. Australian Journal of Audiology 14: 28–40.

Plant, G. and Moore, A. (1992b) The Common Objects Token (COT) Test: A sentence test for profoundly hearing-impaired children. Australian Journal of Audiology 14: 76–83.

Plant, G. and Moore, A. (1993) The Plott Screening Test and the Plott Sentence Test. Australian Hearing Services, Sydney.

Plant, G. and Westcott, C.S. (1982) A speech intelligibility test for deaf children. Paper presented at the Audiological Society of Australia Conference, Leura.

Plant, G. and Westcott, C.S. (1983) The Plott Test. NAL, Sydney.

Thielmeir, M.A., Tonokawa, L.L., Petersen, B. and Eisenberg, L.S. (1985) Audiological results in children with a cochlear implant. Ear and Hearing 6(Supplement): 27S–35S.

Quinn, S. (1983) Aboriginal hearing loss and ear disease in the Australian Northern Territory. Australian Journal of Audiology 5: 41–6.

Stewart, J.L. (1992) Native American populations. ASHA 40–2.

Tonisson, W. (1976) Australian standardisation of the CID Everyday Sentence Lists. Proceeding of the Second National Conference of the Audiological Society of (1982) Australian Aboriginal Languages. London: Andre Deutsch.

18

What Makes a Skilled Speechreader?

JERKER RÖNNBERG

Introduction

In this chapter the term speechreading is used to indicate that visual speech perception is not only a matter of reading lips; it often involves perception of accompanying facial expressions and body language. Speechreading may also be combined with other types of sensory information: acoustic input from residual hearing (Summerfield, 1987), tactual stimulation (Plant, 1992), or electrical stimulation of the cochlea (Blamey and Cowan, 1992).

The general argument of this chapter is that many of the successes and failures in rehabilitation with sensory aids for adventitiously hard-of-hearing and deaf adults can be traced to (a) individual variations in the cognitive architecture underlying speechreading skill, (b) how effectively the speech signal can be picked up and processed by the cognitive system, and (c) how effectively the individual capitalizes on contextual and social constraints. This area is relatively neglected in speech and hearing sciences. This chapter attempts to introduce and remedy some of these problems.

In common with chess playing, wine tasting, and downhill skiing, everyday observation suggests that there are many levels of skill in speechreading. For many speechreaders, however, speechreading is often difficult and attention-demanding. There are ample reasons for this state of affairs. These include; (a) Phoneme visibility is low (Dodd, 1977; Jeffers and Barley, 1977; Woodward and Barber, 1960), (b) the roles of vision in speech perception are of a relatively automatic nature (e.g., fusion illusions; McGurk and McDonald, 1976) and have been observed in early childhood (Massaro, 1987), constraining the ways in which visual information can be used by the speechreader, and (c) speechreading is an 'on-line' rather than 'off-line' communicative form, and hence, more time-pressured. Despite these constraints, there exist cases of extreme speechreading skill.

The purpose of this chapter is to address the problem of speechreading skill from a cognitive perspective, with particular reference to the architecture underlying the skill. To this end, three issues are discussed, primarily with reference to data from our laboratory, but the general results and conclusions are also evaluated in the light of other pertinent studies. The issues are:

1. Do adventitiously hard-of-hearing or deaf adults compensate for their hearing loss by becoming better speechreaders compared to matched normal-hearing controls, or do they improve in cognitive abilities that are important to the skill?
2. What are the main components in the cognitive architecture underlying general speechreading skill, and how do they relate to each other?
3. What is the architecture behind cases of extreme speechreading skill?

The general discussion is concerned with speechreading from the perspective of working memory, with particular emphasis on the role played by phonology. The chapter concludes by addressing the clinical consequences of these findings.

Compensation

The general theoretical description of the speechreading process that we assumed as the point of departure for our initial series of studies took the following form. During speechreading (visual or audiovisual), fragments of a message must be decoded and temporarily stored, simultaneously, with successive decoding of new information. At a given point, the fragments are used for inference-making/interpretation of the message. The understanding of a message is also governed by social premises for communication (Rönnberg and Lyxell, 1986).

From this description we hypothesized that speechreaders who had been hearing-impaired for a large part of their adult lives would compensate spontaneously by becoming more skilled than matched controls. The simple and straightforward rationale was that the daily dependence on speechreading in a variety of social situations would lead to improved speechreading skills. However, in a series of experimental studies by me and my colleagues (Lyxell and Rönnberg, 1989; Rönnberg, Öhngren and Nilsson, 1982; 1983; Rönnberg, 1990), we have found no evidence to substantiate the claim that adventitiously hearing-impaired individuals compensate for their hearing loss by becoming better speechreaders. This held true irrespective of test materials (digits, words, or sentences), test form (live vs recorded materials), average hearing loss and 'handicap age'. It has also been shown, in a recent study of subjects' ability to follow conversation in various kinds of noise, that the benefit of speechreading support, measured in gains in signal-to-noise ratio, is constant across normal-hearing and hearing-impaired subjects (Hygge *et al.*, 1992).

In summary: we have not seen any systematic signs of spontaneous compensation in speechreading skill for adventitiously hard-of-hearing and deaf adults (see also Cowie and Douglas-Cowie, 1992; Mogford, 1987). It should be noted, however, that the lack of compensation refers to average group performance, not to skill variability within each group. Typically, this variation around the mean group performance is larger for deafened adults than normal-hearing controls. This suggests that there are a few very skilled individuals and a few individuals with very little skill in each group of deafened adults. As such, this constitutes interesting information from an individual difference perspective and this will be addressed later in the chapter.

Although speechreading skill seems *generally* unrelated to various aspects of impairment, there is another possible route to compensation, viz., if the adventitiously hearing-impaired adult compensates via perceptual and cognitive components that underlie various aspects of the skill. Again, there is no support for such an hypothesis. Lyxell and Rönnberg (1987a) demonstrated that both speechreading skill and various indices of cognitive function, such as word- and sentence completion, working memory, and vocabulary, did not differ between an adult hearing-impaired and a matched normal-hearing group. In those cases where compensation has been found for cognitive testing in deafened adults, for example for visual short-term memory (Rönnberg and Nilsson, 1982, 1987; Rönnberg *et al.*, 1982) and for linguistic abstraction (Rönnberg, Öhngren and Lyxell, 1987), this cognitive compensation has not been proven to mediate speechreading skill. There is one deviation from the pattern. It seems that deafened adults' internal speech functions (cf. Conrad, 1979) deteriorate significantly compared to a control group, which in its turn is associated with lower levels of speechreading performance (Lyxell, Rönnberg and Samuelsson, 1994). But the general conclusion still holds true: neither speechreading skill nor cognitive compensations potentially relevant to *improve* the skill seem to develop with long periods of hearing loss in adults.

Accepting the null hypothesis that no compensation exists puts extra demands on the variety of research efforts that must be undertaken to convince the critic. To accomplish this, we have in another, but related, line of research studied the potential impact of facial expressions, body language, and emotional content on the intelligibility of speechread messages (Johansson and Rönnberg, in press 1993). This set of variables is interesting because it adds information to an already difficult perceptual task. It also represents information which is naturally present in everyday conversation.

However, the results give no indication as to any systematic effects of facial expression (Johansson and Rönnberg, in press) or body-language (Johansson and Rönnberg, 1993) on speechreadability. What is important is the emotional content of the message and how it is related to the scenario/script in which it is embedded (e.g. Schank and Abelson, 1977). For example, 'sad' messages (obtained via ratings) within the cognitive script of a 'visit-to-a-doctor', and 'happy' messages within the script of a 'visit-to-a-restaurant' optimize performance, whereas the reverse is not true. This demonstrates that predictability of actions within a cognitive script has a more powerful effect on speechreadability than emotional content or emotional expressions as such. Emotionally neutral messages that are *typical* of a particular script are the most powerful (Johansson and Rönnberg, in press; Samuelsson and Rönnberg, 1991). Thus, this set of data suggests to us that one very important reason why deafened adults do not compensate by becoming better speechreaders is that the information that might be potentially useful such as facial expression and body language is subordinated to content and script – and scripts are important to cognitive processing of speechread information (Samuelsson and Rönnberg, 1991, 1993).

Nevertheless, facial expression and body language do seem to play another equally important role in speech communication. Instead of improving speechreadability per se, facial expression and gestures seem to make message perception easier in that accompanying exralinguistic gestures make the process less attention demanding (Lyxell *et al.*, 1993). From a disability perspective, consumption of attentional resources might be as handicapping as a lack of ability to speechread efficiently. The fact that subjective and objective aspects of communicative competence can be dissociated (cf. Johansson, Rönnberg and Lyxell, 1991), and the fact that extralinguistic gestures affect the subjective, but not the objective aspect of communication, must be taken seriously in evaluating compensatory and rehabilitative efforts (for example, Binnie, 1977).

Finally, there is yet another possibility where compensation can be detected. The individual might have developed another speechreading strategy. The hearing-impaired adult might, for example, evidence a greater sensitivity to visual cues. However, the net effect of this qualitative change in coding strategy (from audiovisual to visual) may prove to be zero. Even though visual (molecular) skills have improved, it does not necessarily imply an improvement in the overall (molar) skill of speechreading (Salthouse, 1987). The reason is that a greater skill in utilizing visual cues per se is counteracted because visual segmental and suprasegmental information are less informative than auditory. Another way of expressing this strategic shift is that it can also be associated with less accurate phonological representations of the observed speech. In partial support of this tenet, Lyxell and Rönnberg (1991a,

1991b) have obtained evidence to suggest that visual word discrimination, involving skill in matching of visual features of two spoken words, does not predict performance in sentence-based speechreading tasks. But, the qualitative change in strategy may provide hints as to how to adjust a sensory aid for an individual, and thus open the way for quantitative improvements and compensation.

In summary: it has been argued that spontaneous compensation in speechreading skill does not occur with adult acquired hearing loss. Although we are now prepared to accept this important null hypothesis, we want to caution that the results do not exclude the possibility that compensation may be discerned in terms of subjective improvements, or by means of qualitative, strategic changes.

Cognitive Architecture: the General Case

These results have more or less forced us to accept the possibility that very little of the (quantitative) variation in speechreading skill can be predicted by impairment-related factors, or by particular psychological compensations induced by the impairment. Instead, a cognitive individual-difference approach to speechreading has been advocated to account for skill variations. The cognitive tests were operationalized with the aforementioned theoretical description of the speechreading process as the point of departure (Rönnberg and Lyxell, 1986). The classes of cognitive tests that seemed to match this general description were: short-term/working memory tests (cf. 'fragments...decoded and temporarily stored, simultaneously, with...'); decoding/discrimination tests ('a message must be decoded'); guessing/inference-making and vocabulary tests ('at a given point in time, the fragments are used for verbal inference-making/interpretation'). In addition, we assumed that various aspects of information-processing speed, notably lexical access speed, would constitute an important component (Hunt, 1985). These were the main classes of tests used in the initial stage of this second phase of our research. The tests are briefly summarized and explained in Table 1 (For greater detail, see Rönnberg et al., 1989).

The results of our different studies indicated that the following picture of predictors of sentence-based speechreading are found with both hearing-impaired and normal-hearing subjects (Figure 1).

In Figure 1, each 'cloud' represents a conceptual 'cloud' which can be operationalized in various ways. The arrows are not causal, rather they suggest structural relations. Our results indicate that there are three *direct* predictors of speechreading skill. Decoding ability and information-processing speed are most important for the population as a whole (Lyxell, 1989; Lyxell and Rönnberg, 1991a, 1991b; Lyxell et al., 1993, in press; Rönnberg, 1990), and are generalizable to different speechreading conditions. Verbal inference-making/guessing ability is

Table 1. Summary description of a core set of tests used

Test	Measurement objective
Speechreading tests	In general, the tests intend to measure individual differences in speechreading with different levels of contextual support.
Context-bound speechreading	The subjects' ability to speechread sentences with varying length and with different levels of contextual support.
Context-free word discrimination test	The subjects' ability to correctly discriminate between lipped words in a context-free word pair as being either similar or dissimilar.
Context-free word decoding test	The subjects' ability to correctly identify the second word, given that the first was audiovisually presented. Naming is required.
Guessing/inference - making tests	In general, the tests intend to measure individual differences in guessing/inference-making with different levels of contextual support, under time pressure.
Sentence completion test	The subjects' ability to fill in (guess/infer) missing words in a sentence, presented with a contextual frame and a contextual cue.
Word completion test	The subjects' ability to fill in (guess/infer) missing letters in a word, presented without a contextual frame.
Vocabulary	The subjects' ability to choose one of four alternatives that constituted a synonym/antonym to each of 70 target items, under time pressure.
Information processing speed *Long - term memory access tests*	In general, the tests intend to measure individual differences in speed of retrieving different kinds of information from long-term memory by means of different judgements.
Physical matching	The subjects' ability to match two letters as being similar or dissimilar in physical shape.
Name matching	The subjects' ability to match two letters as having the same or a different name.
Lexical access	The subjects' ability to decide whether or not a string of letters constitutes a real word.
Semantic access	The subjects' ability to decide whether or not a presented word belongs to a predefined category of words.
Rehearsal operation speed Asymptote	The asymptote (i.e., the middle section) in the serial position curve in free recall of words is assumed to reflect rehearsal operation speed.

Table 1. (Contd)

Short-term/working memory tests	In general, the tests intend to measure individual differences in short-term/working memory tasks of different complexity.
Digit span	The subjects' ability to recall a string of digits in the correct serial order.
Word span	The subjects' ability to recall a string of words in the correct serial order.
Reading span	The subjects' ability to read and comprehend a sequence of short sentences, and to recall the final word of each presented sentence in the correct serial order.
Recency	The subjects' ability to recall the last four words in a list of 12 words irrespective of order.

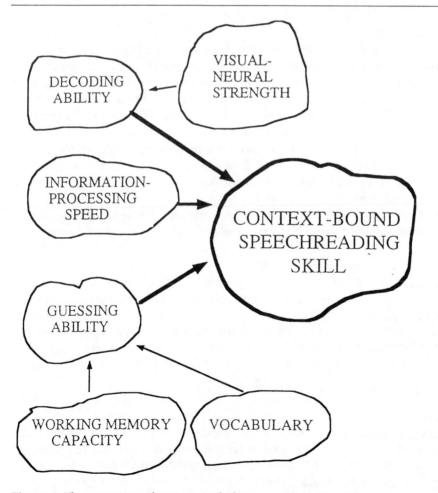

Figure 1. The cognitive architecture underlying speechreading skill.

important in specific situations such as when contextual support is relatively low (Lyxell and Rönnberg, 1987b, 1989).

At a more detailed test level, the results are most prominent when the decoding task triggers lexical activation, mediated by a phonological access route (Rönnberg, 1987; Öhngren, 1992), as opposed to mere visual discrimination of lip movements (Lyxell and Rönnberg, 1991a). Recoding from the visual perception of lip movements to an inner auditory or phonological representation may be achieved in different ways (i.e., audiovisual priming of visual decoding, Lyxell and Rönnberg, 1991a; visual-tactile decoding, Lyxell *et al.*, 1993; Öhngren, 1992). The putative speed component is especially important when text-based reaction-time tasks emphasize lexical and semantic access speed as opposed to physical and name matching (Lyxell, 1989; Rönnberg, 1987, 1990), and, when verbal inference-making is operationalized by a sentence completion test rather than a word completion test, it represents a more relevant skill promoting sentence-based speechreading (Lyxell and Rönnberg, 1989).

Indirectly important predictors of sentence-based speechreading are as follows. (a) The VN 130/P200 peak-to-peak amplitude measure in the visual evoked potential which is related to word decoding. This suggests that the strength of a short-lived visual-neural memory trace plays a role (Rönnberg *et al.*, 1989). (b) Working memory, especially the dual reading span task, constitutes an important measure of storage and processing capacity necessary for inference-making/guessing (Lyxell and Rönnberg, 1989). (c) The ability to solve synonyms/antonyms also represents an important prerequisite for guessing (Rönnberg, 1987; see also Lyxell and Rönnberg, 1992).

In two discriminant analyses, one aimed at discriminating skilled from less skilled speechreaders, and one which aimed to discriminate old (mean = 62 years) from young (mean = 37 years), Rönnberg (1990) discovered that there was an interesting communality in that both analyses involved word decoding and one speed measure as significant predictors (i.e., the asymptote, assumed to reflect rehearsal operation speed) among a large set of cognitive predictors. Summarizing much of the earlier research, for example, a study showing that skilled speechreaders rely heavily on the initial phoneme in word decoding (Lyxell and Rönnberg, 1991a), it was concluded that (a) an age-dependent model of speechreading must take as a point of departure the argument that a temporally early lexical access system is crucial to decoding (cf. Marslen-Wilson, 1987), and (b) a high rate of rehearsal operations represents a further aspect important to the bottom-up character of the task. The general suggestion was that (a) and (b) converge on a basic cognitive speed function that will be troublesome for the old speechreader (Salthouse, 1985).

In summary: what is clear from a cognitive analysis of speechreading skill is that it represents a multicomponential skill not predicted by a single predictor, nor by a simple structure of direct predictors (cf. De Filippo, 1982; Gailey, 1987). As a rule of thumb, low-level processes such as decoding and speed (or simply general speed) account for twice as much of the variance in a sentence-based speechreading criterion compared to high-level processes (i.e., guessing and working memory). Old speechreaders are facing the challenge of mastering a communicative form which demands cognitive resources that typically are very sensitive to chronological age: cognitive speed (Salthouse, 1985).

Cognitive Architecture: the Extreme Case

Given this set of background data, I will now turn to the issue of *extreme* speechreading skill. I will briefly present the cases of three subjects who vary in their approaches to communication, but all are very skilled speechreaders. They have been tested using our cognitive test battery (see Table 1) and on several speechreading tests.

Case 1: GS

GS is a 54-year-old male (for details, see Rönnberg, 1993a). He holds a masters degree in biochemistry and works at University of Uppsala, Sweden. GS was deafened by meningitis at the age of 8 years. His hearing loss is complete for the frequencies 125–4000 Hz (Plant and Spens, 1986). His communication method, Tactiling, involves placing the hand on the shoulder of the talker with the thumb on the neck, combining this information with speechreading. Using this method, he outperforms controls by a factor of two to three in a sentence-based task (Lyxell and Rönnberg, 1989) and in speech tracking (De Filippo and Scott, 1978). In low-level speech perception tasks, such a visual consonant discrimination (Öhngren, Kassling and Risberg, in press), he is, in a relative sense, less proficient.

Cognitive testing reveals that, compared to an age-matched control, GS is outstanding in a complex working memory task (i.e., reading span), whereas for simpler forms of short-term memory testing (i.e., recency, digit and word span) he performs within normal ranges, his ability to make verbal inferences in sentence completion is extremely good, and his access speed from long-term memory is normal (Rönnberg, 1993a). GS appears to excel in the ability to store and process information in working memory, as assessed by the more complex 'high-level' reading span test. This implies that his cognitive capacity is optimal for dealing with large meaningful linguistic units simultaneously in working memory. Taken together with other performance characteristics of GS, it is quite reasonable that verbal inference-making and complex working memory capacity are mutually dependent, constituting cognitive prerequisites for an information-processing strategy aimed at Tactiling and inferencing larger chunks of meaningful information.

This strategy seems to presuppose that the information provided by Tactiling, combined with perception of lip movements, patterns the speech information in a way which is compatible with chunking. The prosody of speech serves this suprasegmental and global function. In the same way that auditory presentation of fundamental frequency greatly aid speechreading (Risberg and Lubker, 1978), it can be argued that tactiling as well as technical tactile aids built on this premise are effective speechreading supplements (Öhngren, 1992; Öhngren et al.., in press; Öhngren, Rönnberg and Lyxell, 1992). Therefore, efficient Tactiling seems to presuppose a perceptual platform for ongoing speech which builds on an effective complementarity of the two streams of sensory information (Summerfield, 1987).

Case 2: SJ

SJ is 56-year-old female engineer (for details see Lyxell, 1994). She became deaf at the age of 14 following meningitis. Audiometric testing reveals no response to sound for the test frequencies 125 to 4000 Hz. She is one of the most skilled speechreaders in a database of 119 subjects (Rönnberg, 1990). She uses a particular speechreading strategy where she attempts to silently mouth the talker's message; she also uses pauses to summarize what has been said and to infer what has not been perceived. Using this method, she outperforms her controls by a factor of two in both sentence-based speechreading and in speech tracking, whereas her visual decoding skill is within normal range. In common with GS, SJ demonstrates a robust superiority for complex working memory functions, as well as a superior rehearsal speed (indexed by the asymptote; Salthouse, 1980), which very well matches her speech perception strategy. SJ also performs relatively, but non-significantly, higher than controls on verbal inference-making (Lyxell, 1994).

Case 3: MJ

MJ is a 25-year-old female who works as a pre-school teacher for deaf children (for details, see Rönnberg, 1993b). Her average hearing loss (at 500, 1000 and 2000 Hz in the better ear), is 50 dB ISO. She is fluent in Swedish sign language, as assessed by standardized tests, has normal speech production, and is extremely proficient in speechreading. MJ performs at ceiling on a range of decoding, sentence-based and discourse-based speechreading tests. Cognitive testing revealed that *only* her complex working memory function, as assessed by the reading span test, was significantly better than controls.

In sum: the results from the three case studies generalize across communicative form and strategic habits. All three subjects demonstrate a robust superiority for complex working memory functions (i.e., the reading span test), whereas simpler forms of short-term memory and speed indices were not significant for any of the three cases. Thus, the general importance of central information processing in working memory and its potential reliance on phonological recoding (cf. the phonological loop, Baddeley, 1990), has led us to expand on and apply the concept of working memory to speechreading (cf. Baddeley *et al.*, 1985).

General Discussion

Extreme speechreading skill is dependent on higher order cognitive functions such as complex verbal working memory. Although lower order functions (i.e., processing speed and decoding) are important in the general case, these components are not as prominent in extreme cases of speechreading skill. There may, therefore, be a threshold as to what can be extracted from the speech signal per se, and the speed with which the lexicon is accessed. Given that these thresholds are reached, a further improvement of speechreading skill must be accounted for by higher order cognitive functions. The inference that can be made from the data presented above on extreme speechreading skill is that complex working memory seems to serve this function. Having a capacious working memory is assumed to help the speechreader by (a) having capacity freed for predicting what is to come in a dialogue, and (b) by having a larger capacity for maintaining previously encountered stimuli/contextual information in an active state, and hence being able to disambiguate speech information retrospectively in the light of new information.

There are some other independent data that attest to the involvement of working memory. Primacy effects are small in speechreading, as opposed to heard word list recall, which may be taken as an indication that working memory is fully occupied with the business of decoding and interpreting lipped speech. Because of this there is not enough capacity freed for engaging in rehearsal operations typically ascribed to account for primacy (Rundus, 1971). Also, inference-making based on lipread short passages was less effective compared to auditory presentation, again suggesting that less capacity in working memory may be deployed for inferencing, rather than decoding (Cowie and Douglas-Cowie, 1992; see also Gailey, 1987).

To the extent that working memory is important both to the skill in general, and to extreme skill in particular, it seems here appropriate to develop and apply the concept of working memory to speechreading. The general idea, which will be defended by independent and our own data, is that in a dialogue or in speech perception tasks like speech tracking, the general capacity of working memory may never be fully realized unless phonological recoding runs smoothly. That is, the recoding process can to varying degrees interfere with, and thus, compete for resources from the ongoing higher level predictions and disambiguation. Three roles of phonology in working memory will be discussed.

In research on the acquisition of reading skill, the role of phonology (in working memory) is typically ascribed to the accessing of lexical or sublexical units (Wagner and Torgesen, 1987). In the following discussion of speechreading, phonology is assumed to be important both to the lexical and supralexical level (i.e., access to scripts). It will also be argued that phonology is a necessary means of recoding during speechreading, and that there is no efficient direct visual to lexical route, as has been argued for adult reading of simple text (Crowder, 1982).

Phonology (or internal speech) is a recoding strategy of speechread items

This statement draws partly on evidence from the suffix-effect in short-term memory, where it can be shown that in recall of a list of items the last items are better recalled (i.e., the recency effect), and where the addition of an immediately following sound (i.e., the suffix) abolishes recency (Crowder and Morton, 1969). Interestingly, suffix effects are present with both mouthed and silently lipread stimuli in normal listeners (Campbell and Dodd, 1980; Greene and Crowder, 1984); concurrent articulation during recall does not show a selective effect when heard and lipread lists are compared (Campbell and Dodd, 1984), and digit span performance is also similar comparing the two presentation modes (Campbell, 1990). At a general level, the memory representations that mediate lipread and heard short-term memory phenomena are phonetic-phonological (cf. McClelland and Elman, 1986) and prelexical in nature. Campbell (1990) suggests in some detail how the phenomena can be interpreted within a structured system of reciprocally connected components (phonetic/phonological input/output and lexical processors) that maintain particular states of activation. Campbell's (1990) general approach to interpreting speech fits with our general notion of working memory in that the speechreader's task is to maintain decoded information (a certain state of activation) for both prospective and retrospective purposes.

One other type of evidence and argument as to why phonological recoding of speechreading items seems to be the case, might derive from the complementary nature of manner and place of articulation on the one hand, and visual and auditory speech perception in noise on the other (Summerfield, 1987). That is, features that can be seen on the lips (place of articulation) are more affected than those features which are not accessible by lipreading alone (manner of articulation). Based on these constraints, it seems reasonable to argue that phonological processing is optimized when audiovisual complementarity is optimized. This is probably also the reason why speechreading is enhanced when F0 information is provided either auditorily or tactually (Risberg and Lubker, 1978; Öhngren, 1992), or, when the lipreader has a strategy which is aimed at optimizing complementarity, for example in the case of SJ, she obviously is 'phonologizing' visible speech explicitly (Lyxell, 1994).

At a more general level, it can also be argued that for communicative forms where stimuli are to a greater or lesser degree degraded, distorted or ambiguous, such as in speechreading, phonology is relatively more important than for example in reading of print. One of the reasons for this is that there is no simple means of conceptualizing an efficient and automatized pattern recognition system based on lip movements which at the kinematic level can specify vocal gestures uniquely. The dynamic variation of lip movements, within individuals and across individuals, and the effects of coarticulation and context, are simply too complex to handle within a pattern recognition system.

For reading of print, however, Crowder (1982) suggests that lexical access is mediated by an abstract phonological representation once a word has been encountered during reading. Here, automatization is quite possible because, typically, print is unambiguous and static. There is the possibility that lexical access may be direct, at least for familiar words (cf. Hardyk and Petrinovitch, 1970). Hence, lexical access is quite possible without even having to deploy working memory resources; working memory and phonological recoding will only become important in the sense that it aids the overall functions of resolving anaphoric referents in discourse by maintaining order of items, by maintaining contextual information to anticipate events, etc.

Phonology is important for continuous accessing of lexical items in working memory

For speechread words in a sentence, which can be accessed directly with only a low probability when out of script context (Samuelsson and Rönnberg, 1991), phonological processing will place a heavy, but necessary, burden on working memory. Unless phonological recoding is accomplished by some means, pattern recognition and lexical access will suffer. That is, phonologically based lexical access is assumed to become a continuous process in working memory (cf. Öhngren, 1992).

Lyxell, Rönnberg and Andersson (1993) suggest that when at least one word in a rhyme task is a non-word, speed of executing rhyme judgements is significantly correlated with both decoding and sentence-based speechreading among deafened adults. Hence, speed and relatively pure estimates of phonology are important prerequisites for the deafened adult. For speech tracking (De Filippo and Scott, 1978), speed is relatively less important, but accurate phonological representations become more prominent. This may be understood on the grounds that, in tracking, the subject can control the rate of speech input, but in sentence-based speechreading the speed demand becomes a focal prerequisite (Rönnberg, 1990).

More general support for this thesis stems, of course, from Conrad's (1979) data, where acoustic confusions in working memory represented an operationalization of internal speech, and where presence or absence of internal speech predicts speechreading skill. What can be seen from our data is that speed and accuracy in phonology play different roles in different speechreading tasks, but that some aspect of phonology is always important. If it were possible to automatize this word decoding process, as it is for reading of print, working memory would be relatively relieved of its burden. This seems rather unlikely, as most data do not lend support to the notion that speech recognition during speechreading can be substantially improved as a function of everyday practice. Again, the problem is one of pattern recognition from dynamic variations in lip movements.

Phonological patterning of the speech signal serves the overall purpose of accessing global, implicit knowledge of the communicative situation

This implies that suprasegmental information such as syllabic stress, word emphasis and intonation directs accessing of information to larger and more abstract, supralexical packages of information stored in the memory of the perceiver, for example to the script (telling the speechreader that the sentence to be speechread involves ordering something at a restaurant; Samuelsson and Rönnberg, 1991; 1993). This possibility compensates for the previously noted potential conflict between points (1) and (2): On one hand the argument is that phonological recoding is a necessary means of accessing the lexical and semantic information during visual speech processing. On the other hand, a continuous phonological recoding places an interfering, but necessary, burden on working memory. The net effect of comparing a visual speechreading strategy with a more phonologically based strategy may therefore be zero.

However, as hypothesized, this can be compensated for if phonological structuring of the visual input provides a means of accessing that knowledge which is most conducive to speech processing; here denoted implicit knowledge. Implicit knowledge structures are characterized by scriptual information which is abstract and typical (cf. Abbot, Black and Smith, 1985; Galambos, 1986). Across different contextual variations, implicit structures are on average more facilitative of the speechreading process; they may also represent those conditions where speechreading skill variations are most prominent (Samuelsson and Rönnberg, 1991, 1993). Thus, working memory is assumed to operate most efficiently with implicit knowledge structures. The main reason is that implicit structures are more predictable and therefore demand less maintenance of information in working memory. And, the accessing of implicit knowledge is assumed to covary with the individual's phonological ability to perceive the rhythm, intonation and stress patterns of the speech signal.

This last conjecture connects well with other types of results. If, instead of patterning the visual, speechread signal by some auditory means, for example auditory F0, heard speech is patterned by means of seeing it, then there is the interesting effect that more cognitively demanding text can be disambiguated (Reisberg, McLean and Goldfield, 1987). Adding lipreading to heard speech may also be useful for some patients with phonological disorders or to patients with cortical deafness (Campbell, 1990). This suggests that lipreading can serve as an extra source of phonetic information which triggers a rather abstract phonological processor. The assumption here is that the processor is abstract and modality-independent; its function can also be triggered by added tactile, laryngeal information (Öhngren, 1992). Possibly, what are perceived are the articulatory dynamics of speech (Studdert-Kennedy, 1983), not its kinematics (cf. Baddeley and Wilson, 1985). Thus, seeing voices (Reisberg et al., 1987) as well as touching voices (Rönnberg, 1993a; Öhngren, 1992) both represent sources of information that contribute to more efficient higher order processing of messages. The general point is that the abstract phonological processor is assumed to interact with the semantic system in a way that capitalizes on implicit packages of knowledge, stored in the perceiver's memory system. This interaction will presumably unload working memory.

To take matters a further, final step before concluding this section, it seems relevant to point out that in a study of perception of connected discourse, by means of sign language, speechreading (seeing plus hearing the speaker), and listening, regional cerebral blood flow patterns were very similar when speechreading and signing conditions were compared (Söderfeldt, Rönnberg and Risberg, 1994; Rönnberg, Söderfeldt and Risberg, 1991). As long as there is a visual component involved, processing of visual languages engages posterior parts of the temporal lobes bilaterally as well as left sylvian areas to a much larger extent than listening. Speculatively, sign language, or some simpler form thereof, may from an evolutionary perspective have been primary, and hence, as a first mode of communication become neurally coupled to lexical-semantic interpretation. This argument would resolve the potential conflict with the fact that these temporal areas traditionally are seen as an auditory association cortex (Seldon, 1985). Given the previous argument with respect to abstract phonology, there is no reason to argue otherwise for sign language. Instead of phonemes that combine to form words, signed languages form signs on the basis of, for example, varying hand configurations, types of arm movements, and facial expressions (Poizner and Kegl, 1992).

To sum up: prospective and retrospective functions of working memory are important for a communicative form such as speechreading. Three aspects of the role of phonology in working memory, as applied to speechreading, have been delineated and discussed. They can be summarized in the following way: (a) Unless speechread information is phonologically recoded, (b) it will not effectively access the lexicon, and (c), it will not unload working memory in the sense that implicit script processing is favoured.

Some Clinical Suggestions

As can be inferred from the data presented on compensation, speechreading training as such does not seem to provide a generally viable avenue to success. After all, the information provided via the visual speech signal and by accompanying gestures is relatively poor, unless complemented with other types of information. And, the empirical picture on this topic is not a success story (Lyxell, 1989).

This does not, of course, exclude the possibility that some individuals may benefit from speechreading training. The potential utility of a tailor-made training programme is assumed to depend on the following rationale: The cognitive architecture of the individual sets constraints on training efficacy. The general assumption is that whenever different aspects of low-level processing such as speed and decoding are involved, and when they do not meet at least some threshold value, the probability of obtaining practice effects is small. This assumption rests on the argument that there is at least some credibility to the claim that such low-level processes are modular in nature (Fodor, 1983; Lyxell and Rönnberg, 1991a), hence representing more obligatory, neurobiologically determined, and from, central processes, encapsulated information processing. Speed and decoding are also most affected by cognitive ageing (Rönnberg, 1990; Salthouse, 1985). Combined, the suggestion is that for adventitiously hearing-impaired adults most room for strategic improvement is to be found in higher order cognitive skills, given that the perceptual input has passed some minimal threshold.

Our suggestion is, that selecting out patients on these grounds would potentially prove to be more cost-effective and psychologically appropriate.

Should training prove to be inefficient, the following logical scheme can be used to improve fitting and training with sensory aids. The scheme is based on the possibility that computerized testing procedures for low-level and high-level cognitive predictors are available (Ausmeel, 1988). From the foregoing, it can be concluded that a minimal test battery should at least assess decoding, phonological (relatively abstract) and working memory capacities. The point to be made is that both decoding and phonology can be viewed as a perceptual–cognitive bottleneck in the whole information-processing system, against which high-level cognitive processing and rehabilitation efforts with a sensory aid could be organized and conceived. It will be important to distinguish four cases, two of which are unambiguous with respect to implementation, and two of which are somewhat debatable.

The first two cases are represented by consistency in assessment across both high- and low-level predictors. When performance on standardized word decoding and phonological recoding tests is below normal, and when this also holds true for working memory, the speechreader would appear to be in a difficult position. In such a case, coping with the impairment must be seen from a broader perspective than the communicative skill per se. His or her cognitive architecture does not allow for efficient rehabilitation with a sensory aid. The second case is also conceptually simple, in that performance on the minimal test battery is at or above normal for each of the main predictors. The profile gives good ground for expecting that the implementation of, and training with a sensory aid should show significant gains – and, given that the aid optimizes phonological recoding (such as the Tactilator), a very high communicative competence could be expected.

In addition to this, we know from reading research that metaphonological skills in kindergarten are important to the development of reading skills in the first years of school (Lundberg, Frost and Petersen, 1988). By extrapolation, this aspect of phonology might serve as a predictor of a child's ability to take advantage of sensory aids designed to improve speech understanding–and, which are based on the premise that recruitment of inner speech is a prerequisite for phonological recoding with the aid. Our guess is that for speechreading, more global metaphonological skills such as rhyming are important, at least initially (Öhngren, 1992), whereas more analytical skills predict reading skill (i.e., phonemic segmentation; Lundberg *et al.*, 1988).

If, however, high- and low-level performances do not match, as is true for the two remaining cases, the implementation strategy of sensory aids is not as clear cut. When low-level processing seems to be at or above threshold, we would still be inclined to suggest a period of training with a sensory aid. This is because the bottleneck of information processing is surpassed, and also because higher-level processing is presumably easier to modify with training. The final case, when higher-order processing seems to be at or above normal level, but where low-level processing is below normal, is tricky. As input through speechreading generally is too poor, working memory based predictions may be totally misleading and really built on wild guesswork. We would be inclined to defer an implementation of sensory aids even in this case.

Except for the above four principal cases with regard to use of a minimal cognitive test battery, there is one general point which is our present concern regarding implementation of sensory aids: *coding of sensory information must be as direct and phonologically relevant as possible.*

When perception is mediated by learning of a coding scheme for the speech signal, cognitive processes come into play. For example, when several tactile channels are used to convey features of the speech signal, one always runs the risk of interference between 'knowing where' on the skin certain acoustic features are represented and 'knowing what' features/information were actually present in a certain channel. Comparisons between single-channel and multichannel systems are not necessarily in favour of the multichannel system, given that cosmetic and engineering disadvantages are accounted for (Summers, 1992), and, sometimes not even in terms of objective performance characteristics (Plant, 1989). We believe that these considerations and data have a bearing on the issue of 'knowing where' and 'knowing what'. This potential problem may in principle also be present with a cochlear implant procedure, but in a more subtle and less obvious way. We know of no research where one has attempted to disentangle the potentially interfering effects of learning place coding with that of optimizing the perceptual qualities of the aid. One aspect of this is, of course, time and effort. Unless the coding scheme is automatized by the individual, perceptual qualities can never be properly evaluated. But how can one really tell?

Related to this is *the issue of whether the aid should be constructed with the philosophy of optimizing the percept, rather than the representation of the signal.* The answer seems obvious. Based on our research, the aid should convey more abstract phonological information (or input that drives phonological processing, i.e., internal speech) rather than phonetic detail, and it should be done with as direct an approach as possible. By this way, working memory is supported with the purpose of optimizing the processing of implicit, scriptual structures. For example, Öhngren´s (1992) research on transmission of laryngeal vibrations to taction by means of the Tactilator, Risberg and

Lubker's (1978) ingenious work on auditory F0 support to speechreading (see also Breeuwer and Plomp, 1986; Plant, 1987; Risberg, 1974; Rosen, Fourcin and Moore, 1981), and Weisenberger and Russel's (1989) evaluation of the one-channel Minivib (Spens, 1984; Spens and Plant, 1983), all seem to show that some aspect of this principle is met. However, we know of no research which explicitly has attempted to address the question of what kind of percept (i.e., relatively abstract phonology) can best be produced with the help of a sensory aid.

Finally, *the subjective aspect of rehabilitation efforts must also be addressed in this context*. It is quite possible that objective assessments via speechreading tests do not show compensation, but that the subjective costs (experienced energy expenditure) of reaching the same level of performance may vary with the individual. Binnie (1977) found that the attitude to speechreading training and its effects became more positive after training, whereas actual performance did not improve. Lyxell and Rönnberg (1993) in a study with normal-hearing subjects found that working memory can be more engaged when speechreading in noise is compared to speechreading in quiet, whereas this does not affect objective speechreading performance in the two conditions. However, one might speculate that the subjective cost associated with the performance levels attained in noise is generally more taxing (of working memory), and hence, draws on attentional resources.

One general methodological problem with subjective measures, or inferences about subjective costs/benefits, is that they can be confounded by a general lack of metacognitive or metaperceptual competence in the individual (Johansson *et al.*, 1991; Schneider, 1985), rather than reflecting true associations or lack of associations between the subjective and the objective. One way of tackling this problem was proposed by Hygge *et al.* (1992), where the subjects adjusted a signal voice (a female reading a short story) to a preset noise masker (a level at which the subject could listen to speech without strain or discomfort) until they could just follow conversation (JFC). That is, they were told to concentrate and to follow the meaning of the text, disregarding whether they occasionally missed a word or two. The signal level dropped three times per condition, and the subjects were to readjust the audiometer (in 1-dB steps) until the JFC criterion was reached. Calculated reliabilities were very high across conditions. Thus, this method (cf. McLeod and Summerfield, 1987) represents one reliable way of assessing a complex subjective experience (i.e., comprehension of discourse) by objective quantities that have a precise meaning for the clinician.

One use of this method for rehabilitation research on different sensory aids would be to use whatever aid X one would wish to evaluate in contrast to Y, and Z, given different kinds of competing noise conditions and silence. This method would allow straightforward estimates of the gains with an aid, its sensitivity to noise, and also open one avenue for fruitful interaction between subjective and objective measures. Such an interaction is necessary to capture the broader, communicative problems which adventitiously hearing-impaired adults face in their everyday lives.

Acknowledgements

The preparation of this chapter was carried out while the author held a research position at the Council for Research in the Humanities and Social Sciences in the area of 'Speech, Sound, and Hearing', during the autumn of 1992. I am very grateful to Arne Risberg for having 'hand-picked' me to this area, for having taught me about many of the problems in the area of speech, sound and hearing, and for always having given generously from his deep knowledge. Needless to say, without my enthusiastic group at Linköping University, the vast amounts of empirical data briefly summarized and put into theoretical perspective in this chapter, would never have been collected.

I am especially indebted to Björn Lyxell, Geoff Plant, and Stefan Samuelsson for various kinds of support in the preparation of this chapter.

References

Abbot, V., Black, J.B. and Smith, E.E. (1985) The representation of scripts in memory. Journal of Memory and Language 24: 179–99.

Ausmeel, H. (1988) Text-Information-Processing-System (TIPS): A user's guide. Ms. Department of Education and Psychology, Linköping University, Sweden.

Baddeley, A.D. (1990) Human Memory: Theory and Practice. Hove: Lawrence Erlbaum.

Baddeley, A.D. and Wilson, B. (1985) Phonological coding and short-term memory in patients without speech. Journal of Memory and Language 24: 490–02.

Baddeley, A., Logie, R., Nimmo-Smith, I. and Brereton, N. (1985) Components of fluent reading. Memory and Language 24: 119-131.

Breeuwer, M. and Plomp, R. (1986) Speechreading supplemented with auditorily presented speech parameters. Journal of Acoustical Society of America 79: 481–99.

Binnie, C.A. (1977) Attitude changes following speechreading training. Scandinavian Audiology 6: 13–19.

Blamey, P.J. and Cowan, R.S. (1992) The potential benefit and cost effectiveness of tactile devices in comparison with cochlear implants. In Summers, I.R. (Ed) Tactile Aids for the Hearing Impaired. London: Whurr Publishers. pp 187–217.

Campbell, R. (1990) Lipreading, neuropsychology, and immediate memory. In Vallar, G. and Shallice, T.(Eds) Neuropsychological Impairments of Short-term Memory. Cambridge: Cambridge University Press. pp 268–86.

Campbell, R. and Dodd, B. (1980) Hearing by eye. Quarterly Journal of Experimental Psychology, Human Learning and Memory 32: 85–100.

Campbell, R. and Dodd, B. (1984) Aspects of hearing by eye. In Bouma, H. and Bouwhuis, D.G. (Eds) Attention and Performance X. Hillsdale, N.J.: Lawrence Erlbaum. Ass. pp 300–11.

Conrad, R. (1979) The Deaf Schoolchild. Harper and Row: London.

Cowie, R. and Douglas-Cowie, E. (1992) Postlingually Acquired Deafness: Speech Deterioration and The Wider Consequences. New York: Mouton de Gruyter.

Crowder, R.G. (1982) The Psychology of Reading: An Introduction. New York: Oxford University Press.

Crowder, R.G. and Morton, J. (1969) Precategorical acoustic storage (PAS) Perception and Psychophysics 5: 365–73.

De Filippo, C.L. (1982) Memory for articulated sequences and lipreading performance of hearing-impaired observers. Volta Review 31: 134–46.

De Filippo, C.L. and Scott, B.L. (1978) A method for training and evaluating the reception of ongoing speech. Journal of the Acoustical Society of America 88: 1186–92.

Dodd, B. (1977) The role of vision in speech perception. Perception 6: 31–40.

Fodor, J. (1983) The Modularity of Mind. Cambridge: MIT Press.

Gailey, L. (1987) Psychological parameters of lipreading skill. In Dodd, B. and Campbell, R.(Eds) Hearing by Eye: the Psychology of Lipreading. London: Lawrence Erlbaum Ass. pp 115–41.

Galambos, J.A. (1986) Knowledge Structures for Common Activities. In Galambos, J.A., Abelson, R.P. and Black, J.B. (Eds) Knowledge Structures. Hillsdale, N.J.: Lawrence Erlbaum Ass.

Greene, R.L. and Crowder, R.G. (1984) Modality and suffix effects in the absence of auditory stimulation. Journal of Verbal Learning and Verbal Behavior 23: 371–82.

Hardyk, C.D. and Petrinovitch, L.R. (1970) Subvocal speech and comprehension level as a function of the difficulty level of the reading material. Journal of Verbal Learning and Verbal Behavior 9: 647–52.

Hunt, E. (1985) Verbal ability. In Sternberg, R.J. (Ed) Human Abilities: An Information Processing Approach. New York: Freeman. pp 31–58.

Hygge, S., Rönnberg, J, Larsby, B and Arlinger, S. (1992) Normal and hearing-impaired subjects' ability to just follow conversation in competing speech, reversed speech, and noise backgrounds. Journal of Speech and Hearing Research 35: 208–15.

Jeffers, J. and Barley, M. (1977) Speechreading (Lipreading) Springfield, Illinois: C.C. Thomas Publ. Co.

Johansson, K. and Rönnberg, J. (in press) The role of emotionality and typicality in speechreading. Scandinavian Journal of Psychology.

Johansson, K. and Rönnberg, J. (1993) The effects of facial expression and body language on speechreadability. Ms. Department of Education and Psychology, Linköping University, Sweden.

Johansson, K., Rönnberg, J. and Lyxell, B. (1991) Contrasting subjective judgement and objective tests in the severely hearing-impaired. Scandinavian Audiology 20: 91–9.

Lundberg, I., Frost, J. and Petersen, O-P. (1988) Effects of an extensive program for stimulating phonological awareness in preschool children. Reading Research Quarterly XXIII/3: 263–84.

Lyxell, B. (1989) Beyond lips: Components of speechreading skill. PhD thesis, Department of Psychology, University of Umea, Sweden.

Lyxell, B. (1994) Skilled speechreading: a single case study. Scandinavian Journal of Psychology 35: 212–19.

Lyxell, B. and Rönnberg, J. (1987a) Necessary cognitive determinants for speechreading skills. In Kyle, J.G. (Ed) Adjustment to Acquired Hearing Loss:

Analysis, Change, and Learning. Chippenham, Wiltshire: Antony Rowe Ltd.

Lyxell, B. and Rönnberg. J. (1987b) Guessing and speechreading. British Journal of Audiology 21: 13–20.

Lyxell, B. and Rönnberg, J. (1989) Information processing skills and speechreading. British Journal of Audiology 23: 339–47.

Lyxell, B. and Rönnberg, J. (1991a) Visual speech processing: Word decoding and word discrimination related to sentence-based speechreading and hearing-impairment. Scandinavian Journal of Psychology 32: 9–17.

Lyxell, B. and Rönnberg, J. (1991b) Word-discrimination and chronological age related to sentence-based speechreading skill. British Journal of Audiology 25: 3–10.

Lyxell, B. and Rönnberg, J. (1992) Verbal ability and speechreading. Scandinavian Audiology 21: 67–72.

Lyxell, B. and Rönnberg, J. (1993) Background noise, working memory capacity, and speechreading performance. Scandinavian Audiology 22: 67–70.

Lyxell, B., Rönnberg, J. and Andersson, J. (1993) Phonological deterioration and speechreading ability in deafened adults. Ms. Department of Education and Psychology, Linköping University, Sweden.

Lyxell, B. Rönnberg, J. and Samuelsson, S. (1994) Internal speech functioning and speechreading performance in deafened adults. Scandinavian Audiology 23: 179–85.

Lyxell, B., Johansson, K., Lidestam, B. and Rönnberg, J. (1993) Facial expression and speechreading. Ms. Department of Education and Psychology, Linköping University, Sweden.

Lyxell, B., Rönnberg, J. Andersson, J. and Linderoth, E. (1993) Vibrotactile support: Initial effects on visual speech perception. Scandinavian Audiology 22: 179–83.

Marslen-Wilson, W. (1987) Functional parallelism in spoken word recognition. Cognition 25: 71–103.

Massaro, D.W. (1987) Speech Perception by Ear and Eye: A Paradigm for Psychological Inquiry. Hillsdale: N.J.: Lawrence Erlbaum Ass.

McClelland, J.L. and Elman, J.L. (1986) The TRACE model of speech perception. Cognitive Psychology 18: 1–86.

McGurk, H. and MacDonald, J.W. (1976) Hearing lips and seeing voices. Nature 264: 746–8.

McLeod, A. and Summerfield, Q. (1987) Quantifying the contribution to speech perception in noise. British Journal of Audiology 21: 131–41.

Mogford, K. (1987) Lipreading in the prelingually deaf. In Dodd, B. and Campbell, R. (Eds) Hearing by Eye: The Psychology of Lipreading. Hillsdale, N.J.: Lawrence Erlbaum Ass.

Öhngren, (1992) Touching voices: Components of direct tactually supported speechreading. PhD thesis, Department of Psychology, Uppsala University, Sweden.

Öhngren, Kassling and Risberg, A. (in press). The hand and the Tactilator: A comparison between two tactile aids to visual speech perception. Scandinavian Journal of Psychology.

Öhngren, G., Rönnberg,J. and Lyxell, B. (1992) Tactiling: A usable support system for speechreading? British Journal of Audiology 26: 167–73.

Plant, G. (1987) A single-transducer vibrotactile aid to lipreading. Speech Communication 6: 335–42.

Plant, G. (1989) A comparison of five commercially available tactile aids. Australian Journal of Audiology 11: 11–19.

Plant, G. (1992) The selection and training of tactile aid users. In Summers, I.R. (Ed) Tactile Aids for the Hearing Impaired. London: Whurr Publishers. pp 146–67.

Plant, G. and Spens, K. (1986) An experienced user of tactile information as a supplement to speechreading: an evaluative study. Speech Transmission Laboratory, Quarterly Progress and Status Report 4: 1–16. Stockholm, KTH.

Poizner, H. and Kegl, J. (1992) Neural basis of language and motor behaviour: perspectives from American Sign Language. Aphasiology 6: 219–56.

Reisberg, D., McLean, J. and Goldfield, A. (1987) Easy to hear but hard to understand: A lipreading advantage with intact auditory stimuli. In Dodd, B. and Campbell, R. (Eds.), Hearing by Eye: The Psychology of Lipreading. London: Erlbaum. pp 97–114.

Risberg, A. (1974) The importance of prosodic speech elements for the lipreader. Scandinavian Audiology (Suppl 4): 153–64.

Risberg, A. and Lubker, J. (1978) Prosody and speechreading. Report STL - QPSR 4/1978, Department of Linguistics, University of Stockholm, Sweden.

Rosen, S.M., Fourcin, A.J. and Moore, B.C.J. (1981) Voice pitch as an aid to lipreading. Nature 291: 150–52.

Rundus, D. (1971) Analysis of rehearsal processes in free recall. Journal of Experimental Psychology 89: 63–77.

Rönnberg, J. (1987, September) The role of lexical speed and working memory capacity in speechreading. Paper presented at the Second Conference of the European Society for Cognitive Psychology, Madrid.

Rönnberg, J. (1990) Cognitive and communicative function: The effects of chronological age and 'handicap age'. European Journal of Cognitive Psychology 2: 253–73 .

Rönnberg, J. (1993a) Cognitive characteristics of skilled Tactiling: The case of GS. European Journal of Cognitive Psychology 5: 19–33.

Rönnberg, J. (1993b) The 'bilingual' enrichment hypothesis: The case of MJ. Ms. Department of Education and Psychology, Linköping University, Sweden.

Rönnberg, J. and Lyxell, B. (1986) Compensatory strategies in speechreading. In Hjelmquist, E. and Nilsson, L-G.(Eds) Communication and Handicap: Aspects of Psychological Compensation and Technical Aids. Amsterdam: North Holland.

Rönnberg, J. and Nilsson, L-G. (1982) Representation of auditory information based on a functionalistic perspective. In Carlsson, R. and Granström, B.(Eds) The Representation of Speech in the Peripheral Auditory System. Amsterdam: Elsevier Biomedical Press.

Rönnberg, J., and Nilsson, L-G. (1987) The modality effect, sensory handicap, and compensatory functions. Acta Psychologica 65: 263–83.

Rönnberg, J., Söderfeldt, B. and Risberg, J. (1991) Sign language perception measured by rCBF. Journal of Cerebral Blood Flow and Metabolism 11(2): 375.

Rönnberg, J., Öhngren, G. and Lyxell, B. (1987) Linguistic abstraction and hearing handicap. Scandinavian Audiology 16: 95–9.

Rönnberg, J., Öhngren, G. and Nilsson, L-G. (1982) Hearing deficiency, speechreading and memory functions. Scandinavian Audiology 11: 261–8.

Rönnberg, J., Öhngren, G. and Nilsson, L-G. (1983) Speechreading performance evaluated by means of TV and real-life presentation: A comparison between a normally hearing, moderately impaired and profoundly hearing-impaired group. Scandinavian Audiology 12: 71–7.

Rönnberg, J., Arlinger, S., Lyxell, B. and Kinnefors, C. (1989) Visual evoked potentials: Relation to adult speechreading and cognitive function. Journal of Speech and Hearing Research 32: 725–35.

Salthouse, T.A. (1980) Age and memory: Strategies for localizing the loss. In Poon, L.W. Fozard, J.L. Cermak, L.S. Arenberg, D. and Thompson, L.W. (Eds) New Directions in Memory and Aging. Hillsdale, N.J.: Lawrence Erlbaum Ass. pp 47–65.

Salthouse, T.A. (1985) A Theory of Cognitive Ageing. Amsterdam: North-Holland.

Salthouse, T.A. (1987) Age, experience, and compensation. In Schooler, C. and Schaie, K.W. (Eds) Cognitive Functioning and Social Structure over the Life Course. New York: Ablex. pp 142–50.

Samuelsson, S. and Rönnberg, J. (1991) Script activation in lipreading. Scandinavian Journal of Psychology 32: 124–43.

Samuelsson, S. and Rönnberg, J. (1993) Implicit and explicit use of scripted constraints in lipreading. European Journal of Cognitive Psychology 5: 201–33.

Schank, R.C. and Abelson, R.P. (1977) Scripts, Plans, Goals, and Understanding. Hillsdale: N.J.: Lawrence Erlbaum Ass.

Schneider, W. (1985) Developmental trends in the metamemory-memory behavior relationship: An integrative review. In Forest-Presley, D.L., McKinnon, G.E. and Waller, T.G. (Eds) Cognition, Metacognition, and Human Performance. New York: Academic Press.

Seldon, H.L. (1985) The anatomy of speech perception: Human auditory cortex. In Peters, A. and Jones, E.G. (Eds) Cerebral Cortex, vol 4. New York: Plenum.

Spens, K-E. (1984) To hear with the skin. Doctoral dissertation, Dept. of Speech Communication and Music Acoustics. Royal Institute of Technology, Stockholm, Sweden.

Spens, K-E. and Plant, G. (1983) A tactual hearing aid for the deaf. STL-QPSR 1/83: 52–6.

Studdert-Kennedy, M. (1983) On learning to speak. Human Neurobiology 2: 191–5.

Summerfield, Q. (1987) Some preliminaries to a comprehensive account of audio-visual speech perception. In Dodd, B. and Campbell, R. (Eds) Hearing by Eye: The Psychology of Lipreading. Hillsdale, N.J.: Lawrence Erlbaum Ass. pp 3–51.

Summers, I.R. (1992) Single-processing strategies for single-channel systems. In Summers, I.R. (Ed) Tactile Aids for the Hearing Impaired. London: Whurr Publ.

Söderfeldt, B, Rönnberg, J. and Risberg, J. (1994) Regional cerebral blood flow in sign-language users. Brain and Language 46: 59–68.

Wagner, R.K. and Torgesen, J.K. (1987) The nature of phonological processing and its causal role in the acquisition of reading skills. Psychological Bulletin 101: 192–212.

Weisenberger, J.M. and Russel, A.F. (1989) Comparison of two single-channel vibrotactile aids for the hearing-impaired. Journal of Speech and Hearing Research 32: 83–92.

Woodward, M.F. and Barber, C.G. (1960) Phoneme perception in lipreading. Journal of Speech and Hearing Research 3: 212–22.

19

Evaluation of Speech Tracking Results: Some Numerical Considerations and Examples

KARL-ERIK SPENS

Introduction

De Filippo and Scott's (1978) speech tracking procedure or connected discourse tracking (CDT) has been used to train and evaluate the effectiveness of a number of different technical aids developed to improve the lipreading ability of profoundly hearing-impaired people (Brooks *et al.*, 1986; Cowan *et al.*, 1988; Grant *et al.*, 1986; Weisenberger, Broadstone and Saunders, 1989, and many other authors). However, the results vary considerably (Figure 1) not only for different aids but also different authors evaluating similar or the very same aids show different results, suggesting that there could also be procedural factors contributing to the variability. The method has been criticized for having many uncontrolled variables (Tye-Murray and Tyler, 1988; Hochberg, Rosen and Ball, 1989). However, there are variables which can be monitored or controlled which will intuitively contribute very much to the variability of CDT results. These factors are related to the speaking rate, the relative number of errors the relative time used for corrected words, scoring metrics and language characteristics. It is felt as important to try to analyse these factors and their relations to CDT results.

In this chapter speech tracking will be described using a numerical model in an attempt to estimate the effects and the internal relations of the mentioned factors that usually are not under control. The chapter is partly related to Spens *et al.* (1992). It also contains some minor corrections and several examples.

In speech tracking, the sender reads from a book phrase by phrase. The receiver is required to repeat back what is said without any errors. If errors are made, the sender repeats the phrase or uses other strategies to enable correct identification. At the completion of a specified

417

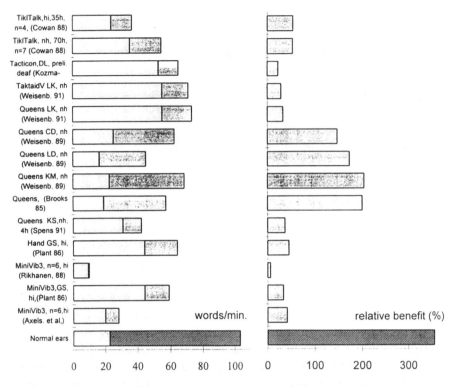

Figure 1. Aided and unaided tracking rates (left) and relative benefit from different tactile aids (right) obtained by different investigators. When known it is indicated if the subject were normal-hearing (nh) or hearing-impaired (hi), hours of training time and number of subjects (n) or initials of single subjects.

time period (usually 5 or 10 minutes), the number of words correctly identified is calculated and divided by the time elapsed to give a word-per-minute (w.p.m.) rate. For example, if a subject is able to correctly repeat back 356 words in a 10-minute speech tracking session she or he has a tracking rate of 35.6 w.p.m.

The method has a number of important advantages.

- The procedure is a straightforward one and requires little training for either the sender or receiver and no special equipment.
- The method of scoring is easy to understand and gives a measure of the fluency with which the receiver can 'track' speech.
- Speech tracking has high face validity as it, in part, replicates every-day communication using connected discourse. As Tye-Murray and Tyler (1988) point out 'specialists desire a test with a high face valid-ity, one that indexes how well a subject recognizes speech encoun-tered in normal everyday life' (page 230).
- Material can be drawn from a virtually unlimited number of sources and can be selected to meet the language skills and lipreading abil-ity of individual subjects.

There are also a number of potential problems with the procedure. Tye-Murray and Tyler (1988) in a critique of the method list such factors as text selection and uncontrolled sender and receiver characteristics.

The following parameters (also sources of variability in the tracking score) will be considered in this chapter:

- Text difficulty.
- Speaking rate.
- Repair strategies.
- Some language characteristics.
- Scoring metric.

Text difficulty

Hochberg, Rosen and Ball (1989) have investigated the effect of the sender–receiver pair and text difficulty on the result and conclude that it is not appropriate to compare tracking results across different sender–receiver pairs. It is intuitively obvious that changing the text difficulty will have an effect on the CDT score. It will be shown later what numerical effects a change in the difficulty of the text material will cause. Another variable related to text difficulty and sender characteristics is the sender's choice of average number of words per phrase. There is a range of words per phrase which is reasonable, not too many and not too few. However, there will always be an influence from the average number of words per phrase. To many words per phrase will increase the probability of errors and to few will increase the proportion of turn taking time. However this parameter can be kept under control by segmenting the text in phrases (lines) of appropriate lengths. The KTH-procedure (Gnosspelius and Spens, 1992) allows for describing the text material in simple statistical terms, average number of words per phrase (line) max, min and distribution. A subject's ability to lipread a certain text could be measured in corrected words per conveyed word. That is a relative measure strongly related to the CDT score, illustrated in Figure 2. If all other parameters could be kept constant a good technical aid should decrease the proportions of corrected words needed to convey a certain text. In this chapter the text difficulty will be regarded as something very closely related to the subject rather than general measures like Flesch Reading Ease, Flesch Grade Level, Flesch–Kincaid, or Gunny–Fog Index.

The mental effort used by the subject is also part of the subject's experienced text difficulty. Much anecdotal evidence exists from subjects stating that a technical aid does not necessarily increase the lipreading (tracking) rate but certainly lowers the mental effort. Such effects are not considered in this chapter.

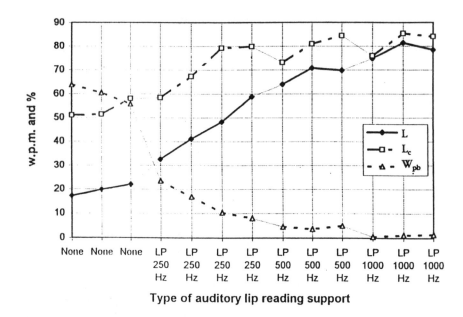

Type of auditory lip reading support

Figure 2. Examples of relations between the CDT score (L), the ceiling rate (L_c – a function of the sender's speaking rate) and the proportion of blocked words (W_{pb}) for a variety of auditive lipreading supports. The relative time loss for each correction is kept almost constant by using the computer-supported tracking system described by Gnosspelius and Spens (1992).

Speaking rate

This is an uncontrolled sender–receiver characteristic, which, as we will show later, numerically affects the tracking score very much. The faster the sender presents the material, the more words are possible to convey per time unit. This will have an increasing effect on the tracking score. However, the presentation rate will also have an effect on the number of blocked words, which will indirectly influence the tracking score. The presentation rate as well as the response rate may to some extent vary at random, by bias, will or motivation (Tye-Murray and Tyler, 1988). The parameter seems difficult to control. However, it can be monitored down to phrase level by using the KTH tracking procedure described by Gnosspelius and Spens (1992). This makes it possible to look at all phrases that are conveyed without any errors and define a maximum tracking rate for a particular session. This will be used in the numerical model. Figures 2, 6, 7 and 8 illustrate examples of relations between the ceiling (maximum) rate, proportion of corrected words and CDT rate.

Repair strategies

The lack of a standardized protocol for dealing with breakdowns or 'blockages' is a great problem (Owens and Teleens, 1981) in understanding, when the receiver is unable to lipread a certain word or a phrase. Schoeplin and Levitt (1991), for example, found large differences in the correction or 'repair' strategies used by experimenters in various studies using CDT as an evaluation method. Consequently, they argued, that the procedure is unstandardized and subject to a number of methodological variables. There have been attempts to specify the procedures to be used when blockages occur but none of these appear to have won wide acceptance.

De Filippo and Scott (1978) in their initial description of the method outlined the protocol they used to resolve blockages. 'If the repetition does not match the text exactly, the talker (a) chooses to present the segment again, making no change, modifying the style of presentation (especially timing and exaggeration of speech movements), shortening the segment to focus on a phrase, word, syllable or sound, or lengthening the segment to review or preview phonetic or linguistic context; (b) chooses to instruct the receiver with context comments by labelling the error, labelling the topic, or paraphrasing the text; or (c) chooses to combine or sequence several strategies. The basis for the talker's decision necessarily depends on the receiver's errors and changes as receiver skill changes' (De Filippo and Scott 1978, page 1187).

Owens and Telleen (1981) and Owens and Raggio, (1987) attempted to shift the responsibility for overcoming blockages to the receiver. In their adaptation of the method, the receiver is trained to use a series of questions or requests when breakdowns occur. This approach has many benefits in training but in practice the receiver's ability to use these strategies varies widely. As a result, the amount of benefit derived will vary widely from receiver to receiver and will greatly influence the tracking rate obtained in experimental studies.

There are other strategies which can be adopted when breakdowns occur. These include writing down, finger spelling and signing the word or words which the receiver cannot lipread. When artificially deafened hearing subjects are used in experimental studies, the sender may choose to present the blocked words to the receiver auditorily. The time taken for each of these correction methods varies considerably. Presenting the words auditorily or via sign is the quickest alternative while writing will probably occupy the most time. Schoeplin and Levitt (1991) found that: 'fewer than 7% of the talker–listener sequences extended beyond five trials' (page 248) before the word or words were recognized correctly.

It can be concluded that the type of correction strategy will have an influence on the tracking score and its variability. Tye-Murray and Tyler

(1988) recommended a limited hierarchy of strategies to reduce talker effects. In the computer controlled tracking procedure described by Gnosspelius and Spens (1992), it is suggested that only repetitions be used. The last resort strategy used is to present the blocked word on a LED screen. That method takes about the same time as a repetition. It is fast and convenient and applies to both deaf and artificially deafened subjects.

Language characteristics

Where studies are conducted in different languages it is most likely that the final result will be influenced by differences in average word length. For example, the average word length in English is 6.09 letters/word (ls/w) while in Swedish the average is 6.43 ls/w, and German has as much as 7.69 ls/w. If phonetic data are more closely considered, these correspond to the time it takes to pronounce a word; the average values are 4.96, 5.94, and 6.78 phonemes/word, respectively (Carlson *et al.*, 1985). In Swedish nouns, for example, all definite articles are indicated by a suffix, such as *en hund* (a dog) and *hunden* (the dog), i.e., it is just one word, while the English language uses two words to convey the same information. If this relation is linear, the use of Swedish in a tracking test would yield a result about 20% lower score than when English is used. A consequence of such language differences will be a need for some scaling factors to be used for across-language comparisons of tracking results. However, we will leave this parameter for analyses in later publications.

Scoring metrics

If different scoring metrics are used this will of course disturb comparisons of CDT results. This will be discussed later in the chapter.

In spite of the factors mentioned that certainly contribute to the variability of CDT scores, the technique is widely used for both evaluation and training purposes. If results are published it is, of course, tempting to make comparisons and forget about all those parameters.

If we look at a cross-study of speech tracking investigations, they show a very large range of results. This is exemplified in Figure 1, which shows tracking rates obtained via lipreading alone and lipreading supported by a number of different tactile aids reported by various researchers. It should be pointed out that probably all authors have used a last resort correction strategy that is based on another modality such as audition, finger spelling etc. The w.p.m. score will then not truly represent the test condition of lipreading (De Filippo, 1992). In some cases, different researchers evaluated the same aid and yet obtained very different results. Therefore, it can be anticipated that the wide range of results is not only an effect of the effectiveness of different aids. Other factors, such as those described above most likely introduce variability. In an attempt to estimate these effects, we will now describe speech tracking using a numerical model.

Numerical Model

Tracking as described by De Filippo (1988) is a composite measure, represented by the relation:

$$L = \frac{W_s}{T_s} \quad \text{w.p.m.}$$

where L = the average w.p.m. score, W_s = the total number of words conveyed during one session, and T_s = the session time in minutes.

In order to include the mentioned components of CDT in the numerical relations, it is necessary to introduce some new parameters.

In CDT, the passage being used is presented in logical linguistic units of appropriate lengths. The receiver has to repeat back exactly what was presented with no deviations from the printed text. Sometimes the receiver is able to repeat the entire phrase or sentence after only one presentation. On other occasions, the receiver may 'block' on a particular word or series of words and require one or more repeats of the word or words that are creating difficulties. Other strategies such as those discussed above may also be used to overcome blockages. However, if the receiver is unable to correctly identify the word or words even after repeats, and the sender is forced to resolve the problem by using a presentation method other than that being evaluated. For example, the sender may be forced to write down or sign the word(s) creating difficulties to the receiver.

We can now divide the words in a particular tracking session into separate categories determined by the number of trials needed to make the receiver respond correctly (Figure 3). The categories used are:

W_0 or W_c – words correctly identified with no corrections, i.e., after the first presentation. Such words error free phrases are on average conveyed at the highest w.p.m. rate or ceiling rate, used in the session under consideration and using the communication system under evaluation. We will use the index 0 or c to indicate this definition of the ceiling rate or no correction rate for the communication system under evaluation.

W_1 – words which are correctly identified after one correction.

W_2 – words which are correctly identified after two correction trials.

W_n – those words in units which cannot be correctly conveyed within the communication system being evaluated. The sender is forced to use another communication mode such as signing, talking or writing

to convey the words. These are words conveyed *outside* the system.
W_s – the total number of words conveyed from the text in a tracking session.

In the same way we can define session time in categories used to convey words corrected from zero to n times (Figure 3). We now have the opportunity to directly compare the time taken to convey non-blocked words (W_c), blocked words resolved inside the system ($W1$, W_2 .... W_{n-1}) and blocked words resolved outside the system (W_n).
These new parameters are:

- k_1 – the average time relation between blocked words resolved after the first correction and non-blocked words.
- k_2 – the average time relation between blocked words resolved after the second correction and non-blocked words.
- $k_{(n-1)}$ – the average time relation between blocked words corrected the last time inside the system and non-blocked words.
- k_n – the average time relation between blocked words corrected outside the system and a non-blocked word.

There will be a relation between k values like: $1 < k1 < k2 .... < kn$. The more unsuccessful trials to correct a blocked word the larger the value

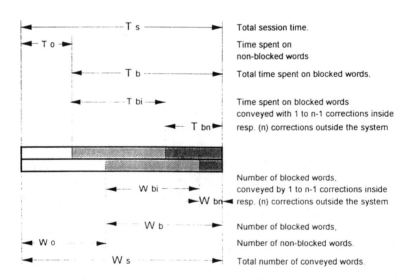

Figure 3. The total number of conveyed words (W_s) in a tracking session (duration T_s) divided into categories of repair strategy and time needed to correctly identify each group. The category repaired inside the system can be further divided into subgroups according to the number of repair efforts needed, see text.

of the average k factor. The values of the k factors will obviously be highly dependent on the strategy chosen to repair blocked words.

Finally, we are able to specify the fastest tracking rate or the *ceiling* rate (L_c) obtained within an individual tracking session when using the communication system under evaluation. This is the average speed (in w.p.m.) for transmission of non-blocked words.

That is

$$L_c = \frac{W_c}{T_c} \quad \text{or} \quad \frac{W_s - W_b}{T_s - T_b} \quad \text{w.p.m.}$$

If there are very few phrases conveyed with no corrections, the precision will be low and a more relevant measure would be the conventional formula where Ws and Ts are reduced by the blocked words and the time spent on corrections.

The definitions could be made otherwise. However, these are chosen because they can be quantified by using an updated version of the computer-assisted tracking procedure described by Gnosspelius and Spens (1992).

Numerical relations

The conventional tracking result is calculated by the relation:

$$L = \frac{W_s}{T_s} \quad \text{w.p.m.}$$

Using the above definitions we can express that as:

$$L = L_c \cdot \frac{\dfrac{W_0}{W_s} + \dfrac{W_1}{W_s} + \cdots \dfrac{W_{(n-1)}}{W_s} + \dfrac{W_n}{W_s}}{1 + (k_1-1)\dfrac{W_1}{W_s} + \cdots (k_{(n-1)}-1)\dfrac{W_{(n-1)}}{W_s} + (k_n-1)\dfrac{W_n}{W_s}} \tag{1}$$

A more detailed derivation of the above expression is given in Spens *et al.* (1992)

The general expression (1) shows that the tracking score (L) is proportionally influenced by the ceiling rate (L_c) for that particular session. It is mentioned before that (L_c) is the tracking rate for all words conveyed without any errors. The sender's presentation rate will also have an effect on the proportion of blocked words. The faster the presentation rate the more corrections will be needed. At very low presentation rates the lipreading patterns will eventually deviate from normal to much and the difficulty may increase again. The proportion of blocked words resolved outside the system W_n/W_s should be only a small fraction of W_s; otherwise the result will deviate too much from a true representation of the subject's lipreading ability (De Filippo, 1992).

The expression also shows that L in a non-linear fashion will depend on the proportion of blocked words and their respective weights (k_i). The weights k_i are related to the repair strategy chosen.

Equation (1) also shows that the conventional tracking score would be as high as the ceiling rate if the terms (W_1/W_s) to (W_n/W_s) were zero, i.e., if there are no blocked words. As soon as there are corrections either inside or outside the system, one or more of the terms ((k_i-1)*W_i/W_s) will increase the denominator and hereby reduce the conventional tracking score (L). The higher the values of the k factors, the faster the score (L) will get reduced by blocked words.

By using p as an index for proportions and the fact that

$$W_{p0} + W_{p1} .... + W_{p(n-1)} + W_{pn} = 1$$

we can simplify the above relation to:

$$L = \frac{L_c}{1 + W_{p1}(k_1-1) + ...W_{p(n-1)}(k_{(n-1)}-1) + W_{pn}(k_n-1)} \qquad (2)$$

If all blocked words are considered to be one category with about the same average k value, we will get an even simpler version (3), which of course is an approximation. The approximation will be valid only if the blocked words have a stable relative distribution of repair efforts. This is only possible if the proportion of blocked words is a small fraction of the total number of conveyed words. A very exaggerated example would be if the text material is so difficult that all words are blocked and cannot become resolved without using the last resort strategy in both the aided and the unaided condition. Then the eventual benefit from the aid will not be reflected at all in the tracking results. To avoid these kind of end-effects it is important to use a text material of reasonable difficulty.

$$L = \frac{L_c}{1 + W_{pb}(k-1)} \quad \text{w.p.m.} \qquad (3)$$

Equation (3) does not show the influence of different strategies to repair words inside or outside the communication system, nor does it show what happens if the scoring metric exclude words resolved outside the system. However, it clearly illustrates the non-linear properties of the tracking score (L). Equation (3) also seems valid for W_{pb} values which are reasonable fractions of W_s (Figures 6 and 7).

Discussion and Some Results

Several sender dependent factors can be kept under control by using methods based on interactive video technique (see Chapter 26) However, some of the natural dialogue situation will then be lost. A solution that keeps the dialogue situation is the one proposed by (Gnosspelius and Spens, 1992) in which the book to read from is substituted for the computer screen. This system will be referred to as the KTH procedure. The text to be read is prompted to the sender phrase by phrase. Each first presentation of text is a full line. Then the text difficulty due to individual choice of phrase lengths will not vary between senders just as when using a video system. The proposed computer-assisted tracking technique also allows for the monitoring or control of the parameters discussed and examples are given in Figures 2, 6, 7 and 8.

In Figure 4 equation (3) is shown graphically. The conventional tracking score (L) is shown for two ceiling rates (conversational speech $L_c = 100$ and clear speech 50 w.p.m. respectively, Picheny et al., 1985) as a function of text difficulty i.e., the proportion of blocked (corrected) words (W_{pn}). The k values 3, 5, 8, and 12. corresponding to the relative losses of 2, 4, 7 and 11 words per correction, are used as parameters. It should be noted that also here W_{pb}/W_s should not approach one; if it does, equation (3) will suffer from end effects.

Speaking rate and text difficulty

There is a strong correlation between the subject's ability to lipread and the sender's speaking rate. Therefore the two parameters' influence on the tracking score will be discussed together. The ceiling rate (L_c) contains both the sender's, the receiver's speaking rate and the turn taking times. It is obviously independent of the repair strategies used, as it is calculated only on non-blocked words. It can vary considerably between different sessions (see Figure 2).

The adaptation of their own speech made by people talking to hearing-impaired persons, as reported by Picheny et al. (1986) is probably reflected in L_c's mentioned dependence of W_{pb}. They found the more well articulated and slower 'clear' speech presented with about half the rate (100 w.p.m.) compared to 'conversational' speech (200 w.p.m.). It is obvious that the experienced communication difficulty in a lipreading situation will make most talkers use the clear speech mode, which has a significantly higher intelligibility (Picheny, Durlach and Braida, 1985; Plant, Gnosspelius and Spens, 1994). The L_c value of 50 w.p.m. obtained in a lipreading situation would correspond to the 'clear' speech talking rate of 100 w.p.m. When the sender detects a lowered W_{pb} he will eventually try to increase his speech rate up to the conversation level of about 200 w.p.m. The receiver may not increase his speed that much, but the corresponding L_c will be in the area of 80 to 100 w.p.m. for a very good communication system like the exemplified LP 1000 Hz condition in Figure 2.

The faster the sender presents the material, the more words are possible to convey per time unit. However, at very low presentation (ceiling) rates lipreading is difficult and sequence of words may be difficult to remember (Plant, Gnosspelius and Spens, 1994). This will cause a high proportion of blocked words. For presentation rates approaching more natural ranges blocked words will decrease and the tracking score will improve both from an increased ceiling rate and the lowered proportion of blocked words. At a certain rate of presentation, the score will stop becoming improved because the proportion of blocked words will also increase to much and cause a negative net change of the tracking score. An important consequence is that there will be a presentation rate for each sender–receiver pair that gives a maximum tracking rate. A maximum of that kind is indicated in Figure 8.

Figure 2 shows the results obtained by a normally-hearing female subject when tracking materials were presented via lipreading alone and lipreading supplemented by auditorily-presented speech which was low-pass filtered (LPF) at 250, 500, and 1,000 Hz. There were three 10-minute tracking sessions in each condition and the KTH-procedure was used. The repair strategy chosen was maximum two repetitions in a little more well articulated manner to solve the blocked words. In this case the average k value is about 5 (= 4 lost words in the final score per blocked word). After two unsuccessful repetitions, the blocked word was given in written form on a LED screen hanging just above the sender's head. The phrases were read from a monitor by the sender. The last resort correction using the orthographic modality was somewhat faster than a repetition. The sender just clicked at the blocked word with the mouse to indicate made repetitions or to advance to the next phrase (line).

The subject's w.p.m. rate increases rapidly with the addition of the LPF speech signal. It can be seen that the subject's tracking rate in the lipreading alone condition is approximately 20 w.p.m. When lipreading was supplemented by the speech LPF at 250 Hz, her tracking rate rose to around 50 w.p.m.. The tracking rate for lipreading plus the speech LPF at 500 Hz was around 65 w.p.m. Finally, when the speech LPF at 1000 Hz supplemented lipreading , the tracking rate was around 85 w.p.m.

A striking change which occur as more auditory information is provided is the decline in the proportion of blocked words. This falls from around 60% for the lipreading alone condition to about 1% in the lipreading plus speech LPF at 1000 Hz condition. This indicates the proportion of blocked words as the factor that mostly mirrors the benefit of an aid.

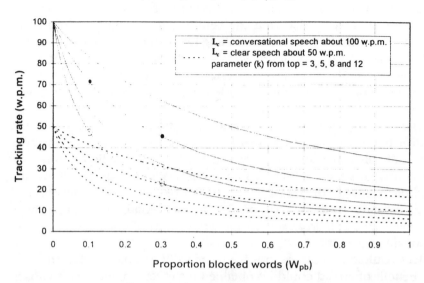

Figure 4. Graph showing the simplified relation for two L_c-values (100 and 50 words/min) and k = 3, 5, 8 or 12. It shows how the tracking rate (L) depends on losses per corrected word (k), the ceiling rate (L_c) and the proportion of corrected words of W_b/W_s.

The ceiling rate (L_c) also increases with added auditory information and training. The ceiling rate of approximately 50–60 w.p.m. in the unaided condition rises to around 80–90 w.p.m.. for each of the aided conditions. It should also be noted that the asymptotic level is reached relatively quick in the aided conditions. This adaptation is a mix of the sender trying to find a speaking rate that gives a reasonable proportion of blocked words and the receiver's performance getting better with training.

The changes in L_c exemplify the possibility to choose a text material which has a level of familiarity to the receiver which makes the sender use 'clear' speech (low L_c) to keep the fluency in the unaided condition. In the aided condition, the sender will eventually approach a more 'conversational' speech rate. The final score will then get the contribution from the increased L_c, and the aided/unaided relation would improve from that. This would not be the case if in both the aided and the unaided conditions, the proportions of corrected words were high enough to make anything other than 'clear' speech inefficient, i.e., L_c would be about the same in both conditions. The same situation could appear if the receiver is a very skilled lipreader. If the material is simple enough to allow the sender to use conversational rate in both conditions, the relative improvement caused by the aid would not get any contribution from an increase in L_c in the aided condition.

How the corrections needed reflects the tracking rate is exemplified in Figure 2 where the ceiling rate is varying according to the preference of the speaker. It is clear that the ceiling rate also has an important influence. In Figure 6 where the ceiling rate is monitored and kept at a rather constant value of about 90 w.p.m (the first 16 data points) it is more obvious. Here the tracking rate almost exactly mirrors the proportion of corrected words. An aided condition should give a lower proportion of corrections and a correspondingly higher tracking rate.

The graph (Figure 4) representing equation (3) indicates that the relative benefit from an aid will be influenced just by changing to a more difficult text material. In Figure 5 this is exemplified graphically. The constraints are a similar ceiling rate in both the aided and unaided conditions and a constant relation of 0.8 between the proportion of blocked words in the aided and the unaided conditions. The relative benefit of an aid increases with the proportion of corrected words in the unaided condition.

This could be an indication that more valid comparisons of the relative benefit of an aid could be obtained if the text material was chosen in such a way that the same unaided baseline was used for across-subject comparisons. Other obvious conditions are constant ceiling rates and k values.

How a small change in the ceiling rate could change the tracking rate is illustrated in Figures 6 and 7. Figure 6 shows several sessions were the ceiling rate (about 88 w.p.m.) is kept rather constant except for the last three sessions where the ceiling rate is only about 76 w.p.m. The CDT score of the first 16 sessions almost exactly mirrors the proportion of corrected words. In Figure 7 the same data as in Figure 6 are plotted using equation (3). In the sessions with a lower ceiling rate the subject found the tracking easier, i.e., fewer corrections per conveyed word. However the CDT score did not change significantly because the two effects of reduced ceiling rate and a lower number of blocked words counteracted each other.

It is not known whether the subject during the three last sessions experienced less stress or mental effort but it seems very likely she did.

Figure 8 also illustrates how the tracking score and proportion of blocked words can vary with ceiling rate for a lipreading alone condition. For very low ceiling (presentation) rates an increase of blocked words is indicated. However the ceiling range of about 55 to 70 w.p.m. corresponding to a natural sender's speaking rate of 110 to 140 w.p.m. the proportion of blocked words seems constant except for its text depending variability. For higher presentation rates the lipreading ability and proportion of blocked words increase. In the range of 50 to 70 w.p.m. range the tracking rate increases because of the L_c factor in equation (3). In the ceiling rate range of 65 to 70 w.p.m. there is a maximum tracking performance of close to 40 w.p.m. For higher ceiling

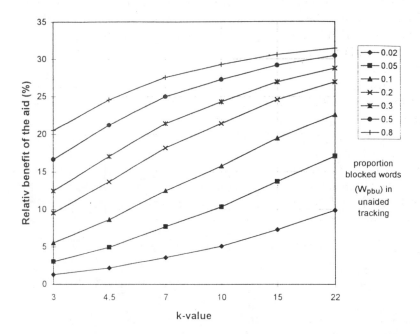

Figure 5. Relative benefit of aid as a function of losses from repair strategy (k) and proportion of blocked words in the unaided situation (W_{pbu}), given the relation (W_{pa}/W_{pu}) is 0.75 and that the presentation rate (L_c) is constant.

rates the increased proportion of blocked words dominate and reduces the tracking rate. It seems that it will always be possible to find a maximum tracking rate by varying the presentation (ceiling) rate. If that maximum tracking rate is optimal in terms of communication convenience, stress or other criteria remains to be discussed.

Considering the effect of varying ceiling rates it seems obvious that interpreting tracking data is difficult without knowing about the ceiling rate. Comparing aided and unaided conditions is even more difficult. The ceiling rate is obviously a sender–receiver characteristic containing the sender's speaking rate, the receiver's turn taking time and speaking rate. These factors could vary at random to some extent, at will or because of bias. When interpreting or comparing CDT results, ceiling rate must be considered a very dangerous factor if not monitored.

The repair strategy

Figure 4 shows how a repair strategy which is fast, i.e., a low k value, will contribute to a high tracking rate.

However, the tracking score will indicate an increased relative benefit from a lipreading aid for higher k values. This is exemplified in

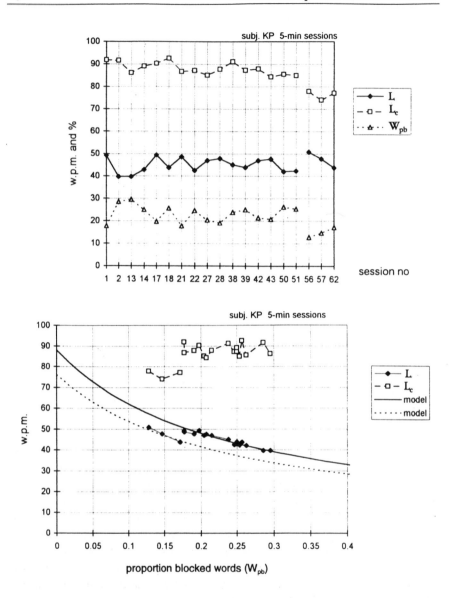

Figures 6 and 7. Illustrations of relation between tracking rate, ceiling rate and proportion of blocked words (subject KP, 5 minute sessions). In Figure 6 data are displayed with the time (session number) as parameter. In Figure 7 the same data are displayed using equation (3) with the proportion of blocked and corrected words as parameter.

Figure 4 where filled circles indicate for 'conversational' speech and a k factor 5, tracking results of 72 w.p.m. and 10% blocked words in the aided condition and 48 w.p.m., 30% blocked words in the unaided. That corresponds to a 50% relative benefit from such an aid. If about three times as much time were spent on each repair (k = 12) the aided

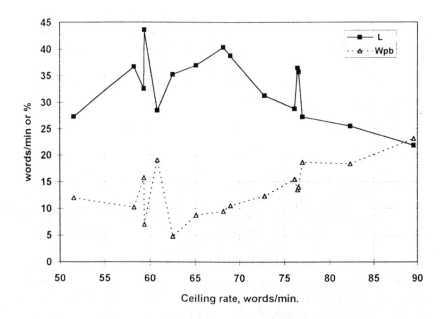

Figure 8. Example of tracking rate (L) and proportion of blocked words (W_{pb}) as function of the ceiling rate. An obvious maximum tracking performance is indicated.

and unaided tracking scores (open circles) would have been only 48 and 24 w.p.m. respectively i.e., a 100% relative benefit from the very same aid.

The relative benefit will increase even more if the k value is high only in the unaided condition. A somewhat exaggerated example would be if the k value is allowed to change from 12 to 5 switching from the unaided to the aided condition. Then the relative benefit would become 72/24, i.e., a performance increase of 200% for again the same aid.

In Figure 5 it is shown how the relative benefit will vary depending on the k value and the unaided proportion of blocked words, considered the ceiling rate is kept constant and that the proportion of blocked words in the aided and the unaided condition has a constant relation of 0.8. The graphic representation in Figure 5 is idealized and as mentioned before not valid if the proportion of blocked words approaches one and there is a large fraction of repairs for which the last resort modality is used. If so the tracking result for even a good aid would show close to zero benefit.

When comparing tracking results, different repair strategies (different average k values) could be compensated for. A compensation for a different k value would correspond to a vertical movement in Figure 4.

However, to make the recalculation using equation (3), a necessary condition is that the ceiling rates used were the same, the text material is of the same difficulty and that the proportion of blocked words is known.

The analysis indicates that the losses caused by the repair strategy used in a tracking procedure will have a considerable influence on the tracking rate.

Scoring metrics

In equation (1) the sum of the terms in the numerator equals one. That makes it possible to simplify the relation but this is only applicable if all the words presented by the sender in one session are included in the relation. Some authors like De Filippo (1988) and Fenn and Smith (1987), specify scoring schemes that will have a modifying effect on the general relation. De Filippo (1988), and others using her procedure, specify a scoring design which does include the time spent on resolving blocked words outside the system i.e., the term $(k_n * W_n / W_s)$, but it does not include the number of words resolved outside the system, i.e., the term (W_n / W_s) in the numerator. This is set to zero. If (W_n / W_s) in the numerator is omitted, that will of course have a negative effect on the resulting CDT score. However, the relative benefit from an aid, i.e., the relation aided/unaided will become increased if the number of words resolved outside the system is lower in the aided situation.

For example, if the result is 50 w.p.m. in an aided condition and 40 w.p.m. in a corresponding unaided, the relative improvement given by the aid would be 25% if all conveyed words are counted. If, somewhat exaggerated, there are 5 blocked w.p.m. resolved outside the system in the unaided condition and only 1 in the aided, the final tracking score would be 49 and 35, respectively, omitting these words, i.e., a somewhat lower result in both conditions. However, the relative improvement would be 49/35, which equals a 40% improvement in the aided condition. Penalty schemes can increase relative improvements even further. In most cases, such schemes can be numerically included in equation (1).

Conclusions

Using the numerical model of the speech tracking procedure it has been shown that the tracking rate and particularly the relative benefit expressed as relative increase in the aided condition will depend very much on the ceiling rate (L_c), the relative number of blocked words (W_{pb}) and the relative loss per blocked word (k). It also depends on language characteristics and scoring metrics. If the text material is too difficult, end effects could introduce unnecessary variability. The only way to circumvent the non-predictable influence of a varying ceiling rate (L_c) is to monitor its constancy. The k values should also be stable or compensated for. The proportion of blocked words (W_{pb}) would then be the only parameter to influence the tracking rate. If the ceiling rate is allowed to vary it still should be monitored. The relative improvement of an aid could then be calculated at a specified ceiling rate or eventually for the respective maximum tracking rates.

It seems likely that some of the variability in results shown in Figure 1 could be explained by the relations described.

The computer-assisted tracking procedure suggested by Gnosspelius and Spens (1992) produces a very detailed protocol. Information about the transmission time for each phrase is given as raw data as well as the average L, L_c, k values and proportion of blocked words (W_{pb}). Other interesting parameters like the total number of first interventions, second interventions etc., up to the last resort resolution and the respective times taken are also given or can easily be calculated. General measures of the text material like average word length, phrase lengths, distributions and standard deviations can be calculated by the programme.

As the text file is stored in the computer, it is also easy to asses the general text difficulty estimated by standardized methods, such as Flesch Reading Ease, Flesch Grade Level, Flesch–Kincaid, or Gunny–Fog Index found in modern word processors.

It would certainly help interpreting speech tracking results if the ceiling rate (or even better the sender's presentation rate), the proportions of corrected words as well as the average k values used, were reported as complementary data to the CDT results.

If this kind of information was frequently published, informal standards of these parameters would probably appear.

It is hoped that the assessment of more data from the tracking session like those mentioned will make the interpretation of tracking results more interesting and informative than today.

References

Axelsson, A., Berenstaf, E. and Spens, K-E. (1986) Erfarenheter av träning med ett vibrotaktilt hjälpmedel. Kursbok för Nordiska Audiologiska Sällskapets möte i Åbo, 167–9.

Brooks, P.L., Frost, B.J., Mason, J.L. and Gibson, D.M. (1986) Continuing evaluation of the Queen's University tactile vocoder. II: Identification of open-set sentences and tracking narrative. Journal of Rehabilitation Research 23(1): 129–38.

Carlson, R., Elenius, K., Granström, B. and Hunnicut, S. (1985) Phonetic and orthographic properties of the basic vocabulary of five European languages. STL-QPSR No. 1, 63–94 (KTH, Stockholm).

Cowan, R.S.C, Alcantara, J.I., Blamey, P.J. and Clark, G.M.(1988) Preliminary evaluation of a multichannel electrotactile speech processor. Journal of the

Acoustical Society of America 83(6): 2328–38.

De Filippo, C.L. (1988) Tracking for speech reading training. Volta Review 90(5): 215–37.

De Filippo, C.L. (1992) The tracking technique: Cautions in generating and inter-preting data. In Proceedings Second Internat. Conf. on Tactile Aids, Hearing Aids and Cochlear Implants (Eds: Risberg, A., Felicetti, S., Plant, G., and Spens, K.-E.) Stockholm, Sweden. TRITA-TöM 1992:5.

De Filippo, C.L. and Scott, B.L. (1978) A method for training the reception of ongo-ing speech. Journal of Acoustical Society of America 63: 1186–92.

Fenn, G. and Smith, B.Z.D. (1987) The assessment of lipreading ability: some prac-tical considerations in the use of the tracking procedure. British Journal of Audiology 21: 253–8.

Gnosspelius, J. and Spens, K-E. (1992) A computer based speech tracking proced-ure. STL-QPSR No. 1, 131–7 (KTH, Stockholm).

Grant, K.W., Ardell, L.A.H., Kuhl, P.K. and Sparks, D.W. (1986) The transmission prosodic information via an electrotactile speech reading aid. Ear and Hearing 7: 328–35.

Hochberg, I., Rosen, S. and Ball, V. (1989) Effect of text complexity on connected discourse tracking rate. Ear and Hearing 10(3): 192–9.

Kozma-Spytek, L. and Weisenberger, J.M. (1987) Evaluation of a multichannel elec-trotactile device for the hearing-impaired. Central Institute for the Deaf, St. Louis, MS, USA.

Matthies, M.L. and Carney, A.E. (1988) A modified speech tracking procedure as a communication performance measure. Journal of Speech and Hearing Research 31: 394–404

Owens, E. and Raggio, M (1987) The UCSF tracking procedure for evaluation and training of reception by hearing impaired adults. Journal of Speech and Hearing Disorders 52: 120–28.

Owens, E. and Teleen, C.C. (1981) Tracking as an aural rehabilitative process. Journal of the Academy of Rehabilitation Audiology 14: 259–73.

Picheny, M.A., Durlach, N.I. and Braida, L.D. (1985) Speaking clearly for the hard of Hearing I: Intelligibility differences between clear and conversational speech. Journal of Speech and Hearing Research 28: 96–103.

Picheny, M.A., Durlach, N.I. and Braida, L.D. (1986) Speaking clearly for the hard of Hearing II: Acoustic Characteristics of clear and conversational speech. Journal of Speech and Hearing Research 29: 434–46.

Plant, G. and Spens, K-E. (1986) An experienced user of tactile information as a supplement to lip-reading. An evaluation study. STL-QPSR No. 1, 87–110 (KTH, Stockholm).

Plant, G., Gnosspelius, J. and Spens, K-E. (1994) Three studies using the KTH speech tracking procedure. STL-QPSR No. 1: 103–34 (KTH, Stockholm).

Rihkanen, H. (1988) Rehabilitation Assessment of Postlingually Deaf Adults Using Single Channel Intracochlear Implants or Vibro-tactile Aids: A Prospective Clinical Study, Diss.

Schoeplin, J.R. and Levitt, H. (1991) Continuous discourse tracking: An analysis of the procedure. Journal of Communication Disorders 24:237–49.

Spens, K.-E.; Gnosspelius, J., Öhngren, G., Plant, G. and Risberg, A. (1992) Numerical aspects of the speech tracking procedure. STL-QPSR No 1, 115–30.

Tye-Murray, N. and Tyler, R.S. (1988) A critique of continuous discourse tracking as a test procedure. Journal of Speech and Hearing Disorder 53: 226–31.

Weisenberger, J.M., Broadstone, S.M. and Saunders, F.A. (1989) Evaluation of two multichannel tactile aids for the hearing-impaired. Journal of the Acoustical Society of America 86: 1764–75.

Weisenberger, J.M. and Kozma-Spytek, L. (1991) Evaluating tactile aids for speech perception and production by the hearing impaired adults and children. The American Journal of Otology 12: suppl.

Part IV
Speech Production

20

Principles for a Complete Description of the Phonological System of Deaf Children as a Basis for Speech Training

ANNE-MARIE ÖSTER

Teaching Methods in the Swedish Education of Deaf Children

The educational method used in Swedish schools for the deaf was, from the turn of the century, predominantly oral. During the 1950s, this changed into a strictly auditory–oral method with intense training of speech and hearing.

During the period of auditory–oral teaching, it was assumed, but never clearly declared, that all deaf children could develop conversational speech. The aim was for children to learn to speak and speechread so well that more or less normal conversations could be held both between deaf persons and between deaf and hearing persons. It is apparent that very few deaf children reached this level.

At the end of the 1960s, an evaluation was made of the speech and language development of children in schools for the deaf in Sweden (Amcoff, 1973). The results of this study showed a large retardation in language development compared to normal-hearing children of the same age. It was also found that the speech of the severely deaf children was rarely intelligible to naive listeners. These results, together with similar results published in other countries, led to an intense discussion about teaching methods. Different manual or combined systems were tested, for example, Cued Speech and Signed Swedish.

Since 1983, Swedish Schools for the Deaf have been bilingual. Swedish Sign Language is the accepted teaching language used, and Swedish is mainly learnt in its written form assisted by sign language. Speech training, based on a child's individual potential, is provided in special speech clinics for about 40 minutes a week. No speech training is practised in the classroom during ordinary lessons.

The purpose of speech training in the present curriculum is for prelingually profoundly deaf children to develop intelligible speech for the purpose of making statements and, more seldom, for the purpose of communication. They should learn 'survival speech' that makes it possible for them to give and to understand simple messages in shops, in the street, etc. Visual and tactile aids are to some extent used as a complement to help the teacher explain what is correct and what is wrong and to train correct production.

Speech Acquisition

The hearing child acquires speech and language spontaneously through a combination of hearing and lipreading. Auditory and visual input control helps the child to compare the vocal output of other speakers with his/her own production. Wundt (1911) called the observation of the talking face 'the impulse to speech'. Young children observe lip movements to find out how to articulate different speech sounds and then imitate these movements. Visual articulatory movements give concrete cues about how to produce speech sounds, while hearing provides a measure of success.

The *blind child* has no access to visual information. It would then seem likely that this will affect his or her phonological development. In fact, some studies (Mills, 1983) have reported that facial movements in blind children are 'muted', and articulation is less distinct. Göllesz (1972) investigated Hungarian vowels articulated by blind children, through electromyography and spectrography. He found less lip movement compared with normal sighted children. However, the spectrograms showed no deviations in the acoustic properties of the productions. According to Mills, 'blind children will follow a different and slightly slower path in earlier phonology compared to sighted children and this is attributed to the absence of lip-read information. The children studied showed no sign of developing a disordered phonological system in the long term.'

Prelingually deaf children very rarely develop speech spontaneously. Speech is almost always developed through training, using the visibility of phonetic features, reading, tactile sensations and, if possible, residual hearing. These inputs severely limit speech perception potential and can cause deaf children to make unavoidable articulatory deviations that affect their ability to signal meaning differences in spoken language. Despite these limitations they may develop systematic phonological rules. Several studies have shown that deaf children possess some kind of abstract and stable phonological systems (West and Weber, 1973; Oller and Kelly, 1974; Dodd, 1976, 1988; Oller and Eilers,

1981; Abberton et al., 1985; Öster, 1989a, 1991, 1992) but these may differ from those of normal-hearing speakers.

The fact that the limited information available in visual aspects of speech may be used to develop a phonological system has been discussed by Dodd (1988). She suggests 'that strong evidence is provided that lip-read and heard speech are processed in a code insensitive to input modality. A phonological system can be derived from hearing by ear or from hearing by eye, but the resulting systems will differ in some respects.'

Intelligibility of Deaf Children's Speech

The speech of deaf children should be looked upon as a special idiolect that is dependent on speech reception capabilities and other factors that children rely upon when learning to speak. To compare the articulatory skill of a deaf child with that of a normal-hearing speaker is inappropriate, since the quality of the articulation is unimportant as long as the speech is intelligible.

The effect of different phonetic deviations on the intelligibility of deaf speech has been studied using different techniques: correlational studies and qualitative studies (Hudgins and Numbers, 1942; John and Howarth, 1965; Monsen, 1983), manipulation by means of digital speech processing (Huggins, 1977; Kruger, Stromberg and Levitt, 1972; Maassen and Powel, 1984, 1985; Osberger and Levitt, 1979), or speech synthesis techniques (Bernstein, 1977). With digital speech-coding techniques, only suprasegmental deviations are easily manipulated, but, in the case of speech synthesis, both segmental and suprasegmental factors can be manipulated.

The effect on the intelligibility of different kinds of deviations from normal production has not been decisively established. Most of the previous studies have not studied the interaction between the deviations and the individual effect of a deviation on intelligibility. Hence, the effect on intelligibility has varied depending on the contribution of deviations that have been examined.

At the Department of Speech Communication and Music Acoustics (KTH) a synthesis-by-rule system has been developed (Carlson and Granström, 1976). The system transforms text to synthetic speech by means of phonological and phonetic rules. The technique was used in a study by Öster (1985) to investigate the effects of segmental and suprasegmental deviations on the intelligibility of three deaf children's speech. The advantage of this technique was that it provides the only possible way to manipulate segmental and/or prosodic deviations, leaving others unchanged, to study the effect on intelligibility and the interaction between them.

The assessment of the speech of the three children was made

through traditional error analysis which did not pay any attention to contrastive function. The transcription was coarse, and the deviations made by the children were translated into simplified phonetic rules. In this study, the intention was not to investigate what the speech of the children did express, but rather to gain an opinion of the relative effect on intelligibility of a specific phonetic deviation.

Normal-hearing subjects estimated the effects of the children's segmental and suprasegmental deviations on intelligibility. A listening test was generated consisting of 96 different sentences: 32 of them mirroring each child's speech behaviour. The relative impact of the deviations and the individual effect on each child's speech intelligibility were established.

This study broadly classified the deviations of each child in an order of precedence according to intelligibility and it indicated which deviations should be corrected first, as they affected the intelligibility to the highest degree. Based on the results of the listening tests, recommendations could be given regarding an individual order for efficient correction. These findings stressed the importance of an individual assessment and an individual speech training programme for speech improvement. The result also showed that a slow tempo might have a positive impact on intelligibility, if the articulation was extremely poor. This was also shown by Osberger and Levitt (1979) and by Maassen and Powel (1985) and was explained by the fact that the listeners had more time available to process and interpret the meaning of the utterance. This was in accordance with an earlier study by Mártony, Tunblad and Öster (1981) where a remarkably slow tempo, but otherwise good articulation, made the speech unnatural but still intelligible.

Factors Affecting the Intelligibility of the Speech of Deaf Children

The intelligibility of the speech of deaf children will depend on to what extent their phonological system and phonetic realization of this system resemble the norm of the language users in general. The deviations in the speech of a deaf person will be influenced by a number of different factors. In the following a brief description is given.

Degree of hearing loss and functional hearing

Several studies have shown that there is a close relationship between degree of hearing impairment and the speech intelligibility of hearing-impaired children. Poor speech usually accompanies increasing hearing loss. Boothroyd (1984) and Levitt (1987) for example, have shown that, on average, speech intelligibility decreased with increasing hearing loss until a loss of about 90 dB. Above that, the degree of correlation was reduced.

The speech intelligibility of a hearing-impaired child depends not only on the amount of hearing, as measured by pure tone audiometry, but also on the quality of the hearing sensation and the use that the child, through training, has been able to make of his/her residual hearing. For a hearing loss above 90 dB, the term 'functional hearing' has been used. The functional hearing of a child, that is, the degree to which a child can use his/her hearing for speech perception and the control of his/her own speech production, will depend on many factors: degree of hearing loss, shape of the audiogram, amount of hearing aid use, amount of auditory training, etc. As pointed out by Monsen (1978) 'a good audiogram may correlate quite consistently with good speech; but, on the other hand, children with more severe hearing losses may commonly span the whole range from very intelligible to quite unintelligible speech'. Hence, the intelligibility of the speech of children with pure tone averages more than 90 dB cannot be predicted from the degree of hearing loss, as measured by pure tone audiometry. In these areas, sound might be perceived through vibrotactile rather than auditory receptors. Vibrotactile perception is mostly limited to speech-envelope features such as duration and intensity (Erber, 1974a). Normal auditory perception also includes the use of spectral features such as small differences in fundamental frequency and vowel formant patterns. The audiogram will not differentiate 'vibrotactile' from 'auditory' children as it provides insufficient information about speech processing capabilities, such as the ability to perceive gap durations and small differences both in frequency and intensity.

Speech processing capabilities and functional hearing are more appropriately measured by means of a speech test than by pure tones (Risberg, 1979). Since the range of speech reception skills in profoundly deaf children is quite limited, and since they are often low-verbal, speech test materials might be difficult to use. Sentences might contain words or difficult grammatical constructions with which they are unfamiliar. Speech tests especially designed for this group must be used. Cramer and Erber (1974) have shown that the result of a simple spondee recognition test provides valuable information about a profoundly deaf child's ability to perceive speech and his/her possibility to develop intelligible speech.

The lack of auditory feedback causes disordered respiratory processes in speech, which also affect the intelligibility of the speech of deaf persons. Whitehead (1983) showed that deaf persons often speak on low lung volumes and even initiate reading and conversation below the residual air capacity without inspiration. The lack of sufficient air is one reason for the poor control and low intelligibility of the speech of deaf children.

Visibility of speech elements

The perception of speech through vision is difficult since many articulatory features of speech are not accessible from visual observation (Woodward and Barber, 1960). Acoustically, each speech sound is unique, but many sounds are hard or impossible to discriminate visually. Some speech sounds have almost identical articulatory movements and others have invisible articulatory positions (Erber, 1974b). Markides (1989) stated that lipreading gives correct identification of about 30–40% of initial consonants and only 20–30% of final consonants.

Any set of speech segments that is visually contrastive from another is called a *viseme* (Fisher, 1968). Confusions in both articulation and perception occur within visemes but not between them. The set of visemes has, according to Owens and Blazek (1985), varied from study to study due to differences between languages, talkers, subjects' response tasks, and effects of vowel contexts. They reported that the vowel /u:/ limited the number of contrastive visual units. However, a certain consistency can be seen. Mártony *et al.* (1970) found three visible groups for Swedish consonants according to place of articulation: bilabials, labiodentals, and 'others'. As much as 82% of the Swedish consonants belong to the group 'others'. With the Swedish vowels, two visemes were identified, rounded and unrounded, due to the visibility of lip rounding and jaw opening. Hence, the articulatory extreme vowels /a:/ and /i:/ are visually contrastive to /u:/ and to each other.

Impact of orthography

Each language has its own sound system and sound pattern, i.e., specific rules of how to combine phonemes to build up meaningful words and utterances. The knowledge of the phonologic system of a specific language includes the knowledge of its pronunciation rules.

The new teaching situation in Swedish schools for the Deaf implies that speech training methods must be based on written Swedish and the use of sign-language for instruction and explanation. This means that it is extremely important for the children to be familiar with the pronunciation rules of Swedish. Insufficient knowledge of these rules causes deviations, which often are found in the speech of deaf children. The various orthographic representations of the phonemes /ʃç o: ε:/ give rise to some deviations and the fact that two, and sometimes three, letters are pronounced as one sound in Swedish is not obvious to some children.

Impact of teaching methods

When teaching deaf children articulation skills, 'clear speech' is often used by the teacher to improve lipreading. This 'over articulation' is not merely a louder version of normal speech, but may also involve an active reorganization of phonetic gestures (Lindblom and Moon, 1988; Moon, 1991). Picheny, Durlach and Braida (1986) reported major differences between conversational speech and clear speech. For example, stop bursts are always released with a higher intensity in clear speech, and the speaking rate decreases. There is an increase in the number of pauses used, and the durations of individual speech sounds and pauses are prolonged. This might cause temporal deviations in the speech of the children as well as a lack of coarticulation, and inappropriate sound insertions.

Other factors

Levitt (1987) has shown that the effect of background variables on the intelligibility of the speech of deaf children is of particular interest. He divided the background variables into three groups: 'etiological' (age at onset of hearing loss, deafness in the family and hearing level), 'educational' (age at onset of special education, age when the hearing aid was first fitted, use of the hearing aid, intelligence quotient, reading score, and syntactic comprehension) and 'other variables' (other handicapping conditions, home language, parental occupation, socio-economic status, and number of siblings). He emphasized the important role of special education and early, effective intervention.

Speech Assessment in a Learning Situation

In a speech teaching programme, it is necessary to continuously assess the speech of a deaf child to measure his/her performance, and any improvements resulting from training. Many assessment methods have been developed over the years.

Speech can be described at two levels: the phonetic and the phonological. A phonetic description is more or less detailed, and shows how consonants and vowels are produced (articulatory phonetics) or what the acoustical signal looks like (acoustic phonetics). A phonetic description does not have to pay attention to a specific language. Phonology on the other hand, is the study of how speech sounds are realized in spoken language. It looks for underlying rules in the child's speech, and specifies any idiosyncratic realization of phonological contrasts through a detailed transcription.

The speech of deaf children and adults contains a large number of deviations in segmental production that can be classified as distortions, substitutions, omissions and insertions. A distortion is a non-standard production. A substitution is when a standard phoneme replaces another phoneme. When a deviation is defined as an omission, a speech sound is not produced at all at a place where it should be. Finally, in the case of insertions, an improper addition of a speech sound is made. A *phonetic deviation* is the result of incorrect phonation or articulatory movements that has no effect on the speaker's ability to signal meaning differences. A phonetic deviation affects the naturalness of the speech. The presence of a phonetic deviation is defined as a *phonological deviation*, if it affects the meaning of the word.

Traditionally, the speech of deaf children has been assessed using phonetic error analyses only. This approach, however, provides insufficient information on which to base an effective speech training programme.

Assessment of phonetic deviations

A number of qualitative and quantitative studies have described the types of segmental and prosodic deviations, which are typical of the speech of the deaf, Calvert, 1961; Mártony, 1971; Calvert and Silverman, 1975; Ling, 1976; and Hochberg *et al.*, 1983. A review of acoustical and perceptual studies dealing with phonetic aspects in the speech of the deaf is given by Gold (1980). These phonetic descriptions did not pay attention to the contrastive function in a specific language.

Early studies were, for the most part, case studies based on diaries. Later, more extensive studies appeared, such as the classic study of Hudgins and Numbers (1942), which documented the speech of 192 deaf children ranging in age from 8 to 20 years. These early studies can be described as phonetic error analyses. They compared the articulation of deaf speakers with that of persons with normal hearing, and provided information on what deaf speakers were not capable of articulating. Unfortunately, the articulation was usually assessed using a coarse phonetic transcription, missing important articulatory details. Phonological aspects, which determined what the speech did express or the effects of different deviations on intelligibility, were seldom investigated.

A traditional error analysis provides information on the sounds that a deaf child is *not* capable of articulating. Hence, only speech sounds that the child never articulates correctly are treated in the speech clinic. The sounds that the child articulates correctly are ignored and it is assumed they are used correctly. The result of a phonetic error analysis provides insufficient information for planning speech training, since it pays no attention to either the usage of the productive knowledge in spoken language or to whether a deviant articulation might signal a 'correct' contrast (Monsen, 1976).

Assessment of phonological deviations

Present work, assessing the speech of deaf children, is concentrated on deeper aspects of speech production. A phonological assessment provides information about the use of a deaf child's productive knowledge, and identifies the phonetic deviations that affect the speaker's ability to signal meaning differences in spoken language. A phonological assessment investigates whether a deviant pronunciation is in fact a realization of signalling a contrast of meaning and, if so, in what way the child's realization differs from the normal model. Furthermore, it provides information about the speech sounds that the child can not yet produce.

Several studies of the phonological systems of hard-of-hearing and deaf children (West and Weber, 1973; Oller and Kelly, 1974; Dodd, 1974, 1976; Oller and Eilers, 1981; Öster, 1989a, 1989b, 1991, 1992) have shown that, although deaf children make deviations in production, they possess some kind of abstract and stable phonological system. They often have well-established speech habits, since they tend to produce a speech sound in the same deviant manner, in similar contexts.

Studies of the phonological systems of hard-of-hearing and deaf children have been inspired by Clinical Phonology (Hodson, 1980; Shriberg and Kwiatkowski, 1980; Grunwell, 1987; Ingram, 1989), which was developed to analyse phonological processes in disordered speech through descriptions of contrasts and processes. According to Grunwell (1987), there are five major clinical assessment procedures which are based on a phonological process analysis:

- Phonological Process Analysis (PPA; Weiner, 1979).
- Natural Process Analysis (NPA; Shriberg and Kwiatkowski ,1980).
- Assessment of Phonological Processes (APP; Hodson, 1980).
- Procedures for the Phonological Analysis of Children's Language (PPACL; Ingram, 1981).
- Phonological Assessment of Child Speech (PACS; Grunwell, 1985).

Linguistic theories such as Taxonomic Phonemics and Generative Phonology, Jakobson's Child Phonology theories (1968) and Stampe's Natural Phonology (1979) have contributed to the development of Clinical Phonology. Taxonomic Phonemics, developed in the 1940s and 1950s, classifies contrasting sound units or phonemes, which cause a difference in meaning. Generative Phonology described by Chomsky and Halle in the 1960s uses distinctive features and formal rules to describe the sound patterns of a language. Jakobson (1968) claimed that children learn contrasts, not individual sounds, in a certain order from maximal to minimal contrast. Stampe (1979) stressed that small children have a tendency to simplify adult speech by innate rules or processes.

Description of a Complete Phonological Assessment of a Deaf Child's Speech

The importance of an efficient and individualized assessment is stressed by, for example, Stoel-Gammon and Dunn (1985) 'It is necessary to identify the unique characteristics of each child's system in order to design the most appropriate treatment plan for each child.' Saben and Ingham (1991) also claimed that it is important to concentrate on the usage, in spoken language, of a child's *productive knowledge*, that is, the speech sounds that the child can produce in isolation, to identify the deviations made by the child.

To ensure that speech training does not become a series of meaningless 'articulatory gymnastic' sessions, the Hearing Technology Group has been involved in a joint project with the Manilla School for Deaf Children in Stockholm over the past 8 years. In this project we have developed a phonologically based assessment method on which to base speech training. This outlines a child's unique phonological system (phonetic and phonemic inventories) and is done in three steps, which are described below. First the individual child's productive knowledge is assessed. Then usage in spoken language and the idiosyncratic realization of phonological contrasts are analysed through a detailed phonetic transcription. The outcome of such a complete assessment provides significant and valuable information, which cannot be obtained if only a traditional phonetic error analysis is used.

As an example, the videorecorded speech of a 15-years-old, prelingually deaf child, educated using sign-language will be phonologically assessed below. His pure tone-average (at 0.5, 1 and 2 kHz) in the better ear was 108 dB ISO. Obviously, speech information was not perceived at all without a hearing aid.

The child was videorecorded saying 58 polysyllabic Swedish words. Within the constraints of the Swedish phonotactic system, these words sampled each Swedish consonant at least twice in the initial, medial and final positions. Consequently, each phoneme was sampled at least six times. The videorecorded speech was transcribed narrowly using IPA symbols and some specific diacritics (see Appendix).

Step 1: Analysis of the productive knowledge

Many children articulate several speech sounds correctly in isolation but have problems in producing them contrastively in various contexts. At first, it is important to concentrate upon those speech sounds which the child can produce in isolation or in syllables, but which are not correctly realized in a linguistic context. These speech sounds should be consolidated before attempts are made to introduce the speech sounds, which are not yet within the child's productive inventory. By assessing the productive knowledge, it is also possible to exclude a motoric disorder as a cause of a phonological deviation.

Table 1 shows the speech sounds that are present (the productive knowledge) and the speech sounds that are absent in the child's inventory (the blank cells). This is done without regard for the accuracy of the child's productions. Although the child has an articulatory knowledge of 8 of the 18 Swedish consonants, some deviations occurred in different positions, due to limited information of phonetic features, limited knowledge of the rules of pronunciation, etc. The table shows that he produced only five of the eight consonants correctly in the initial position, six of them in the medial position and five of them in the final position. The consonants which caused deviations were /g, ç, m/.

Table 1. Productive knowledge of a prelingually deaf child (in bold style), the word position where the consonant was correctly articulated (X) and the word position where a deviation occurred (blank cells).

IPA	Productive knowledge	Used correctly		
		Initial	Medial	Final
p				
t				
k	X	X	X	X
b	X	X	X	X
d	X	X	X	X
g	X			
f	X	X	X	X
v				
s				
ʃ				
ç	X			
j				
h				
m	X		X	
n				
ŋ				
l				
r	X	X	X	X
=	8 18	5 17	6 16	5 16

Step 2: Assessment of the usage of the productive knowledge through a detailed phonetic analysis

The assessment of the usage of the child's productive knowledge must be based on a detailed phonetic analysis that forms the 'raw data'.

Many peculiarities and fusions occur in prelingually deaf children's speech. These make an expansion of IPA symbols and diacritics necessary. We have used some of those which Bush *et al..* (1973); Grunwell (1987); Roug, Landberg and Lundberg (1987) have developed to transcribe babbling and phonetic development in early infancy.

In Table 2 the deviations made by the child in the initial, medial and final positions are shown. Special attention should be paid to the consonants /g, ç, m/. The child has an articulatory knowledge of these sounds, but his productions always (except /m/ in medial position) involve substitutions of other phonemes. It can be seen that [g] is used for /ŋ/ but when asked to produce /g/ it is realized as [k]. Similarly [ç] is substituted for /s/ and /ʃ/ but when the child is asked to produce /ç/ he substitutes a [k]. The nasal /m/ is produced correctly in the medial position but in the initial and final position it is phonetically similar to /b/.

Table 2. Phonetic deviations made in various word positions in a prelingually deaf child's speech. The productive knowledge is shown in bold style.

IPA	Initial	Medial	Final
p	b	b	b ə
t	d	d	d ˺
k			
b	**b**	**b**	**b**˺
d			
g	k	k	k
f			
v	f K	f K	f K
s	ç	ç	ç
ʃ	ç k	ç	ç ə
ç	k		
j	ɖ F	ɖ F	ɖ F
h	Ø		
m	b̃	**m** b	b̃ ə
n	d̃	d̃	d̃
ŋ		g	g ə
l	ɖ	ɖ	ɖ
r			

In training, the child needs to develop the ability to use these existing sounds appropriately. Only when these sounds can be produced in all word positions should new speech sounds be taught.

Step 3: Assessment of idiosyncratic realizations of phonological contrasts through a detailed transcription

The phonetic deviations which may affect the child's ability to signal meaning differences in spoken language, must be established and corrected to improve intelligibility. Such an analysis compares a deaf child's system with the adult standard Swedish system, and describes the child's deviations through a detailed phonetic transcription, and diacritics to specify the phonetic elements used.

By studying Table 2 closely it is possible to determine whether a deviant pronunciation is, in fact, an attempt by the child to realize a phonological contrast. Some of the deviant phone types represent different phonemes despite the phonetic similarity. For example, many of the deviant phone types are similar to /b/ and /d/. It can be assumed that the child, despite the phonetic similarity to [b], makes contrasts between /p/, /b/ and /m/ in the initial position through voicing for /p/, lip protrusion for /b/ and nasal air emission for /m/. It is also very likely that the child, despite the phonetic similarity to [d], contrasts /t, d, j, n, l/ in the final position, through a non-audible release for /t/, retroflexion and frication for /j/, nasal air emission for /n/ and retroflexion for /l/. Obviously, the child understands the phonological contrasts between these visually similar consonants, but has difficulties in realizing them correctly.

Table 3. The outcome of a coarse and a detailed phonetic transcription of some of a prelingually deaf child's phonetic deviations.

The importance of a detailed phonetic transcription

Table 3 shows the different outcomes from a coarse or a detailed phonetic transcription of the child's speech.

A coarse phonetic transcription would have missed the important articulatory details that the child uses, trying to realize the contrasts discussed above.

The result of the coarse phonetic transcription would have been that /p, m/ were substituted by /b/ and /t, j, n, l/ by /d/, i.e., that the child was missing /p, m, t, j, n and l/ in his phonetic inventory. Articulatory training of each of these consonants in isolation might dissolve the unique phonological system of the child. Instead, the articulatory training must be directed to deal with all these contrasting consonants simultaneously.

Conclusions

Prelingually deaf children very rarely develop speech spontaneously. Speech is almost always developed through training using the visibility of phonetic features, reading, tactile sensations and, if possible, residual hearing. These inputs severely limit speech perception potential and cause deaf children to make unavoidable articulatory deviations. These phonetic deviations may affect the child's ability to signal meaning differences in spoken language.

The speech therapist must be aware that the input limitations, the impact of orthography and teaching methods cause deviant phonological processes in deaf children's speech. If training is made without an awareness of a child's phonological system, this may destroy already established couplings between the abstract entities and articulation. To increase the intelligibility of his/her speech, the child must first be made aware of his/her deviant way of expressing phonological contrasts. The articulatory training must then be directed to deal with all contrasting consonants simultaneously. Otherwise, the result might be that the child's phonological system will be disturbed and the intelligibility of his/her speech will decrease after training.

As a basis for an effective speech training, only a thorough phonological assessment can provide the answers to questions such as: How successfully can the child produce speech contrasts? Might a deviant production in fact be a realization of a phonological contrast? In what ways do the phonetic elements used for contrastive function differ from those used in normal speech? Speech training which is based only on a phonetic error analysis will not take account of the individual deaf child's phonological system.

It is important that the speech therapist is aware of which level, phonetic or phonological, he or she is working on in a specific situation. If an assessment shows that the child understands a phonological contrast, but has difficulties in realizing it correctly, the therapist can concentrate on articulatory training. However, the child must first be made aware of the deviant way he/she expresses the contrast in different contexts. If, on the other hand, the assessment shows that the child does not understand a phonological contrast, it must be learned simultaneously with articulatory training in how to realize it.

Acknowledgements

The work has been supported by grants from the Bank of Sweden Tercentenary Foundation.

References

Abberton, E., Fourcin, A.J. and Hazan, V. (1985) Phonological competence with profound hearing loss. Paper presented at the Int. Congr. on Education of the Deaf, Manchester, United Kingdom.

Amcoff, S. (1973) Relationer mellan sprakliga uttrycksformer. En undersökning av elever i specialskolan för hörselskadade. Pedagogisk forskning, Uppsala, No.1.

Bernstein, J. (1977) Intelligibility and simulated deaf-like segmental and timing errors. Record IEEE Int. Conf. Acoust. Speech and Signal Processing, Hartford.

Boothroyd, A. (1984) Auditory perception of speech contrasts by subjects with sensorineural hearing loss. Journal of Speech and Hearing Research 27: 128-134.

Bush, C.N., Edwards, M.L., Luckau, J.M., Stoel, C.M., Macken, M.A. and Petersen, J.D. (1973) On specifying a system for transcribing consonants in child language: A working paper with examples from American English and Mexican Spanish. Report, Dept. of Linguistics, Stanford University.

Calvert, D. (1961) Some Acoustic Characteristics of the Speech of Profoundly Deaf Individuals. Ph.D. thesis, Stanford University, Palo Alto, CA.

Calvert, D.R. and Silverman, S.R. (1975) Speech and Deafness. Washington: Alexander Graham Bell Association for the Deaf.

Carlson, R. and Granström, B. (1976) A Text-to-Speech System Based Entirely on rules. Conf. Record. 1976 IEEE Int. Conf. on Acoustics, Speech and Signal Processing, April, Philadelphia, PA., pp 686–9.

Cramer, K.D. and Erber, N.P. (1974) A spondee recognition test for young hearing-impaired children. Journal of Speech and Hearing Disorders 39: 304–11.

Dodd, B. (1974) The acquisition of phonological skills in normal, severely subnormal and deaf children. Doctoral dissertation, Univ. of London.

Dodd, B. (1976) The phonological systems of deaf children. Journal of Speech and Hearing Disorders 41: 185–97.

Dodd, B. (1988) Lip-Reading, Phonological Coding and Deafness. In Dodd and Campell (Eds) Hearing By Eye: The Psychology of Lip-Reading, pp 177–89.

Erber, N.P. (1974a) Pure-tone thresholds and word-recognition abilities of hearing-impaired children. Journal of Speech and Hearing Research 17: 194–202.

Erber, N.P. (1974b) Visual perception of speech by deaf children: recent developments and continuing needs. Journal of Speech and Hearing Disorders 39: 178–85.

Fisher, C.G. (1968) Confusions among visually perceived consonants. Journal of Speech and Hearing Research 11: 796–804.

Gold, T. (1980) Speech production in hearing-impaired children, Journal of Communication Disorders 13: 397–418.

Göllesz. (1972) Uber die Lippernartikulation der von Geburt an Blinden. In Interdisciplinary Speech Research, Proceedings of the Speech Symposium, 1971, Szeged, Budapest: Akademiai Kiado, pp. 85–91.

Grunwell, P. (1985) Phonological assessment of child speech (PACS). Windsor: INFER-Nelson. San Diego, CA: UK/College-Hill Press.

Grunwell, P. 1987. Clinical Phonology. Baltimore: Williams and Wilkins.

Hochberg, I., Levitt, H. and Osberger, M.J. (1983) Speech of the Hearing-Impaired, Research, Training and Personal Preparation. Baltimore, MD: University Park Press.

Hodson, B.W. (1980) The Assessment of Phonological Processes. Danville, IL.: Interstate Inc.

Hudgins, C. and Numbers, F. (1942) An Investigation of the Intelligibility of the Speech of the Deaf. Genet. Psychol. Monographs 25: 289–392.

Huggins, A.W.F. (1977) Timing and speech intelligibility. In Requin, J.(Ed) Attention and Performance, VII. Hillsdale, N.J.: Lawrence Erlbaum.

Ingram, D. (1989) Phonological Disability in Children. (2nd edn). London: Cole and Whurr.

Jakobson, R. 1968. Child Language, Aphasia and Phonological Universals. The Hague: Mouton and Co.

John, J.E.J. and Howarth, J. (1965) The Effect of Time Distortions on the Intelligibility of Deaf Children's Speech. Language and Speech 8:127–34.

Kruger, F., Stromberg, H. and Levitt, H. (1972) Synthetic speech as a diagnostic tool. CSL Research Report No. 2, June.

Levitt, H. (1987) Interrelationship among the speech and language measures, in Development of language and communication skills in hearing-impaired children. ASHA Monograph, 26: 123–58.

Lindblom, B. and Moon, S-J. (1988) Formant undershoot in clear and citation form speech. Perilus VIII (Phonetic Experimental Research, Institute of Linguistics, University of Stockholm), 20–32.

Ling, D. (1976) Speech and the Hearing-Impaired Child: Theory and Practice. The Alexander Graham Bell Association for the Deaf, Inc. Washington, D.C. 20007, USA.

Maassen, B. and Powel, D.J. (1984) The effect of correcting temporal structure on the intelligibility of deaf speech, Speech and Communication 3: 123–35.

Maassen, B. and Powel, D.J.(1985) The effect of segmental and suprasegmental corrections on the intelligibility of deaf speech. Journal of the Acoustical Society of America 78: 877–86.

Markides, A. (1989) Lipreading: Theory and practice. Journal of the British Association of Teachers of the Deaf 13(2): 29–47.

Mártony, J. (1971) Om gravt hörselskadades tal, Fillic. avhandling, Inst. för Talöverföring, KTH, Stockholm.

Mártony, J., Tunblad, T. and Öster, A-M. (1981) Talets naturlighet. In Talfel och dess effekter, Technical report, TRITA-TLF-81-3

Mártony, J., Risberg, A., Agelfors, E. and Boberg, G. (1970) Om talavläsning med elektronisk avläsningshjälp, Intern rapport, Inst. för Talöverföring, KTH.

Mills, A. (1983) The development of phonology in the blind child. In Dodd, B. and Campbell, R. (Eds) Hearing by Eye: The Psychology of Lip-Reading, Hillsdale, N.J.: Lawrence Erlbaum, pp 145–61.

Monsen, R.B. (1976) The production of English stop consonants in the speech of deaf children. Journal of Phonetics 4: 29–41.

Monsen, R.B. (1978) Toward measuring how well hearing-impaired children speak. Journal of Speech and Hearing Research 21: 197–219.

Monsen; R.B. (1983) Voice quality and speech intelligibility among deaf children. American Annals for the Deaf 128: 12–19.

Moon, S-J. (1991) An acoustic and perceptual study of undershoot in clear and citation-form speech. Perilus XIV, 153–6 (Phonetic Experimental Research, Institute of Linguistics, University of Stockholm).

Oller, D.K. and Kelly, C.A. (1974) Phonological substitution processes of a hard-of-hearing child. Journal of Speech and Hearing Disorders 39: 65–74.

Oller, D.K. and Eilers, R.E. (1981) A pragmatic approach to phonological systems of deaf speakers. Speech and Language, Advances in basic research and practice. Academic Press. pp 103–41.

Osberger, M.J. and Levitt, H. 1979. The Effect of Timing Errors on the Intelligibility of Deaf Children's Speech. Journal of the Acoustical Society of America 66: 1316–24.

Öster, A-M. (1985) The Use of a Synthesis-by-Rule-System in a Study of Deaf Speech. STL-QPSR 1/1985, pp 95–107. Stockholm: Dept. of Speech Communication and Music Acoustics.

Öster, A-M. (1989a) Studies on phonological rules in the speech of the deaf. STL/QPSR 1/89: 159–62.

Öster, A-M. (1989b) Applications and experiences of computer-based speech training. STL/QPSR 4/89: 37–44,

Öster, A-M. (1991) Phonological assessment of eleven prelingually deaf children's consonant production. STL-QPSR 2-3/91: 11–18.

Öster, A-M. (1992) Phonological assessment of deaf children's productive knowledge as a basis for speech training. Proceedings of ICSLP 92, october 12-16, Banff, Alberta, Canada, pp 955-958.

Owens, E. and Blazek, B. (1985) Visemes observed by hearing-impaired and normal hearing adult viewers. Journal of Speech and Hearing Research 28: 381–93.

Picheny, M.A., Durlach, N.I. and Braida, L.D. (1986) Speaking clearly for the hard of hearing II: Acoustic characteristics of clear and conversational speech. Journal of Speech and Hearing Research 29: 434–46

Risberg, A(1979) Bestämning av hörkapacitet och talperceptionsförmaga vid svara hörsel skador, Rapport TRITA-TLF-79-2, Doktorsavhandling, Inst. för Talöverföring, KTH, Stockholm.

Roug, L., Landberg, I.and Lundberg, L-J. (1987) Phonetic development in early infancy. A study of four Swedish children during the first 18 months of life. Report from Dep. of Linguistics, Stockholm University.

Saben, C.B. and Ingham, J.C. (1991) The effects of minimal pairs treatment on the speech-sound production of two children with phonologic disorders. Journal of Speech and Hearing Research 34: 1023–40.

Shriberg, L.D. and Kwiatkowski, J. (1980) Natural Process Analysis (NPA). New York: John Wiley.

Stampe, D. 1979. A Dissertation on Natural Phonology. In Hankamer, I. (Ed) New York: Garland.

Stoel-Gammon, C. and Dunn, C. (1985) Normal and Disordered Phonology in Children. Baltimore, Md.: University Park Press.

Weiner, F.F. (1979) Phonological Process Analysis (PPA), University Park Press, Baltimore, Md.

West, J.J. and Weber, J.L. (1973) A phonological analysis of the spontaneous language of a four-year-old, hard-of-hearing child. Journal of Speech and Hearing Disorders 38: 25–35.

Whitehead, R.L. (1983) Some respiratory and aerodynamic patterns in the speech of the hearing impaired. In Hochberg, Levitt, Osberger (Eds) Speech of the Hearing Impaired; Research, Training and Personal Preparation, Maryland, MD: University Park Press. pp 97–116.

Woodward, M.F. and Barber, C.G. (1960) Phoneme perception in lipreading, Journal of Speech and Hearing Research 3: 212–22.

Wundt (1911) Volkerpsychologie Band I: Die Sprache, 3rd edn, Leipzig: Engelman.

Appendix: Diacritics to assess the speech of deaf children

(Inspired by C.N. Bush *et al*. L. Roug *et al*., P.Grunwell)

Modification of manner of articulation:

Symbol	Example	
~	ã:	Nasalized
≈	≈̃a:	Heavily nasalized
ω	$\overset{s}{\omega}$	Labialization
~	ɫ	Velarization
↑	tɪt↑a	Inhalation
↓	tɪt↓a	Expiration
⧣	kɔma⧣	Very weak production
( )	(f)⧣	Silent articulation; absence of air-stream but articulation present
⌐	t⌐	Stop with non-audible release
F	Fp	Stop with unspecified frication
᷈	p̃	Nasal air emission
O	⑦	Inadequately realized; doubtful symbol
(( ))	((ɑ:))	Masked by noise
←	ḇ̱	Lip-protrusion
K	fK	Fricative with explosive release

Modification of place of articulation:

Symbol	Example	
⊥	e⊥:	Tight variant
⟂	e⟂:	Loose variant

⊢	k:	Advanced variant
⊢	k:	Retracted variant
⩯	e:	Instability between base and tight
⩦	i:	Instability between base and loose
⊓	s	Interdental articulation
⌒	i:	Markedly spread lips
L1	s L1	Apex part of tongue
L2	s L2	Blade part of tongue
L3	s L3	Mid part of tongue
L4	s L4	Back part of tongue
L5	s L5	Root part of tongue

Modification of vocal fold activity:

Symbol	Example	
o	b o	Voiceless
∨	s ∨	Voiced
∨	∨s s∨	Pre/post-voiced
h	p h	Aspiration
h	h p	Preaspiration
=	p=	Unaspiration
∧∧∧	a: ∧∧∧	Laryngealization

Modification of duration:

Symbol	Example	
∪	mb ∪	Coarticulation

		Absence of coarticulation: short silence between
—	mIn−nɛ:sa	segments or words
=	mIn=nɛ:sa	long silence between segments or words
≡	mIn≡nɛ:sa	extra long silence between segments or words
:	ɑ:	Long production
::	ɑ::	Very long production
ⱽ	t̬	Very clipped
|	bɔ|j	Long break
||	bɔ||j	Very long break
:|	ɔ:|	Repitition of a segment
|::|	|:ɔm:|	Repitition of a word

Modification of pitch:

Symbol	Example	
—	ā	High tone
_	a̲	Low tone
/	ᐟa	Rising tone
\	aˋ	Falling tone
/\	a̍	Rising - falling tone
\/	a̍	Falling - rising tone
_ _	ab̄āba̲	Sequence tones
⌒⌒	ababa	Continuous tones

21

The Use of Sensory Aids for Teaching Speech to Children who are Deaf

JAMES MAHSHIE

Teaching children who are deaf[1] to speak is a formidable task for both teacher and child. Even with amplification, reliance on residual hearing to mediate speech learning may not be adequate for many deaf or hard-of-hearing children. With limited auditory capability, the deaf child often lacks both accurate auditory models of speech targets and auditory feedback with which to achieve accurate productions. Alternative sources of speech production information are thus desirable, or in some cases, necessary for speech to develop.

Sensory aids are devices and procedures designed to supplement or replace hearing as the sensory modality for speech. Sensory aids have long been a part of the armaments available to speech teachers[2] in their quest to facilitate speech development in deaf children. Among the non-electronic sensory aids historically used to facilitate deaf children's speech development are visual depictions of the speech mechanism, tactile manipulation of non-visible articulators (such as the tongue or soft palate) to convey shape and position information, feathers or tissue to depict air flow patterns, and devices such as the manometric flame (Scripture, 1902).

More recently, electronic and digital devices have replaced these more rudimentary sources of speech information. There are currently dozens of devices designed specifically to help deaf and hard-of-hearing children acquire speech skills. It is hard to find an educational or school programme for deaf children that does not have (or that is not trying to obtain) a speech training aid. In addition, sophisticated tactile devices, and the rapid appearance of cochlear implants as sensory supplements or alternatives to hearing, are having a significant impact on the form of speech instruction provided to deaf children.

While sensory aids have long been used for speech teaching (Coyne, 1938; Hudgins, 1935) not all agree that these devices benefit speech learning. For example, Ling (1976, 1977) suggests that sensory aids may delay the internalization of production patterns and thus actually

461

limit the acquisition of speech skills by deaf children. Ling further suggests that sensory aids should be used only when it is clear that the skill cannot be taught using residual hearing or speechreading (Ling, 1976, 1977).

Despite these concerns, the limited research evaluating the effectiveness of devices for facilitating speech development (see reviews by Bernstein, Goldstein and Mahshie, 1988; Braeges and Houde, 1981) suggests that sensory aids can contribute to deaf children's speech improvement.

It is clear that sensory aids will continue to be developed and used for teaching speech. Refinements in signal processing, the availability of different types of sensors, the relative accessibility of low-cost computers, refinements in tactile and visual displays, and other innovations have contributed to the development of many appealing and potentially useful devices to promote speech development.

However, questions exist about how available devices can best be used to yield optimal speech gains. Current clinical models, such as that developed by Ling (1976), are widely accepted among clinicians. In addition, there is considerable knowledge available about pedagogical factors (such as the nature and timing of cues and feedback presented to the learner) and their importance for speech teaching (Ruscello, 1984). Examination of existing devices, however, suggests there is not always a good match between speech teaching practices and the capabilities of existing sensory aids designed for teaching speech (Granzin and Morganstern, 1980).

In the present chapter, the pedagogical issues involved in teaching speech will be used as a framework within which to examine the development, evaluation, and use of existing technologies. More specifically, this chapter will: (1) examine the issues inherent in developing speech in children with minimal auditory capability; (2) describe pedagogical issues associated with using sensory aids for speech training with deaf children; (3) examine existing technologies and the evidence for their clinical efficacy; and (4) discuss future needs.

Issues Involved in Acquiring Speech

The following section will describe the process of speech learning for hearing children, and will examine ways in which that process may differ for a deaf or hard-of-hearing child.

Normal-hearing children and speech development

From their earliest experiences with the auditory world, children begin to organize their mental impressions of what they hear in ways that ultimately contribute to future development of both auditory and speech skills. While our understanding of the relationship between what is heard and what is produced is incomplete, the following series of steps are the likely sequence involved in acquiring speech skills:

1. As the child hears speech, an auditory pattern is stored in memory. These auditory patterns serve as both the directors of motor productions, and as the reference of correctness (Schmidt, 1988) for learning the motor patterns.[3]
2. The child attempts to produce speech that he/she hears.
3. Awareness of the speech patterns produced is not concurrent with production, but rather occurs after the production. The child obtains information about the outcome of the production attempt through auditory feedback and then compares the auditory pattern associated with his/her imitations to the stored reference patterns. This comparison acts as an error detection mechanism whereby the production accuracy is assessed.
4. Subsequent attempts are adapted to reduce the 'error' in the production, and comparisons are again made.
5. Through repeated attempts to produce the pattern, the child establishes the sensory-motor transforms required to produce that pattern.
6. The outcome is development of learned transformations between the auditory patterns and the motor patterns (sensory-motor association) (Risberg, 1968).

Speech acquisition thus relies on, and is mediated by, hearing. Among the particular motor tasks involved in speaking that the child must learn through audition are:

1. Placement of articulators
2. Control of the breathstream
3. Coordination of articulators
4. Coordination of articulatory, phonatory and respiratory elements of speaking
5. Production of adequate phonation (pitch and quality)
6. Accurate articulatory patterns of the larynx responsible for the production of voice vs voiceless contrast, together with appropriate coordination of the patterns
7. Breath support

Speech development and the deaf child

Traditional approaches to facilitating development of speech in deaf children typically attempt to mimic hearing children's speech acquisition, albeit with a little help through amplification and instruction.

Where a child has the ability to extract usable information from what is heard, this approach can be beneficial. These deaf or hard-of hearing children, through amplified audition, receive early auditory input of spoken language in the environment, and speech feedback from their own productions. While appropriate for some, not all deaf children will develop speech automatically merely by providing them with amplification. Limited auditory capabilities result in both difficulty detecting and difficulty processing speech. As a result, residual hearing alone is not sufficient to enable many (perhaps most) deaf children to develop speech.[4]

For some deaf children, alternative sensory information is needed for skills to develop. This has involved providing the child either with alternative auditory input in the form of a cochlear implant (Osberger, Chapter 11), or a supplemental or alternative input in the form of vibrotactile input (Vergara *et al.*, 1993). For these children the goal is to facilitate natural speech production and sensory development via a prosthetic device, one that is worn all the time. Discussion of how these devices can impact on speech development is discussed elsewhere in this volume.

Teaching speech to deaf children

Development of speech for the vast majority of deaf children in programmes in the United States, Sweden, and elsewhere requires speech instruction; these children are typically not expected to develop speech on their own (or with minimal specific intervention directed toward speech improvement), but rather they are provided specific (and for some intensive) speech teaching. Increasingly, sensory aids, both visual and tactual, are being used in speech therapy to either supplement amplified audition, or in some cases, to replace it. The speech-learning process for a deaf child who does not benefit greatly from amplification, and who must be taught speech skills, differs significantly from speech-learning of a hearing child or a deaf child whose speech development can be facilitated through the prosthetic use of amplification or other sensory aids (Risberg, 1968).

Pedagogical Factors Involved in Teaching Speech

Teaching speech skills to deaf and hard-of-hearing children typically requires consideration of at least three major factors: (1) the tasks and target skill to be taught; (2) the cues presented to the child to elicit the production; and (3) the feedback provided to the child about his/her production attempt. The following discussion will examine issues associated with each of these factors and describe ways that existing technologies address each issue.

Skill areas and tasks

To establish the precise speech areas to be taught to a young deaf child, the teacher typically evaluates the child to determine skills that are present or lacking. By systematically examining the speech patterns the child is capable (or not capable) of producing, the teacher can determine whether or not segmental and suprasegmental production patterns are present that might be expected given the child's previously acquired speech capabilities, age, auditory skills, etc. In the US and Canada, many clinicians rely on the teaching sequence described by Ling (1976) to determine the production skills that should be taught, and in what order. While the sequence described by Ling is arguably based on the patterns observed in normal-hearing children's speech development, this framework does provide both a useful model for selecting speech skills to be taught and useful tools for evaluating deaf children's speech.

Once skill areas are selected, speech teaching is initiated. While the specific structure of teaching speech to deaf children may vary somewhat from clinician to clinician, there are generally four identifiable steps involved: elicit, automate, generalize, and facilitate linguistic use (Ling, 1976; Risberg, 1968).

An initial step for all speech skill teaching involves *eliciting* production of a target. For example, teaching production of the nasal consonant /m/ involves demonstrating to the child the target sound (through audition, taction, or vision) and then having the child attempt the utterance until it is produced acceptably. This can often be a time intensive task for the child, and requires that the teacher have a good understanding of the respiratory, phonatory and articulatory bases of the speech unit being taught.

Following an acceptable production, the pattern is drilled and practised so that it is achieved without the speaker having to attend to details of the production. This is referred to as *automaticity* (Ling, 1976; Schmidt, 1988) and is considered necessary for speech to be produced smoothly and effortlessly.

Once the target can be produced easily and automatically, the child is taught to *generalize* the production pattern to different contexts and syllable locations. Such generalization training is an important component of teaching the child to use a developing skill for communication.

Finally, the child is taught to produce the target pattern in meaningful words or phrases. *Facilitating linguistic use* involves the transfer of skills from imitated and practised utterances to communicative speech. Activities directed at promoting linguistic use typically start with easier tasks (such as monosyllabic words in limited contexts) and become less structured and rehearsed as the child demonstrates mastery. The desired end-point of this teaching step is the spontaneous use of the skill in conversational speech.

Each of these four major steps can be further subdivided into smaller steps or subskills that are achievable for the child. For example, generalization of the nasal consonant /m/ production might initially involve production in isolation, followed by production of the consonant after the neutral vowel /e/. Subsequent attempts might vary vowel context, and syllable context. Similarly, promoting linguistic use might initially involve production of the target segment in words, followed by practice in phrases, sentences, and finally, conversational speech. There are thus numerous 'small' steps involved as sub-components of these four major steps.

Many devices have been designed to facilitate production of suprasegmental patterns. Many of these devices also permit limited work on consonant and vowel articulation, although there are no currently available devices that permit extensive work on both suprasegmentals and segmentals.

Not all devices are equally suited to facilitating productions at the four steps described above. For example, the Indiana Speech Training and Evaluation Aid (ISTRA) (Watson *et al.*, 1989) is designed to promote drill and practice of syllables and words by providing feedback based on the match between a production attempt and a stored template. The system uses speaker-dependent speech recognition technology and so the templates are based on acceptable production attempts that have been facilitated by the teacher. The system is thus designed to promote automaticity, generalization and early stages of promoting linguistic use. ISTRA contains only limited functions directed at eliciting productions, and the system was not designed to provide feedback during connected speech. Conversely, the electropalatograph (EPG) (Fletcher and Hasegawa, 1983) provides direct feedback of contact between the tongue and palate. While useful for eliciting initial productions and automaticity, it appears less optimal for promoting generalization or linguistic use.

Cues or targets

The cue or target comprises the information that is provided to the child to signal the production goal to be achieved. The strength and specificity of cues provided to the child interact with the task (Mower, 1977). Cues will be very specific during earlier tasks associated with a particular skill area. As the learner obtains greater proficiency with the task, cue strength is reduced. The task level will subsequently be made more demanding, and cues will again be made stronger. Cues and tasks are thus related, and are adapted by clinicians to match the performance level of the learner.

For speech training devices, the cues provided are typically in the form of models or templates, with or without explanations provided by the teacher. Currently available devices permit only limited adaptation of cues to the performance level of the child. However, an experimental system developed at Johns Hopkins University (Ferguson, Bernstein and Goldstein, 1988; Mahshie *et al.*, 1988) explored graded cuing for teaching loudness control. During earlier training steps, the intended intensity target was cued by a vertically oriented bar. The bar was divided into blocks of three different colors, each representing a different intended intensity level. Blue, at the bottom, signalled low-intensity speech, green, in the middle, corresponded to conversational levels and red, at the top, corresponded to loud speech. During later tasks, a clown holding different colored balloons was used to signal different intensity targets to be produced. The spatial orientation was eliminated so that only colors were used to signal a desired intensity level. When the balloon having a particular color started flashing, the student was required to produce a vocalization whose intensity corresponded to the target color. While the Hopkins system demonstrated the feasibility of graded cuing in a computer based training device, no currently available commercial device provides the user with the ability to alter the level of cuing provided.

Feedback

The third factor that a clinician considers in teaching a particular speech pattern is the feedback that will be given. Like the cues provided to the child, the feedback will vary depending on the level of skill acquisition demonstrated by the child. Ultimately, the goal of all intervention will be for the child to self-monitor his/her productions so that he/she is able to detect better and poorer productions without external mediation. However, such internal feedback develops only after considerable drill and practice of a particular skill. Consequently, the child will depend on external feedback to develop this more useful internal feedback.

There are a number of factors the teacher considers (either explicitly or implicitly) in providing feedback to the speech learner. Each of these factors is briefly described below, along with a brief examination of how the factor is implemented in existing speech teaching technologies.

Sources of feedback information

In traditional speech teaching, the teacher will listen to the child's attempt and provide feedback about the accuracy of the production. This feedback is most often verbal (or signed) and is based on what is heard. As suggested earlier, however, teachers have long relied on tactile or visual information as an additional source of feedback. For example, children are often taught a nasal/oral sound contrast by touching the nose and feeling the presence or absence of vibration.

Feedback provided by sensory aids can be obtained from a number of acoustic or physiological transducers. Among possible signals that have been employed in speech teaching aids are microphones (for example, Watson and Kewley-Port, 1990, aerodynamic measuring devices such as the pneumotachograph (Mahshie and Yadav, 1990), accelerometers (Stevens, Kalikow and Willemain, 1975), and specialized devices such as the electropalatograph (EPG) that monitor the extent and pattern of contact between the tongue and palate (Fletcher and Hasegawa, 1983). While the majority of computer-based systems use a single transducer (for example, IBM SpeechViewer II, there are some devices that employ multiple transducers. For example, a system developed by Matsushita Electronic Industries of Japan uses a microphone, accelerometer, an airflow measuring sensor, and an electropalatograph (Murata *et al.*, 1986). Another device, the Nasometer (Seaver *et al.*, 1991) employs a special arrangement of microphones that permits separate monitoring of acoustic energy from the oral and nasal tracts. Comparison of these signals provides an objective measure of the degree of oral and nasal coupling during speech.

Feedback timing

The clinician typically manipulates both the timing and nature of external feedback to match the level of performance demonstrated by the child. The timing of feedback can be concurrent with, or immediately following, the production attempt (immediate feedback), or it can be given somewhat after the production attempt (delayed feedback). Feedback can also be given after each attempt (separated feedback), or after a group of attempts (accumulated feedback) (Schmidt, 1988). Operant-conditioning literature (for example, Mowrer, 1977) suggests that during earlier stages of teaching a new skill, continuous feedback is normally provided. Maximum learning will subsequently occur when feedback is provided on an irregular basis. As the child begins to acquire a skill, the schedule of reinforcement should be varied so that learners have an opportunity to internalize the means of evaluating their production patterns. It has been suggested that this process can be enhanced when external feedback is given less frequently and on an irregular schedule.

Few currently available devices permit manipulation of feedback timing.[5] An exception is the experimental system developed at Johns Hopkins (Ferguson *et al.*, 1988; Mahshie *et al.*, 1988), which systematically altered the timing of feedback for a series of lessons designed to teach deaf children to control vocal intensity. During early activities feedback was immediate – occurring during the production attempt. For later activities, feedback was delayed, occurring after the production attempt was completed. Only one commercially available system, the Indiana Speech Training Aid (ISTRA), is reported to provide the teacher with the ability to vary feedback schedule depending on the student's performance level (Kewley-Port and Watson, 1991).

Knowledge of results vs knowledge of performance

The nature of feedback can also vary. In some cases, it is desirable to provide the learner with information about the outcome of the attempt. In this case, the child is provided *knowledge of results* (Schmidt, 1988) of his/her production attempt with respect to the training goal. This type of feedback can convey information about the magnitude of accuracy (right vs wrong, 80% correct, etc.) and about the direction of the attempt (undershoot, over-occluded, etc.)

The majority of currently available devices present knowledge of results as the primary form of feedback. For example, the Video Voice, an acoustically based training device, presents patterns corresponding to a Formant 2 vs Formant 1 (F2-F1) plot of the target word. The template and an attempt are shown on the same screen, with the extent of 'overlap' (and a numerical score corresponding to the degree of overlap) providing the learner with knowledge of results of the production attempt.

In contrast to knowledge of results, *knowledge of performance* is feedback about the actual movement patterns that were used by the individual. Providing the child with knowledge of performance would involve conveying information about how closely his/her articulatory pattern matched the desired goal, or information about the time course of a particular articulatory pattern. Devices such as the EPG (Fletcher and Hasegawa, 1983) or systems relying on the pneumotachograph (Mahshie, Herbert and Hasegawa, 1984) provide knowledge of performance.

There is little empirical data available about the relative importance of these two forms of feedback for speech learning. For the acquisition of other motor behaviours, knowledge of performance is extremely useful feedback when a skill is being elicited (Schmidt, 1988). It has been suggested that speech learning can be enhanced by presenting physiologic feedback that provides an explicit view of how the speech mechanisms move for production of a target segment (Bernstein, 1989; Mahshie *et al.*, 1984). This type of feedback would seem particularly useful for early stages of skill development, such as during the elicitation stage. During later stages, providing knowledge of results feedback would appear most beneficial, since such feedback would probably lead to less dependence on the visual display, and together with varied feedback schedules, would facilitate internalization of the task.

The majority of existing systems offer little flexibility in the type of feedback that can be provided. Generally, devices that provide feedback from physiological sensors (such as the EPG) provide knowledge of performance, while the majority of acoustically-based devices provide knowledge of results.

It is possible to obtain knowledge of performance (that is articulatory information) from the acoustic signal. For example, a number of computer-based devices offer programmes that display speech spectrograms, spectral displays, or F2 vs F1 formant displays (such as the SpeechViewer II and the Video Voice) . However, obtaining knowledge of performance from such displays is not always a simple task (Bernstein, 1988) and often requires that the teacher be able to provide an articulatory interpretation to the displayed acoustic pattern.

Standards

Whether knowledge of results or performance is provided to the learner, feedback requires a comparison of the production attempt to a reference. In traditional therapy, the standard against which the production attempt is compared resides in the teacher. Watson and Kewley-Port (1989) suggest that the reference for a sensory aid (particularly a computer-based device) can be a teacher, a reference group, or the learner. In addition, the comparison can be accomplished automatically (by the system) or by judgements about the visual display made by the teacher or student.

The reference

Finding an appropriate reference is not always a straightforward task. When the standard for comparison is produced by the learner, then it is necessary for an acceptable production to be obtained and stored so that it can be compared to subsequent production attempts. While this is reasonable for some task levels (such as automaticity) it is less likely when elicitation is the goal. Although a model can be developed by manually 'correcting' a pattern associated with a student's production, few systems currently available permit such editing of targets. The one exception to this is a commercially available EPG (the Palatometer) that enables the instructor to manually edit a target screen to include or eliminate specific target points. The resultant 'synthesized' target can then be used as the comparison for subsequent attempts.

Sometimes the standard used is a teacher's production (for example, the Video Voice), or is derived from productions of the target utterance by a number of speakers (for example, SpeechViewer II). Use of productions by other speakers can be problematic, however, since there is considerable variability in articulatory and acoustic patterns between speakers. Moreover, motor equivalence and coarticulatory effects introduce considerable articulatory variability, making invariant 'templates' somewhat inaccurate for any particular production.

Nonetheless, the use of templates derived from speakers other than the learner as a standard and model appears to be beneficial for teaching skills to deaf individuals. It is likely that the use of generalized models and comparison of productions to these models enables the learner to develop a pattern of their own that is similar, but not identical, to that used to produce the model. This view is supported by Fletcher, Dagenis and Critz-Crosby's (1991) who examined gains associated with speech teaching using the EPG. Recall that the EPG utilizes sensors that monitor the amount of contact between the tongue and various portions of the palate. Fletcher *et al.* (1991) found that the largest gains were in children using the EPG for speech learning when their productions were grossly different than normal. When their productions were close approximations prior to therapy, gains were often minimal. This suggests that the feedback based on generalized standards may be less useful for refinement required to improve close approximations to the correct production than for facilitating production of gross approximations to the target pattern.

Comparisons

In many cases, computerized devices are involved primarily with displaying a target and an attempt, and the teacher or user must evaluate the similarity or differences between them (for example, the Palatometer and Visipitch). The teacher thus plays an important role both by evaluating the closeness of the attempt to the standard, and by providing an explanation of what should be done to more closely approximate the target.

A few devices are able to compare the speaker's attempt to a standard and provide a proximity metric. These devices typically give the learner a proximity score (or graphic display based on this score) reflecting the extent of match between the attempt and target. Examples of devices capable of such comparisons are the ISTRA system (Watson *et al.*, 1989), the SpeechViewer II, and the Video Voice.

Most devices capable of providing proximity scores based on automatic comparisons of attempts and targets provide the learner with knowledge of results. To date, no devices have been reported that provide knowledge of performance by automatically evaluating attempts and comparing those attempts to a standard. This is understandable since the task of discerning the elements of signals that are important for production from those that are not, may be a difficult one. For example, in using the EPG, it may not be clear from subject to subject which electrodes must be contacted for articulation of a particular sequence and which electrodes are not essential for accurate production (Fletcher, Dagenis and Critz-Crosby, 1991).

Tactile feedback

Much of the discussion thus far has focused on devices that provide visual displays of models, speech attempts and feedback. Alternatively, tactile devices have been used to facilitate speech development. Systematic exploration of tactile sensation for speech reception began with the pioneering work of Gault (1924). Since that time various approaches have been explored for transforming and encoding speech for tactile presentation. Devices have been developed and studied that use single-channel (Carney, 1988) or multichannel (Friel-Patti and Roeser, 1983) stimulation, vibrotactile (Geers, 1986) or electrotactile (Lynch *et al.*, 1988) stimulation, and that present the skin with information about the speech spectra (Lynch, *et al.*, 1988) or about selected speech parameters such as fundamental frequency (Boothroyd, 1983; Mahshie *et al.*, 1993). Miniaturized electronics have led to development of portable devices that can be worn outside of laboratory/clinical settings. As a consequence, all tactile aids are not the same (see Sherrick, 1984, for a review).

In most cases, tactile devices used to teach production were designed primarily as aids to assist in speech reception. Some of these devices have been aimed at providing the child with information about a single speech parameter, such as fundamental frequency (Youdelman, MacEachron and Behrman, 1988; McGarr *et al.*, 1986). Other tactile devices provide information about the entire speech signal, and are thus potentially useful for facilitating production of specific articulation patterns (for example, Friel-Patti and Roeser, 1983).

Summary

There are three elements of teaching speech skills that the speech teacher must consider: (1) the task, (2) the cues used to elicit production, and (3) the feedback provided. The task selected results from an interaction among the particular skill being taught (determined by current speech abilities, existence of antecedent or prerequisite skills, developmental readiness, etc.), the general steps involved in teaching any oral sensory motor skill (elicitation, automaticity, generalization, and facilitation of linguistic usage), and the level of success achieved by the child as he/she moves from initial attempts to mastery. Production cues are the instruction or demonstration provided to the learner in order to evoke a pattern. Cues can range from being extremely detailed descriptions of what the speaker is to do, to very abstract signals. Feedback refers to the information provided to the child concerning his/her production attempts. Feedback can vary both in timing (immediate vs delayed, concurrent vs terminal, accumulated vs separated) and nature (knowledge of performance vs knowledge of results). Furthermore, feedback can be presented either visually or tactually. While task, cues and feedback are designated for every aspect of speech teaching, they are interrelated and dependent upon each other.

The majority of existing sensory aids used for speech teaching appear to be most useful for teaching automaticity and generalization of productions. Additionally, many devices focus either exclusively, or primarily on suprasegmental aspects of speech (for example, the Visipitch). However, many of the most popular speech teaching devices in the US do provided activities directed at drill and practice of vowel or limited consonant production (for example, the SpeechViewer), or production of whole words or phrases (for example, ISTRA, and the Video Voice). These devices typically provide feedback about the proximity of the attempted production to a target (knowledge of results).

Because computer-based devices can potentially be used independently and often motivate children to work on speech activities, they are in many ways optimal for automaticity training which requires significant amounts of drill and practice. While there are some devices that can aid in eliciting productions, they are not as commonly used, and often require use of sensors able to detect physiological, rather than acoustic signals. No devices are currently available that are optimal for facilitating linguistic usage. While experimental systems have been developed that permit clinicians to control cue and feedback parameters during instruction, only limited manipulation of these parameters is possible with popular technologies available in the marketplace.

Efficacy Studies

The previous section examined the extent that existing sensory aids designed to facilitate speech development support and expand current speech teaching practice. Perhaps the most significant questions impacting on the value of existing technologies are those relating to their effectiveness and usefulness in improving speech skills. While numerous devices have been developed to assist deaf children learning to speak, there is a significant lack of research examining the effectiveness and usefulness of these devices (for example, Bernstein, Goldstein and Mahshie, 1988; Bernstein, 1989; Watson and Kewley-Port, 1989). Nonetheless, there is a body of literature emerging that examines the effectiveness of various speech teaching technologies.

Assessment of systems and devices typically involves two somewhat distinct types of evaluations, formative and summative (Dick and Carey, 1990). Formative evaluations are designed to establish both how well the system does what it purports to do and how easily the end-user is able to use the features built into the system. Summative evaluations, on the other hand, examine how effective the system is in promoting accurate speech production. Each of these types of evaluation will be discussed below.

Formative evaluation

Formative evaluations of speech training aids are typically designed to address two questions: (1) how accurately does the device do what it is supposed to do? and (2) how acceptable and desirable is the device to clinicians and children?

Accuracy

As suggested above, computer-based devices for speech teaching not only provide models and cues, but must also accurately and reliably present feedback. This latter aspect is particularly important in systems that provide criterion-based feedback of results, since the feedback must be consistent from trial to trial and also correspond closely with the clinician's perceptions.

Evaluation of the accuracy of speech training devices, and calibration of such device decisions against clinician perceptions, has been limited. The ISTRA system uses speaker dependent speech recognition technology to permit practice and drill of syllables and sentences (Watson *et al.*, 1989). Several evaluations were conducted to determine how well the speech recognition system would substitute for human judgements on the goodness of articulation of whole words. Five clinicians rated the overall accuracy of a series of words produced by two normal-hearing speakers who intentionally varied the intelligibility of their utterances. The judges rated the overall articulatory goodness of the utterances using a six point scale. The three productions of each utterance that were perceived by the listeners as most intelligible were subsequently used to generate a template for the computer-based recognizer. The computer-based recognizer was then used to evaluate the proximity of each utterance to the template. Correlational analyses of these data indicated that the experienced human listeners' judgements were in somewhat greater agreement about the intelligibility of these utterances than were the computer-based judgements, but the computer judgements were in general agreement with the human jurors.

A basic requirement of a speech teaching device is that it provide reliable feedback; the feedback must be consistent for similar attempts at a production. To establish their system's reliability, Watson *et al.* (1989) had judges listen to and score twice a series of recorded utterances produced by a deaf speaker. Additionally, the utterances were twice scored by the computer-based system. Results showed that the device was considerably more consistent than were clinicians in rating the same utterances twice. This is understandable since the computer-based system would not be susceptible to varying criteria, speaker familiarity, or other factors that might affect the human judge's reliability.

These findings suggest that this computer-based system provided a reasonable substitute for human judgements of acceptability, and somewhat more reliable judgements than those obtained from human judges. This latter point is important for demonstrating the potential utility of a device to be used for independent drill, since inconsistent, unreliable responses are clearly undesirable in a device designed to provide feedback during independent practice of speech skills.

Clinical acceptability

Often device development results from an engineering solution looking for a problem rather than from the needs of clinicians and students. For this reason, it is extremely important that end-user input be a part of the development, and that reaction of end-users be evaluated. Devices that are complex to operate and calibrate, that fail to address skills that are clinically important, or that fail to grade tasks and cues adequately, are not likely to be used.

Mahshie *et al.* (1988) examined a number of human factor issues for the Hopkins speech training device by having two clinicians keep records during an extended period of trial clinical use. The device was part of a larger project to develop two related computer-based systems, one for use in a clinical setting and the other for drill and practice at home. This approach to evaluating human factors revealed a number of features of the system relating to ease of use, reliability, children's reactions to the device, and perceived clinical benefit.

An alternative approach was used to evaluate the acceptability of a system developed at Gallaudet University that provided the learner with feedback derived from aerodynamic sensors (Mahshie *et al.*, 1991). The system (the Feedback of Aerodynamic Information for Speech Learning or FAISL) was placed at a school for deaf children where teachers and children used the system during therapy. Following a brief evaluation period, a focus group was convened and the teachers were asked a series of questions aimed at evaluating such factors as user friendliness, value of feedback provided, and children's reactions to using the device. Many of the recommendations served as the basis for subsequent changes to the system.

Kewley-Port and Watson (1991) point out the importance of these types of formative evaluations, but stress that they are not substitutes for substantive evaluation of clinical effectiveness. Summative evaluations of clinical efficacy constitute a different type of device evaluation.

Summative evaluation

Summative evaluation studies are directed at the central question of how effective the devices are for teaching speech to deaf children. This, of course, is the ultimate question that needs to be addressed for all systems. In general, efficacy experiments examine the clinical value of speech teaching devices either by comparing the progress made with the device with that associated with alternative intervention methods, or by examining changes that occur as a consequence of intervention (Watson and Kewley-Port, 1989).

While questions of clinical efficacy are most important, few systems currently on the market have undergone rigorous evaluation of clinical effectiveness. For example, Watson and Kewley-Port (1989) reported that only 5% to 10% of the commercially available or prototype computer-based speech teaching systems that have been reported in the literature have been tested in controlled experiments.

Below is a brief description of speech teaching technologies whose clinical efficacy has been reported. While other systems and devices exist, the limited data available concerning their clinical benefit makes it difficult (if not impossible) to ascertain their clinical value. The description that follows is organized according to three major categories of devices: (1) non-computerized devices, (2) computer-based devices, and (3) tactile devices.

Non-computerized devices

Since the beginning of the modern electronic era, instruments and procedures designed to analyse speech have been applied to the task of providing visual representations of speech to deaf children (Braeges and Houde, 1981). As the field of electronics has matured, there has been continued development of devices intended to facilitate deaf children's speech development. Some devices have focused on single speech parameters (for example, /s/ indicators, nasality indicators, and pitch meters), while other devices have provided visual representations of the entire speech signal (for example, the speech spectrograph).

One of the earlier studies of sensory aid use for speech teaching examined whether or not devices could be used by deaf children to modify aspects of their speech production. Boothroyd (1973) conducted a series of experiments on the control of voice by profoundly deaf children using a pitch extractor and storage oscilloscope display for feedback. The device was used to teach 20 severely to profoundly deaf children (ages 6–17) to modify their vocal fundamental frequency. The teaching sequence ranged from matching pitch levels, to producing rising and falling intonation patterns. The children were divided into two groups, with each group receiving an initial four weeks of instruction either through traditional means, or through use of the experimental display system. The following 4 week period involved instruction using the alternative approach.

Regardless of the source of feedback, the children's productions improved during the initial four weeks, with the older children showing greater improvement than the younger children. The older group also demonstrated continued improvement following the termination of training. Boothroyd noted, however, that while gains were observed in the therapy sessions, little improvement was noted in conversational speech.

Risberg (1968) examined the speech improvements for two-hard-of-hearing children using a visual /s/ indicator. The results showed that both children demonstrated improved /s/ when monitoring their production with the /s/ indicator, and that production of practised words continued to improve as a result of training using the device. One of the two children also showed significant carry-over from trained stimuli to those that were not trained. Risberg pointed out that these children both had residual hearing and they seemed to use audition to internally monitor their productions. A brief experiment with three children having less residual hearing revealed diminished 'self-corrective' behavior. While additional experience with visual feedback might have resulted in further speech improvement, it is also likely that degree of hearing and other subject attributes had a significant impact on benefits derived from such feedback.

While there were positive results of teaching speech using these single parameter devices, limited carry-over was noted. Carry-over continues to be a central concern of speech teaching using sensory aids (for example, Fletcher, Dagenis and Critz-Crosby, 1991; Ling, 1976; Mahshie et al., 1991; Nickerson et al., 1983).

In contrast to the single parameter devices evaluated by Boothroyd (1973) and Risberg (1968), other devices have been designed to provide speech learners with spectrographic representations of the entire speech signal (Stark, 1971). The spectrograph provides a display of the acoustic properties of speech as a function of time, and has been used extensively for analysing speech. Earlier studies with spectrographic display devices revealed that it was possible for individuals to perceive syllabic distinctions based on the spectrographic display (House, Goldstein and Hughes, 1968). Only limited research has examined the utility of this technology for teaching deaf individuals to speak (Braeges and Houde, 1983; Maki et al., 1981; Stark, 1971).

Maki et al. (1981) examined the ability of deaf adults to judge the accuracy of their speech by using visual feedback from a real-time speech spectrographic device called the SSD. The results of their work demonstrated that when subjects used the SSD, they were better able to judge the accuracy of their speech production. Houde and Braeges

(1983) examined the efficacy of the SSD for drill and practice of articulation by a group of deaf children ranging from 6 to 13 years of age. Fifty-one children were assigned to two experimental groups, one using the SSD for independent drill and practice, and the other receiving teacher mediated drill. The results showed gains by both groups, suggesting that the SSD mediated drill was at least as useful to the children as was teacher mediated drill and practice.

These earlier findings suggest that teacher independent, computer-mediated drill and practice can be of value. This points to an important consideration in light of currently inadequate speech teaching resources common in many schools and programmes for deaf children (Watson and Kewley-Port, 1989). Devices could be used to enable children to practise their speech skills independently, and thus permit more quality practice than might be otherwise possible. However, reliable and accurate operation of such systems is necessary if they are to supplement human listeners.

Computer-based devices

The majority of recently designed devices for facilitating speech learning are computer-based. The following section examines separately devices that rely on physiological, or acoustical sources for models and feedback.

Physiological devices

It was suggested above that earlier stages of speech teaching are aimed at providing the learner with an awareness of how to control the articulatory gestures for production of a particular speech pattern. It would thus seem that providing direct, physiologically relevant feedback would be most optimal for earlier stages of teaching speech skills. Accordingly, a number of devices and systems have been evaluated that provide feedback obtained from physiological sensors, and that provide models and cues about appropriate patterns to be achieved.

The electropalatograph (EPG) has been used to teach certain aspects of articulation to deaf individuals (Fletcher and Hasegawa, 1983; Fletcher et al., 1991). This is a computer-based physiological monitoring system that provides visual information about tongue and palate contact during speech. The results of the earliest training study (Fletcher et al., 1979) showed significant improvement in a deaf adult's production of /s ð t k/ in conjunction with training using the EPG. Two noteworthy aspects of the study were that the improvements were also observed in segments not actually trained (a cross-over effect) and improvements were maintained for 10 months following teaching using the device. Fletcher et al. (1991) examined the benefit of teaching lingual consonants (/t d k g s z ð/) to five profoundly hearing-impaired children (ages 10 to 16) using electropalatography. They examined both change toward contacting critical electrodes (those considered essential for production) and listener-perceived changes in the consonant–vowel (CV) syllables. The children were seen twice a week for 4 weeks, during which they drilled CV syllables containing the target consonants in /i/ and /a/ contexts. Statistically significant improvements following training were observed in the perceived accuracy of target segments produced by all children. Four subjects showed significant perceived improvements in the majority of segments, while all of the children demonstrated some improvement in contact of critical areas of the palatal region for articulation of the target segments.

Fletcher *et al.* (1991) noted that the gains associated with EPG use were particularly remarkable because the children had not been able to improve production of these segments despite significant period of speech therapy during their lives. They concluded that physiologically based visual displays can be of benefit.

It was earlier noted that Fletcher *et al.* (1991) found the greatest gains in students whose productions were grossly different from normal. It would appear that the primary benefit of the feedback provided by the EPG (and possibly other physiologically-based feedback devices) is in facilitating awareness of articulation. Thus these devices are probably most beneficial during earlier stages of speech learning because they provide the learner with a generalized pattern of what is to be achieved, and feedback about how well they have attained that goal.

The pneumotachograph (PTG) is a somewhat less invasive device that provides information about articulatory gestures (Mahshie, Herbert and Hasegawa, 1984). The PTG has been used in the laboratory to examine oral and nasal airflow patterns associated with production of various segments. Such patterns can provide useful information about the manner of production and voicing categories of consonant segments. Since aerodynamic patterns result from an ensemble of articulatory effects, the absolute articulatory patterns used (such as the precise placement of the articulators) becomes less important than production of the overall aerodynamic pattern required of a particular segment or sequence. It has also been suggested that the aerodynamic properties of the vocal tract represent significant speech goals (Abbs, 1986). Visual displays of aerodynamic targets and feedback would thus seem potentially useful for both practical and theoretical reasons.

To examine the clinical value of the PTG, a visual display of the airflow signal was used to teach accurate consonant voicing to two deaf adults (Mahshie, Herbert and Hasegawa, 1984; Mahshie, 1987). As shown in Figure 1A, more normal aerodynamic patterns resulted from training using the PTG (Mahshie, Herbert and Hasegawa, 1984). In addition (and more importantly), listeners perceived notable improvements in consonant voicing accuracy in conjunction with training using the device (Mahshie, 1987) (Figure 1B). Although results were encouraging, the system was not designed for use with young children; nor was it practical to replicate for use outside of the laboratory.

A second generation system was subsequently developed. This system (Mahshie and Yadav, 1990) provides feedback of aerodynamic and limited kinematic speech parameters obtained from oral and nasal airflow, oral air pressure, electroglottograph, and accelerometer signals. This PC-based system permitted easy selection and storage of templates, multi-parameter display, and other improvements that enabled its use with children.

Efficacy of the device was examined through a series of multiple

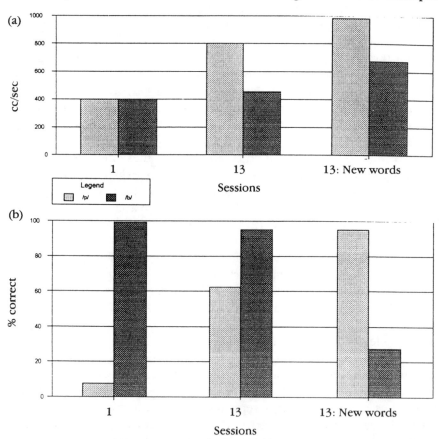

Figure 1. Changes associated with training a young deaf adult to modify voicing status of intervocalic bilabial plosives using aerodynamic feedback. Shown are data for the trained words during the first and last training session, and data for untrained words. A: mean peak airflow associated with /p/ and /b/ production before the initial training session (1), following the final training session (13) and for a set words not trained. Hearing speakers produce /p with greater than 600 cc/s and /b/ with less than 300 cc/s mean peak airflow. B: listener perceived accuracy for words in each of these sessions.

baseline, single subject studies involving four profoundly deaf children (Mahshie *et al.*, 1990). The children, age 11;8 to 12;5, were taught to produce one or two consonant segments that were error productions prior to teaching. The device was used to present targets and to display the aerodynamic patterns associated with each trial.

Results showed that the children using the training system made appreciable gains in production of the target segments in the words that were trained, and that the skill generalized to correct production of these segments in words not trained (Figure 2). The rate of improvement varied for different children and for different segments and contexts. One of the encouraging findings of this work was that correct production of the target segments was generalized to new words without specific generalization teaching for three of the four children. The remaining child required a brief period of teaching about how to use the newly acquired articulatory skill before generalization was observed.

These limited studies point to the potential usefulness of physiologically based feedback for teaching speech skills to deaf individuals. Both significant improvements and notable carry-over have been observed. However, existing devices do not enable the teacher to control many of the pedagogical features that were discussed above. Moreover, although feedback of actual articulatory patterns is probably beneficial for effectively eliciting production patterns, it may not be optimal for all stages of skill learning. Thus these learning patterns may represent minimal, rather than optimal, gains associated with such feedback.

Acoustical devices

Whilst physiologically based devices appear to have a role in speech teaching, the vast majority of devices rely on feedback obtained from a microphone. One of the first computer-based speech training (CBST) systems (Nickerson, Kalikow and Stevens, 1976) employed a PDP-8E laboratory computer system, and utilized a voice microphone and accelerometers on the throat and nose. The system provided four different types of visual displays to teach production of various timing, pitch, voice quality and articulation skills .

To examine system efficacy, 42 orally educated deaf students between 8 and 18 years of age (mean = 11) used the system in conjunction with a series of speech tutorials (Boothroyd *et al.*, 1975). Each child received between 11 and 96 tutorial sessions. The students using the device showed gains in isolated speech skills and in rehearsed speech, with the most improvements observed in production of suprasegmentals. Boothroyd *et al.* (1975) concluded that 'the system, as evaluated, lent itself to work on suprasegmentals rather than articulatory features. Moreover, (while) it was relatively easy for students to use the display for the acquisition of vocal gymnastics skills and the

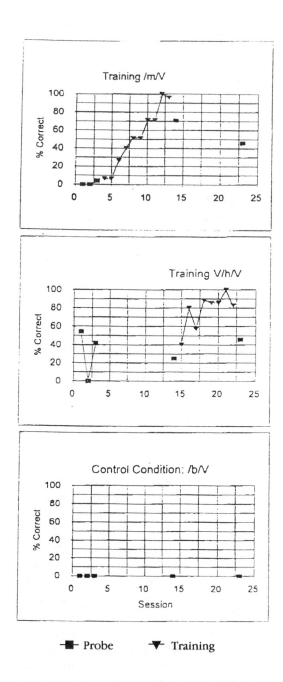

Figure 2. Results for one of four deaf children using aerodynamic feedback from FAISL to improve production of initial /m/ and medial /h/ segments. Also shown is data for a control segment (/b/) that was not trained. Given are the per cent correct for the baseline/probe sessions (squares) and the training sessions (triangles). Different stimuli sets were used for the baseline/probe sessions and traing sessions.

improvement of rehearsed voice...less than half of (the children) showed significant generalization to unrehearsed or spontaneous speech' (page 189). The investigators suggested, however, that the limited carry-over observed was likely because the device was used for only a limited number of sessions and there was little focus during the therapy sessions on generalization to spontaneous speech.

Most studies of clinical efficacy of CBST technologies examine device use for fairly limited periods of time. Arends *et al.* (1991) evaluated the efficacy of a CBST device during an entire school year. The system, the Visual Speech Apparatus or VSA, was developed in Holland and provides visual feedback of various speech parameters. The investigators examined speech improvement associated with device use by comparing gains in performance by an experimental group (receiving instruction using the VSA) and a control group (receiving traditional therapy).

Among other evidence of gains associated with use of the VSA, Arends *et al.* (1991) observed significant improvements in skills associated with extended use of the device.[6] Moreover, these differences between traditional and VSA based training were not observed in performance evaluated at the middle of the academic year following a more limited use of the VSA. While these results were promising, most of the gains observed, like those reported by Boothroyd *et al.* (1975), were in isolated and rehearsed speech, particularly suprasegmentals.

The IBM SpeechViewer[7] is perhaps one of the most popular commercial devices currently available. This device, relying on a microphone signal, offers games and activities for facilitating awareness, 'skill-building' and patterning of selected speech features, including intensity and fundamental frequency control, and vowel contrasting. There are also a number of graphic displays that present acoustic parameters against time.

Despite its popularity in schools and clinics, there is a dearth of research evaluating the clinical value of the SpeechViewer. One exception to this statement is a study conducted by Öster (1989) in which two Swedish deaf children were taught to alter consonant duration (Child I) and plosive consonant voicing (Child II) using the device. Gains were observed in association with teaching these two skills using the SpeechViewer. Öster suggested that the primary benefit offered by this device derived from its ability to provide the learner with 'objective, meaningful, non-verbal' feedback.

More recently Pratt, Heintzelman and Deming (1993) explored the efficacy of the IBM SpeechViewer's Vowel Accuracy Module for the improvement of vowel production. They examined the extent of progress made by six deaf children who used the device for a 4-month period to learn production of the vowels /i/ /a/ and/u/. The investigators found that the device did promote more accurate production, but noted that a number of difficulties were encountered, including inaccuracies in the feedback provided by certain voice qualities and pitches, inability to sustain the children's interest, and non-linearity in the criterion adjustment control.[8]

As noted above, computer-based devices are particularly appealing because they can be used for unsupervised speech training. Boothroyd et al. (1975) saw this potential nearly 20 years ago, but expressed two concerns: (1) a lack of adequate graded drill and practice activities, and (2) the tendency for children to develop bad speech habits that are related to skills for which the computer does not provide feedback. These same concerns continue today with current technologies.

Only limited research has examined the use of speech training devices in the home. The Johns Hopkins Speech Training Aid (Mahshie et al., 1988) consisted of two systems, one designed for use in the clinic (the Speech Training System or STS), and the other designed for use in the home (the Speech Practice System or SPS). The STS used both physiological and acoustical transducers while the SPS used only acoustic signals (Ferguson et al., 1988).

To evaluate the SPS, it was placed in the homes of five profoundly deaf children for a 1–2 week period. The children used the device for an average of 8 to 25 minutes each day, usually under the supervision of a parent or sibling. Parents kept detailed logs of the amount of time their children used the device, as well as observations about interest, ease of operation, and overall reaction to the system. The parents reported that the device was used with interest by the children, and that the activities and games seemed appropriate. Clearly the most significant outcome of this preliminary evaluation was the increased practice the device permitted outside the therapy room. In addition, having the device served as a focal point for speech activity.

An alternative approach to independent drill and practice was employed in the ISTRA system (Kewley-Port et al., 1987). ISTRA uses a speaker-dependent speech recognition board in which productions are compared to a stored template, and a proximity metric is generated. The developers suggest using the student's best production as the standard used to evaluate accuracy. This approach is somewhat different from others because analytical work involved in teaching particular articulatory patterns is left to the clinician, while enabling the learner to drill and practise independently of the teacher. Thus the targets for speech teaching are syllables, words or phrases that the child has produced adequately (at least a few times). The primary virtue of the ISTRA system is that it facilitates development of automaticity by providing directed and monitored feedback that appears valid and reliable.

Limited evaluation of the clinical value of the ISTRA has been reported, in which three children (two deaf, one normal-hearing) were studied during a series of tutorial sessions in which ISTRA was used to mediate speech drill. The authors concluded that 'there is evidence that the changes that occurred in production and generalization of speech sounds can be directly attributed to the treatment provided and not extraneous variables' (page 36).

Tactile devices

The majority of studies examining the impact that tactile devices have on speech learning have addressed the long-term effects of tactile aid use on hearing-impaired children's speech production (for example, Proctor and Goldstein, 1983). In most cases, wear-time is for circumscribed periods of each day, most often during speech therapy, and the devices are used as prostheses for speech reception. For example, Oller *et al.*, (1986) looked at speech reception and production of 13 hearing-impaired children who wore multichannel tactile devices (the Teletactor or Oregon Vocorder) for approximately 70 hours distributed over approximately 200 sessions in a 4 month period. They found gains in speech production and reception associated with the period of aid use, although there were considerable differences among their subjects.

Proctor and Goldstein (1983) looked at a hearing-impaired child's receptive vocabulary acquisition associated with 10 months of training using a single-channel vibrotactile aid. While the total amount of wear-time was not reported, their findings revealed that the most rapid increase in vocabulary development occurred after 3 to 4 months of aid use. More recently Geers (1986) replicated this study with a second hearing-impaired child and obtained similar results.

Friel-Patti and Roeser (1983) attempted to look at broader aspects of communication associated with aid use. They studied four children who wore a multichannel device (the SRA-10 multichannel device) for approximately 10–11 hours per week over a 3 to 4 month period. They evaluated various general and structural characteristics of the children's signed and spoken communication. The researchers concluded that the children exhibited improved communication skills during the period the aid was being used, while there was a decrease in these skills during the period the aids were not used.

Few studies have attempted to compare the use of sensory aids to other approaches for teaching a particular speech skill. Inherent in such comparisons is the need to attend to instruction as a significant variable, and hence to address some of the pedagogical issues discussed earlier. One such comparison was initiated at the Lexington School for the Deaf in which the relative merit of auditory, visual and tactile feedback of fundamental frequency for teaching fundamental frequency control was examined (McGarr, Youdelman and Head, 1989; Youdelman, MacCeachron and McGarr, 1989; McGarr *et al.*, 1988). A similar curriculum was used to teach fundamental frequency control to four groups of children: a control group receiving traditional therapy, a group receiving auditory only feedback, a group receiving visual feedback from the Visipitch and a group receiving tactile feedback from an 8-channel vibrotactile aid. Their findings indicated that the children whose speech lessons included a sensory aid showed significantly greater gains than did the children who received traditional therapy. In addition, the visual display appeared more effective for teach appropriate average pitch, while the tactile display was particularly helpful for teaching dynamic intonation patterns. These findings are supported by research by Mahshie, Vari-Alquist, Hilley and Brandt (1993).

Although tactile aids appear useful for teaching some speech skills, it is clear that there are significant questions that remain concerning when they are the most optimal source of feedback. Additional research is needed to examine both optimal sensory modalities for different tasks, learner attributes that might suggest the merit of one modality over another, and the relative value of using combined sensory modalities for teaching various speech skills.

Summary and Future Needs

This chapter has described a number of issues inherent in teaching speech skills to deaf children, and has examined various sensory aids that have been developed to facilitate speech learning. It has been suggested here that sensory information plays a key role in acquisition of speech by permitting development of models and by enabling after-the-fact feedback to mediate speech change. For many deaf children, reliance on audition as the primary source of feedback may be inadequate and alternative sensory information may need to be provided. In addition, there is a trend in many schools and programmes in the US toward reduced resources directed at speech development. Reduced time available for speech development activities requires that speech teaching be as efficient as possible. The demonstrated effectiveness of sensory aids, and the likelihood that reported gains represent minimal, rather than optimal, gains possible with such devices, suggest that sensory aids can play an important role in the speech development of deaf children. A particularly promising aspect of CBST devices is their potential use for independent drill and practice. As devices become more reliable and easier to use, they can prove useful as extensions of speech teaching classes.

While teacher-independent use continues to be an important aim of these devices, consideration of the inherent limits of computer-based feedback must be considered and safeguards taken to limit development of inappropriate speech behaviours resulting from extensive drill and practice of incorrect patterns not monitored by the device.

However, there is a need to examine how sensory aids are to be used, and to urge developers of these aids to consider significant peda-gogical factors. Clinicians typically consider a number of factors in determining a particular course of speech teaching, including the task to be taught, the order and sequencing of instruction, and the grading of cues and feedback. A major premise of this chapter has been that devices should permit clinicians to continue to adapt the important parameters of speech teaching to the changing level of mastery of the student. Device use should not result in suspension of concern about these normally important issues.

Research addressing specific devices has provided insight into the general utility of sensory aids for teaching speech. Earlier summative evaluation studies examining non-computerized devices suggest that device-mediated therapy can be as effective as more traditional, clini-cian-mediated approaches. However, caution was expressed about the prognoses for carry-over, and the importance of developing appropri-ate pedagogy for incorporating the devices into speech teaching.

More recent studies suggest that devices providing feedback and models from either physiological or acoustic sources can result in sig-nificant gains in speech skills. However, there has been little considera-tion of pedagogical issues associated with their use. This is probably the result of evaluation studies that are device oriented, rather than learner oriented. It is likely that optimal gains would be realized by incorporating attributes of some devices during earlier aspects of skill development, and attributes of other devices during later stages of acquisition and mastery. Reported gains are therefore suggestive of minimal, rather than optimal, improvements. Moreover, incorporation of graded cues and feedback might further enhance speech learning using these devices.

Despite the obvious importance of evaluative research, there are a dearth of studies examining the most commonly used commercially-available devices. Both formative studies and summative evaluation of clinical efficacy of these devices are needed.

The efficacy of tactile sensory devices for teaching prosodic speech skills has been studied, and the results suggest that such displays can be most beneficial for teaching certain dynamic aspects of speech pro-duction (such as production of intonation patterns). An additional ben-efit of tactile devices resides in their ability to be worn, and thus to serve as a prosthesis or outside of therapy room aid to speech monitor-ing. As additional wearable devices are developed, this aspect of their use needs to be considered.

Notes

1. The primary target group discussed in this chapter are those children whose pri-mary contact with the hearing world is through vision rather than audition. This

term is used irrespective of any audiometric criterion that would place children in the categories deaf or hard-of-hearing.

2. The term *speech teacher* will be used to describe the professional who works with deaf children to promote speech development. In various countries and settings this person may be a speech–language pathologist, logopedist, audiologist, or teacher of the deaf.

3. While recognizing the important role that language plays in this process, the discussion here will focus on the more limited area of speech development.

4. For children with limited auditory capabilities and for whom there is no other language access (such as through native sign languages), there is also likely to be a language deficit that will further hamper speech development.

5. Clinicians often vary feedback timing by manipulating the display screen – turning the screen away from the student or asking the child to close his/her eyes is often the easiest way of controlling the delay between the production and presentation of feedback.

6. It will later be pointed out that an important consideration in comparing computer-based and conventional speech teaching procedures is that instruction be developed that permits comparison by being able to be implemented using both approaches. This was not addressed in this study.

7 While the most recent version of this device is the SpeechViewer II, to the author's knowledge there is no published research on its efficacy.

8. This study was conducted using the predecessor of the current, IBM SpeechViewer II device. The current system may have addressed some of the difficulties encountered in this study (for example, more varied activities are available that might maintain children's interest).

References

Abbs, J. (1986) Invariance and variability in speech production: A distinction between linguistic intent and its neuromotor implementation. In Perkell, J. and Klatt, D.(Eds) Invariance and Variability in Speech Processes. Hillsdale, New Jersey: Lawrence Erlbaum Associates, Publishers.

Arends, N., Povel, D.J., van Os, D., Michielson, S., Claassen, J. and Feiter, I. (1991) An evaluation of the visual speech apparatus. Speech Communication 10: 405–14.

Bernstein, L., Goldstein, M. and Mahshie, J. (1988) Speech training aids for hearing-impaired individuals I: Overview and Aims. Journal of Rehabilitation Research and Development 25(4): 53–62.

Bernstein, L. (1989) Computer-based speech training for profoundly hearing-impaired children: Some design considerations. Volta Review , 19-28.

Boothroyd, A. (1973) Some experiments on the control of voice in the profoundly deaf using a pitch extractor and storage oscilloscope display. IEEE Transactions on audio and electroacoustics AU-21,3, 274-8.

Boothroyd, A. (1983) A tactile display of pitch period for use in sensory substitution. Journal of the Acoustical Society of America 73: S27.

Boothroyd, A., Archambault, P., Robb, A. and Storm, R. (1975) Use of computer-based systems for speech training aids for deaf persons. Volta Review 77 (3): 178-193.

Braeges, J. and Houde, R. (1981) Use of speech training aids. In Sims, D., Walter, G. and Whitehead, R. (Eds) Deafness and Communication, Assessment and Training: 222-44.

Carney, A. (1988) Vibrotactile perception of segmental features of speech: A comparison of single-channel and multichannel instruments. Journal of Speech and Hearing Research 31: 438–48.

Coyne, A.E. (1938) Description and practical application of voice pitch indicator. Volta Review 40: 549–552.

Dick, W. and Carey, L. (1990) The Systematic Design of Instruction. Harper Collins: New York:

Ferguson, J., Bernstein, L. and Goldstein, M. (1988) Speech training aids for hearing-impaired individuals: II. Configuration of the Johns Hopkins Aids. Journal of Rehabilitation Research and Development 25(4): 63–8.

Fletcher, S., Dagenis, P. and Critz-Crosby, P. (1991)Teaching consonants to profoundly hearing-impaired speakers using palatometry. Journal of Speech and Hearing Research 34: 929–42.

Fletcher, S. and Hasegawa, A. (1983) Speech modification by a deaf adult through dynamic orometric modelling and feedback. Journal of Speech and Hearing Disorders 48: 178–85.

Friel-Patti, S. and Roeser, R. (1983) Evaluation of changes in communication skills of deaf children using vibrotactile stimulation. Ear and Hearing 1: 31–40.

Gault, R. (1924) Progress in experiments on tactual interpretation of oral speech. Journal of Abnormal Psychology 14: 155–9

Geers, A. (1986). Vibrotactile stimulation: Case study with a profoundly deaf child. Journal of Rehabilitation Research and Development 23(1): 111–17. Houde, R. and Braeges, J., (1983) Independent Drill: A role for speech training aids in the speech development of the deaf. In Hochberg, I., Levitt, H. and Osberger, M.J. (Eds) Speech of the Hearing Impaired. Baltimore,: University Park Press. pp 283–96.

Granzin, A. and Morganstern, K. (1980) Instruction: The forgotten variable? A discussion of methodological issues in the investigation of sensory communication aids. American Annals of the Deaf, 21–6.

Houde, R. and Braeges, J., (1983) Independent Drill: A role for speech training aids in the speech development of the deaf. In Hochberg, I., Levitt, H. and Osberger, M.J. (Eds) Speech of the Hearing Impaired. Baltimore,: University Park Press. pp 283–96.

House, A., Goldstein, D. and Hughes, G. (1968) Perception of visual transforms of speech stimuli: Learning simple syllables. American Annals of the Deaf 113: 215–21.

Hudgins, C. (1935) Visual aids for the correction of speech. Volta Review 637–43.

IBM Personal system/2 Æ SpeechViewer Four Case studies. (undated manuscript).

Kewley-Port D. and Watson, C. (1991) Computer assisted speech training: Practical considerations. In Dyrdal, A., Bennett, R. and Greenspan, S. (Eds) Behavioral aspects of speech technology: Theory and Application.

Kewley-Port, D., Watson, C., Maki, D. and Reed, D. (1987) Speaker-dependent speech recognition as the basis for a speech training aid. Proceedings of the 1987 IEEE International Conference on Acoustics, Speech and Signal Processing, Dallas, pp. 372-375.

Kewley-Port, D., Watson, C., Elbert, M., Maki, D. and Reed, D. (1990) The Indiana Speech Training Aid (ISTRA) II: Training curriculum and selected cases. Clinical Linguistics and Phonetics 5(1): 13-38.

Levitt, H. (1989) Technology and speech training. Volta Review 1-5.

Ling, D. (1976) Speech and the Hearing Impaired Child: Theory and Practice. Washington: A.G. Bell Association for the Deaf.

Ling, D. (1977). Models for speech training with non-auditory feedback. Unpublished manuscript.

Lynch, M., Eilers, R., Oller, D.K. and LaVoie, L. (1988) Speech perception by congenitally deaf subjects using an electrocutaneous vocoder. Journal of Rehabilitation Research and Development 25(3): 41–50.

McGarr, N., Head, J., Friedman, M., Behrman, A.M. and Youdelman, K. (1986) The Use of Visual and Tactile Sensory Aids in Speech Production Training: A Preliminary Report. Journal of Rehabilitation Research and Development 23(1): 101-9.

McGarr, N., Youdelman, K. and Head, J. (1989) Remediation of phonation problems in hearing-impaired children: Speech training and sensory aids. Volta Review 7-17.

Mahshie, J. (1987) Modifying deaf individuals' speech using visual feedback of airflow. Asha 29: 10.

Mahshie, J. (1989) Issues in Development of Speech Training Aids. Proceedings of Speech Tech '89, 2: 209–11.

Mahshie, J. (1992) Using computers to improve the speech of hearing-impaired children. Asha 34:19, p. 221.

Mahshie, J. and Yadav, P. (1990) The Gallaudet University Speech Training and Evaluation System (GUSTES) for deaf children. Asha 32: 10, p.75.

Mahshie, J., Herbert, E. and Hasegawa, A. (1984) Use of airflow feedback to modify deaf speakers' consonant voicing errors. Asha 26: 10.

Mahshie, J., Vari-Alquist, D., Waddy-Smith, B. and Bernstein, L. (1988) Speech training aids for hearing-impaired individuals III: Preliminary observations in the clinic and children' homes. Journal of Rehabilitation Research and Development 25(4): 69–82.

Mahshie, J., Wilson-Favors, V., Schneider, D. and Brandt, F. (1991) Computer-based speech training with deaf children. Asha 33:10, p.211.

Mahshie, J., Vari-Alquist, D., Hilley, C. and Brandt, F. (1993) Using a tactile device to teach intonation production to deaf children. In Risberg, A. and Spens, K.-E. (Eds) Tactile Aids, Hearing Aids, and Cochlear Implants. Stockholm, Sweden.

Maki, J., Streff-Gustason, M., Conklin, J. and Humphrey-Whitehead. (1981). The speech spectrograph display: Interpretation of visual patterns by hearing-impaired adults. Journal of Speech and Hearing Disorders 46: 379–87.

Mowrer, D.E. (1977) Methods of Modifying Speech Behaviors: Learning Theory in Speech Pathology. Columbus, OH: Charles E. Merrill Publishing Company.

Murata, N., Yamada, Y., Sugimoto, T., Hirosawa, K., Shibata, S. and Yamashita, S. (1986) Speech training aid for people with impaired speaking ability. In Proceedings of the International Congress on Acoustics, Speech and Signal Processing, New York: IEE Press.

Nickerson, R., Kalikow and Stevens, K. (1976) Computer aided speech training for the deaf. Journal of Speech and Hearing Disorders 41: 120–32.

Nickerson, R., Stevens, K., Rollins, A. and Zue, V. (1983) Computers and speech aids. In Hochberg, I., Levitt, H. and Osberger, M.J.,(Eds) Speech of the Hearing Impaired. Baltimore: University Park Press. pp 313–26.

Oller, K., Eilers, R., Vergara, K. and LaVoie, E. (1986) Tactual vocorders in a multisensory program training speech production and reception. Volta Review 21–36.

Osberger, M.J. (this volume).

Oster, M-A. (1989) Applications of computer-based speech training. In STL-QPSR 4: 37–44.

Pratt, S., Heintzelman, A. and Deming, S. (1993).The efficacy of using the IBM SpeechViewer Vowel Accuracy Module to treat young children with hearing impairment. Journal of Speech and Hearing Research 36: 1063-4.

Proctor, A. and Goldstein, M. (1983) Development of lexical comprehension in a profoundly deaf child using a wearable vibrotactile communication aid. Language, Speech and Hearing Services in the Schools 14: 138-49.

Risberg, A. (1968) Visual aids for speech correction. American Annals of the Deaf 113(2): 178–94.

Ruscello, D. (1984) Motor learning as a model for articulation instruction. In Costello, J. (Ed) Speech Disorders in Children, 120–56.

Schmidt, R. (1988). Motor Control and Learning: A behavioral emphasis. Second edition. Champaign, IL: Human Kinetics Publishers, Inc.

Scripture, E.W. (1902) The Elements of Phonetics. New York: Charles Scribner.

Seaver, E., Dalston, R., Leeper, H. and Adams, L. (1991) A study of nasometric values for normal nasal resonance. Journal of Speech and Hearing Research 34: 715–21.

Sherrick, C. (1984) Basic and Applied Research on Tactile Aids for Deaf People: Progress and Prospects. Journal of Acoustical Society of America 75(5): 1325–42.

Stevens, K., Kalikow and Willemain, T. (1975) A miniature accelerometer for detecting glottal wave forms and nasalization. Journal of Speech and Hearing Research 18: 594.

Stark, R.E. (1971) The use of real-time visual displays of speech in the training of a profoundly deaf, non-speaking child: A case report. Journal of Speech and Hearing Disorders 36(3): 397–408.

Vergara, K., Miskiel, L., Oller, D.K., Eilers, R. and Balkany, T. (1993) Hierarchy of goals and objectives for tactual vocorder training with hearing-impaired children. In Risberg, A. and Spens, K.-E. (Eds), Tactile Aids, Hearing Aids and Cochlear Implants. Stockholm, Sweden.

Watson, C. and Kewley-Port, D. (1989) Advances in computer-based speech training: Aids for the profoundly hearing impaired. Volta Review 4: 29–45.

Watson, C., Reed, D., Kewley-Port, D. and Maki, D. (1989) Indiana Speech Training Aid (ISTRA). I: Comparisons between human and computer-based evaluations of speech quality. Journal of Speech and Hearing Research 32: 245–51.

Youdelman, K., MacEachron, M. and McGarr, N. (1989) Using visual and tactile sensory aids to remediate monotone voice in hearing impaired speakers. Volta Review 197–207.

Youdelman K., MacEachron, M. and Behrman, A.M.(1988) Visual and Tactile Sensory Aids: Integration into an Ongoing Speech Training Program. Volta Review 197–207.

Dedication

In 1967, Arne Risberg spoke at a conference on Speech-Analysing Devices for the Deaf that was held at Gallaudet. In his talk he spoke of the important differences between hearing and deaf speakers who are developing speech skills, and reflected on the important role that sensory aids might have. Twenty-five years later, those insights continue to be relevant, and his observations have proven quite accurate.

22

Speech Pattern Elements in Assessment, Training and Prosthetic Provision

ADRIAN FOURCIN AND EVELYN ABBERTON

Introduction

The aim of this chapter is briefly to review past and ongoing work which has been inspired by common lines of thought but which in the ordinary course of conferences and publications is never brought together. We and our colleagues[1] have especially benefited from our links with Arne Risberg and our other friends at KTH and in the fifth decade of interaction (AF), this occasion for a conspectus is especially welcome.

The particular advantages of an analytic speech-based approach to the design of hearing aids and the provision of training and assessment for the profoundly deaf are discussed. The relation with the sequence of speech development in the normally-hearing child is used as a guide to the definition of important speech dimensions. Special importance is attached to the possibility of signal analysis motivated by these perceptually related dimensions and to the prospect of a 'naturally' structured basis for work in both perception and speech production with post-speech deaf adults and deaf children in the early stages of acquisition.

Major Problems and Possible Solutions

The three main areas of supporting work for the hearing impaired involve: assessment of need; the provision of effective assistance for hearing and communication; and training and education both in regard to the use of prosthetic assistance and in the development of associated cognitive skills. Although progress has been made in all of these areas the new work has uncovered new problems and even, in some cases, made the climate of support less helpful than it has been in the past. The aim here is briefly to review some of the outstanding and substantial problems which are very well recognized as in need of solution and to discuss how some advantages can come from the adoption of a structured approach which is based on the course of natural development at the first stages of normal speech acquisition. Although the emphasis is on profound and near total deafness, the approach is intended to contribute to a much broader range of need.

Familiar problems in working with the hearing impaired arise, for both adults and children, from the influence of environmental noise which, when profound deafness is associated with marked reduction in analytic ability, produces a very marked influence on speech receptive processing ability. In the extreme case of electro-cochlear stimulation for total deafness, inability to combat noise has led to developments in the encoding of the speech pattern presentations so as to give a degree of preference to the use of the whole speech signal via band-pass filters. In effect this shifts the burden of signal analysis from the level of signal processing in the aid itself to the auditory system of the user. It is now more than four decades since the major advance which accompanied the introduction of miniature and effective hearing aids for use with children provided a substantial change in the ways in which the hearing-impaired child could be accommodated within the educational system. Moderate or even severe deafness is not now the primary obstacle to success at school that it once was and it is quite customary for a hearing-impaired child to be accommodated within classes composed of normally-hearing children. For the profoundly hearing-impaired child the situation is, however, quite different. The real difficulties associated with the use of even the most powerful hearing aids in the oral educational environment can lead to the development of speech skills which, to the ears of the outside world and the parents in particular, are inadequate. In some countries the now established situation is that the profoundly hearing-impaired child will automatically be assigned to a school in which manual signing is the primary vehicle of education and communication. This relative lack of progress in the utilization of acoustic aids has led to interest in the provision of electro-cochlear stimulation even for children who have potentially useful residual hearing for acoustic aids. The suggestion here is that the implementation of new methods of speech analysis by micro-electronic engineering will provide a basic contribution to the solution of this problem when allied with a phonetically motivated approach to the provision of training and the design of supporting hearing aids.

A Reference Structure

In the first stages of our work in the EPI group, we have concentrated on the provision of larynx period information provided on a larynx closure by closure basis both by electrical stimulation in work with cochlear implants and via acoustic stimulation for patients with profound or total hearing impairment. This was designed to assist in the patients' use of lipreading by the provision of the essential prosodic information which is not visible on the lips of the speaker but which is essential for many lipreaders in regard to their receptive ability in the conversational situation. It is also, as is discussed below, capable of providing useful supportive information for the better production and control both of voicing and of some aspects of articulatory activity. The use of period by period larynx synchronous pulsing enables auditory ability, even in profound deafness, to distinguish a voice with poor intonation and hoarse quality from one whose larynx activity is well controlled.

This provision of voicing was intended, however, not as an end in itself but simply as the first step in a structured approach towards the presentation of a complete set of speech pattern element components which, taken together, would provide a complete coverage of all of the essential needs for both receptive and productive spoken language abilities.

The right hand column of Figure 1 lists these essential acoustic elemental components of speech with an ordering which is directly related to their relative importance in the successive stages of speech development of normal children (Fourcin, 1978). Although the emphasis in regard to phonological use for contrastive communication is different from one language environment to another, this broad pattern of successive emphases on acoustic element component groupings appears to be substantially language independent.

Speech acquisition in normal children across languages
and the needs of the profoundly deaf child — and adult

stage	percept	quantity	element
CRY	Loudness Regularity	intensity periodicity	Ax Tx
BABBLE	Timing Coordination	sequence	t
INTONATION SYLLABIC TONE	Pitch Rhythm	fundamental frequency	Fx
VOWEL SYSTEM	Timbre	resonance	F1 then F1 & F2
CONSONANTAL SYSTEM	Timbre Nasality Friction	transience	F nasality F friction F1 F2 F3

Figure 1. Stages of speech acquisition and speech pattern elements.

In parallel with the introduction of increasingly complex pattern combinations of the basic acoustic elements in speech, normal phonological development has an overlapping progression from the prosodic to the vocalic and then the consonantal systems, with the most complex and difficult to perceive consonants being incorporated into the contrastive system last. The idea that there might be a component of auditory/acoustic complexity which was basic to the ordering of the sequence of acquisition led to early experiments in which the aim was to study the development of speech receptive ability over the period of development from 3 to 14 years of age (Simon and Fourcin, 1978). This work showed a very consistent process of evolution and development in both British and French children with the establishment of categorization ability progressing in a systematic fashion from an ability to identify only the extremes of a minimal pair range with reliability to an ability to categorize the test stimuli from a continuum into contrastive groups.

Speech Elements and Stages of Development

Figure 2(a) gives an example of the sequence of developmental stages in regard to the ability to categorize voiced/voiceless contrasts for groups of English children of 3, 5 and 14 years of age. The stimulus continuum here is synthesized on the basis of the speech of a woman producing a voiced/voiceless contrast (goat versus coat). In the lower half of Figure 2 a somewhat similar sequence of labelling abilities is shown for a single profoundly hearing-impaired child (Hazan, Fourcin and Abberton, 1991). The stimulus continuum in this case is based on the much simpler situation of contrastive vowels during a critical period of one year in the child's life between 8 and 9 years. The broad pattern of development is very similar to that which is shown for normal children for the much more complex voiced/voiceless velar consonantal contrast and spans a sequence of development which goes effectively from random categorization to progressive through to essentially well established categorization. In contrast to this work with normal children, different investigations (Eimas *et al.*, 1971) based on the sucking responses of neonates appeared to show that receptive categorization ability for phonologically relevant speech contrasts was already established within the first months of life. A simple explanation is now beginning to be widely accepted for the apparent divergence of these experimental results in which, on the one hand for infants, the ability was essentially innate and on the other, for older children, required a long process of apprenticeship based on the development of increasingly complex cognitive processing. A gradually increasing ability to categorize which develops over the first decade of life has now been also been shown in subsequent experiments (Burnham, Earnshaw and

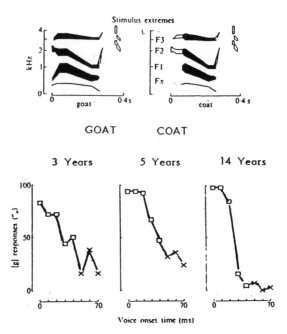

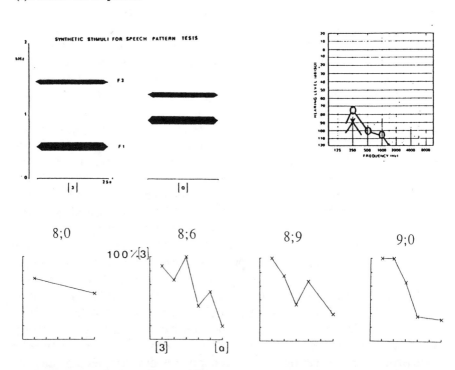

(a) Normal development

(b) receptive vowel contrastive development in a profoundly hearing impaired child

Figure 2. The development of labelling abilities in (a) normal children and for (b) an individual deaf child (work by Claude Simon).

Quinn, 1987). There are simple psychoacoustic explanations for the early ability shown by very young children less than 6 months of age to categorize speech like stimuli. The sounds used in these experiments are acoustically distinct and could be categorized by machine or by animals (chinchilla) as well as human neonates. Phonetic and phonological processes which are essentially concerned with the communication of meaningful utterances do not have a primary contribution to make at this early stage of development. Repeated meaningful exposure to particular contrastive token types does appear to have an influence in regard to a development of categorization ability after the age of 6 months which is not motivated simply by psychoacoustic differences (Tsushima *et al.*, 1994). The picture now beginning to emerge is one in which successive layers of perceptual processing ability progressing from the psychoacoustic to the phonetic and phonological components of speech communication ability have their correlates in the levels of ability shown by normally developing neonates, infants and children. The essential dimensions that should be used as a guiding framework in the structuring of speech habilitation and rehabilitation work for the hearing impaired must, however, be drawn from what is primarily of phonetic and phonological importance. This is what has been attempted in Figure 1, where voice skills are shown as basic to all others.

Voice Production and Perception

Figure 3 illustrates two aspects of the development of voice/prosodic processing ability in a profoundly deaf child. The progression from random labelling to the first establishment of a good approximation to categorical labelling, shown in the top half of the figure, has taken place over a period of 2 months. The acquisition of this receptive ability by this 9-year-old child has been possible (work by Ann Parker and Angela King) as the result of daily training with an interactive visual display showing an intonation contour derived from the laryngographic sensing of vocal fold vibration (Fourcin, 1989). The laryngographic data acquired in this way has also made it possible to analyse the child's fundamental frequency range, and the histograms associated with these analyses are shown directly below each of the labelling functions which are based on the range of stimuli shown at the top of the figure — both increased range and reduced vocal fold irregularity are typical. Figue 4 illustrates another related feature of skill aquisition (coming from the work of Yvonnne Paris, at Mary Hare Grannar School) by a profoundly deaf boy of 14 years. Here, there is a more complete picture of the gradual process of transition from random through progressive labelling to the stage of contrastive labelling ability.

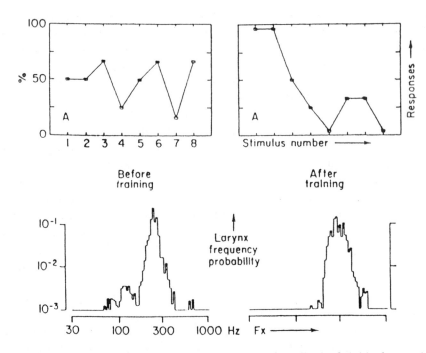

Figure 3. An example of the improvement by a profoundly deaf child of prosodic perception and production with interactive auditory and visual Fx pattern training (work by Ann Parker and Angela King, stimulus 5 below omitted).

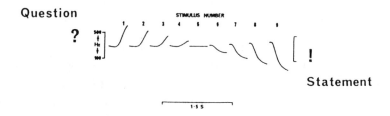

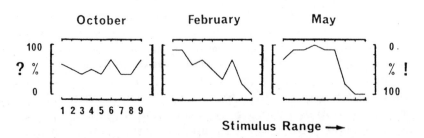

Figure 4. The stages of random, progressive and categorical labelling as the result of auditory and visual interactive Fx training (work by Yvonne Paris).

A fundamental issue in this work is in regard to the basic processes that make it feasible for speech skills, which are essential to efficient phonological development, to be appropriately developed and appropriately measured. The key to success lies in the perception and production of clearly defined speech element targets which are relevant to the child's stage of development.

Figure 5 shows another aspect of the benefit in the control of speech production that can come from interactive training (work by Ginny Wilson, nee Ball) with a speech pattern element display (displays manufactured and distributed by Laryngograph Ltd[2]; Bootle, Fourcin and Smith, 1988; Fourcin, Abberton and Ball, 1993).

The rehabilitation work here is with a profoundly deaf adult. The histogram, Dx, plots in the lower half of the figure, show as before the advantage, in regard to the better control of range, which is associated with this type of therapy whilst the Cx (larynx period to period scatterplot) analysis shows clearly the reduction in vocal fold irregularity which is associated with better control. At the top of the figure the speech and laryngograph waveforms, Sp and Lx, give a more detailed indication of the ways in which the improvement in the control of vocal fold regularity changes not only the nature of the excitation but also, of course, the nature of the acoustic response of the whole vocal tract itself. This type of improvement is based on the use of cross-modal transfer in so far as the visual presentation has a direct influence on the possibility of controlling the acoustic level of speech production and it also has an important influence on the development of better perceptual monitoring skills.

Normalization — in Perception, Production and Prostheses

There is, however, another aspect of receptive processing which is basic to the success of all of this work — this is normalization which is intrinsically related to the fundamental mechanisms of speech communication at all levels, from perception to cognition, and essentially involves inference from context. Figure 6 gives a particular illustration, at the top of the figure, of typical differences in range between two speakers of the same English dialect, a man and a woman. Receptive normalization makes it possible for quite different sized vocal tracts to be used for the production of identical phonetic outputs and the process of normalization is important in every aspect of the physical nature of the control of speech. In Figure 7 this principle has been applied to a training display (work by Colin Bootle; Bootle, Fourcin and Smith, 1988), both for the control of fundamental frequency and amplitude and also in regard to the presentation of frication information. Normally frication exists in the region of frequencies essentially

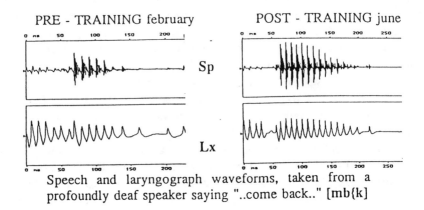

PRE - TRAINING february   POST - TRAINING june

Speech and laryngograph waveforms, taken from a profoundly deaf speaker saying "..come back.." [mb{k]

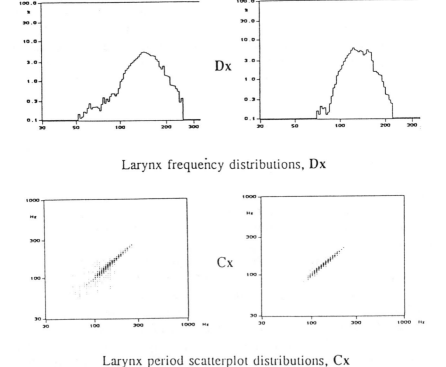

Larynx frequency distributions, Dx

Larynx period scatterplot distributions, Cx

Figure 5. Speech production improvement by a profoundly deaf adult as the result of interactive training (work by Ginny Wilson).

up to 10 kHz but here, using the principle of normalization, a specially synthesized sound is used to encode the original fricatives within a range which corresponds to the user's hearing area. This combination of frication, intensity and fundamental frequency in a composite display (Fourcin, Abberton and Ball, 1993) can also be used as the basis for a corresponding auditory presentation in which the individual acoustic elements are matched to the auditory ability of the user.

The association of assessment, training and prosthetic facilities which is made possible by this analytic approach groups together the components of a common structured framework in the solution of problems for the individual hearing-impaired user. Our present work in this area has been directed towards providing help for those who have become profoundly hearing-impaired and who are not able to make sufficiently satisfactory use of the very best commercial aids in lipreading. Figure 8 shows the acoustic output of a SiVo ('Sine Voice') hearing aid in which the same principles have been applied to the produce an acoustic output as have been used in regard to the provision of an interactive visual display in Figure 7.

Figure 9 shows a group of thresholds of detection and discomfort for profoundly hearing impaired people who have contributed to recent experimental work using this type of hearing aid as a take home device (Faulkner et al., 1992).

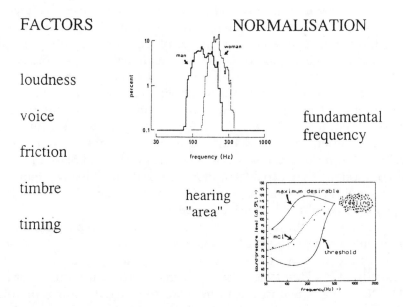

Figure 6. Perceptually important speech factors and the associated normalisation of speech elements related to voice.

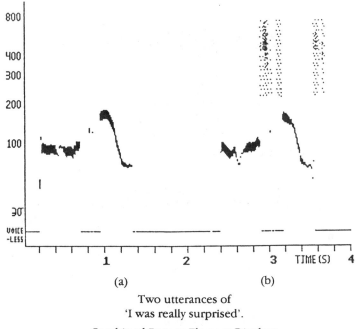

(a)   (b)

Two utterances of
'I was really surprised'.

Combined Pattern Element Displays

Figure 7. Real-time interactive displays: (a) period by period fundamental frequency and amplitude; (b) with the addition of voiceless frication (work by Colin Bootle).

The term 'Mapitch' (Fourcin *et al.*, 1983) has been used to refer to the use of normalization in mapping a speaker's larynx frequency range into the listener's auditory range of frequencies. This principle can be used for all speech dimensions (including time (Nejime *et al.*, 1994)). In this fashion the complex spectrogram of the complete speech signal has been substantially simplified in the output of the SiVo aid (Faulkner et al., 1992) so that only fundamental frequency and intensity together with frication, are presented together within the range of frequencies below 1 kHz. For the purposes of training, of course, each one of these separate elements Fx, Ax and Sx — the frication component — is capable of being utilized individually. Figure 10 gives an indication of one aspect of the effect of using the SiVo aid on the productive ability of a particular patient.

In many cases the use of a hearing aid of this type may have a marked influence on the quality of speech production ability and here the use of the aid gives the patient the ability more closely to monitor the quality of his laryngeal voice vocal tract excitation (Fourcin *et al.*, 1993). Not only is it possible to improve the overall control of voice frequency range but also, as for visually based training, the periodicity and regularity of vocal fold vibration. An important point regarding the results shown in Figure 10, for this particular patient, is that they can

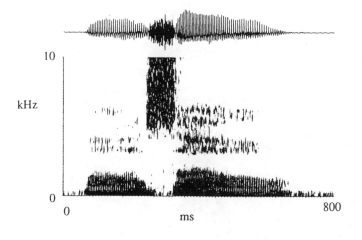

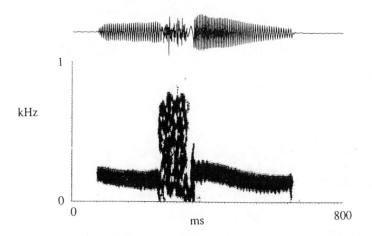

Figure 8. Real-time spectrograms of an original speech signal and the corresponding pattern element ouput from the SiVo aid — both voice and frication information are mapped into the available hearing area (work by the EPI group and the STRIDE project).

be obtained whenever the SiVo hearing aid is used and in this particular comparison the mere change from the conventional hearing aid which the patient is ordinarily using to the SiVo aid results in an improvement, and changing back results in a degradation in any recording session no matter in which order the changes are made. Figure 11 gives a brief indication of the results of using the SiVo aid for a group of subjects in respect of the change in their receptive processing abilities; the particular histograms shown relate to success in respect to a consonant identification test in which both lipreading and

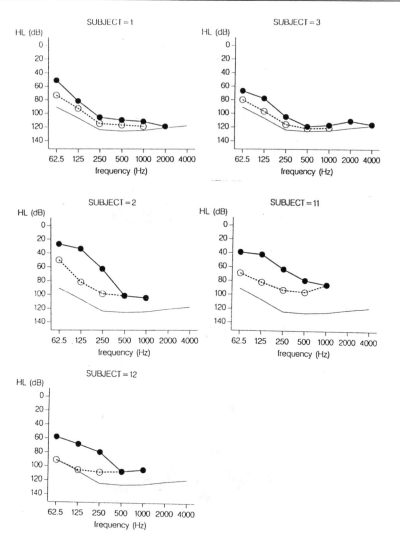

Figure 9. Typical hearing areas for users of the basic SiVo aid (see Faulkner et al., 1992).

the acoustic signal are employed. For each member of this group the combination of the elements relating to fundamental periodicity, amplitude and frication gives better receptive performance than is obtained with the commercial hearing aids which the subjects ordinarily have been employing (Faulkner *et al.*,1992).

Future Prospects

This brief discussion has concentrated on particular aspects of the ways in which the use of an analytic approach to the provision of information regarding essential speech contrasts can result in both perceptual

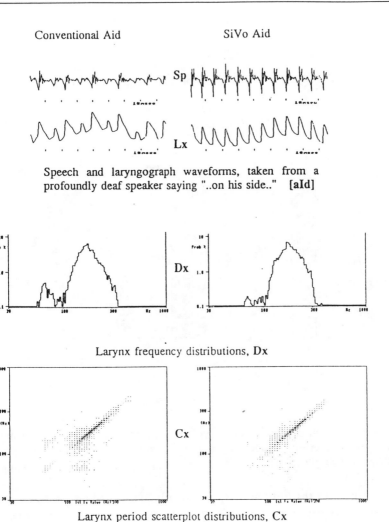

Conventional Aid   SiVo Aid

Speech and laryngograph waveforms, taken from a
profoundly deaf speaker saying "..on his side.."   [aɪd]

Larynx frequency distributions, Dx

Larynx period scatterplot distributions, Cx

Speech Improvement with a SiVo hearing aid

Figure 10. Speech production improvement by a profoundly deaf person (work by
Ginny Wilson and the EPI group — repeatable results within a single session).

and productive improvements. There are, however more intangible,
and yet more important, aspects of this type of work. It has been our
experience that patients who profit from this approach are not only
able to improve their measurable performance with regard to speaking
and hearing but are also more relaxed and are more confident than
when using a conventional hearing aid. We are conscious, however,
that the particular speech elements, Ax, Fx and Sx discussed here, are
rather basic and of use when the patient's condition is one which
involves considerable receptive difficulty — a condition which in many

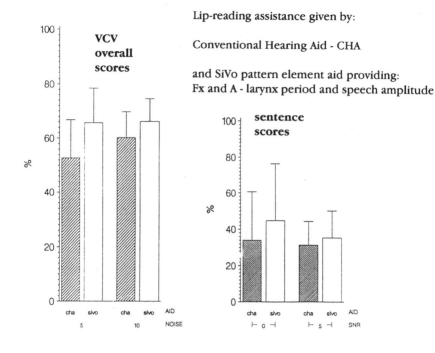

Figure 11. Speech receptive improvement by profoundly deaf adults using the SiVo aid with different speech to noise ratios (from the STRIDE project work, see Faulkner et al., 1992).

cases might be thought to require an electro-cochlear implant rather than an acoustic prosthesis. The same principles can, however, be applied to a full range of acoustic pattern element presentations, and the same methods of basic analysis can be implemented in regard to these further factors, particularly timbre. Figure 12 (prepared by Jianing Wei to illustrate the algorithm developed by her in conjunction with David Howells, John Walliker and Ian Howard (Walliker et al., 1993)) shows the essence of the way in which our present speech analytic techniques are being applied.

A neural net processing system has been trained to produce a satisfactory noise resistant analysis of fundamental voice period, by the use of a target derived from the electrolaryngograph signal, Lx, which has been simultaneously acquired during the production of the speech signal itself. In this fashion, it is possible to arrange that the neural network can be trained to deal with signals which are both reverberant and noisy. We are developing similar techniques for the analysis of frication and timbre. The use of an analytic approach of the type discussed

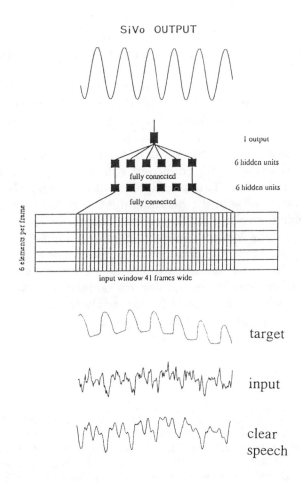

Figure 12. Essential stages in the training of a neural net algorithm — a noisy speech signal is processed with reference to the target information provided from the speaker by a simultaneously derived laryngographic, Lx,waveform (prepared by Jianing Wei — work by her and John Walliker, Ian Howard and David Howells).

here not only makes it possible to provide for selective analysis capable of giving excellent noise resistance but also makes it feasible for individual speech element characteristics to be used over the whole range of work for the hearing impaired as a function of research investment.

The discussion so far has concentrated largely on the provision of analytic speech element aids for adults, but the first part of this chapter was concerned with ways in which one could use the natural sequence of developmental stages as a guide in order to define essential dimensions of analysis. In the longer term this may well be one of the greatest benefits that can come from an analytic speech element approach. In work for children the initial stages of plasticity which are always associated in the first decade of life with an enhanced ability for the acquisition of spoken language skills, both of one's own and of other languages, could be made great use of if it were feasible to support this vital period of cognitive development with appropriate speech analytic and teaching tools. In work with adults (E. Fresnel-Elbaz, personal communication: results from the STRIDE project (European TIDE Programme: Technology Initiative for the Disables and Elderly in Europe)) our colleagues have found that the use of the SiVo aid can help very substantially in the acquisition of skills which make it feasible for the conventional aid to be employed with much greater success than is otherwise feasible. This principle would certainly also be of great assistance in work with the hearing-impaired child. At each stage of spoken language development appropriate interactive visual speech displays, and especially acoustic analytic wearable behind the ear hearing aids focusing auditory attention on salient aspects of importance at that stage of development, would be of crucial assistance in the development first of voice productive and control skills, then of skills relating to frication and timbre. In this way analytic support can be provided for a full range of speech components so as to serve the stages of spoken language acquisition from the most simple to the most complete and complex.

Notes

1. The External Pattern Input Group: Evelyn Abberton*, Barbara Cadge**, Julian Daley*+, Ellis Douek+, Andrew Faulkner*, Adrian Fourcin*, Kerensa Smith*, Deborah Vickers*, John Walliker*+, Jianing Wei*, Ginny Wilson*. * University College London. ** Royal National Throat, Nose and Ear Hospital, London. + Guy's Hospital, London. and David Miller and David Howells, Laryngograph Ltd. Related research has also been carried out in the European STRIDE Project in collaboration with partners in Denmark (Oticon), France (CCA, Paris; Fondation Rothschild, Paris; CNRS, Université de Provence at Aix-en-Provence), The Netherlands (University Hospital (AZU), Utrecht; Instituut voor Doven, St Michielsgestel), Sweden (KTH, Stockholm).
2. Displays supplied by Laryngograph Ltd., I Foundry Mews, Tolmers Square, London NW1 2PE.

References

Bootle, C., Fourcin, A. and Smith, J. (1988) Speech Pattern Element Display. In Proceedings of Speech '88, 7th FASE Symposium, Edinburgh: Institute of Acoustics, pp. 179–185.

Burnham, D.K., Earnshaw, L.J. and Quinn, M.C. (1987) The development of categorical identification of speech. In McKenzie, B. and Day, R.H.(Eds) Perceptual Development in Early Infancy. Hillsdale, New Jersey and London: Lawrence Erlbaum Associates

Eimas, P. D., Siqueland, E.R., Jusczyk,P. and Vigorito, J. (1971) Speech perception in infants. Science 171: 303–6

Faulkner. A. (in press) Paper presented at the Autumn Meeting of the British Society of Audiology, September 1994.

Faulkner, A., Ball, V., Rosen, S., Moore, B.C.J. and Fourcin, A.J. (1992) Speech pattern hearing aids for the profoundly hearing-impaired; speech perception and auditory abilities. Journal of the Acoustical Society of America 91: 2136–55.

Fourcin, A.J. (1978) Acoustic patterns and speech acquisition. In Snow, C. and Waterson, N. (Eds) The Development of Communication. Chichester: John Wiley. Fourcin, A.J. (1989) Links between voice pattern perception and production. In. Elsendoorn, B.A.G and Bouma, H.(Eds) Working Models of Human Perception. Academic Press. pp 67–91.

Fourcin, A.J., Abberton, E. and Ball, V. (1993) Voice and intonation: analysis, presentation and training. in B.A.G. Elsendoorn and F. Coninx, (Eds.) Interactive Learning Technology for the Deaf NATO-ASI Series, Springer Verlag, 137-150.

Fourcin, A.J., Douek, E.E., Moore, B.C.J., Rosen, S., Walliker, J.R., Howard, D.M., Abberton, E. and Frampton, S. (1983) Speech perception with promontory stimulation. In Parkins, C. and Anderson, S. (Eds) Cochlear Prostheses: an International Symposium, Annals of the New York Academy of Sciences, 405: 280–94.

Hazan, V., Fourcin, A.J. and Abberton, E. (1991) Development of phonetic labelling in hearing-impaired children. Ear and Hearing 12: 71–84.

Nejime, Y., Aritsuka, T., Imamura, Y., Ifukube, T. and Matsushima, J. (1994) A portable digital speech-rate converter and its evaluation by hearing-impaired listeners. Proceedings of the 1994 International Conference on Spoken Language Processing 4: 2055–8.

Simon, C. and Fourcin, A.J. (1978) A cross language study of speech pattern learning. J.A.S.A. 63: 925–39

Tsushima, T., Takizawa, O., Sasaki, M., Shiraki, S., Nishi, K., Kohno, M., Menyuk, P. and Best. C. (1994) Discrimination of English /r-l/ and /w-y/ by Japanese infants at 6-12 months: language-specific developmental changes in speech perception abilities. Proceedings of the 1994 International Conference on Spoken Language Processing Vol. 4, 1695–8.

23

Speakers and Hearers are People: Reflections on Speech Deterioration as a Consequence of Acquired Deafness

RODDY COWIE AND ELLEN DOUGLAS-COWIE

Scandinavia has produced a long line of distinguished linguists. Fifteen years ago we were invited to contribute to a festschrift for one of them, Professor Paul Christopherson. We searched for a topic which would interest both of us (a linguist and a cognitive psychologist), and one which came to mind was what happens to people's speech when they become deaf. That began a collaboration which has continued to the present. We take the opportunity in this chapter to review its current state.

Our aim is not to present data. Our findings are described at length elsewhere (Cowie and Douglas-Cowie, 1992). Although we need to say something about them, there is no gain in simply repackaging them. Instead our aim is to articulate some significant general lessons that we have learned from our research on deafness. To many people they will be no news at all. However, speech research is sustained by a continual flow of incomers, and at the start some may be as naive as we were 15 years ago. It seems fair that those who have lost rough edges painfully should do what they can to ease the process for those who come after.

Our central point is that the ideal speech researcher needs to embrace two disparate ideals: to be highly sophisticated in technical matters and to be thoroughly humane. These two have often fragmented. However, a few figures have consistently shown that they can be held together. We have regarded research in Stockholm as an example in this respect, and it seems a fitting tribute to acknowledge the lesson.

The Scope of Research on Deafened People's Speech

The term 'deafened' refers to people who suffer a profound hearing loss after acquiring spoken language. Both linguistically and in other respects, their situation is very different from that of 'the Deaf', whose hearing loss originates at birth or at any rate early enough to have a profound effect on their acquisition of language. It is not clear how sharp a distinction there is between people whose acquired loss is profound and those with less severe acquired losses: certainly many of the points that we make do apply to the latter group.

Our experience with deafened speakers repeatedly highlighted unconscious assumptions about the scope of research on speech. Two examples may illustrate the point.

The first example involves an event which occurred during experiments on the intelligibility of our deafened speakers. We asked subjects to 'shadow' passages which the speakers had read, i.e. to repeat what they heard word by word as they heard it. We took the number of words correctly repeated as a measure of intelligibility. We believed, and we still believe, that this measure of intelligibility is one of the most fundamentally valid that exists. It measures ordinary people's ability to understand the words somebody says in real time. That is what communication in the real world is like. It is an advantage, not a disadvantage, that part of the listener's attention is directed elsewhere (i.e. to repeating the speaker's words). It is the norm for attention to be divided among multiple tasks, and creating a situation which allows total concentration is false purism.

Some of our subjects broke off in mid-experiment to laugh. Like good experimenters we stopped the tape until they had settled down, and then began again. But on reflection, we saw that the truer measure would have been to leave the tape running. Humans are not emotionless robots, and in a human listener the quality of speech can provoke emotions which interfere with pure signal processing. Concealing that by meticulous procedure is not being scientific. It is better described as scientism, devotion to the surface forms of science without the guiding grasp of reality.

The second example arose from a discussion with our editor, Dr M-L. Liebe-Harkort. We doubted whether a linguistic series was the right outlet for our research on the quality of deafened people's lives. She replied that linguistics deserved to die if it dissociated itself from understanding the impact of disordered speech, and that the impact of disordered speech is very much a function of the speaker's life. A secure and fluent person may suffer very little when a visit to the dentist leaves her/his fricatives slushy. However, a disorder which is objectively similar may be a major burden to someone whose social confidence barely exists, and whose difficulties centre on flawed communication. For her/him, the listener's puzzled look and restrained giggle may seem a barrier too high to cross: and to believe that the barrier is too high can mean encasement in a private world.

These experiences, and a great many others like them, made us aware that a full understanding of speech in acquired deafness involved a far wider range of issues than we had initially assumed. Figure 1 is an attempt to pull together the issues that now seem relevant, and to set them in a reasonably compact framework. It is loosely based on the sequence of events involved in part of an interchange, but that is a device to give it coherence: in no way does it pretend to be a psychological model.

The general point of the model is to make explicit the context in which two basic types of judgement are made. One is whether a particular speech disorder, or a particular aspect of a speech disorder, matters to the person who has it; the other is whether a particular attempt at treatment meets a person's need. These are not the only questions to be asked about speech disorders, but they are fundamental questions, and it is important that they should be brought into the open and addressed seriously and consciously. On them hang a series of other questions: whether particular ways of describing speech disorders are inherently better than others; whether particular ways of measuring speech disorders are complete, partial, or downright inappropriate; whether particular theories about the process of speech production or speech comprehension are adequate or not; and so on.

The need to make these issues explicit is a function of success. Speech science has amassed a dazzling range of techniques for studying the physiological events involved in speech, measuring acoustic effects, rating perceptual qualities of the voice, categorizing linguistically significant events, providing feedback and training to clients, etc. Beside all this technical expertise the question 'does it matter?' can easily seem a crude, perhaps slightly disreputable relic of a less sophisticated generation.

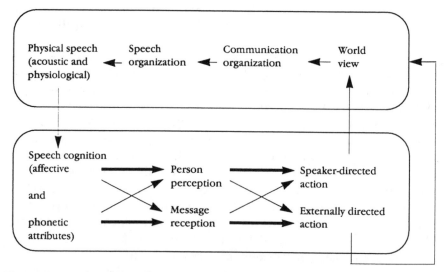

Figure 1: An aide-memoire for the study of disordered speech.

We want to counter that idea by highlighting the rich body of issues and established knowledge which surrounds the question 'does it matter?'.

It seems best to begin by considering the lower block in Figure 1, which summarizes issues related to a listener interacting with someone whose speech is disordered.

The block involves two broad streams. They are not wholly separate, but they are worth distinguishing in the first instance. The lower stream deals with transmitting propositional information and getting the listener to perform actions which are practically significant (these may include verbal actions). The upper one deals with forming impressions of the speaker, and with gestures on the part of the listener which convey these impressions (again, these may include verbal gestures). Speech is significant because it triggers these streams, and so understanding them is the background to rational research on speech.

Message reception

The lower stream hinges on message reception. It has been the traditional focus of scientific research on speech and language. Phonetics deals with the elements of speech signals that can convey propositional messages (hence the thick arrow from phonetic attributes to message reception), research on syntax and semantics deal with the way these elements may be combined, psycholinguistics deals (in practice) with the mental process of receiving a message or transmitting one, communications theory deals with the transmission of messages, and so on.

If one focuses narrowly on the lower stream, deafened people's speech can seem not too bad a problem. The extreme illustration is a paper by Goehl and Kaufman (1984). They argued against speech conservation training for deafened people on the grounds that their speech showed few segmental errors and was relatively intelligible – 'perfectly functional speech', as they put it. That description is factually incorrect for some deafened people, notably those who suffer a profound loss in adolescence or earlier. They do tend to have substantial losses in intelligibility (Cowie and Douglas-Cowie, 1992, Chapter 4). But even when the description is true so far as it goes, it does not go far enough to serve as a basis for judgements about therapy. It ignores the upper stream, not to mention the rest of Figure 1.

Person perception

By comparison with message reception, the upper stream is on the fringes of speech research. Yet everyone knows the song

It ain't what you say, it's the way that you say it
That's what gets results.

A string of famous examples suggest that the song is at least close to the mark. Richard Burton's career rested on the impression his voice created, not on his words: Ronald Reagan won two presidential terms on the strength of delivery as much as content – as, for example, in the way he made 'there you go again' a mortal blow to Michael Dukakis: Margaret Thatcher is said to have invested great efforts in mellowing her voice to create an image that the British people could accept: and so on. Our experience of listeners laughing at deafened speakers represents the negative side of this coin.

These examples run together points which the figure separates out. On one side, they suggest that person perception is particularly affected by variables of speech which are not central to message reception (this is reflected in the use of dark and light arrows): and on the other side, they suggest that person perception has a major bearing on the way listeners respond to an utterance. Both of these suggestions are backed by ample evidence.

A mass of research supports the intuition that perceptions of the speaker are a major factor in reactions to the messages that he or she conveys. A widely cited example comes from Giles (1973), who showed that an argument couched in standard words was more able to sway listeners if it was presented in an accent like the listeners' own. Figure 2 (after Douglas-Cowie and Cowie, 1984) summarizes the outcome of a range of studies reviewed by Bradac, Bowers and Courtright (1980) on the general topic of what makes communications effective. The point which is immediately relevant is that in half of the cells (the lightly shaded ones) the listener's perceived status critically affects whether the communication achieves its goals.

Impressions of the speaker matter. It would wrong to assume that they were unimportant so long as the speaker managed to transmit the words which conveyed his or her message, because impressions of the speaker determine whether the words achieve their intended effect. Given that, it matters to know whether speech makes a major contribution to person perception.

From speech variables to person perception

Research into person perception identifies a multitude of relevant factors. Appearance and non-verbal behaviour are well known to be important (for example, Knapp, 1972). Verbal messages are also important, both at the level of content and at the level of style – a second point which is apparent from Figure 2. Speech variables appear to play no less a role.

Dialect is the most intensively studied of these variables. It involves primarily phonetic variables of speech – the same ones that dominate message transmission. It is one of the major cues to social status,

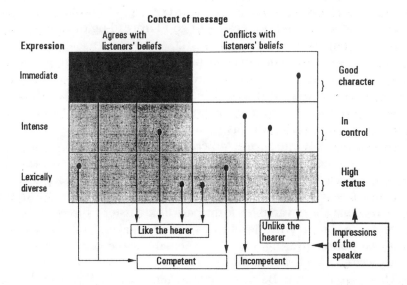

Figure 2. Factors which make messages effective (dark shading), effective for high status speakers (light shading), or ineffective (no shading).

whose effect is shown in Figure 2. Dialect has also been shown to affect a range of other judgements about a speaker, such as his or her perceived integrity, expertise, intelligence, and educational attainment (Giles and Powesland, 1975). These effects have been a central concern of sociolinguistics.

It tends to be assumed that dialect effects are irrelevant to clinical research. The argument is presumably along these lines. Dialect affects work by signalling that speakers belong to groups – geographical or socio-economic – for which listeners have preconceived stereotypes. The characteristics listeners attribute to a speaker are the stereotypical characteristics of these group. Clinical speech disorders are not associated with known social groups, and so dialect effects are not a relevant issue.

This argument is dubious for at least four reasons.

1. Apparently one of the major effects of dialect is to create a sense that the speaker and the listener are similar or dissimilar (Giles and Powesland, 1975; Berger and Bradac, 1982). Whatever else deafened people's speech does, it marks the speaker as different from the listener. We have shown that deafened people's speech does stand out as different from normal in a variety of respects. This is true in face-to-face contact as well as in studies with recordings (Cowie and

Douglas-Cowie, 1992, Chapter 9). Note that speech may stand out as distinctive when interactants have not registered that the speaker has a hearing problem (because of good lipreading or skilful interaction strategies).

2. There is some evidence that people who listen to deafened speakers find them difficult to place within a standard socio-economic framework (Cowie and Douglas-Cowie, 1983). This may be a problem in itself if, as some authors argue, knowing what to expect of a speaker has a strong bearing on his or her ability to persuade the listener (for example, Burgoon and Miller, 1985).

3. We have studied how people who listen to deafened speakers rate them on status-related variables – presumed level of occupation and education (Cowie and Douglas-Cowie, 1992, Chapter 8). Analysis shows that these variables form part of a cluster of items related to competence. Hearing level does affect speakers' ratings on these items: poorer hearing, like lower actual socio-economic status, was associated with lower ratings.

4. There does seem to be a stereotype which deafened people's speech evokes apart from the socio-economic dimension. It may be best described as 'neurological damage'. This is suggested by another cluster of items in the analysis which dealt with status. Deafened speakers were rated likelier than controls to suffer a range of disabilities, most of all to be stroke victims. This kind of rating had a particularly strong association with judgements that speech was abnormal, and with the level of loss that speakers suffered. We do not know the implications of having speech which evokes that stereotype.

In short, there is doubt about the way deafened people are affected by the mechanisms studied in sociolinguistics, but there seems to be little doubt that they are affected.

A second set of speech-related variables with a major effect on person perception may be classed under the broad heading 'prosodic'.

Some of the clearest evidence in this area relates to rate. Brown and Bradshaw (1985) have reviewed a series of studies showing that decreasing speech rate decreases the speaker's perceived competence. However, there is a balance involved: if speech rate becomes too fast, it lowers speakers' perceived benevolence. Non-fluencies – in the form of pauses and repetitions – may be considered here: several studies suggest that they relate to perceived competence and dominance (for example, Miller and Hewgill, 1964; Scherer, 1979). There is good evidence that deafened people's speech tends to be too slow (Leder *et al.*, 1987a) and that some speakers pause too often (Plant and Hammarberg 1983) and too long (Plant and Hammarberg, 1983; Lane and Webster, 1991).

Speakers' emotions seem to be inferred from a complex of prosodic variables, including rate, but also volume and pitch. Frick (1985) reviews the evidence and concludes that activity is signalled by increases in pitch height, pitch change, loudness, and rate; aggression by low pitch; happiness, and perhaps fear and grief, by cues involving high pitch. There have also been attempts to link prosody to the perception of enduring personal traits rather than transient emotions, but they have been less successful (see, for example, Brown and Bradshaw, 1985). Abnormalities of pitch height, pitch change, and loudness are among the most widely reported attributes of deafened people's speech (Cowie and Douglas-Cowie, 1992, Chapter 2).

Another category of vocal cues is broadly described as voice quality. Voice quality has long been linked to judgements about personality. A study by Addington (1968) is widely cited. He presented recordings of speakers simulating voice qualities defined by Heinberg (1964) and asked listeners to rate the speakers on a range of variables. His main findings are summarized in Table 1. It would be unwise to take these data at face value, as Addington himself points out. But one of the reasons why the study is so widely cited is presumably because one can sense, perhaps uncomfortably, what the ratings mean. Deafened speakers have been described as having qualities of voice which at least may correspond to the first five cues in the list (see Douglas-Cowie and Cowie, 1992, Chapter 2, for a review).

Table 1. Vocal cues and inferred personality (after Addington, 1968)

Simulated vocal cue	Sex of speaker	Stereotyped perception
Breathiness	Males	Young; artistic
	Females	Feminine; pretty; petite; effervescent; highly strung; shallow
Flatness	Males	Masculine; sluggish; cold; withdrawn
	Females	Masculine; sluggish; cold; withdrawn
Nasality	Males and females	Wide array of undesirable characteristics
Tenseness	Males	Older; unyielding; cantankerous
	Females	Younger; emotional, feminine, highly strung; less intelligent
Throatiness	Males	Older; realistic, mature; sophisticated; well adjusted
	Females	Less intelligent; masculine; lazy; boorish; unemotional; ugly; sickly; careless; inartistic; naive; humble; neurotic; quiet; uninteresting; apathetic
Thinness	Males	None
	Females	Immaturity; sense of humour; sensitivity
Orotundity	Males	'Hardy and aesthetically inclined'
	Females	Lively, gregarious; aesthetically sensitive; proud; humourless

A final attribute of speech which affects person perception is clarity. Sebastian and Ryan (1985) obtained personality ratings for the same speakers under two conditions: one, with ordinary recordings, and the other for the same recordings with noise added. Ratings were more negative for every aspect of personality in the second condition, even though the listeners knew consciously that their difficulties with comprehension were due to the tape rather than the speaker. Given that intelligibility is seriously impaired for some deafened speakers, and somewhat impaired for most, this is a finding worth considering.

From person perception to practical consequences

Our case so far is that many speech variables appear be important because of the effect that they have on person perception, and that many variables in that category at least may be affected by acquired deafness. Person perception is important because it in turn affects a wide variety of behaviours towards the speaker. We have mentioned its impact on persuasion, but the literature suggests a wide variety of contexts where speakers are practically affected by perceptions of them which rest on speech variables. Scherer (1979) and Lind and O'Barr (1979) have reported on the effects of speech variables in courtroom situations; Edwards (1979) studied their effect in education; Giles and Powesland (1975) discussed their effect in the context of employment; Fielding and Evered (1977) examined the way they affected medical diagnosis of the speaker. We have reported a case involving interaction between a deafened speaker and the police: one of our informants carried a letter explaining that his speech was slurred because he was deaf, not because he was drunk (Cowie and Douglas-Cowie, 1983).

World view and the meaning of actions

At this point we move from the bottom half of Figure 1 to the top. What a speaker says may result in various actions which impinge on him or her. Some of these actions, including the ones suggested above, are likely to be significant for anyone. But even their impact depends on what we have called the world view of the person involved: his or her self-image, his or her image of other people in the world, his or her image of the pressures and potentials involved in their interaction. Many other gestures that an interactant makes may be trivial to someone with a robust world view, but overwhelming to someone who is barely able to face the world as he or she knows it.

Systematic information about deafened people's worlds has been accumulating gradually over a decade or so. The simplest summary is provided in a landmark study by Thomas (1984). In a reasonably representative sample of hearing-impaired people, he found that 18% were clinically depressed at the time of interview. An earlier study (Thomas and Gilhome-Herbst, 1980) suggested that the figure was much higher among people with profound losses.

Stewart-Kerr (1992) has provided a fuller picture, and in particular she has clarified the things that deafened people feel affect their quality of life. The emotional charge which communication has for deafened people is a dominant theme. The experiences which most respondents felt had a very bad effect on their lives were feeling embarrassed or stupid after failing to understand a conversation, and feeling that hearing people ignored them in conversation and could not be bothered with them because of their deafness.

In that context, speech problems have a wholly unusual charge. One of Stewart-Kerr's informants reported:

> People who have known me before I was deaf, the first thing they said to me was, 'Have you a cold? You seem to talk through your nose.' and then someone told me my voice was weak. That upset me more than anything. (page 328)

Another informant expressed dread at the thought that as well as losing his hearing, he would 'maybe lose my speech altogether' (loc cit.). Abrahams (1972), a deafened person herself, writes that incidents where people do not understand her speech happen 'all the time', and that 'hundreds of incidents add up as hundreds of bricks add up to a wall'. These views are not atypical: 30% of Stewart-Kerr's informants reported that their lives were badly or very badly affected by incidents where others did not understand what they said.

It is almost a reflex to discount this kind of point as tear-jerking and unscientific. However it is anything but that if these emotional experiences affect the quality of people's lives. Stewart-Kerr shows that they do: they predict reported quality of life, and vulnerability to depression, much better than audiological variables. The point which emerges is that communicative problems are massively and specially significant for deafened people. What would be unscientific would be to assume that their difficulties with speech could be judged according to the viewpoint beloved of English law, 'the man on the Clapham omnibus'.

From world view to the organization of communication

A person's world view in turn shapes his or her next communication. One extreme is simply to avoid communicating. This is commonplace among deafened people. One of Stewart-Kerr's informants says

> It just put me off. I didn't want to mix with company or friends. You just feel you want to come home and sit on your own.

Another says

> I avoid people like the plague. It embarrasses them, it embarrasses me. (page 249).

Those who do not withdraw may develop strategies which cope with some problems but aggravate others. One is to dominate conversation:

> I have to dominate the meeting, I make myself the artificial centre of attention so that people will just speak to me ... instead of speaking to the chairman they would be speaking to me. (Cowie, Douglas-Cowie and Stewart-Kerr, 1992, page 269).

Another is to bypass communication by taking action without consulting others who would normally expect to be asked. Various other moves, from pretending to understand to enforcing a blunt question-and-answer pattern of interaction, have been reported (Cowie and Douglas-Cowie, 1992, Chapter 10).

Relatively little is known about these moves, and it would be wrong to dwell on them. The point, however, is that they combine with speech to provide the immediately accessible evidence a hearer may use to assess the kind of person he or she is meeting. Non-verbal behaviours could in principle offset the effects of anomalous speech, but in practice deafened people's hearing loss may lead to non-verbal behaviours which are more likely to aggravate the impact of speech disorders than to override them.

Organizing speech

We move now from the global level of organizing communication to the specific level of organizing speech. Historically this level has been pivotal for research on deafened people's speech. Ideas about the way that deafness could possibly affect speech production have been at least as influential as evidence on the way it does. In particular, one hypothetical mechanism has dominated theoretical work in the area.

The issue which has captured centre stage is whether auditory feedback is used to guide articulatory gestures during the course of their execution – see, for example, Cowie and Douglas-Cowie (1983). It seems unlikely that the fine detail of speech involves this kind of control, on the theoretical grounds that the auditory loop is too slow and on the empirical grounds that articulation does not disintegrate when auditory feedback is manipulated experimentally (Gammon et al., 1971; Garber et al., 1980; Siegel et al., 1980).

That, however, is only one of the mechanisms by which hearing could impinge on speech production. Removing it from centre stage opens the way to look at a great variety of other mechanisms which have a better claim to significance.

The oldest candidates involve control over comparatively slow-changing variables such as pitch, volume and possibly nasality. Leder and his colleagues have confirmed that these variables are generally affected in acquired deafness (Leder *et al.*, 1987b; Leder and Spitzer, 1990). It is worth noting that one of the best known features of deafened speech, volume which is grossly inappropriate to the context, may be only partly to do with feedback in a classical sense: the other contributor is plain lack of information about background level, which could be an input to feedforward mechanisms as much as an element in feedback.

Recent work has highlighted subtler possibilities which are related to these. We proposed in 1983 that auditory feedback might contribute to maintaining coordination in the multi-element systems that speech typically involves, but through off-line 'tuning' rather than instant on-line adjustments. Our hypothesis dealt with the upper vocal tract: there is no direct evidence on it, but it still seems plausible. However, Lane and Webster (1991) have produced good evidence that hearing contributes to maintaining long-term coordination among the structures involved in breath control for speech.

Another refinement raised by Lane and Webster is that precise calibration may be particularly important when the system has to cope with a wide space of possibilities. Transitions between stock units are an obvious example: transitions within a unit such as a word or a syllable may be comparatively rehearsed and stereotyped, but transitions between them involve an immense space of possibilities. This may explain a feature of our data: errors of articulation tended to cluster at word boundaries (Cowie and Douglas-Cowie, 1992, Chapter 7).

So far we have considered speech organization as a mechanical task. However, it is a great deal more than that. It is an integral part of normal speech to vary it for effect in multiple ways. These stylistic changes involve almost every aspect of speech – vocabulary, phonemic and phonetic realization, rate, volume, pitch, intonation, syntax, phrasing. They are deeply implicated in signalling the speaker's attitude to the topic and to the listener (see, for example, Giles and Powesland, 1975) and in projecting an appropriate self image. It is common experience that these changes are acoustically monitored, as witness phrases like 'that came out all wrong' or 'I didn't mean to sound like that'.

Our data indicate that deafened speakers have difficulties with these stylistic transitions and with the types of information they convey. The difficulties take various forms. In terms of pitch change, deafened speakers 'gravitate too much to a basic pattern of rise followed by fall' (Cowie, Douglas-Cowie and Rahilly 1992, page 131): the same pattern is common among controls, but they vary it much more. In terms of stress, deafened speakers tend to use multiple heavily accented syllables in a single phrase: that would be unusual in a normal-hearing English speaker, and would be associated with a style which was emphatic to the point of hectoring (Cowie, Douglas-Cowie and Rahilly, 1992). When they are reading, deafened females go too far in a family of shifts which are normally associated with adopting a reading style, whereas deafened males tend to underplay them (Cowie and Douglas-Cowie, 1992, Chapter 5).

These are still not the most complex effects that we might expect to depend on auditory feedback. People create their own speech styles to reflect themselves – by imitating mannerisms of people they admire, by accommodating to prevailing (and perhaps changing) norms, by searching for tones of voice that convey the way that they feel or would like to be seen. Very little is known about this academically, but there is no reason to believe that the process can be switched off when hearing ceases to signal whether attempted self-creations work. This may well be related to a striking fact about deafened speech: although there are general trends, different individuals may show very different patterns of abnormality.

Against this background, it is small wonder that acquired deafness changes the physical and acoustic expression of speech.

Speakers and listeners as people

We have tried to convey in outline the issues that we see as relevant to a proper understanding of deafened people's speech. The root point is that speech is thoroughly entangled with so many of the things it means to be a person. It is all too easy to imagine we are studying a mouth transmitting sound waves to an ear, as diagrams in textbooks often show. Of course there are times when it is right to blank out complications and focus on part of a complex system. However, in the context of acquired deafness, and perhaps in the context of many other speech problems, there are high risks attached to doing that without first firmly setting an image of the people in our minds.

Potential Developments

The kind of description we have given often meets a sceptical response: 'This is all very interesting, but what does it achieve in practice?' We accept that analysing issues is only useful if it leads to practical developments. We also accept that there is no global solution to the whole package of problems we have outlined. However, we believe that given the will and the imagination, it is perfectly possible to identify specific developments which take up some of the points we have made. This section illustrates that point by outlining briefly two areas where developments seem to be possible, one technical and the other non-technical.

The social/instrumental axis

The technical area involves developing new forms of measurement. Awareness of human interactions may, so to speak, be embedded in techniques designed to capture speech variables that are relevant to interactions. In particular, there would be many applications for methods of measuring the aspects of deafened people's speech which affect its social acceptability. They include:

1. Establishing whether a particular individual has appreciable speech problems. This kind of test has two sides. It is worthwhile reassuring those who do not have speech problems as well as identifying those who do.
2. Targeting treatment. Abnormality is not a cause for treatment in and of itself: a person should not be subjected to treatment for an abnormality which is measurable, but has no adverse effect on listeners. Hence it is worthwhile knowing which abnormalities have a significant effect, both in order to motivate the general development of treatments and in order to design appropriate programmes for individuals.
3. Evaluating treatments. Technology has produced a rapid development in two types of device which may be relevant to deafened people's speech: sensory transducers (such as cochlear implants and vibrotactile aids) and feedback displays (such as the laryngograph and its descendants). It is worthwhile knowing whether particular variants on these themes, with or without particular types of supporting therapy, produce appreciable benefits.

Phonetics has studied the acoustic variables which underpin message reception, and it is clear that they are subtle and resistant to automatic measurement. However, it seems possible that some of the variables which contribute to person perception may be easier to capture at least roughly.

Some of the work we have cited illustrates the general theme. Rate and pausing, which are exceptionally easy to measure, seem to be socially significant. Pitch and pitch change are also highly accessible to automatic measurement. Some aspects of voice quality, though not all, can also be recovered. In particular, there have been intriguing studies linking perceived voice quality to the distribution of energy across the spectrum (Hammarberg *et al.*, 1980).

We have begun to explore links between these variables and the judgements that listeners make about deafened speakers. Listeners made their judgements by rating speakers on a list of social and personal qualities after listening to a tape of their speech. These ratings were subjected to factor analysis in order to identify the main themes underlying individual responses. A range of acoustic measurements were then extracted from the speech recordings, and regressions were used to establish which acoustic measurements were statistically related to the major themes extracted from the ratings. Table 2 (after Cowie and Douglas-Cowie, 1992, page 177) summarizes the main connections which emerged.

Table 2. Relations between instrumental measures of deafened people's speech and listeners' judgements of their attributes

Quality judged	Attribute associated with negative judgement
Competence	Rises in amplitude drawn out rather than abrupt
Warmth	Change in the spectrum concentrated in a narrow band, few instances where F0 inflects more than once between pauses
Poise	Narrow F0 range, highly variable volume
Stability	Excessive amplitude change low in the spectrum
Neurological impairment	Lack of defined peaks high in the spectrum

This is a crude preliminary step. It would be unreasonable to expect more in a short time. However, it illustrates the point that there are some reasonably clear technical lines of progress from the outline of issues presented in the first part of this chapter. We are currently developing systems which deliver a far more extensive battery of speech variables that may be relevant to the social evaluation of speech, and we will study their ability to predict reactions to a far more extensive sample of speakers.

Style therapy

We have pointed to evidence that style shifting poses problems for deafened people. Style shifting is not a variable that traditional speech science pays a great deal of attention to: witness the fact that speech evaluations rarely include any explicit comparison of performance in different styles (research on stuttering is the exception, for rather special reasons). However, theories of communication suggest it is an extremely important variable. Accommodation theory argues that shifting our speech to converge with the speaker's or diverge from it is a key signal of the way we perceive our relationship to the speaker, and a key element in the speaker's relationship to us (for example, Giles and Powesland, 1975; Ball, Giles and Hewstone, 1985). It may be worth incorporating checks on style shift more generally into speech assessment techniques.

Deafened people often receive training in communication strategies. We suspect that training related to style shifts could be a useful part of that kind of provision. It may not be difficult to alert people to the basic norms of accommodation, and to practise them in adopting appropriate styles. We suspect that simple practice, and building confidence that it is possible to manage at least some stylistic variation, would go a long way. This would appear to be a useful component of training concerned with self-presentation.

Initial development of this approach probably depends on people with specialist knowledge about speech. However it may well be that once appropriate routines had been established, they could be delivered by non-specialists – perhaps therapists with a more general remit, or quite possibly the client's close friends or relatives.

Conclusion

We have presented a view of deafened people's speech which emphasizes its social functions and personal impact. We will make no complaint if readers feel most of the points we have made are obvious. However, it is a talent worth cultivating to keep the obvious clearly in view. To do that consistently, and master the techniques of a modern scientific discipline, is no small challenge. We believe that it is a challenge at the centre of speech science. The motto of the Royal Institute of Technology puts it more briefly: 'Science and art'.

References

Abrahams, P. (1972) The effects of deafness. Hearing 27: 260–3.

Addington, D.W. (1968) The relationship of selected vocal characteristics to personality perception. Speech Monographs 35: 292-503.

Ball, P., Giles, H. and Hewstone, M. (1985) Interpersonal accommodation and situational construals: An integrative formalisation. In Giles, H. and St Clair, R.N. (Eds) Recent Advances in Language, Communication, and Social Psychology. London: Lawrence Erlbaum Associates. pp 263–86.

Berger, C.R. and Bradac, J.J. (1982) Language and Social Knowledge: Uncertainty in interpersonal relations. London: Edward Arnold.

Bradac, J.J, Bowers, J.W. and Courtright, J.A. (1980) Lexical variations in intensity, immediacy, and diversity: an axiomatic theory and a causal model. In St Clair, R.N. and Giles, H. (Eds) The Social and Psychological Contexts of Language. Hillsdale, N.J.: Lawrence Erlbaum Associates. pp 193–223.

Brown, B. and Bradshaw, J. (1985) Towards a social psychology of voice variation. In Giles, H. and St Clair, R.N. (Eds) Recent Advances in Language, Communication, and Social Psychology. London: Lawrence Erlbaum Associates. pp 263–86.

Burgoon, M. and Miller, G.R. (1985) An expectancy interpretation of language and persuasion. In Giles, H. and St. Clair R.N. (Eds) Recent Advances in Language, Communication, and Social Psychology. London: Lawrence Erlbaum Associates. pp 199–229.

Cowie, R. and Douglas-Cowie, E. (1983) Speech production in profound postlingual deafness. In Lutman, M.E. and Haggard, M.P.(Eds) Hearing Science and Hearing Disorders. London: Academic Press. pp 183–230.

Cowie, R. and Douglas-Cowie, E. (1992) Postlingually Acquired Deafness: Speech deterioration and the wider consequences. Trends in Linguistics: Studies and Monographs 62. Berlin: Mouton de Gruyter.

Cowie, R., Douglas-Cowie, E. and Rahilly, J. (1992) Intonation In R. Cowie and E. Douglas-Cowie Postlingually Acquired Deafness: Speech deterioration and the wider consequences. Trends in Linguistics: Studies and Monographs 62. Berlin: Mouton de Gruyter. pp 115-137.

Cowie, R., Douglas-Cowie, E. and Stewart-Kerr, P. (1992) Understanding the quality of deafened people's lives. In R. Cowie and E. Douglas-Cowie Postlingually Acquired Deafness: Speech deterioration and the wider consequences. Trends in Linguistics: Studies and Monographs 62. Berlin: Mouton de Gruyter. pp 259–78.

Douglas-Cowie, E.E. and Cowie, R.I.D. (1984) Sociolinguistics: A frame of reference. Journal of the Northern Ireland Speech and Language Forum 10: 89–104.

Edwards, J. (1979) Judgements and confidence reactions to disadvantaged speech. In Giles, H. and St. Clair R. (Eds) Language and Social Psychology. Oxford: Blackwell. pp 22–44.

Fielding, G. and Evered, C. (1977) The influences of patient's speech style on doctors' decisions in the diagnostic interview. Unpublished ms., Social Psychology Department, University of Bristol.

Frick, R. (1985) Communicating emotion: the role of prosodic features. Psychological Review 97: 412–19.

Gammon, S., Smith, P., Daniloff, R. and Kim., C. (1971) Articulation and stress/juncture production under oral anaesthetization and masking. Journal of Speech and Hearing Research 14: 271–82.

Garber, S., Speigel, T., Siegel, G., Miller, G. and Glass, L. (1980) The effects of presentation of noise and dental appliances on speech. Journal of Speech and Hearing Research 23: 823–52.

Giles, H. (1973) Communicative effectiveness as a function of accented speech. Speech Monographs 40: 330–1.

Giles, H. and Powesland, P. (1975) Speech Style and Social Evaluation. London: Academic Press.

Goehl, H. and Kaufman, D. (1984) Do the effects of adventitious deafness include disordered speech? Journal of Speech and Hearing Disorders 49: 58–64.

Hammarberg, B., Fritzell, B., Gauffin, J., Sundberg, J. and Wedin, L. (1980) Perceptual and acoustic correlates of abnormal voice qualities. Acta Otolaryngologica 90: 441–51.

Heinberg, P. (1964) Voice training for Speaking and Reading Aloud. New York: Ronald Press.

Knapp, M.L. (1972) Nonverbal Communication in Human Interaction. New York: Holt, Rinehart and Winston.

Lane, H. and Webster, J. (1991) Speech deterioration in postlingually deafened adults. Journal of the Acoustical Society of America 89(2): 859–66.

Leder, S., Spitzer, J., Kirchner, C., Flevaris-Phillips, C., Milner, P. And Richardson, F. (1987a) Speaking rate of adventitiously deaf male cochlear implant candidates and normal-hearing adult males. Journal of the Acoustical Society of America 82: 843–6.

Leder, S., Spitzer, J., Milner, P., Flevaris-Phillips, C., Kirchner, C. and Richardson, F. (1987b) Voice intensity of prospective cochlear-implant candidates and normal-hearing adult males. Laryngoscope 97: 224–7.

Leder, S. and Spitzer, J. (1990) A perceptual evaluation of the speech of adventitiously deaf adult males. Ear and Hearing 11(3): 169–75.

Lind, E. and O'Barr, W. (1979) The social significance of speech in the courtroom. In Giles, H. and St. Clair, R. (Eds) Language and Social Psychology. Oxford: Blackwell. pp 66-87.

Miller, G.R. and Hewgill, M.A. (1964) The effect of variations in non-fluency on audience ratings of source credibility. Quarterly Journal of Speech 50: 36–44

Plant, G. and Hammarberg, B. (1983) Acoustic and perceptual analysis of the speech of the deafened. Speech Transmission Laboratory Stockholm, Quarterly Progress and Status Report 2-3/1983, 85–107.

Scherer, K. (1979) Voice and speech correlates of perceived social influence in simulated juries. In Giles, H. And St. Clair, R. (Eds) Language and Social Psychology. Oxford: Blackwell. pp 88–120.

Sebastian, R. and Ryan, E. (1985) Speech cues and social evaluation: Markers of ethnicity, social class, and age. In Giles, H. and St. Clair R.N. (Eds) Recent Advances in Language, Communication, and Social Psychology. London: Lawrence Erlbaum Associates. pp 112–43.

Siegel, G., Fehst, C., Garber, S and Pick, H. (1980) Delayed auditory feedback with children. Journal of Speech and Hearing Research 23: 802–13.

Stewart-Kerr (1992) The experience of acquired deafness: A psychological perspective. Unpublished PhD thesis, Queen's University, Belfast.

Thomas, A. (1984) Acquired Hearing Loss: Psychological and Psychosocial Implications. London: Academic Press.

Thomas, A. and Gilhome-Herbst, K. (1980) Social and psychological implications of acquired deafness for adults of employment age. British Journal of Audiology 14: 76–85.

24

Speech Visualization System as a Basis for Speech Training and Communication Aids

AKIRA WATANABE

Introduction

One receives much more information through a visual sense than through a tactile one. However, most visual aids for hearing-impaired persons are not wearable because it is difficult to make them compact and it is not a best way to mask always their vision. Therefore, it seems that most visual aids have been restricted to use for speech training (Risberg, 1968; Levitt, 1973).

Development of personal computers and application software gave rise to many speech training aids, in which speech elements are represented with beautiful colours and one can enjoy a game (Nickerson and Stevens, 1973; Bernstein, Ferguson and Goldstein, 1986)).

In such trainers, only one or two speech features are individually represented on the display. Although many acoustical features of speech form an integrated image in normal hearing, visual representations in which many features are integrated as a pattern have never been devised. We are interested in integrating speech features as a visual pattern by which one can intuitively understand not only continuous speech but also individual speech elements included in it. If it is possible, such visual aids will be useful for communication aids as well as speech training ones even if they are not wearable.

Generally, it is difficult to get the integrated patterns by a single mathematical transform of signals, such as a Fourier transform (Liberman *et al.*, 1968). In order to obtain the integrated pattern, speech parameters should be carefully extracted by an analysis according as each parameter, and a visual pattern, which can intuitively be understood by anyone, must be synthesized from them. Successful integration of speech parameters will never disturb understanding of individual features, so that the system can be used for speech training and communication.

One of the situations in which the non-wearable system is useful for communication is in understanding telephonic speech because the system will be used on the side of a telephone.

Speech analysis and visualization methods described in this chapter provide a basis for speech training and communication aids which represent the integrated-visual patterns in real time.

Speech Visualization System for Ordinary Speech and its Characteristics

System

As a prototype of a speech visualization system, a colour display system for connected speech has been developed using analogue hardware (Watanabe, Ueda and Shigenaga, 1985; Watanabe and Ueda, 1988). In the system, four parameters, that is the lowest three formant frequencies (F1-F3) and pitch (F0) are used to control the image displayed. The lowest three formant frequencies decide the colour of a speech sound in voiced portions and the pitch signal restricts the horizontal length in the colour pattern. In unvoiced portions which are extracted with a ratio of high to low frequency components, a colourless and dapple pattern can be seen. The patterns are represented as spatial patterns whose time axis is given vertically on the CRT screen.

After the realization of this system, spectrum analysis by 64 point fast fourier transform (FFT) was made with a fixed point digital signal processor (DSP) chip and added to it. The normalized spectrum is overlapped to whole patterns. In this case, the spectral channel (frequency) corresponds to the horizontal position and the intensity to luminance.

A block schematic diagram of the speech visualization system is shown in Figure 1. In principle, the lowest three formant frequencies are converted into three primary colour signals as follows:

$$R = 5F1/F3$$
$$B = F2/3F1$$
$$G = 3F3/5F2 \tag{1}$$

It can be expected from equation (1) that the circular ratios of the formant frequencies normalize influence of vocal tract lengths on the formant frequencies and that the coefficients of 1/3, 3/5 etc., make a neutral vowel colourless.

Therefore, it will be possible in the system to display the five Japanese vowels as five different colours independently of vocal tract lengths due to age and sex of speakers. However, R-G-B balance may not make a perfect grey as a result of the biased characteristics in the

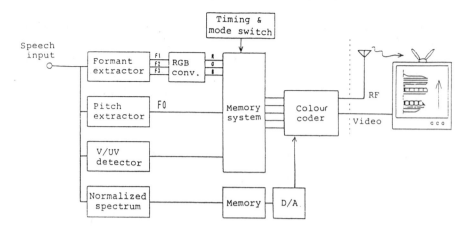

Figure 1. Real-time visualization system for connected speech.

colour display. In such cases, the coefficients of equation (1) should be corrected slightly.

The memory system in Figure 1 has a role in converting speech signals into a spatial pattern in which the time axis of speech is vertically represented. The colour coder shown in Figure 1 generates a composite colour video signal from the three primary colour signals according to the national television standard colour (NTSC) system.

Why is colour representation needed?

As described in the above section, the colours are naturally decided by equation (1) from speech parameters, that is the lowest three formant frequencies. In a perceptual meaning this is quite different from how automatic speech recognition results would be assigned to a corresponding colour.

Why is such colour representation needed? One of the answers is in the correspondence between auditory and visual perception.

Many speech researchers have argued that individuality of speakers and the complicated coarticulation make automatic recognition of connected speech difficult. These difficulties can also pose serious obstacles when subjects understand connected speech through other senses than hearing.

A prominent property of hearing in perceiving connected speech is in compensation for a coarticulation effect caused by continuous movement of speech organs with different response speeds.

In the speech visualization system described in this chapter, the conversion from the lowest three formant frequencies into colours in equation (1) normalizes talkers' individual vocal tract sizes. The chromaticity of five Japanese vowels can be estimated by simple calculation based on NTSC system from the three primary colours in equation (1). Figure

2 shows the distribution of five Japanese vowels on a Commission Internationale d'Eclairage (CIE) chromaticity diagram, which has been uttered by 213 speakers (age 6–23, males and females). Five vowels distribute as different colours around the colourless point (white).

As connected vowels are represented by changes of chromaticity, the coarticulation effect may show insufficient changes. However, if the

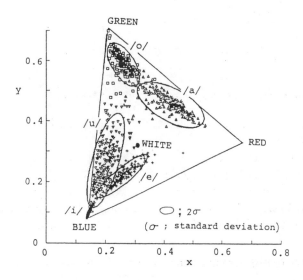

Figure 2. Distribution of five Japanese vowels on CIE chromaticity diagram (213 speakers, males and females, age 6–23).

proposed colour representation is used, it is expected that the contrast effect of colours compensates for the coarticulation effect to appear in the changes of chromaticity.

To verify this characteristic, an experiment using synthetic vowels has been conducted (Ueda and Watanabe, 1987). First, three connected vowels, shown in Figure 3, are synthesized by a terminal analogue synthesizer. In the connected vowels, the first and the third vowels are the same, that is /V1V2V1/ and the pitch frequency is constant (130 Hz). The formant frequencies whose stimulus is judged to be a typical vowel by listening tests are chosen for the first and third vowels (V1). And another typical vowel is used for a target of the second vowel.

A straight line on the F1-F2 plane is divided into ten equal parts from V1 to the target and each point is used as V2 shown in Figure 3. The stimuli are transmitted to subjects in three ways: by sounds, colours and formant patterns. The formant patterns mean a frequency-time representation for only the lowest three formant frequencies on a visual display.

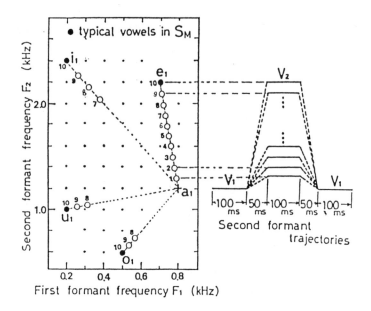

Figure 3. Formant frequencies selected for three connected vowels and examples of F2 trajectory.

Four subjects were required to say what the second vowel was in the three connected vowels which were presented at random. Prior to the tests, the subjects learned all isolated vowels by receiving visual (colours or formants) and auditory (sounds) information simultaneously. But connected vowels were not trained at all.

The identification rate of /e/ in the judgement of /a(e1)a/ which is indicated in Figure 3 is shown in Figure 4 together with those of isolated vowels given between /a1/ and /e1/. The stimulus numbers in Figure 4 correspond to those in Figure 3. Thus, the shift of the phoneme boundary from the isolated vowel to the connected ones indicates the compensation for coarticulation effect.

According to these examples, the shift is largest in the auditory judgement and appears in V-colour (colour representation) also. But it does not exist in V-formant (formant representation).

To evaluate the general tendencies in all connected vowels, total rates of V2 identified as the target vowel were determined, as shown in Figure 5, by changes to the stimulus number. Since coarticulation effects do not appear in the isolated vowels, the falling tendency in the identification rates are almost the same in any condition of auditory, V-colour or V-formant.

If coarticulation effect is compensated by judgement of connected vowels, the categorical boundary will shift to expand the area of the tar-

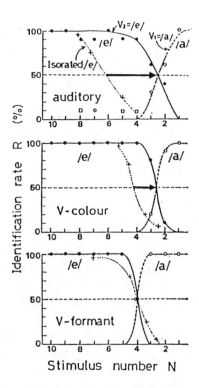

Figure 4. Identification rates in the judgement of V2 in /a V2 a/. (Arrows show the shifts of categorical boundaries from the isolated vowel to the connected ones).

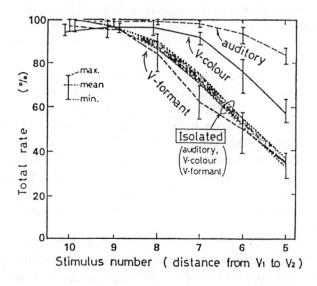

Figure 5. Total rates of V2 identified as the target vowel. (All of the five typical vowels are combined as V1 and the target of V2 in /V1 V2 V1/.)

get vowel. Such compensation is most intensive in auditory information (sounds) and appears considerably in V-colour too. But it does not appear in V-formant at all. It is verified by another visual experiment showing that the compensation in V-colour is caused by contrast effect between colours (Watanabe et al., 1985; Watanabe and Ueda, 1981). The visual tests demonstrate that in reading real isolated and connected vowels, V-colour is greatly superior to V-formant in connected vowels while both representations give high performance with isolated vowels (Watanabe et al.,1985).

Thus the colour representation given by equation (1) is very useful in transmitting vowel information.

Tests for reading a group of words (Watanabe and Ueda, 1988)

The speech visualization system represents voiced segments by colours and overlaps the normalized spectrographic patterns as luminance changes on the whole pattern. Thus the black-and-white pattern in unvoiced portions gives a clear image in contrast with the vivid colours of voiced portions.

The spectral patterns will perhaps be insufficient to transmit perfect consonantal information. However, various complementary information such as redundancy in a context, voiced/unvoiced timing and intonation etc., may promote understanding of words.

With this in mind, possibilities for reading a group of words have been investigated by simple tracking tests. Speech materials used were 40 adjectives and 50 nouns (average 3.2 syllables/word). Visual patterns were presented repeatedly together with speech sounds recorded by an adult male speaker until the correct response in temporary tests reached 100%. In the tests, one of the two or three speakers pronounced directly towards a microphone and only the visual patterns were displayed. While the pattern of each word kept stopping at the centre of the screen, the subjects (with normal hearing) were required to read it. If the answer was wrong or not readable, the same word was pronounced repeatedly up to five times. The number of presentations and the response time were recorded.

The cumulative correct rates and the response time corresponding to the number of repetitions are shown in Figure 6. Figure 6(a) is the result of 90 isolated words and (b) 100 compound words comprising an adjective plus a noun. The compounds had not been trained at all before the test.

The correct rate for the isolated words is 83% in the first presentation and the improved scores reach 94% and 98% in the second and third presentations, respectively. Figure 6(b)shows that 85% of 100 compounds are understandable within two trials. Of 200 individual words which are included in the compounds, 78% are readable in the

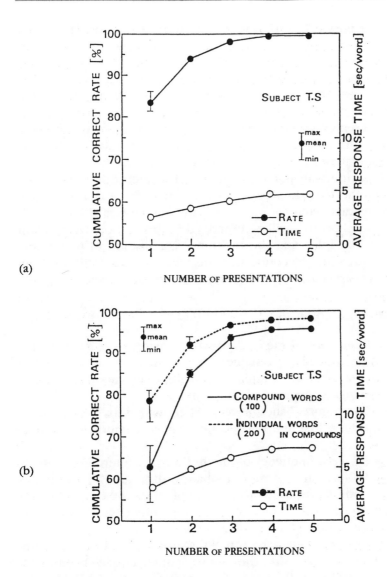

Figure 6. Correct response rates. (a) 90 isolated words (two male speakers). (b) 100 compound words (three male speakers)

first presentation and 92% in the second one. These results indicate that understanding of words in the compounds is a little lower than for isolated words.

Although the time necessary to read patterns is relatively long because of the lack of consonantal information, the speech visualization system makes it possible to read words if they are pronounced slowly, putting in intervals.

Speech Visualization for Telephonic Speech

Introduction

The visual patterns may not be good enough yet to transmit continuous speech information as described in the previous section. However, if they are presented together with auditory information by a hearing aid, they will help understanding in telephone communication.

In order to extend the speech visualization system to communication by telephone, the parameter extraction methods need to be improved for the band-limited signals in a telephone channel. New methods to extract pitch (F0) and formant frequencies (F1-F3) from telephonic speech signals will be described in this section. Next, it will be shown by examples that the real-time visualization of telephonic speech can be realized by connecting this parameter extraction system with the other parts in the system (Figure 1) for ordinary speech.

Formant extraction method

The inverse filter control method which is basically the same as for ordinary speech is used for a stable and real-time formant extraction for telephonic speech. The system which has been modified for the band-limited signal is constructed as shown in Figure 7.

IF1 and IF2 in Figure 7 show inverse filters with a fixed bandwidth, which eliminate the first and the second formant component, respectively.

In the system, zero frequency of the third inverse filter IF3 is initially set to be of 3000 Hz and likewise its bandwidth, 200 Hz. The bandwidths of IF1 and IF2 are always fixed to be of 50 Hz (80 Hz) and 80 Hz (120 Hz) in male (female) voice, respectively. Initial zero frequencies are 500 Hz in IF1 and 1500 Hz in IF2.

Telephonic speech signals are, initially, sampled at 12 kHz and quantified into 12 bits/sample. After the sample sequences have been band-limited in 300–3000 Hz, they are decimated to a half (6 kHz) in the sampling frequency. (But the signals are used without decimating for pitch extraction.) Next, a root-mean square (RMS) value of the signals is calculated in a frame of 20 ms and weights are decided by linearly interpolating the RMS values between two sequential frames. Each sample in a frame is divided by the corresponding weight so that the signal levels are normalized.

Thus, the band-limited and normalized signals are processed by the inverse filter control system shown in Figure 7. The zero frequency of IF1 is controlled by the mean frequency obtained from the output of IF2 and likewise, IF2 by the output of IF1.

The FRQ in Figure 7, which has been improved for this digital

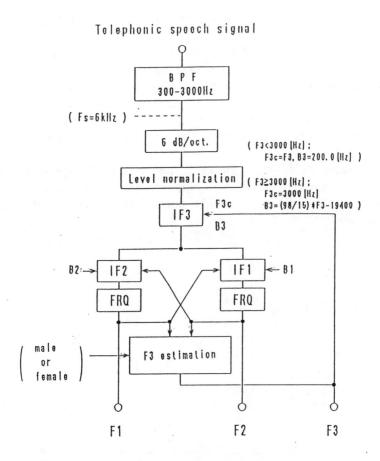

Figure 7. Formant extraction system for telephonic speech

processing, is a routine to compute the mean frequency from the output of the inverse filter. This routine has two steps in the approximation. In the first step, a mean frequency of the power spectrum is calculated in the time domain by the following equation:

$$\bar{f} = \frac{1}{2\Pi T} \cdot \cos^{-1}\left(\frac{\sum\limits_{i=1}^{N} X_i X_{i-1}}{\sum\limits_{i=1}^{N} X_i^2}\right) \tag{2}$$

where xi, T and N represent the speech sample, the sampling period and the number of samples in a frame, respectively.

As the bandwidth of signals is limited to 3000 Hz, the mean frequency of equation (2) must be computed in the sampling frequency of 6 kHz. This computation is simple and can be executed at a high speed.

Second step of the computation FRQ is somewhat more complicated. A weighted mean of the zero-crossing frequency distribution in each frame is computed in the time domain. The weighting function has the shape of a symmetrical triangle as a function of frequency as shown in Figure 8.

The centre frequency of the triangle shows the mean frequency which is initially given by the first approximation (mean frequency of the power spectrum). If the weighted mean changes from the first approximation, the centre is moved to the new frequency. This operation is repeated three times reducing the base of the triangle and the final mean frequency is extracted. The final base reaches 30% of the starting one.

Furthermore, as shown in Figure 8, the frequency range of the base is also given as a function of the centre frequency, which is a linear function between +300 Hz at 180 Hz and +3000 Hz at 4500 Hz in the first computation.

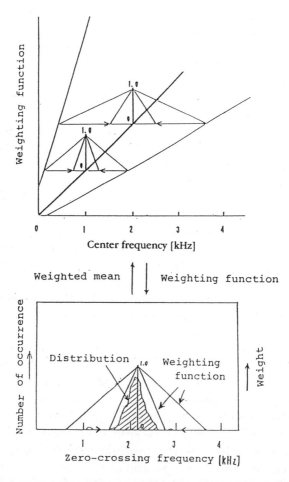

Figure 8. Schematic diagram of weighted mean computation based on zero-crossing frequency distribution (2nd approximation in the computation of formant frequencies).

The control loop of the formant extraction system is executed twice in each of the two FRQ computations. Thus, the first and the second formant frequencies (F1 and F2) are extracted and the third formant frequency, which may be outside the limited frequency band, is estimated from the lowest two formant frequencies by a regression equation (Watanabe, Hamasaki and Ueda, 1991) that was statistically determined.

Two regression equations are prepared for male and female (including child's) voice, respectively. The speaker sex of the input speech is judged by a majority decision of the past pitch sequence which continues in a voiced segment. That is, if the majority of the past pitch values is beyond a threshold (192.4 Hz), the voice is judged to be female and otherwise male. The threshold separates statistically the Japanese voice into male or female voice by a pitch frequency.

If the estimated third formant frequency is beyond 3000 Hz, the zero frequency of IF3 is fixed at 3000 Hz and its bandwidth is controlled by estimated frequency as shown in the equations of Figure 7.

Figure 9 (a) shows an example of the convergent process of the lowest two formant frequencies. In the first four control times, zero frequencies of IF1 and IF2 are controlled by the mean frequency of power spectrum in equation (2). Likewise, in the fifth to twelfth control times, they are controlled by the weighted mean of zero-crossing frequency distributions. The vertical bars in Figure 9 (a) indicate a standard deviation of the zero-crossing frequency distributions.

The mean of the zero-crossing frequency distribution is also represented for the first four control times in which the control is conducted by the mean frequency of the power spectrum.

Figure 9(b) shows the spectrum in the same example in Figure 9(a) and the normalized zero-crossing frequency distributions after convergence. In this case, as the lowest two formant frequencies are close to each other and to the centre of the frequency range, the first mean frequencies of the power spectra give a good approximation to the last means of zero-crossing frequencies. On the other hand, in the widely spread spectrum shown in Figure 10(a), the mean frequency of the spectrum indicates a low value in F2 because of band-limited signals. But, in spite of the inverse filter's mismatch, the zero-crossing frequency distributions are localized sharply and the mean frequencies show constantly stable values.

These results indicate that zero-crossing frequency distribution is a very good parameter for estimating a formant frequency. It may play an important role not only in the formant analysis but also in auditory perception.

Finally, the accuracy of the formant extraction has been examined using the Monte Carlo method. In other words, synthetic speech whose parameters are decided at random is used as an input for the formant

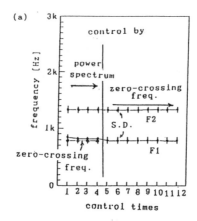

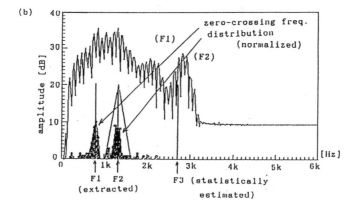

Figure 9. An example of convergent process and zero-crossing frequency distribution after convergence. (a) Convergent process of two formant frequencies. (b) Amplitude spectrum and zero-crossing frequency distributions after convergence

extraction system. First, a pitch frequency is chosen in the range of 80–200 Hz for male voice or 150–350 Hz for female voice by a random number, and likewise F1-F4 are decided at random in their respective ranges.

The signals with these parameters were synthesized by a simulation of a terminal analogue synthesizer. The bandwidths of the resonant filters have been given as a function of the formant frequencies as proposed by G. Fant.

This extraction scheme is very stable and there was no large-error sample in spite of 300 trials. The standard deviations of errors are +/–28.9 Hz in F1, +/–34.0 Hz in F2 for male voice and +/–57.0 Hz in F1, +/–46.5 Hz in F2 for female voice.

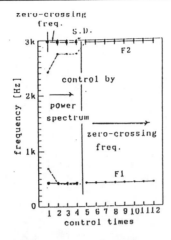

(a) Convergent process of two formant frequencies

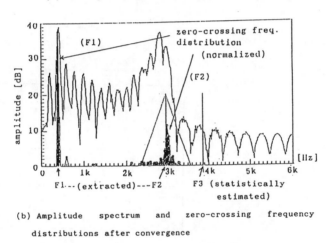

(b) Amplitude   spectrum   and   zero-crossing   frequency

distributions after convergence

Figure 10. As for Figure 9.

This demonstrates that the proposed system is very reliable for practical use.

Pitch extraction method

In telephonic speech, since there are no signal components below
300 Hz, pitch (F0) information must be estimated from the harmonic
components.

Figure 11 shows the pitch extractor proposed for telephonic speech.
In the pre-processing, first of all, band-limited (300–3000 Hz) signals
are processed by the cascade-type-inverse-filters whose zero frequencies equal the respective formants (F1-F3).

Next, the resultant signals are converted into square amplitude ones
with the same sign as that of the originals to restore the fundamental

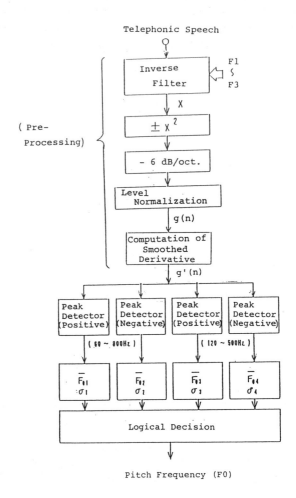

Figure 11. Pitch extractor for telephonic speech.

component. Finally, the signals are integrated to give greater emphasis to the fundamental component and normalized by the RMS level interpolated between frames.

Through this operation, the amplitude spectrum decreases monotonously in frequency and the dynamic range reduces. This shows that the waveform would typically be a train of peaked pulses which synchronize with the fundamental component.

Based on these sequences, a robust method has been devised to decide pitch (F0). Since the resolving power of the pitch periods which are estimated from the peak points is restricted by the sampling period, linear interpolation between samples in the smoothed derivative of waveforms has been adopted. The principle of the interpolation is illustrated in Figure 12. It is assumed that the waveform g(n) in Figure 12 has been extracted after the pre-processing.

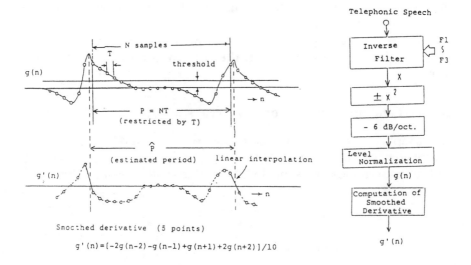

Figure 12. Estimation method of pitch periods by interpolation of the smoothed derivative.

If the interval between peaks is decided by the sample sequences, the pitch period becomes integer multiplication of the sampling period T. Better approximation for pitch estimation is obtained from the smoothed derivative, g['](n) in Figure 12. The smoothed derivative of 5 points is simply calculated in the following equation (Savitsky and Golay, 1964).

$$g['](n) = (-2g(n-2)-g(n-1)+g(n+1)+2g(n+2))/10$$

In the sample sequences of g['](n), if the linear interpolation function between two samples intersects the zero level, the intersecting point will be a better approximation of the peak in g(n). If the linear function has a negative slope, the peak is a positive and if a positive slope, the peak is a negative.

Therefore, the more exact period between peaks will be estimated by searching the zero-crossing points where the linear function intersects the zero level and which exist near the peaks of g(n).

As shown in Figure 11, the positive and negative peaks in the meaning described above are searched for in two ranges of time-intervals, for the male and female voice. Thus, the four sequences of instantaneous periods are detected in a frame of 40 ms, so that a true pitch can be estimated from them.

First, a mean period and a standard deviation are computed from each of the sequences in the frame, and then the pitch (F0) is determined as the reciprocal of the mean period in the sequence with the minimal standard deviation. However, since a second or third harmonic is sometimes chosen as the true pitch in the nasals or liquids etc., a logical decision based on the pattern continuity is also performed.

Formant and pitch extraction from real speech

An example of formant and pitch trajectories extracted by the methods described above is shown in Figure 13. There is no large-error sample and the pattern looks reasonable in the values and the continuity.

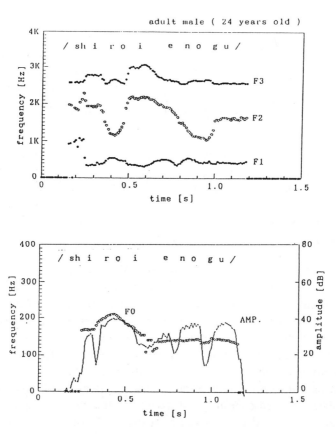

Figure 13. An example of formant and pitch trajectories (adult male, 24 years old).

Visualization examples

If the parameter extraction methods mentioned above are applied to the speech visualization system already described, telephonic speech will be visualized. This has been tested by computer simulation.

The visualization examples are shown in Figure 14. In the pictures, the colour pattern represents voiced segments and the black-and-white patterns only the unvoiced portions. The horizontal length of the colour pattern is restricted by pitch, so that the change in length indicates intonation of utterances. The horizontal position of the white pattern corresponds to the spectral channel.

The vertical axis corresponds to time and the pattern flows from the bottom to the top on the screen. The pattern of two seconds is always represented. Almost the same pattern as that for ordinary speech can be seen in spite of the special processing in the band-limited signals.

Problems to be Solved for the Completed Systems

As described above in the section on speech visualization systems, although the developed system is basically successful in understanding words and compounds, it is desirable to read the patterns more quickly and more accurately. For that, consonants, especially voiced consonants, should be represented to give clear images. Generally, as it is difficult to recognize the consonants automatically by an algorithm in continuous speech, other methods are required.

In the visual representation of speech, the aim will be achieved if consonants can be recognized visually. Therefore, if some acoustical features related to consonants are extracted and the visual image is generated by overlapping the patterns peculiar to the features, one may be able to understand visually what the consonant is. This concept must be natural in the meaning that it resembles auditory perception of acoustic features of speech.

Even if individual features do not perfectly correspond with individual consonants, it seems likely that the consonantal image as a whole is revealed as the overlapped pattern of some features. Therefore, the detection of acoustic features in consonants and their visualization should be attempted.

Neural networks may be appropriate for extracting many acoustical features simultaneously. This is an attractive idea because neural networks can be constructed naturally by learning and researchers do not have to devise the algorithms to extract every feature.

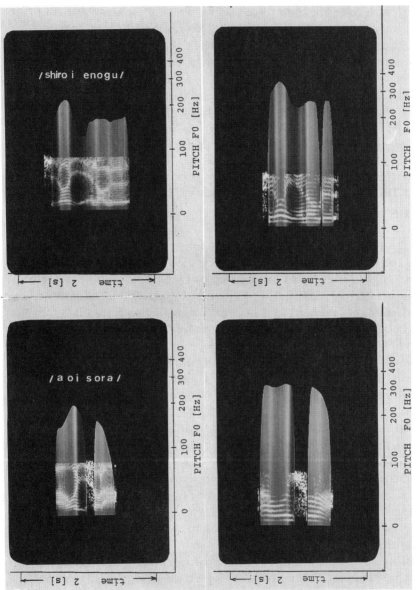

Figure 14. Examples of visualized speech. (a) /aoi sora/ (male, 21 years old); (b) /aoi sora/ (male 7 years old); (c) /shiroi enogu/ (male, 21 years old); (d) /shiroi enogu/ (female, 22 years old). It should be noted that the black and white photographs cannot do justice to the chromaticity dimension on which vowel quality is mapped.

Application Systems for Speech Training and Communication Aids

The speech visualization system described above will be useful as a prototype of aids for the deaf. The hardware system for real-time processing using 32 bit floating-point DSP chips (TMS320C31) has been developed. The real-time system has been successful in extracting the lowest three formant frequencies and pitch from telephonic speech. The extracted values are similar to those obtained by computer simulation.

However, it is desirable for the practical aids that the speech visualization system is expanded by connecting with other devices which give additive functions. Two kinds of application systems are being developed on the basis of the speech visualization system.

Speech training aid

One of the applications for the speech visualization system is as a speech training aid.

The speech training system consists of the visualization system and a personal computer as shown in Figure 15. The computer controls the speech visualization system and a hearing aid. In the computer system, a database for standard utterances which has been collected from normal-hearing persons, is put on the hard disc. The utterances are isolated vowels, monosyllables and words. The speech parameters and signal itself are stored.

Prior to the speech training, the parameters are read out of the database and displayed on the left half of the TV screen as a colour pattern in slow motion. Meanwhile, speech signals by which the visual pattern is generated are provided to the hearing aid from the computer, and the sounds are reproduced repeatedly by pushing a button.

During training, a hearing-impaired person tries to imitate the standard utterances looking at the visual pattern and listening to its speech sounds. Thus, he/she can look at his/her own utterance on the right half of the screen in real time. At the same time, it will be easy to feedback his/her own voice through the hearing aid.

Menus from which a word for the training can easily be selected have a hierarchical structure. The simplest choice requires at least three menus, that is, speaker's sex (male, female or child), word groups and words in a group.

The parameters and the signals are drawn out from the database by assigning a word in the final menu. Since each word in the selected word group is always used in a training session, it must be transmitted fast to the visualization system and the hearing aid.

Adding some intelligent functions to this system will make it more useful in practice.

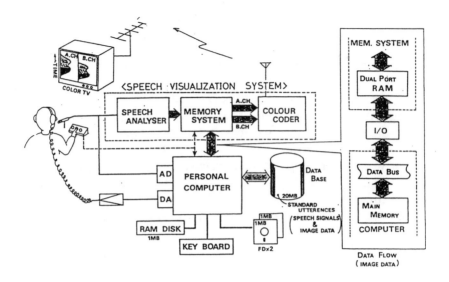

Figure 15. Speech training system using the speech visualization system.

Aid to understanding telephonic speech

As another application, a total system, which transmits telephonic speech to hard-of-hearing persons through visual and auditory senses, is being developed. The telephonic speech receiving aid is constructed as shown in Figure 16.

In this system, first of all, telephonic speech is obtained as electric signals by a telephone talk free adapter and some speech parameters such as formants, pitch etc., are extracted from it. Next, using these

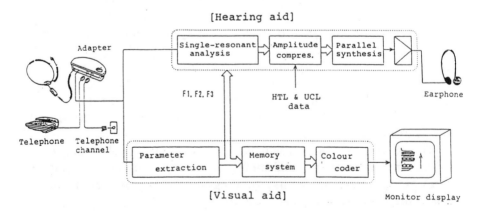

Figure 16. Communication aid for telephonic speech.

parameters, two kinds of signals are synthesized, one for a hearing aid and the other for the visual aid described in the previous sections.

In this hearing aid, speech signals are separated into approximate single-resonant waves by inverse filters, whose anti-resonance is controlled by the extracted formant frequencies. Each single-resonant component is quasi-linearly amplified with slowly varying gain to normalize the level between frames according to their effective values so that the amplitude of the formant always reaches the audible signal region of the hearing-impaired person.

Finally, the two amplified components are added after weighting in the same way as a parallel synthesizer. By this operation, only the components near the formant frequencies are clearly compressed into the audible region. Thus, the compressed signals have little distortion and good quality.

It is expected by using this system that hearing-impaired persons will be able to understand telephonic speech by complementary information in visual and auditory patterns. On the other hand, some techniques peculiar to the telephone might be necessary for practical use. One is a measure against channel noise. For example, average noise level and spectrum can be automatically measured for 50 ms from the instant after the hearing-impaired person picks up the receiver because the sender perhaps does not talk immediately. So this information will be used for deciding on a threshold to detect signal segments or for more active processing to reduce noise.

Conclusion

Our goal for speech visualization is essentially perfect translation from auditory (normal) to visual information to understand speech. In this research and its future extension, the aim is to be able to see phonemic and prosodic information by the integrated patterns of many acoustic features so that continuous speech can be understood intuitively by visual patterns.

Achievement of this aim depends on matching between human factors in vision and the integrated patterns.

Acknowledgement

The author wishes to thank Dr Y. Ueda and A. Shigenaga who collaborated on the development of the analogue-type visualization system and conducted its evaluation. He would also like to thank T. Ikeda, N. Frasherei, K. Tasaki and T. Yamamoto, who designed and assembled the speech-parameter extraction system using a 32 bit floating-point DSP chips.

References

Bernstein, L.E., Ferguson, J.B. and Goldstein, Jr, M.H. (1986) Speech training devices for profoundly deaf children. Proceedings of ICASSP 86: 633–6.

Levitt, H. (1973) Speech processing aids for the deaf: An overview. IEEE Transactions , Audio. Electroacoust., AU-21: 269–73.

Liberman, A.M., Cooper, F.S., Shankweiler, D.P. and Studdert-Kennedy, M. (1968) Why are speech spectrograms hard to read? American Annals of the Deaf 113: 127–33.

Nickerson, R.S. and Stevens, K.N. (1973) Teaching speech to the deaf: Can a computer help? IEEE Transactions AU-21: 445–55.

Risberg, A. (1968) Visual aids for speech correction. American Annals of the Deaf 113: 178–94.

Savitzky, A. and Golay, M.J.E. (1964) Smoothing and differentiation of data by simplified least squares procedures. Analytical Chemistry 36: 1627–39.

Ueda, Y. and Watanabe, A. (1987) Visible/tactile vowel information to be transmitted to the hearing impaired. Journal of the Acoustic Society of Japan (E) 8: 99–108.

Watanabe, A. and Ueda, Y. (1981) Visual image of connected vowels for color display system of connected speech (in Japanese). Transactions IECE, J64-A: 574–81.

Watanabe, A. and Ueda, Y. (1988) Speech visualization and its application for the hearing impaired. Journal of the Acoustical society of America Suppl. 1, 84: 542.

Watanabe, A., Ueda, Y. and Shigenaga, A. (1985) Color display system for connected speech to be used for the hearing impaired. IEEE Transactions, ASSP-33: 164–73.

Watanabe, A., Hamasaki, R. and Ueda, Y. (1991) Parameters' extraction and estimation methods for visualization of telephonic speech (in Japanese). Journal of the Institute of TV Engineers of Japan 45: 233–43.

Part V
Computer - based Training

25

A Multi-media Program Exercising the Basics in Lipreading, Cued Speech and Sign Language Vocabulary

BIRGIT COOK

Introduction

A hearing impairment often results in the need to learn new communication methods such as lipreading, with or without the support of signals from hearing aids, cochlear implants or tactile aids, the sign language of the deaf or different forms of manually supported speech, such as cued speech or the Danish mouth–hand system.

When it comes to fundamentals and routines, the whole teaching/learning process tends to be very tedious and time-consuming for both therapist and trainee (Jeffers and Barely, 1977). It would be more effective and rewarding if the therapist could be released from such basic routines to be able to devote time to more complex matters.

Since the 1960s, researchers in different countries have been engaged in developing self-instruction training programs for use in the rehabilitation of the hearing-impaired and the deaf. Donald G. Sims (1988), when describing the background, evaluation and instruction methods in this field, concludes that it has been clearly demonstrated that self-instruction programs improve proficiency significantly and further, that training with the interactive system is quite up to the standard of teacher-led lessons, judging from the pre- and post-test results achieved.

In the field of hearing rehabilitation in Sweden, computer-supported visual, auditory and audio/visual training (the ACTIVE system (Mizuno and Risberg, 1984) has been used for some time in various forms and combinations at selected centres.

The user response has been wholly positive, which has encouraged us to proceed with the development of a fully interactive multi-media program. The system is currently being test-run at certain Swedish hospitals.

Equipment

The equipment we are using currently consists of an ordinary Macintosh computer and a laser video-disc player. We use a two-screen solution with a separate TV screen which is used to display the stimulus materials – for example, the speaker's face for lipreading or the sign-movements.

The ordinary PC screen displays the text used for instructions, response alternatives, feedback information, etc. The laser-disc provides us with access to 35 minutes of recorded words, phrases and continuous speech.

The Program

Through the menu of the program the trainees are given the responsibility of charting their progress through the program. They sign in at the beginning of each training session and log out at the end.

Results are automatically recorded under the user's individual name. The system also plots the user's progress and may highlight any area of difficulty. Any difficulties revealed will assist in the diagnosis of additional training required, therapist-led where necessary.

The program consists of

1. Familiarization – training by self-selection of stimuli.
2. Recognition training – using randomly computer-selected stimuli.
3. Self-testing.

All three parts contain the same choices of exercises, which appear under the main headings of Vowels/Consonants/Questions requiring one word response/Different groups of subjects/Cued speech/Sign language. Each heading has its own sub-menu of exercises – all according to the user's preference. For example, if the user starts by selecting Vowels, another menu of choices will appear, from which can be selected vowels in nonsense words, in actual words and in sentences.

In the familiarization and recognition training programs the stimulus can be repeated at normal speed or in slow motion. This is one of the program's most popular features as many hard-of-hearing persons find it embarrassing to ask for repetition of the same word over and over again.

All programs can be exercised visually, audiovisually and, by turning off the TV screen, auditively. When desired, varying levels of background noise can be added.

The familiarization training session provides the user with an opportunity of going through the stimuli in the selected menu, with pre-knowledge of what will appear.

Having gained sufficient familiarity with the stimuli the user moves on to the recognition training. In this program and the test program stimuli are randomly presented by the computer.

A list of up to 12 response alternatives will appear on the screen as all programs use a forced choice paradigm with 3 to 12 alternatives. When the stimulus appears on the TV screen the user has to select the answer and the screen will show whether or not the answer given was correct. If correct, the user asks for the next stimulus. If incorrect, the stimulus can either be repeated – in slow motion if desired – or the correct answer can be asked for, which will be displayed together with the incorrect answer given. Both can be repeated to allow for comparison.

For feedback, results of every recognition training exercise will be shown before leaving the program.

After every exercise, the user has the opportunity of undergoing a self-test – without the advantage of the repetition and slow motion function. The results are displayed in numerical, percentage and confusion matrix form. This data is stored in the user's personal file.

Evaluation and User Reaction

The program and equipment was lent out on field trial in the spring of 1993 to the audiological clinics at Karolinska and Danderyd hospitals and to AMI-S (a labour market institute for adults with acquired hearing impairment and adult deafness) in both Uppsala and Sollentuna. The equipment was test-used at these units during rehabilitation courses for hearing-impaired adults.

As an outcome, some seventy persons took the opportunity of complementing their group training sessions in lipreading by working with the program on their own. Their individual views, given in response to a written questionnaire, were also discussed in group session, out of which a consensus report was prepared which showed a universally positive response to this additional training aid.

All the therapists concerned had the same positive reaction. One therapist who has been conducting such courses for many years wrote, 'furthermore, this development has been the greatest thing that has happened since I started working in this field' (Tilberg, 1993)

The opportunity given of exercising on their own was much praised by the participants. Having to ask frequently for words to be repeated is a very common source of embarrassment, now avoidable by use of the program which allows for words to be repeated audiovisually or visually as many times as wanted, even in slow motion, merely by pressing a button.

All involved in this field test wished to see the present program further developed so as to include more exercises and more difficult programs, where the use of openlist answers would be possible. We plan now to go ahead in developing a realistic basic course in lipreading contained on five different laser-disc records.

Conclusion

The potential offered by systems for self-instruction training would seem to be very great. 'In finding ways to integrate new technology into aural rehabilitation, we need only to tap our imaginations' (Tye-Murray, 1992).

Training programs developed in one country can easily be adapted to other languages by recording the stimulus material and storing the response alternatives in the computer program.

The amount of training that can be given in the clinic is often very limited. It would therefore be very positive if equipment for self-instructive training could be used at home, both for training adults and children. The present equipment is prohibitively expensive but we hope that the ongoing development of home video techniques will soon make it possible to develop less expensive systems.

Experience in training of cochlear-implant patients indicates that there is a great need for an interactive multi-media training program of the type described.

Some cochlear implanted patients need only a short familiarization period before the new sounds function while others need an extended and time consuming period of training which may only show full results after a number of years. In both cases, but particularly the latter, the equipment described, capable of providing tailor-made training, would make a significant contribution.

References

Jeffers, J. and Barley, M. (1977) Speechreading (Lipreading), Springfield, Illinois: C.C. Thomas.

Mizuno, C. and Risberg, A. (1984) Computer-aided speechreading training program, STL – QPSR (Dept. of Speech Communication and Music Acoustics, KTH, Stockholm), 2- 3: 109–18.

Sims, D.G. (1988) Video methods for speechreading instruction. Volta Review 90: 273–88.

Tilberg, I. (1993) Written submission, August.

Tye-Murray, N. (1992) Laser Videodisc Technology in the Aural Rehabilitation Setting: Good News for People With Severe and Profound Hearing Impairments, Clinical Focus – Innovation, 33–6, March.

26

Computer-Assisted Interactive Video Methods for Speechreading Instruction: A Review

DONALD G. SIMS AND LINDA GOTTERMEIER

Contrary to the mythology of hearing impairment, speechreading skills can be taught (Walden *et al.*, 1977, 1981; van Uden, 1983; Gesi, Massaro and Cohen, 1992; Massaro, Cohen and Gesi, 1993; De Filippo, Sims and Gottermeier, 1995). However, speechreading skill improvement as measured in these recent studies was accomplished with at least 5 hours of face-to face, intensive drill and practice. Over the past decade, fewer clinicians and clients have found it practical or desirable to undertake this kind of drill and practice because such practice (one-on-one or in small groups) can be inherently tedious. Instead, aural rehabilitation programmes have emphasized conversational repair strategies and the use of assistive listening devices (Abrahamson, 1991). Such a focus may be denying clients the benefits of training to improve visual and auditory speech discrimination skills. Current video related technology, such as computer-assisted interactive video (CAIV), can make speechreading drill both practical and pleasant for client and clinician. Further, interactive video technology enables detailed assessment of instructional benefit and improved research capabilities. According to Gagné, Dinon and Parsons (1991), 'A major advantage of interactive video systems is that they make it possible to control the variability associated with the sender, the stimuli and the environment. Thus it is possible to isolate parameters related to the variable of interest (i.e., the performance of the receiver).' This chapter will (a) focus on studies and programmes which have employed interactive video in various ways to teach speechreading, (b) outline techniques for determining the general pedagogical strengths and weaknesses of computer applications for speechreading instruction, and (c) examine some of the strengths and weaknesses of current CAIV methods for determining speechreading skill acquisition *during* training as opposed to traditional pre- and post-test methods.

Definition and Design of CAIV Systems

The interactive video system consists of a 'library' of video images or sequences for which any number of different programs can be accessed by the host computer. Any segment of video information can be used in different combinations depending upon the needs of the learner and the content selected by the instructor. The interactive system consists of: (a) a video storage/retrieval system, for example, a video cassette recorder or videodisc; (b) a computer system with a video monitor; and (c) the built-in or accessory interface that permits the computer to locate and playback the prerecorded video (Mahshie, 1987).

Another hardware and software approach on the educational horizon is called Digital Video Interactive (DVI). This combination of desktop, high-speed computer, video processing board and optical read/write disc drive is the functional equivalent of a digital production studio containing mixers, tape decks, monitoring systems, effects processors and other items that connect together to record, modify and playback audio and video tracks (Green, 1992). Current low-cost DVI systems have limited frame-rate and/or picture size; and, therefore, are less desirable for speechreading. However, the newest DVI systems could enable school-based, interactive video producers to bypass expensive, conventional videodisc mastering procedures by digitally recording high-quality video and audio, editing and/or graphically enhancing the recording, and then storing programs on optical disc drives. (See Appendix G of the 'Guideline for producing accessible multimedia for deaf and hard-of-hearing students' (Mazaik, 1993) for a discussion of current IBM and Macintosh hard and software for DVI.)

History of CAIV for Speechreading

What is reported below represents an effort to abstract the methodologies and conclusions related to efficacy of training. Studies are presented in a roughly chronological order which shows the increasing sophistication of CAIV design. An effort was made to report on data-based conclusions where they existed.

DAVID

Sims *et al.* (1979) first reported using a Dynamic Audio Video Interactive Device (DAVID) which consisted of a Wang 32K (and later an Apple ll) microcomputer interfaced to a 3/4 inch VCR with a separate microprocessor controller. Students viewed various talkers speaking single sentences. Depending upon the speechreading skill of the student, the instructor chose one of four levels of speechreading practice.

The first level required the student to respond by selecting an appropriate sentence from multiple choice items. The second level required the student to fill in the missing words in a sentence. A key word or two was given in the appropriate place with the blanks to be completed by the student; the number of words and phonemes in the sentence were indicated by underlining on the computer monitor. The third level had the key word given outside the context of the sentence as an advanced organizer but the computer screen for student response did not give any clues as to the length of the words or sentence. The fourth method required the student to speechread and then keyboard, verbatim, the entire sentence. Students could obtain repetitions of the entire sentence on demand. Also, hints about the sentence topic and 'fill-ins' of missing letters or words were supplied by the computer program to prevent frustration.

Assessment of speechreading gains was accomplished by taking key words from the practised materials, embedding them in novel sentences, and measuring pre- and post-test performance. In addition, the CID Sentences (Jeffers and Barley, 1971) and Jacobs' (1982) speechreading tests were administered. Performance was compared to a matched group of students who used conventional videotape instruction with paper-and-pencil, write-down responses. For this pilot study, gains on the pre- and post-test measures were similar to conventional, non-computer, videotape drill and practice. A later study (Sims *et al.*, 1982b) replicated these results but found that when students were exposed to both methods they preferred CAIV as providing (a) better use of their time and (b) increased instructional benefit. Programmatically CAIV freed instructors from daily management of self-instruction and provided summarized performance data to inform future lesson revisions.

Recently, videodiscs have been produced on DAVID for college-aged deaf students to practise speechreading everyday sentences, job interview sentences, and college-related social sentences. Videodisc materials are presented with a Macintosh SE-30/Hyper Card and C-based software with a Sony LDV 1500 videodisc player. Talkers are interpreters and teachers from the National Technical Institute for the Deaf (NTID) who have been rated for overall visibility by speechreading instructors. Materials are used in conjunction with several 10-week instructional courses that focus on communication strategies, viseme perception, and sentence- or paragraph-length drill and practice exercises. Videodisc playback enables students to view the whole sentence or re-articulated isolated words from the target sentence. Slow or fast speeds for viewing can be selected as well as playback with front or side views of the talker's face (45-degree azimuth). If the sentence is not understood, written hints are provided on the monitor regarding the topic of the sentence. In order to eventually achieve the required verbatim responses, letters and words can be filled in by the computer, upon student request, one at a time after each answer attempt.

Performance is measured by counting the time in seconds required until the student keyboards a verbatim identification response for the target sentence. It is assumed that if a sequence of training items are generally equivalent and the instruction is effective, then response times should decrease as skills improve (Tatsouka and Tatsouka, 1978). Sims, Snell and Clymer (1984) have found this expected trend for response times averaged across subjects using time series and regression analyses.

ALVIS

Kopra *et al.* (1986) first described the use of Sony View videodisc system for speechreading training. The Auditory-visual Laser Videodisc Interactive System (ALVIS) was designed to provide supplementary drill and practice to postlingually hearing-impaired adults. The three hundred sentences with previously established item difficulty levels were arranged in 12 lists with 25 sentences each. There were two different drill conditions: (a) 'ALVIS/cluewords' with word clues printed on the screen accompanying the visual stimuli (no sound), and (b) 'ALVIS/hear' with accompanying auditory clues gradually faded in (2 dB steps per sentence repetition). Additionally, the program progressed from sentences which were 'easy' to 'medium' to 'difficult'. Since the ALVIS programs were short sentences composed of common words, minimal typing and spelling skills were needed. Gains from pre-test to post-test training were comparable to speechreading drill and practice with a clinician conducting small group speechreading therapy. Kopra *et al.* (1986) indicated that presentation technique (i.e., ALVIS/cluewords or ALVIS/hear) needed further research to determine whether the audio fade-in method provided optimal learning for a given subject.

CASPER

Computer Assisted Speech Perception Evaluation and Training (CASPER) is an IBM PC based CAIV system (Boothroyd, 1981; Boothroyd *et al.*, 1987) which has provided multi-level assessment and training. The six laser discs produced included the following:

1. The THRIFT (Three Interval Forced Choice Test) measured detection of one suprasegmental and eight segmental speech pattern contrasts in a varying phonetic contexts within nonsense syllables.
2. The SPAC (Speech Pattern Contrast Test) measured identification of two suprasegmental and eight segmental speech pattern contrasts in varying phonetic context within words and phrases.
3. The AB Word Lists included 15 lists of 10 consonant-vowel-consonant words in a carrier phrase. Each list contained the same 30

phonemes which permitted the estimation of phoneme and word recognition probability.

4. The CUNY Topic-Related Sentence Sets 1–60 contained 12 everyday sentences in each set. Sentences varied in length from 3 to 12 words. The same 12 'everyday living' topics appeared in each of the sets which attempted to emulate conversations.

5. The Continuous Discourse Test included 17 short stories which were used to estimate word recognition performance and semi-automated connected discourse tracking.

Each videodisc could be used for testing and/or training. These materials were used with adult users of the Nucleus cochlear implant. Three subjects were catagorized as 'highly successful' in terms of speech perception performance improvement, post-implant; while three others were considered to be 'less successful'. The introduction of formal training using the videodisc at 4 months vs 6 months post-implant had a significant effect on sentence perception by implant alone for 'successful subjects'. Boothroyd *et al.*. inferred that 'time on task' added significantly to the improvements in performance.

Iowa Cochlear Implant Program

Tye-Murray *et al.* (1988) developed three laser videodisc programs using the IBM Info-Window touch-screen videodisc system for training the communication skills of new hearing aid users and cochlear implant clients. Program 1 consisted of eight audio visual exercises that required the client to discriminate and identify different consonants. Program 2 focused on (a) synthetic audiovisual training, (b) the development of 'assertive communication skills, and (c) various conversational repair strategies. Program 3 consisted of 11 exercises for communication practice in home and school settings.

Tye-Murray (1992) listed some benefits of CAIV for adult cochlear implant users as follows: (a) concentrated learning led to faster learning and helped to maintain the client's interest, (b) different versions of training software allowed the training difficulty to be adjusted for clients with poor language and/or speech recognition by daily monitoring of progress, (c) speechreading practice occurred with many different talkers without leaving the clinical setting, and (d) CAIV lessons were successfully used with family members in the rehabilitation process to improve appropriate speaking behaviours and repair strategies for communication breakdowns.

CAST

Pinchora-Fuller and Benguerel (1991) developed and implemented a Computer-Aided Speechreading Training system (CAST) using a PC platform with a videocassette playback. Their system was designed as a component in a comprehensive aural rehabilitation programme for pre-retirement adults with acquired mild-to-moderate hearing loss. Eight lessons provided practice with consonant visemes. Each lesson had four components consisting of review of: a) previously taught visemes, b) training for a new viseme, c) practice identifying visemes in segments of discourse, and d) a recapitulation.

Paragraph texts contained high proportions of a target viseme. These texts were recorded as a continuous paragraph and as phrase-length utterances. The instructor pre-selected the speaking rate, the phrase length, and the modality of presentation. In CAST, the speechreader was allowed to elicit feedback by typing a guess, replaying the videotape, or moving to another phrase with the option to return later. There was a ceiling on the number of times that the message could be replayed before the answer was given. After all the phrases of the lesson had been completed, the entire paragraph was played at the slow presentation rate and then at the normal presentation rate to allow the speechreader to see the phrase integrated in an uninterrupted presentation.

With two groups of eight normal-hearing adults, Gagné, Dinon and Parsons (1991) reported improvement in the experimental group in developing synthetic visual speech perception skills using CAST. Both the control group and the experimental groups were given a Visual Consonant Recognition Test, a test of Sentence Understanding Without Context (key-word and total word recognition were scored), a test of Sentence Understanding With Context (key-word recognition score) and a semi-automated Continuous Discourse Tracking (CDT) activity. The experimental groups received on average 25–30 hours of training with the eight training lessons of CAST. Two weeks after the experimental group completed the CAST training program, a post-test protocol was administered. Significant differences between the control and experimental groups were found for total word recognition scores on the Sentence Understanding With Context test and the semiautomated CDT activity. Given that other measures did not show improvement, Gagné *et al.* (1991) indicate that the potential benefits of CAST for hearing-impaired individuals 'remains to be determined'. While the subjects who participated in the CAST training enjoyed the activities, they felt the lessons were too lengthy (i.e., about 76 minutes). Additionally, many subjects reported that the learner–computer interactions were cumbersome and suggested the need for an assistant to enter commands into the computer.

Interactive training program for speechreading and hearing skills

Ijsseldijk and Elsendoorn (1991) reported on interactive programs developed for orally-educated Dutch children who were severely and profoundly hearing-impaired. The programs operated with the Amiga 2300 computer and a Philips VP406 videodisc player. The speech materials consisted of words, phrases, and segments spoken by three different talkers. Students responded to multiple-choice formats. The videodisc practice was meant to be used in conjunction with classroom language instruction. The following choices would be made by the student: (a) which theme of the practice lesson (i.e., 'Living,' ' Nutrition', or 'Fairy tale'), (b) whether the lesson would be speechreading or auditory training, (c) which language level (i.e., phoneme, word, phrase or sentence level), and (d) which speaker presentation (full face, profile, lips only, or mouth covered). In training, if the answers were incorrect, the right answer was presented, sometimes with the first answer repeated incorrectly to make the student aware of contrasting differences. During practice the student could ask for repetition, slow-speech, and answer corrections.

The videodisc also had a reference section that allowed the student to play 'games' to become familiar with the mouse and a 'telephone alphabet' to help develop an understanding of the different phoneme and viseme groups. With this 'Extra-Training', the instructor was able to tailor the lesson to the needs of an individual student.

To document the effectiveness of the videodisc, 20 students of the Sint-Michielsgestel Institute for the Deaf, ranging in age from 14 to 20 years, participated in training programs where the goal was independent practice. Subjects trained in 30–45 minutes sessions over a 6-month period. The total training time ranged from 24 to 36 hours. Later a second videodisc was developed consisting of two tests of speechreading, one test for vowel recognition, and one for consonant recognition. The training programs did not yield significant differences between hearing and speechreading pre- and post-tests for the complete group of subjects. Ijsseldijk and Elsendoorn attribute the findings to the 'relatively short' training period. Further, subjects were known to have previous 'learning problems'. They suggested the need for more detailed analysis of the results and a determination of whether different training programs have different results for students with various pre-training, speechreading skill levels.

French cued speech/speechreading

Vanden-Bemden et al. (1990) reported on a speechreading and cued speech interactive video course made up of 17 lessons aimed at building receptive skills for parents of French deaf children and the children themselves. Using an IBM 386 PC and Sony 7000 U-matic VCR, Vanden-Bemden et al. have experimented with (a) automated conversion of text responses into a phonetic transcription that is independent of spelling mistakes with several mathematical models, and (b) providing an 'expert system' approach for a student's trajectory through the training experience based on fuzzy-set logic. For example, the lesson might proceed to either a 'review of a segment of a lesson', 'review the whole lesson', 'go to the next segment or lesson', 'give help', or 'give the answer' depending on an analysis of the current answer, the student's skills, and student performance history. No experimental results of this approach have been reported.

This review is not exhaustive but does indicate the range of sophistication and types of validation data collected for interactive video speechreading training programs.

Related Studies

The following studies have utilized interactive video for research and should inform the design of future CAIV speechreading lessons.

Scoring of responses

Since English orthography is irregular and because the language contains homophenes that are spelled differently, scoring of speechreaders' responses is not straightforward and should not only be confined to a percentage sentence-correct score. More detail concerning the within viseme responses would be useful for the researcher and for more specific feedback to the learner within a CAIV lesson. Demorest and Bernstein (1991) and Bernstein, Demorest and Eberhardt (1993) used elements of the DECtalk software (Version 2.0, a computerized text to-speech synthesizer) to transcribe CID Everyday Sentences Test sentences into a phonetic-like code. The test sentence phonetic code was then compared to the similarly coded phonetic elements of the subjects' responses. The program aligned the response elements with the target sentence by the use of the Kruskal and Sankoff (1983) algorithm for sequence comparisons. The program maximized the visual similarity of response phonemes using a distance matrix based on previous data for multidimensional scaling of nonsense-syllable confusions. The output scoring provided not only the percentage correct for sentences, words and phonemes, but also an estimation of the overall visual distance between the stimulus and the response. The 'visual distance score' corresponds to the sum of the values in the distance matrix for each pair of elements in the alignment of a given sentence item. Correct phonemes have a visual distance of zero. Visually similar phonemes have a small distance, and dissimilar phonemes have large distances. Visual distance may be a more useful measure of performance because it does *not* have the moderate-to-severe, skewed distribution which percent correct speechreading performance distributions typically exhibit. As a result, the visual distance score can be 'more sensitive to individual differences throughout the performance range' (Demorest and Bernstein, 1991).

They also calculate an 'uncertainty function' in bits which is derived from the proportion of subjects' correct responses for each phoneme (re. the 47 possible phonetic responses in the DECtalk software). 'Response uncertainty is high when subjects make many different types of errors and it is low when there is a high percentage of correct responses and/or when errors are concentrated in a small number of categories. When response uncertainty is low, it reflects unanimity among subjects and thus may be related to the operation of a stimulus-driven and/or linguistic processes' (Demorest and Bernstein, 1991, page 106). When response uncertainty is high, i.e., subjects are making many different responses, the disparity may be attributable to, 'idiosyncratic speechreading strategies or guessing' (Demorest and Bernstein, 1991, page 106).

Demorest and Bernstein (1991) believe that examination of these various scores can provide valuable information to enable improved speechreading modelling. Future versions of CAIV for speechreading might well incorporate similar procedures.

Video standards for CAIV

Ijsseldijk (1992) reported speechreading performance under different conditions of video image, repetition and speech which are pertinent to how CAIV lessons must be recorded. Three experiments with deaf children ranging in age from 8 to 16 years were completed. In Experiment One, 33 subjects viewed either the talker's entire face, two-thirds profile, or lips-only for words, phrases and sentences tests. There were no significantly different test scores across the three different viewing conditions when analysing the number of syllables that were perceived correctly. Experiment Two examined which form of repetition after a frontal (entire face) presentation was most effective for improving speechreading results with various stimuli. Twenty-four deaf children viewed an entire-face presentation of the words, phrases and sentences test. However, each item of the test was *repeated*. The repetition showed either the talker's entire face, two-thirds profile, or enlarged lips only view. The three types of repetitions all resulted in significant improvements in percentage syllable recognition compared to the frontal view without repetition. Thus, the question as to which type of repetition was best remained unanswered. In Experiment Three, 23 deaf children viewed various speechreading stimuli at four videodisc playback rates (100%, 50%, 33% and 25% of the normal, 25 images per second rate). The four rates did not significantly influence speechreading scores. Ijsseldijk (1992) concluded that there is a wide range within which speaker-sender variables may differ without affecting the overall speechreading results.

CAIV teaching methods

Massaro, Cohen and Gesi (1993) have used syllable stimuli in a variety of CAIV discrimination and recognition training tasks with either visual or bimodal presentation (i.e., auditory and visual modalities combined) and achieved significant improvement in lipreading performance for syllables, words and sentences with six hearing subjects. Gesi, Massaro and Cohen (1992) concluded from their studies that it does not seem to be clear what aspects of the training and experience account for this improved performance. They found that an 'expository method of teaching in which subjects were told *where* to look and *what* to look for had no advantage over a discovery method in which subjects were given no explicit instructions ...' (Massaro *et al.*., 1993, page 560). In addition, they stated 'nor was it necessary to train lipreading with bimodal syllable stimuli as visual training carried over to facilitate auditory *and* bimodal speech perception' (Massaro *et al.*, 1993, page 560). Additionally, they found that the rate of presentation of test items (by altering the playback speed of the videodisc) was important for word but not for syllable recognition.

Thus, there appears to be little evidence that various rates of presentation, viewing angles, and/or accompanying instruction sets are conclusively linked to differential improvement of training results. However, much additional work should be done to assess adult learner preferences and requirements. For example, regarding the 'rate' of stimulus presentation, Ijsseldijk (1992) found no performance changes with slow video *playback* rates. But speechreaders would soon tire of the jerky images resulting from slow video frame *recording* rates as seen in the current 'Quicktime' © video software. On the other hand, the preliminary findings described above suggest that a broad range of lesson parameters may be effective. Thus, creativity can be encouraged in lesson design without predicted penalties in performance.

Time-based performance measures

In CAIV speechreading studies there have been several approaches using time as a performance measure, for example, Continuous Discourse Tracking's words-per-minute score (De Filippo, 1988) and DAVID's sentence response time (Sims, Scott and Myers, 1982a). In both cases, the time necessary to achieve verbatim sentence recognition is the dependent variable.

Tracking

Tracking has been set up with CAIV in order to improve experimental control of the method and to enable detailed analysis of results. For example, Spens *et al.* (1992) found that although connected discourse tracking (CDT) is often used in speechreading training, especially for cochlear implant users, the conventional words per minute score is not enough to document changes in subject performance. Presenting materials live-voice and using a computer to present segments to the talker, they gathered information about the transmission time for a single unit or phrase as well as the proportion of words that were not understood in phrases. Parameters such as the total number of first interventions (repetitions of words in a more well articulated manner), second interventions (words written on an LED-screen) and last resort interventions were numerically documented. Spens *et al.* contend that such numerical documentation helped to eliminate some of the variability in CDT to make it a more valid measure of pre- and post-test gains after training.

Dempsey *et al.* (1992) reported on the use of computer-assisted interactive tracking simulation (CATS) in which a laser videodisc is used in conjunction with an observer. Ten short stories of one paragraph each were created. Each story contained six sentences with vocabulary items and syntactic structures found in reading texts for students in fifth to seventh grades. For each trial, the observer coded the subject's tracking response as: CC – both parts of the test utterance were repeated correctly; CE – the first half was repeated correctly, but there was error in the second half; EC – error in first half, second half repeated correctly; and EE – errors in both halves, or no response. The initial presentation of the utterance occurred at a normal conversational speed. If errors persisted, another recorded version of the target sentence was presented at a very slow speed, with exaggerated articulation. CATS was compared with a similar technique using a live speaker. While live tracking was 65% faster than CATS, Dempsey *et al.* (1992) indicated that computer-assisted tracking allowed greater control of the experimental treatment because the same set of tracking intervention rules was used throughout the practice. This improved test–retest variability as compared to live tracking even when the talker was trained to use the same rules as CATS. Dempsey *et al..* concluded that CATS could be made more efficient by increasing the number of possible correction strategies and by programming a more complex set of rules for their usage.

Coninx *et al.* (1993) reported open paragraph tracking (OPT) where a subject is asked to repeat, verbatim, prerecorded sentence material. Each sentence could be presented up to a pre-set maximum number of trials with the words that were correctly repeated appearing in subtitles on the video screen (through an observer's keyboarding). After a pre-set maximum number of presentations (determined by the instructor) or all the words were repeated correctly, the full sentence appeared on the screen. Pre- and post-test results were reported as the percentage of words repeated correctly. The OPT procedure used bimodal sentence stimuli and repetition controlled by the examiner as the single repair strategy.

Twelve normal-hearing subjects lipread sentences with the support of 500 Hz low-pass filtered speech. Subjects practised with OPT and connected discourse tracking (CDT) using a live talker. They were given two tests immediately after practice, 3 to 4 days later and again in 7 to 8 days. Results showed that OPT and CDT produced the same learning effect. However, as expected, there was more variability with the live talker in the CDT procedure. Coninx *et al.* (1993) indicate that future work will focus on training with severely and profoundly hearing-impaired subjects.

DAVID response time

This method of measuring time as the dependent performance variable is the inverse of tracking; where tracking measures words-per-minute over a paragraph, DAVID measures seconds per sentence. In both cases, the procedure allows for significant intervening help to enable the learner enter a 100% correct response. As expertise and skills are gained, less help is required and learners may begin to recognize the stimuli more quickly.

However, there are two threats to the validity of a response time (RT) measure of performance in CAIV. First, there is some unquantified improvement in RT in the initial stages of instruction as a result of learning the mechanics of the human–computer interaction. The computer-assisted tracking procedures used human observers to score verbal responses and thus help minimize subjects' need to interact directly with the computer. DAVID was developed more for self-instruction laboratory usage as part of speechreading rehabilitation; consequently subjects were required to work independently with the system. In our experiments we provided at least 50 minutes of practice with the system which was supervised by laboratory proctors or speechreading instructors. Most of the mechanical issues were resolved by this training. However, the instructor also received individual, weekly tallies of each student's use of the 'helps' provided by the computer, and a complete history of interactions to items that exceeded a set RT limit beyond the mean for the sentence set. The teacher then reinstructed students as to needed changes in program interaction strategy.

To further examine student–computer interactions, we studied changes in typing skill during the course of speechreading training.

Experimental and control groups (with and without DAVID instruction) were not significantly different on pre- and post-test measures of typing skill change, and it was concluded that keyboarding skill changes are not of sufficient magnitude to influence RT measures significantly (Sims and Mumford, 1994).

The second and most important threat to the validity of RT performance measures is variation in the difficulty of training items. Item difficulty can greatly influence response time. For example, Sims, Snell and Clymer (1984) found that ostensibly small differences in the vocabulary and grammatical complexity used for test/training sentence-length stimuli were correlated to their dependent variable of speechreading RT. This result with deaf, college-aged speechreaders may be importantly related to subjects' variation in English language development. However, for hard-of-hearing persons *without* language deficits, Boothroyd (1988), in a study of auditory speech perception, confirmed that thresholds for sentences in noise were significantly influenced by linguistic 'entropy' (i.e., word frequency, lexical density, and ambiguity of the stimuli). Thus, when training tasks are studied, language-related properties of the stimuli could cause the variability in RT to be larger than the training effects to be measured (Kazdin, 1984).

Thus, item difficulty level must be controlled in some manner. When it is not, performance histories for individual and for groups of subjects is very 'noisy' as large variations in RT are seen (Sims, Snell and Clymer, 1984) across a time-series plot of RT versus the sequence of training items.

Thus, in order to analyse RT, item-by-item difficulty level needs to be established and controlled. A detailed description of the steps to establish an item-difficulty index is provided in the Appendix. This index is used to select pairs of items of equal difficulty and then to compare response times as a function of the amount of intervening training. When a pair of item RTs are separated by only a few intervening training sentences, the difference between the RTs for the pair should not be very great. However, if a considerable amount of training has occurred, one would expect the pair's RT to be much different and the item of the pair from the *second* in order of occurrence in the training sequence should have a reduction in RT. Results of this approach were encouraging as they suggested the expected RT relationships.

Specification of item difficulty and subsequent regression on RT will enable closer predictions of performance as a function of practice. In the future, on-line analysis of an individual student's RT trajectory could be used for predictions of benefit from further training. Also, RT may be explored as a means to study variations in training methodologies or learner characteristics which may impact on lipreading skill acquisition.

CAIV Program Evaluation

Reeves (1990) critiques traditional comparative media studies of, for example, CAIV versus live one-on-one instruction as providing little basis 'for meaningful interpretation of why one treatment was more effective than another' (p. 120). Instead he describes a six level approach as seen in Figure 1. This multilevel evaluation has as its goal a 'process of providing the designers and users of interactive video with timely, accurate information which will contribute to decisions about the improvement, continuance, and/or expansion of their programs' (Reeves, 1990, page 120).

Sample Questions	Levels	Sample Decisions
What are the delivery costs per unit of interactive video instruction? What are the costs of interactive video? What are the costs associated with different levels of achievement?	Cost-Effectiveness Evaluation	Should interactive video training be disseminated? How should it be priced? How should interactive video development proposals be budgeted?
What learning is transferred to workplace? What performance changes are reported by the trainees? What performance changes are observed by supervisors? What is the impact on client services?	Impact Evaluation	Should job aids be developed? Should additional training be developed? Should training priorities be revised? Is liability insurance adequate?
What learning can be measured? What learning is reported by trainees? What learning is observed by instructors?	Immediate Effectiveness Evaluation	Should certification be awarded? How should interactive video be marketed? Should instructor manuals be expanded?
How can the interactive video be improved? How can the interactive video delivery system be improved? How can the interactive video design process be improved?	Formative Evaluation	Which colors should be used for screen commands? Text? Feedback? Which user interface should be adopted? Should staff development retreat be initiated?
What are the relationships between interactive video objectives and institutional needs? Who will benefit from accomplishment of the interactive video objectives? Who will not benefit?	Assessment of the Worth of Objectives	Should the project continue, expand, or terminate design activities? Which clients should be represented in needs assessment and planning? Should interactive video be released?
What activities are accomplished? By whom? When? At what costs? Who was trained? When? At what cost? What is the interactive video reliability?	Project Documentation	Which team members should be assigned to which tasks? Should additional staff be hired? Should additional funding be solicited? Should another delivery system be adopted?

Figure 1. Six levels of evaluation for interactive video with sample questions and decisions (from Reeves, 1990).

Most often, CAIV is evaluated only on the 'Immediate Impact Level' which is a determination of the gains in learner skills. Reeves recommends that multiple assessment instruments of proven reliability, validity and sensitivity be used. Self-assessment and peer assessment of the perceived benefit of the instruction should also be used to provide convergence on the training effects. To further study the impact of the instruction, he suggests the use of computer modelling to relate instructional treatment inputs (student skills at the onset of instruction) and processes (training) to outcomes of the training in an effort to explain the effects of the interactive video. Program components as well as input and output measures can be analysed using statistical procedures such as commonalty analysis (Kenny, 1979, Wang and Walberg, 1983). Another computer modelling approach by Marlino (1989) has studied elements of classical theories of instruction as adapted to CAIV by using a variety of path analysis and 'soft' modelling approaches (Cooley and Lohnes, 1976). These analyses can test the overall predictability of an instructional model and estimate the relative effectiveness of each of the model elements.

Greyerbiehl *et al.* (1986) have developed more informal written survey and rating procedures for describing and judging the merits of software in the fields of speech and hearing. For example, evaluation of the 'purpose' of the software is done with the following items by rating on a five-point scale with descriptors, 'strongly agree' to 'strongly disagree':

1. The program purpose is clearly defined.
2. The treatment/instructional objectives are clearly defined.
3. The objectives state the conditions under which the communication-disordered individual is expected to learn.
4. Based on the task analysis, objectives are presented in a sequence of small steps that move from easy to difficult.
5. The objectives are ordered according to established developmental sequences in communication research.

Several other parameters such as technical quality, foundation for instruction, lesson initiation process and lesson progression are also evaluated in a similar manner.

Conclusions

Examination of the many CAIV speechreading projects leads to the realization of the numerous advantages and potential for this 15-year-old methodology. As in the hearing aid industry, the equipment is now easy to use, relatively inexpensive and has more capability than we know how to use effectively. Perhaps the greatest advantage of CAIV is its capability to gather the much needed learner data during the training to enable rehabilitators to more easily study basic perception of speech, the methods for teaching lipreading and the interaction of learner-related variables with perception and methodology.

The future of CAIV will rest with the DVI technology that is now at hand and promises to make CAIV production easily accomplished in-house and therefore less expensive and more flexible. It is time for us to move into this next generation of equipment. It is conceivable that in a few minutes time, client and clinician could generate their own CAIV lesson and make it closely related to an individual's situational communication problems.

Further, the capability to record the client *during* the CAIV lesson has not been explored. Video feedback has been shown to enhance speechreading skill acquisition, for example, van Uden (1983); De Filippo, Sims and Gottermeier (1994).

As progress is made in the programming and design of interactive video, perhaps greater gains in speechreading performance can be made by hearing-impaired persons. It must be understood, however, that like teaching, CAIV applications benefit from *continuous* improvement made through observations and analysis of student data and lesson trajectories. For CAIV to be effective it must be viewed as an ongoing process of incremental improvement as the analysis of learner data builds the expertise over time. There is no such thing as a teacher who cannot improve on pedagogy and content; and, there is no such thing as a CAIV lesson that cannot be made more effective, interesting and adaptable to student needs.

Appendix

To study a prototype item difficulty measure, response time was examined with a sample population of normal-hearing, college-aged students. Twelve undergraduate subjects completed the DAVID speechreading training in the same manner as the deaf subjects except that the order of the items was randomized for each subject to ensure that training and fatigue effects were equally distributed. Normal-hearing college students were used to enable comparisons to deaf subjects of the same age in subsequent studies. Presumably, English language skills of the deaf subjects (mean 8th grade reading, Michigan Test, Tiegs and Clark (1957)) were different from the hearing subjects. This may have influenced the absolute response time values, making the response times shorter for the normal-hearing persons. However, with regard to general lipreading skills (apart from language differences) hearing-impaired and normal-hearing persons have been shown to be equivalent for viseme perception (Owens and Blazek, 1985; Benguerel and Pinchora-Fuller, 1982).

The data used for establishing item difficulty was the mean response time (MRT) for each sentence across all normal-hearing subjects. The mean of the mean response times for all 175 items $\bar{D}$ was 53.2 seconds with a standard deviation of 47.5 (minimum 7, maximum 434). This mean response time (i.e., item difficulty index) was used to establish a standardized difficulty score for each sentence by equation (1).

$$d_i' = \frac{d_i - \bar{D}}{\sigma_d} \qquad (1)$$

Where d_i' is the standardized item difficulty of items i (i = 1, 2,..175); $\bar{D}$ is the mean item difficulty (i.e., mean response time across all normally-hearing subjects and items) and d_i is the mean response time across all subjects for a *single* item of the series, The σ_d is the standard deviation of $\bar{D}$. With the assumption of normal distribution of item difficulty, d_i should (and did) therefore, fall in the range of –3 to +3 or an absolute value interval of 0 to 6.

Then these results were transformed to the range (0,1) by equation (2).

$$z_i = 1 - \frac{d_i' + 3}{6} \qquad (2)$$

where d_i = standardized item difficulty (see above).

As such, Z_i is similar to the traditional pass-rate item difficulty measure. Higher values of Z_i, indicate easy items. Using these transformed estimates, we hypothesized that for items of equal difficulty, training on the DAVID system should result in decreased response times for an item near the end of the CAIV lesson, i.e., subject should use less time to respond correctly if skills have improved. To determine which items to compare, the following process was completed for the lesson set of 175 sentences (the first 20 were omitted from analysis as they were used for familiarization with the use of the computer program and perceptual task).

1. Using the standardized, transformed item-difficulty measure, Z_i, we selected 143 item pairs with a difference of item difficulty of <0.01. Thus, the items in every pair were about the same difficulty; though each pair could be quite different in difficulty level from another pair.
2. For every selected item-pair, we calculated the difference of mean response time for all deaf subjects by subtracting the mean response time of the second item (the item that was practised later in the lesson) of the pair from the mean response time of the first item to be practised. Thus, a positive value indicated that the mean response time of the second item was less than that of the first item; i.e., the hypothesized effect of reduced response time for items which were

encountered later in the lesson sequence. This is denoted below as (D_i).

3. For every item pair, e.g., pair i, the distance (L_i) (also known as Lag) for the item pair was determined. The distance (L_i) referred to the number of intervening training sentences that were practised between the selected item pairs. For example, if the 130th sentence and 162nd sentence in the lesson sequence were selected as an item pair (as equal in difficulty) then the distance $L_i = 162 - 130 = 32$, which is the intervening number of items between these two training events.

4. Then for every different distance j, (j = 1, 2,...155) we selected all item pairs whose distance equalled j and calculated the mean of the D_{ij}s denoted as R_j. Statistically, this R_j represents the improvement in RT (i.e., speechreading skill) through the training of j items.

5. Using linear regression, the relationship of distance j and R_j was determined and is shown in Figure 2.

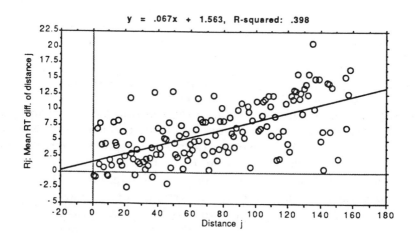

Figure 2. Regression plot for item pair distance and mean response time.

As can be seen, the expected relationship was obtained with a significant correlation between the item distance and the average reduction in response time, R_j. That is, the greater the number of intervening training items, the larger the reduction of response time.

We feel that this item analysis procedure and the R_{ij} metric enables the use of RT as a means of instructional benefit as a result of CAIV sentence drill and practice. However, this data should be considered preliminary as the item difficulty Z transform which we used was based on a sample of 12; a larger sample estimate would be used conventionally. Further, item difficulty index work would best be completed with separate samples of the target populations who have basic, intermediate, and advanced speechreading skills as the psychometric properties of each group are likely to be different (Sims, 1982).

References

Abrahamson, J. (1991) Teaching coping strategies: A client education approach to aural rehabilitation. Journal of the Academy of Rehabilitative Audiology 24: 43–53.

Benguerel, A.P. and Pichora-Fuller, M.K. (1982) Coarticulation effects in lipreading. Journal of Speech and Hearing Research 25: 600-607.

Bernstein, L.E., Demorest, M.E. and Eberhardt, S.P. (1993) A computational approach to analyzing sentential speech perception: Phoneme-to-phoneme stimulus response alignment. Manuscript submitted for publication.

Boothroyd, A. (1981) CASPER: a user friendly computer assisted speech perception and training system. Unpublished internal report, City University of New York.

Boothroyd, A. (1987) CASPER computer-assisted speech perception evaluation and training. in Proceedings of the 10th Annual Conference of the Society of North America, Washington DC: Association for Advancement of Rehabilitation Technology, pp. 134–136.

Boothroyd, A. (1988) Linguistic factors in speechreading. In DeFilippo, C.L. and Sims, D.G. (Eds), New Reflections on Speechreading Monograph, 90(5).

Boothroyd, A., Yeung, E., Hanin, L., Hnath-Chisolm, T., Kishon-Rabin, L., Medwetsky, L., Broeker, B., Eran, O. and Plant, N. (1988) Application of interactive videodisc technology to speech perception testing and training. A scientific exhibit at the annual convention of the American Speech, Language, Hearing Association, Boston, MA.

Coninx, F., Wermers, J., Rasing E., Vermeulen, A. and Elsendoorn, B. (1993) The open paragraph tracking procedure as an assessment tool for speech perception skills at the test level. A technical presentation at the Cochlear Implant Conference, Innsbruck, Austria.

Cooley, W. and Lohnes, R. (1976) Evaluation Research in Education: Theory . Principles and Practice. New York: Irvington.

Cronin, B. (1979) The DAVID system: The development of an interactive video system at the National Technical Institute for the Deaf. American Annals of the Deaf 124: 616–18.

De Filippo, C. (1988) Tracking for speech reading training. Volta Review 90 (5): 215–37.

De Filippo, C., Sims, D. and Gottermeier, L. (1995) Linking Visual and Kinesthetic Imagery in Lipreading Instruction. Journal of Speech and Hearing Research 38: 244, 256.

Demorest, M. and Bernstein, L. (1991) Computational explorations of speechreading. Journal of the Academy of Rehabilitative Audiology 24: 97–111.

Dempsey, J., Levitt, H., Josephson, J. and Porrazzo, J. (1992) Computer-assisted tracking simulation (CATS) Journal of the Acoustical Society of America 92: 701–10.

Floyd, S. and Floyd, B. (1982) Handbook of Interactive Video. White Plains, New York: Knowledge Industry Publications.

Gagné, J., Dinon, D. and Parsons, J. (1991) An evaluation of CAST: a computer-aided speechreading training program. Journal of Speech and Hearing Research 34: 213–21.

Gesi, A.T., Massaro, D.W. and Cohen, M.M. (1992) Discovery and expository methods in teaching visual consonant and word identification. Journal of Speech and Hearing Research 35: 1180–8.

Green, J.L. (1992) The evolution of DVI system software. Communications of the ACM 35: 53.

Greyerbiehl, D., Chial, M., Schwartz, A., Owens, A. and Blackstone, S. (1986) User System for Evaluating and Reviewing Software Users II: Indepth Review. American Speech-Language-Hearing Association: Silver Springs, Maryland.

Ijsseldijk, F. (1992) Speechreading performance under different conditions of video image, repetition and speech rate. Journal of Speech and Hearing Research 35: 466–71.

Ijsseldijk, F. and Elsendoorn, B. (1991) Design and evaluation of interactive training programs for speech reading and hearing skills (ISEG) for children and adolescents with profound hearing impairment. Interactive Learning Technology for the Deaf. NATO Advanced Research Workshop. Sint-Michielsgestel, Netherlands.

Jacobs, M. (1982) Visual communication (Speechreading) for the severely and profoundly hearing-impaired young adult. In Sims, D. Walter, G. and Whitehead, R. (Eds) Deafness and Communication: Assessment and Training. Baltimore: Williams and Wilkins.

Jeffers, J. and Barley, M.(1971) Speechreading (lipreading). Springfield, Illinois: C.C. Thomas.

Kazdin, A. (1984) Statistical Analyses for single-case experimental designs. In Barlow, D. and Herson, M. (Eds) Single-case Experimental Design: Strategies for Studying Behavior Change (2nd Ed) .New York: Pergamon Press.

Kenny, D. (1979) Correlation and Causality. New York: Wiley

Kopra, L., Kopra, M., Abrahamson, J. and Dunlop, R. (1987) Lipreading drill and practice software for an auditory-visual interactive system. Journal for Computer Users in Speech and Hearing 3: 58–68.

Kruskal, J. and Sankoff, D. (1983) An anthology of algorithms and concepts for sequence comparison. In Sankoff, D. and Kruskal, J. (Eds) Time Warps. String Edits and Macromolecules: The Theory and Practice of Sequence Comparison. Reading, MA: Addison-Wesley. pp 265–310.

Mahshie, J. (1987) A primer on interactive video. Journal for Computer Users in Speech and Hearing 3: 39–57.

Marlino, M (1989) An exploration of a process modeling approach in the evaluation of interactive videodisc-based instruction. (Doctoral dissertation, University of Georgia, 1989). Dissertation Abstracts International.

Massaro, D.W., Cohen, M.M. and Gesi, A.T. (1993) Long-term training, transfer and retention in learning to lipread. Perception and Psychophysics 53(5): 549–62.

Mazaik, C. (1993) Guidelines for producing accessible multimedia for deaf and hard-of hearing students. The CPB/WGBH National Center for Accessible Media, WGBH Educational Foundation. 125 Western Ave. Boston, MA 02134.

McReynolds, L. and Kearns, K. (1983) Single-Subject Experimental Designs in Communicative Disorders. Baltimore: University Park Press.

Owens, E. and Blazek, B. (1985) Visemes observed by hearing-impaired and normal hearing adult viewers. Journal of Speech and Hearing Research 28: 381–393.

Pichora-Fuller, M. and Benguerel, A. (1991) The design of CAST (Computer-aided speechreading training). Journal of Speech and Hearing Research 34: 202–12.

Reeves, T. (1990) Redirecting evaluation of interactive video: The case for complexity. Studies in Educational Evaluation 16: 115–31.

Sims, D. (1982) Hearing and speechreading evaluation for the deaf adult. In Sims, D., Walter, G. and Whitehead, R. (Eds) Deafness and Communication: Assessment and Training. Baltimore: Williams and Wilkins.

Sims, D. and Mumford, B. (1994) Response rate measures of learning for an inter-active-video speechreading lesson: The influence of keyboarding skill. (Submitted).

Sims, D., Von Feldt, J., Dowaliby, F., Hutchinson, K. and Myers, T. (1979) A pilot experiment in computer assisted speechreading instruction utilizing the data analysis video interactive device (DAVID). American Annals of the Deaf 124: 618–23.

Sims, D., Scott, L. and Myers, T (1982a) Past, present and future computer assisted communication at NTID. Journal of the Academy of Rehabilitative Audiology 15: 103–115.

Sims, D. Myers, T, Jacobs, M. and Rosen, S. (1982b) Computer Assisted Communication Training. Scientific Exhibit at the American Speech and Hearing Association Annual Convention, November, Toronto.

Sims, D., Snell, K. and Clymer, W. (1984, June) Computer based interactive video-tape communication instruction: Auditory training. speechreading and sign lan-guage. Paper presented at the Summer Institute of the Academy of Rehabilitative Audiology, Watts Bar, TN.

Spens, K., Gnosspelius, J., Öhngren, G., Plant, G. and Risberg, A. (1992) Numerical aspects of the speech tracking procedure. Speech Transmission Laboratory-Quarterly Progress Report. 1992 (1): 115–30.

Tatsouka, K. and Tatsouka, M. (1978) Time Score Analysis in Criterion Referenced Tests, Plato Education Group, CERL Report E-1. Champaign, IL: University of Illinois.

Tiegs, E. and Clark, W. (1957) California Achievement Test – Junior High Level. Monterey: California Test Bureau.

Tye-Murray, N. (1992) Laser videodisc technology in the aural rehabilitation set-ting: good news for people with severe and profound hearing impairments. American Journal of Audiology 33–5.

Tye-Murray, N., Tyler, R., Bong, B. and Nares, T. (1988) Using laser videodisc tech-nology to train speechreading and assertive listening skills. Journal of the Academy of Rehabilitative Audiology 21: 143–52.

Vanden-Bemden, G., Durfour, P. and Marco, C. (1990) French lip-reading and cued-speech training by interactive video. Journal of Microcomputer Applications 13: 193–200.

van Uden, A. (1983) Diagnostic Testing of Deaf Children: The Syndrome of Dyspraxia. Lisse: Swets and Zeitlinger.

Walden, B.E., Prosek, R., Montgomery, A.A., Scherr, C.K. and Jones, C.J. (1977) Effects of training on the visual recognition of consonants. Journal of Speech and Hearing Research 20: 130–145.

Walden, B.E., Erdman, S.A., Montgomery, A.A., Schwartz, D.M. and Prosek, R.A. (1981) Some effects of training on speech recognition by hearing-impaired adults. Journal of Speech and Hearing Research 24: 207–16.

Wang. M.C. and Walberg. H.J. (1983) Evaluating educational programs: An integra-tive causal modeling approach. Educational Evaluation and Policy Analysis 5: 347–66.

Index